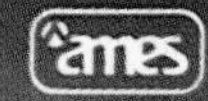

COLOR CHART

Multistix®

10 SG

Reagent Strips for Urinalysis

For In Vitro Diagnostic Use

READ PRODUCT INSERT BEFORE USE.

IMPORTANT: Do not touch test areas. Store at temperatures under 30°C (86°F). Do not store in refrigerator. Do not remove desiccants. Remove only enough strips for immediate use. Replace cap immediately and tightly.

TESTS AND READING TIME							
LEUKOCYTES 2 minutes	NEGATIVE		TRACE	SMALL +	MODERATE ++	LARGE +++	
NITRITE 60 seconds	NEGATIVE		POSITIVE	POSITIVE	(Any degree of uniform pink color is positive)		
UROBILINOGEN 60 seconds	NORMAL 0.2	NORMAL 1	mg/dL 2	4	8	(1 mg = approx. 1 EU)	
PROTEIN 60 seconds	NEGATIVE	TRACE	mg/dL 30 +	100 ++	300 +++	2000 or more ++++	
pH 60 seconds	5.0	6.0	6.5	7.0	7.5	8.0	8.5
BLOOD 50 seconds	NEGATIVE		NON-HEMOLYZED TRACE	HEMOLYZED TRACE	SMALL +	MODERATE ++	LARGE +++
SPECIFIC GRAVITY 45 seconds	1.000	1.005	1.010	1.015	1.020	1.025	1.030
KETONE 40 seconds	NEGATIVE	mg/dL	TRACE 5	SMALL 15	MODERATE 40	LARGE 80	LARGE 160
BILIRUBIN 30 seconds	NEGATIVE		SMALL +	MODERATE ++	LARGE +++		
GLUCOSE 30 seconds	NEGATIVE	g/dL (%) mg/dL	1/10 (tr.) 100	1/4 250	1/2 500	1 1000	2 or more 2000 or more

Ames Division MILES *Ames Division, Miles Laboratories, Inc., Elkhart, Indiana 46515* 2 160510

Reagent strips are the most commonly used diagnostic urine testing kit in the medical office. Multistix 10 SG contains ten reagent areas for testing pH, protein, glucose, ketone bodies, bilirubin, blood, urobilinogen, nitrite, specific gravity and leukocytes. (Courtesy of Ames Corporation, Elkhart, Indiana.)

(The color reproductions on these pages are for illustrative purposes only and must not be used to analyze actual test results.)

INTERPRETING THE HEMOCCULT® TEST

Negative Smears

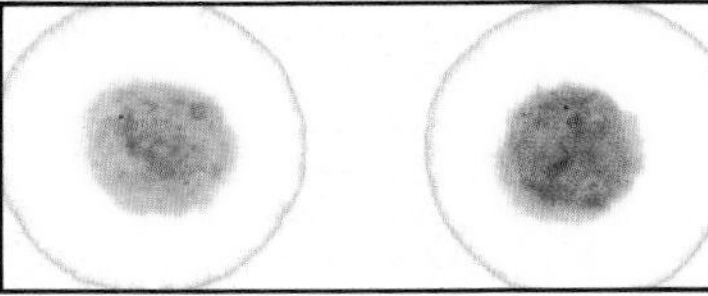

Sample report: negative
No detectable blue on or at the edge of the smears indicates the test is negative for occult blood. (See **LIMITATIONS OF PROCEDURE**.)

Negative and Positive Smears

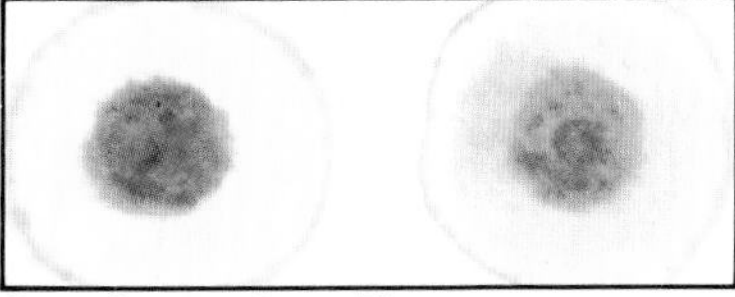

Positive Smears

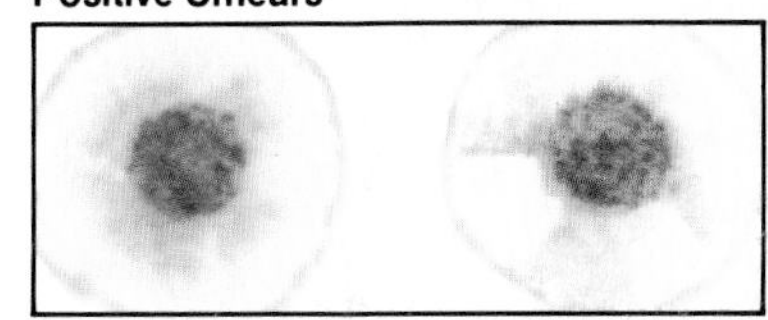

Sample report: positive
Any trace of blue on or at the edge of one or more of the smears indicates the test is positive for occult blood.

SKD **SmithKline Diagnostics, Inc.**
A SMITHKLINE BECKMAN COMPANY
San Jose, CA 95134-1622

CLINICAL PROCEDURES *for* MEDICAL ASSISTANTS

Third Edition

KATHY BONEWIT,
B.S., M.Ed., CMA-C

Coordinator and Instructor,
Medical Assistant Technology,
Hocking Technical College,
Nelsonville, Ohio

Member, Curriculum Review Board
of the American Association
of Medical Assistants

1990
W. B. SAUNDERS COMPANY
Harcourt Brace Jovanovich, Inc.

Philadelphia London Toronto
Montreal Sydney Tokyo

W. B. SAUNDERS COMPANY
Harcourt Brace Jovanovich, Inc.

The Curtis Center
Independence Square West
Philadelphia, PA 19106-3399

Editor: Margaret M. Biblis
Developmental Editors: Lisa Konoplisky & Shirley Kuhn
Designer: Paul Fry
Production Manager: Carolyn Naylor
Manuscript Editor: Leslie Fenton
Illustration Coordinator: Brett MacNaughton
Page Layout Artist: Kristina Hartzell
Indexer: Kathleen Cole
Cover Designer: Paul Fry

Photograph on inside back cover courtesy of SmithKline Diagnostics, Inc.

CLINICAL PROCEDURES FOR MEDICAL ASSISTANTS, Third Edition ISBN 0-7216-2895-8

Printed in U.S.A.

Last digit is the print number: 9 8 7 6 5 4 3 2

To my brother

Bobby,

for showing me the
magic of carousels

Preface

Medical assistants, for many years an integral part of most physician's staffs, now fulfill an ever expanding and varied role in the medical office, both clinically and administratively. With increased responsibilities has come a greater need for professional knowledge and skills. This text has been designed to meet that need.

The underlying principal of the text is to provide a format for the achievement of professional competency in clinical skills performed in the medical office and the understanding of their application to real-life or on-the-job situations. When professional competency is achieved in the classroom, there should be less of a gap between the academic and real worlds, and thus the transition from student to practicing medical assistant will be made more easily.

Although we have emphasized the book's usefulness to students in medical assisting training programs, the practicing medical assistant who has not had an opportunity to receive formal training will also find this text helpful as a learning and reference source. The organization of the text lends itself well to individualized instruction and convenient reference use.

In this third edition, the text has been expanded to encompass additional clinical procedures as well as the theory relating to each. This additional material will help students and instructors meet the demand for the increasing number and variety of clinical skills required of the practicing medical assistant by providing the most current and up-to-date procedures performed in the medical office. The reader will find that nearly every chapter incorporates new information and illustrations to assist in the educational process. Important additions include AIDS infection control guidelines, instructions on the use of electronic thermometers, detailed information on taking a health history, crutch and cane walking, types of surgeries performed in the medical office, application and removal of a Holter monitor, identification of cardiac arrhythmias, measurement of blood glucose using a glucose meter, rapid strep testing, PKU testing, and Hemoccult testing.

Two appendices have been added to the third edition. Appendix A presents the 1984 DACUM Analysis of the Medical Assisting Profession. The DACUM chart (Developing a Curriculum) is included to assist educators in identifying entry-level competencies for a medical assistant. It can also be used by students to help them become familiar with the role and function of the medical assistant. Appendix B is a comprehensive list of medical terms meant to serve as a valuable reference for the student both during and after formal training.

The third edition has been organized to better meet the needs of both educators and students. Presented at the beginning of each chapter are a chapter outline, competencies, learning objectives, and vocabulary. The chapter outline provides a quick reference for review of the cognitive knowledge included in that chapter. Competencies follow to delineate the task or skill to be mastered by the student. (In the student manual, each competency is expanded into a detailed performance objective including conditions and standards of acceptable performance.) The learning objectives address the cognitive knowledge required to perform the competencies. The vocabulary list designates the terms and definitions that should be mastered for each chapter and includes the phonetic spelling of each.

The knowledge or theory that the student must acquire in order to perform each skill is presented in a clear and concise manner. Numerous illustrations accompany the theory section to aid the student in acquiring the knowledge relating to each skill. The procedure for each skill follows the theory section and is designed to help the student perform the skill with the level of competency required on the job. Each procedure is presented in an organized step-by-step format, with underlying principles and illustrations accompanying the techniques. The refined organizational format should facilitate the learning process by providing students and educators with detailed objectives and an in-depth study of the most current and up-to-date clinical procedures performed in the medical office.

Perhaps the most significant improvement to this edition is the development of a competency-based student manual to accompany the textbook. The preface of the manual identifies and thoroughly explains its components. Briefly stated, they include: performance objectives for each clinical procedure; practice worksheets; performance evaluation checklists; vocabulary assessment of the medical terms relating to each chapter; self-evaluation questions; critical thinking skills; and two supplemental educational chapters (Taking Patient Symptoms and Calculation of Drug Dosage).

The student manual greatly enhances the learning value of the textbook. In addition, its competency-based approach meets the criteria required for competency-based program accreditation as stipulated by the Curriculum Review Board of the American Association of Medical Assistants.

Continuing education is of utmost importance in such a rapidly changing profession. New techniques and developments in the field of medicine have a direct influence on the medical assisting profession. Continuing education helps the medical assistant maintain and improve existing skills and learn new skills. The American Association of Medical Assistants is a professional organization for medical assistants that is dedicated to continuing education. Information on the AAMA can be obtained by writing to:

American Association of Medical Assistants
20 North Wacker Drive
Chicago, Illinois 60606

It is the author's hope that individuals using this approach to medical assisting will view this text not as a stopping place but as a means of opening doors to new paths to be explored and enjoyed in the medical assisting profession.

KATHY BONEWIT

Acknowledgments

The completion of the third edition of this text permits the opportunity to relay appreciation to the medical assisting educators who so eagerly and enthusiastically use and enjoy this text. To them I am also indebted for their helpful assistance and suggestions for the third edition.

The following professionals served as invaluable consultants and reviewers and deserve special recognition and appreciation:

Diana Bennett, RN, B.S.N., M.A.T., Indiana Vocational Technical College, Indianapolis, Indiana.

Carol S. Champagne, RMA, CMA-C, ICEA CCE, Clearwater Family Practice Clinic, Clearwater, Kansas; Chairperson, RMA, Continuing Education Committee; Certified Childbirth Education, Private Practice.

Gary A. Clarke, Ph.D., Assistant Professor of Biology, Roanoke College, Salem, Virginia.

Henry G. Croci, M.D., Ophthalmology, Riverside Professional Building, Athens, Ohio.

Larry S. Dansky, M.D., Family Practice, Athens, Ohio.

Julie D. Franklin, MT(ASCP), M.H.E., Former Program Director, Medical Office Assisting, Chattanooga State Technical Community College, Chattanooga, Tennessee.

Cathy Goodwin, CMA-AC, Medical Assistant, San Diego, California.

Jeanne Howard, CMA, AAS, Medical Assisting Technology, El Paso Community College, El Paso, Texas.

Gail I. Jones, M.S., MT(ASCP), Dettman-Connell School of Medical Technology, Fort Worth, Texas.

Richard W. Kocon, Ph.D., Laboratory Director, Damon Medical Laboratory, Inc., Needham Heights, Massachusetts.

Louis Komarmy, M.D., Clinical Pathologist, Children's Hospital, San Francisco, California.

Miriam Lineberger, RN, BSN, M.Ed., Instructor of Pharmacology, Hocking Technical College, Nelsonville, Ohio.

Albert B. Lowenfels, M.D., Associate Director of Surgery, Westchester County Medical Center, Valhalla, New York.

Susan J. Matthews, RN, B.S.N., M.Ed., Watterson College, Louisville, Kentucky.

Jean Moquin, Ohio University Osteopathic Medical Center, Athens, Ohio.

Sally A. Murdock, B.S.N., M.S., RN, California Public Health Nursing Certification, Medical Assisting, San Diego Mesa College, San Diego, California.

Raymond E. Phillips, M.D., FACP, Senior Attending Physician, Phelps Memorial Hospital, North Tarrytown, New York.

Marjorie R. Reif, PA-C, CMA, Rochester Community College, Rochester, Minnesota.

Alan M. Rosich, Instructor of Radiologic Technology, Lorain County Community College, Elvira, Ohio.

Sandra E. Sterling, MT(ASCP), Boulder Valley Vocational-Technical School, Boulder, Colorado.

Joan K. Werner, PT, Ph.D., Director, Physical Therapy Program, University of Wisconsin, Madison, Wisconsin.

Kenneth D. Woods, D.O., Orthopedic Surgery, Athens, Ohio.

The photographs in the third edition have been expanded through the efforts of Brian E. Blauser, professional photographer. I am especially indebted to Brian for his careful precision and patience in taking and developing them, thus greatly enhancing the learning value of this text.

I would like to gratefully acknowledge Rita Burgess, a student in the Medical Assistant Program at Hocking Technical College, for generously contributing many hours to be photographed for demonstration of the procedural steps in many of the chapters.

I would like to express warm appreciation to the following individuals who consented to the use of their photographs in the third edition: Hope A. Fauber, Andrea and Derek Fauber, Diana Moore, Steven Sakadales, Charon Smith, and Barbara Tulodzieski.

I would like to extend my appreciation to the authors, publishers, and equipment companies who have granted me permission to use their illustrations.

The publication of the third edition was accomplished through the capable guidance of many talented individuals at the W. B. Saunders Company. Many thanks to Lisa Konoplisky and Shirley Kuhn for their patience and exceptional developmental editing abilities, to Leslie Fenton for her careful and excellent editing of the manuscript, and to Robert Butler and Carolyn Naylor for their outstanding production work. I want to relay a very special thank you to Margaret Biblis, Editor, Health-Related Professions, for her perseverance, her dedication to quality medical assisting education, and for helping me achieve my best in this edition.

Last, but not least, without the support of my family, this work would not have been possible nor would it have been worthwhile. I relay my warmest thanks and love to my children, Rob and Holly, for their endless patience and understanding. I also want to lovingly acknowledge the memory of my father, Robert Joseph Drummond, who so enjoyed the simple pleasures of life.

With warm regard, I would like to recognize those very important individuals—the medical assisting students, graduates, and practicing medical assistants—who continually strive for excellence in meeting the demands and ever-increasing requirements of such a challenging profession. A quote by an unknown author really says it better: "Celebrate your talents, for they are what make you unique."

KATHY BONEWIT

Contents

1 MEDICAL ASEPSIS AND INFECTION CONTROL

Growth Requirements for Microorganisms ... 2
The Infection Process Cycle ... 4
Protective Mechanisms of the Body ... 4
Application of Medical Asepsis in the Medical Office ... 5
Procedure 1-1: Handwashing ... 6
Acquired Immunodeficiency Syndrome (AIDS) ... 8
Transmission of AIDS ... 9
AIDS Infection Precautions ... 9

2 VITAL SIGNS ... 14

Body Temperature ... 17
How Body Temperature is Maintained ... 17
Methods for Taking Body Temperature ... 17
Body Temperature Range ... 18
Variations in Body Temperature ... 18
Pyrexia ... 19
Glass Thermometers ... 19
Temperature Sheaths ... 21
Cleaning Glass Thermometers ... 21
Procedure 2-1: Taking Body Temperature—Oral ... 22
Procedure 2-2: Taking Body Temperature—Rectal ... 24
Procedure 2-3: Taking Body Temperature—Axillary ... 26
Electronic Thermometer ... 28
Procedure 2-4: Using Electronic Thermometers ... 28

Pulse ... 32
Mechanism of the Pulse ... 32
Sites for Taking Pulse ... 32
Pulse Rate ... 33
Rhythm and Volume ... 34
Procedure 2-5: Measuring Radial Pulse ... 35
Procedure 2-6: Measuring Apical Pulse ... 36

Respiration ... 39
Mechanism of Respiration ... 39
Control of Respiration ... 39
Respiratory Rate ... 39
Rhythm and Depth of Respiration ... 40
Respiratory Abnormalities ... 40
Color of the Patient ... 40
Procedure 2-7: Measuring Respiration ... 41

Blood Pressure ... 43
Mechanism of Blood Pressure ... 43
Normal Blood Pressure ... 43
Equipment to Measure Blood Pressure ... 43
Factors Affecting Blood Pressure ... 45

The Korotkoff Sounds 45
Procedure 2-8: Measuring Blood Pressure 46
Procedure 2-9: Determining Systolic Pressure by Palpation 49

3 THE PATIENT EXAMINATION 50
The Health History 52
Charting in the Medical Record 60
Symptoms 63
Integumentary System 64
Circulatory System 64
Gastrointestinal System 65
Respiratory System 65
Nervous System 65
Weight and Height 66
Positioning and Draping 66
Procedure 3-1: Measuring Weight and Height 67
Preparation of the Examining Room 70
Preparation of the Patient 71
Procedure 3-2: Assisting with the Physical Examination 76

4 THE EYE AND EAR 78
The Eye 81
Structure of the Eye 81
Visual Acuity 81
Measuring Distance Visual Acuity 82
Procedure 4-1: Measuring Distance Visual Acuity 86
Measuring Distance Visual Acuity in Preschoolers 88
Measuring Near Visual Acuity 88
Assessment of Color Vision 90
Procedure 4-2: Assessing Color Vision 91
Procedure 4-3: Eye Irrigation 93
Eye Instillation 95
Procedure 4-4: Eye Instillation 95
The Ear 98
Structure of the Ear 98
Ear Irrigation 98
Procedure 4-5: Ear Irrigation 99
Procedure 4-6: Ear Instillation 102

5 PROMOTING TISSUE HEALING THROUGH PHYSICAL THERAPY 104
Heat 106
Cold 107
Factors Affecting the Application of Heat and Cold 108
Procedure 5-1: Applying a Hot Water Bag 109
Procedure 5-2: Applying a Heating Pad 111
Procedure 5-3: Applying a Hot Soak 112
Procedure 5-4: Applying a Hot Compress 114
Procedure 5-5: Applying an Ice Bag 116
Procedure 5-6: Applying a Cold Compress 118
Procedure 5-7: Applying a Chemical Cold Pack 119

Ultrasound ... 120
Procedure 5-8: Administering an Ultrasound Treatment ... 122
Assistive Devices for Ambulation ... 124
Crutches ... 124
Axillary Crutch Measurement ... 125
Procedure 5-9: Measuring for Axillary Crutches ... 126
Crutch Guidelines ... 127
Crutch Gaits ... 127
Procedure 5-10: Instructing the Patient in Crutch Gaits ... 128
Canes ... 134
Procedure 5-11: Instructing the Patient in Use of a Cane ... 135
Walkers ... 136
Procedure 5-12: Instructing the Patient in Use of a Walker ... 137

6 STERILIZATION AND DISINFECTION ... 138
The General Sanitization Procedure ... 140
Procedure 6-1: Sanitizing Instruments ... 141
Procedure 6-2: Sanitizing Reusable Syringes ... 142
Procedure 6-3: Sanitizing Reusable Needles ... 143
Procedure 6-4: Sanitizing Rubber Goods ... 144
Physical Agents Used to Control Microorganisms ... 146
Moist Heat ... 146
Procedure 6-5: Sterilizing Articles in the Autoclave ... 156
Dry Heat ... 158
Chemical Agents Used to Control Microorganisms ... 159

7 MINOR OFFICE SURGERY ... 162
Surgical Asepsis ... 165
Instruments Used in Minor Office Surgery ... 167
Procedure 7-1: Applying Sterile Gloves ... 174
Procedure 7-2: Removing Sterile Gloves ... 175
Procedure 7-3: Opening a Sterile Package ... 176
Sterile Transfer Forceps ... 179
Procedure 7-4: Utilizing Sterile Transfer Forceps ... 180
Procedure 7-5: Pouring a Sterile Solution ... 181
Wounds ... 182
The Healing Process ... 182
Procedure 7-6: Changing a Sterile Dressing ... 184
Insertion of Sutures ... 187
Suture Removal ... 191
Assisting with Minor Office Surgery ... 192
Procedure 7-7: Assisting with Minor Office Surgery ... 195
Medical Office Surgical Procedures ... 199
Bandaging ... 208
Procedure 7-8: Applying a Tubular Gauze Bandage ... 213

8 ADMINISTRATION OF MEDICATION ... 216
Classification of Drugs Based on Preparation ... 218
Classification of Drugs Based on Action ... 221
Systems of Measurement Used to Administer Medication ... 222

The Metric System 223
Conversion Between Units of Measurement 227
The Prescription 229
Factors Affecting the Action of Drugs in the Body 231
Basic Guidelines for the Preparation and Administration of Medication . 232
Procedure 8-1: Administering Oral Medication 234
Parenteral Administration 236
Procedure 8-2: Reconstituting Powdered Drugs (General Procedure) 242
Procedure 8-3: Preparing the Injection 243
Procedure 8-4: Administering an Intradermal Injection 248
Procedure 8-5: Administering a Subcutaneous Injection 251
Procedure 8-6: Administering an Intramuscular Injection 256
Procedure 8-7: Z-Track Intramuscular Injection Technique 259
Tuberculin Skin Testing 260
Procedure 8-8: Administering a Tine Test 262
Procedure 8-9: Reading the Tine Test Results 264

9 INTRODUCTION TO THE CLINICAL LABORATORY 266
Laboratory Tests 268
Purpose of Laboratory Testing 269
Relationship Between the Medical Office and the Clinical Laboratory 270
Laboratory Requests 271
Laboratory Reports 278
Patient Preparation and Instructions 278
Collecting, Handling, and Transporting Specimens 280
Procedure 9-1: Collecting Specimen for Transport to an Outside Laboratory 284
Testing the Specimen 286
Quality Control 289
Laboratory Safety 290

10 URINALYSIS 292
Structure and Function of the Urinary System 294
Composition of Urine 294
Terms Relating to the Urinary System 295
Methods of Urine Collection 295
Procedure 10-1: Clear-Catch Midstream Specimen Collection Instructions 297
Analysis of Urine 300
Procedure 10-2: Measuring the Specific Gravity of Urine—Urinometer Method 304
Procedure 10-3: Chemical Testing of Urine Using the Multistix 10 SG Reagent Strip 314
Procedure 10-4: Measuring Urine Glucose Using Clinitest 316
Urine Pregnancy Testing 326
Serum Pregnancy Test 328
Procedure 10-5: Urine Pregnancy Test—Slide Agglutination Method 329

11 VENIPUNCTURE 332
Venipuncture Methods 334
Types of Blood Specimens 336

Procedure 11-1: Venipuncture Using the Vacuum Tube Method 337
Procedure 11-2: Venipuncture Using the Syringe Method 342
Separating Serum from Whole Blood 347
Procedure 11-3: Separating Serum from Whole Blood 349

12 BLOOD BANKING 352
The Components and Function of Blood 354
Blood Antigens 354
Blood Antibodies 355
The Rh Blood Group System 356
Antigen and Antibody Reactions 356
Agglutination and Blood Typing 356
Procedure 12-1: Blood Typing (Slide Test Method) 357

13 HEMATOLOGY AND BLOOD CHEMISTRY 362
Hematologic Laboratory Tests 365
Hematology 365
Erythrocytes 368
Leukocytes 368
Thrombocytes 369
Plasma 369
Capillary Blood Specimen 369
Procedure 13-1: Lancet Method to Obtain a Capillary Blood Specimen 371
Procedure 13-2: Autolet Method to Obtain a Capillary Blood Specimen 372
Hematocrit 373
Procedure 13-3: Hematocrit (Michrohematocrit Method) 374
Procedure 13-4: White Blood Cell Count (Manual Method) 377
White Blood Cell Count 376
Red Blood Cell Count 380
White Blood Cell Differential Count 380
Procedure 13-5: Differential Cell Count 382
Hemoglobin 386
Blood Chemistry Tests 389
Blood Chemistry 389
Cholesterol 389
Blood Urea Nitrogen 393
Blood Glucose 393
Fasting Blood Sugar 393
Two-Hour Postprandial Blood Sugar 393
Glucose Tolerance Test 394
Blood Glucose Measurement with a Glucose Meter 395
Procedure 13-6: Blood Glucose Measurement Using the Accu-Chek II Glucose Meter 396
Procedure 13-7: Blood Glucose Measurement Using the Glucometer II Glucose Meter 401
Self Monitoring of Blood Glucose 403

14 MICROBIOLOGY AND DISEASE 406
The Normal Flora 410
Infection 410

Microorganisms and Disease 411
The Microscope 413
Procedure 14-1: Using the Microscope 417
Microbiologic Specimen Collection 419
Procedure 14-2: Taking a Specimen for a Throat Culture 422
Cultures 425
Streptococcus Testing 426
Sensitivity Testing 429
Microscopic Examination of Microorganisms 430
Procedure 14-3: Preparing a Hanging Drop Slide 431
Procedure 14-4: Preparing a Smear 432
Procedure 14-5: Gram Staining 435
Prevention and Control of Infectious Diseases 439

15 ELECTROCARDIOGRAPHY 440
Structure of the Heart 442
Conduction System of the Heart 443
Cardiac Cycle 444
Electrocardiograph Paper 445
Standardization of the Electrocardiograph 446
Electrocardiograph Leads 447
Electrocardiographic Capabilities 450
Artifacts 453
Marking and Mounting the Electrocardiogram 457
Procedure 15-1: Running a 12-Lead Electrocardiogram 458
Holter Monitor Electrocardiography 462
Procedure 15-2: Applying a Holter Monitor 466
Cardiac Arrhythmias 469

16 X-RAY EXAMINATIONS 474
X-rays 477
The X-ray Machine 477
Contrast Media 479
Fluoroscopy 481
Positioning the Patient 481
X-ray Precautions 482
The Darkroom 485
Procedure 16-1: Producing a Radiograph (General Procedure) 486
Specific Radiographic Examinations 488

17 SPECIALTY EXAMINATIONS AND PROCEDURES 494
The Pediatric Examination 497
Pediatric Office Visits 497
Understanding the Child 497
Carrying the Infant 497
Growth Patterns 500
Procedure 17-1: Measuring the Weight of an Infant 504
Procedure 17-2: Measuring the Length of an Infant 505
Procedure 17-3: Applying a Pediatric Urine Collector 506
Pediatric Intramuscular Injections 508
Immunizations 510

The PKU Screening Test ... 511
Procedure 17-4: PKU Screening Test ... 513
The Gynecologic Examination ... 517
Gynecology ... 517
The Breast Examination ... 517
The Pelvic Examination ... 517
The Papanicolaou Test ... 518
Vaginal Infections ... 523
Bimanual Pelvic Examination ... 527
Procedure 17-5: Assisting with a Gynecologic Examination ... 528
Prenatal Care ... 533
Obstetrics ... 533
The First Prenatal Visit ... 533
The Prenatal Record ... 533
Initial Prenatal Examination ... 538
Return Prenatal Visits ... 543
Procedure 17-6: Assisting with a Return Prenatal Examination ... 548
Six-Weeks Postpartum Visit ... 551
Colon Procedures ... 554
Fecal Occult Blood Testing ... 554
Procedure 17-7: Patient Instructions for the Hemoccult Slide Test ... 556
Procedure 17-8: Developing the Hemoccult Slide Test ... 559
Quality Control for the Guaiac Slide Test ... 561
Proctoscopy and Sigmoidoscopy ... 561
Procedure 17-9: Assisting with a Proctoscopy and Sigmoidoscopy ... 564
Glossary ... 569
Appendix A
1984 Dacum Analysis of the Medical Assisting Profession ... 579
Appendix B
Medical Abbreviations ... 581
Suggestions for Further Reading ... 590
Index ... 595

CLINICAL PROCEDURES *for* MEDICAL ASSISTANTS

1

MEDICAL ASEPSIS AND INFECTION CONTROL

CHAPTER OUTLINE

Growth Requirements for Microorganisms
Infection Process Cycle
Protective Mechanisms of the Body
Application of Medical Asepsis in the Medical Office
Acquired Immunodeficiency Syndrome (AIDS)

COMPETENCIES

After completing this chapter, you should be able to demonstrate the proper procedure to perform the following:

Demonstrate the proper procedure for handwashing.

LEARNING OBJECTIVES

After completing this chapter, you should be able to do the following:

1. Define the terms listed in the vocabulary.
2. Define a microorganism, and give examples of types of microorganisms.
3. Explain the difference between a nonpathogen and a pathogen.
4. List the six basic requirements needed for growth and multiplication of microorganisms.
5. Outline the Infection Process Cycle, including the following:
   a. Give examples of the means of entry of microorganisms into the body.
   b. Give examples of the means of transmission of microorganisms from one person to another.
   c. Give examples of the means of exit of microorganisms from the body.
   d. List and explain three protective devices the body uses to prevent the entrance of microorganisms.
6. Define medical asepsis.
7. Identify ten medical aseptic practices that should be followed in the medical office.
8. Explain how proper handwashing helps to prevent the transmission of microorganisms.
9. Explain the principles underlying each step in the handwashing procedure.
10. List the symptoms of each of the following: human immunodeficiency virus (HIV) infection, AIDS-related complex (ARC), and acquired immunodeficiency syndrome (AIDS).
11. Explain how HIV is transmitted.
12. State the AIDS infection precautions included under the following categories: Universal Precautions, Sterilization and Disinfection, and Infective Waste.

• VOCABULARY •

aerobe (a' er-ōb)—An organism that needs oxygen in order to live and grow.

anaerobe (an-a' er-ōb)—An organism that grows best in the absence of oxygen.

asepsis (a-sep' sis)—Free from infection or pathogens.

cilia (sil' e-ah)—Slender hairlike processes.

contaminate (kon-tam' i-nāt)—To soil or to make impure. An aseptic object is contaminated when it touches something that is not clean.

host (hōst)—An animal or plant that provides nourishment for a microorganism to grow and multiply.

infection (in-fek' shun)—The condition in which the body, or part of it, is invaded by a pathogen.

microorganism (mi" kro-or' gah-nizm)—A microscopic plant or animal.

nonpathogen (non-path' o-jen)—A microorganism that does not normally produce disease.

optimum growth temperature (op' ti-mum grōth tem' per-ah-tūr)—The temperature at which an organism grows best.

pathogen (path' o-jen)—A disease-producing microorganism.

perinatal (per" i-na' tal)—Relating to the period shortly before and after birth.

pH—The degree to which a solution is acidic or basic.

reservoir host (rez' er-vwar hōst)—The organism that becomes infected by a pathogen and also serves as a source of transfer of the pathogen to others.

susceptible (sus-sep' ti-b'l)—Easily affected; lacking resistance.

Introduction

Microorganisms are tiny living plants or animals that cannot be seen with the naked eye but must be viewed with the aid of a microscope. Examples of common types of microorganisms include bacteria, viruses, protozoa, fungi, and animal parasites. Most microorganisms are harmless and do not cause disease. They are termed *nonpathogens.* Other microorganisms, known as *pathogens,* are harmful to the body and can cause disease.

Growth Requirements for Microorganisms

In order for microorganisms to survive, certain growth requirements must be present in the environment. These include the following:

Proper nutrition	Microorganisms that use inorganic or nonliving substances as a source of food are known as *autotrophs.* Microorganisms that use organic or living substances for food are known as *heterotrophs.*
Oxygen	Most microorganisms need oxygen to grow and multiply and are termed *aerobes.* Other microorganisms, known as *anaerobes,* grow best in the absence of oxygen.
Temperature	Each microorganism has a temperature at which it grows best, known as the *optimum growth temperature.* Most microorganisms grow best at 98.6°F (37°C), or body temperature.
Darkness	Microorganisms grow best in darkness.
Moisture	Microorganisms need moisture for cell metabolism and to carry away wastes.
pH	Most microorganisms prefer a neutral pH. If the environment of the microorganisms becomes too acidic or basic, they die.

If growth requirements are taken away from the environment of microorganisms, they are unable to survive. This is one way to reduce the growth and transmission of pathogens in the medical office.

The Infection Process Cycle

In order for a pathogen to survive and produce disease, a continuous cycle must be followed; this is known as the Infection Process Cycle (Fig. 1–1). If the cycle is broken at any point, the pathogen dies. The medical assistant has a responsibility to help break this cycle in the medical office by practicing good techniques of medical asepsis. These techniques are discussed in the next section.

Protective Mechanisms of the Body

The body has protective mechanisms to help prevent the entrance of pathogens. These help to break the Infection Process Cycle. Protective mechanisms of the body include:

1. The hairlike cilia in the nose and respiratory tract. Cilia trap microorganisms and help prevent them from entering the body. The cilia constantly beat toward the outside of the body to help remove pathogens from the body.
2. Coughing and sneezing are defense mechanisms of the body. Coughing and sneezing help to force pathogens from the body.
3. Tears and sweat are secretions that aid in the removal of pathogens from the body.

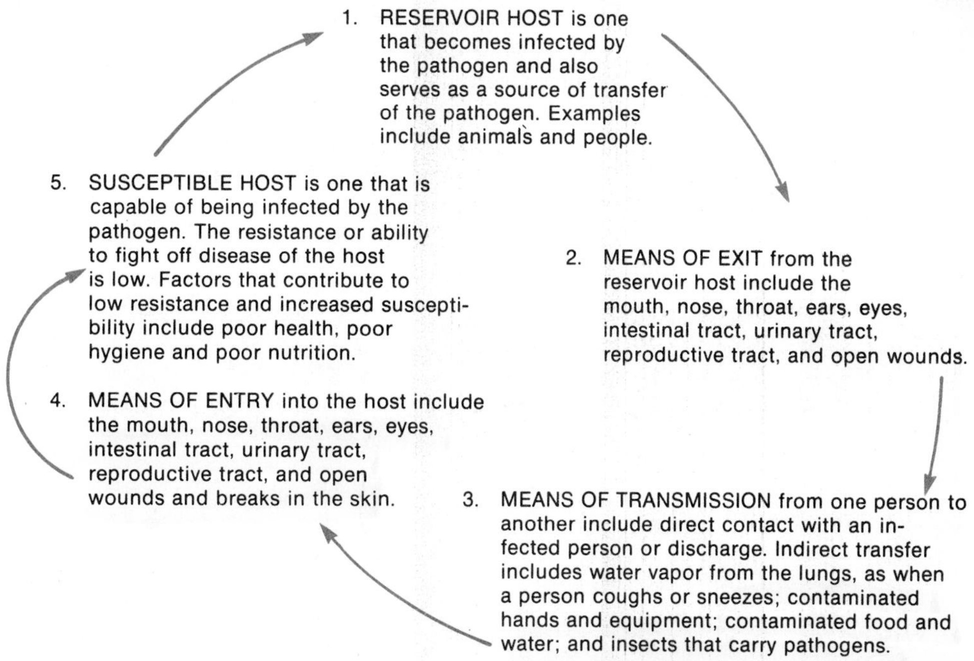

1. RESERVOIR HOST is one that becomes infected by the pathogen and also serves as a source of transfer of the pathogen. Examples include animals and people.

2. MEANS OF EXIT from the reservoir host include the mouth, nose, throat, ears, eyes, intestinal tract, urinary tract, reproductive tract, and open wounds.

3. MEANS OF TRANSMISSION from one person to another include direct contact with an infected person or discharge. Indirect transfer includes water vapor from the lungs, as when a person coughs or sneezes; contaminated hands and equipment; contaminated food and water; and insects that carry pathogens.

4. MEANS OF ENTRY into the host include the mouth, nose, throat, ears, eyes, intestinal tract, urinary tract, reproductive tract, and open wounds and breaks in the skin.

5. SUSCEPTIBLE HOST is one that is capable of being infected by the pathogen. The resistance or ability to fight off disease of the host is low. Factors that contribute to low resistance and increased susceptibility include poor health, poor hygiene and poor nutrition.

FIGURE 1–1. The Infection Process Cycle.

4. The urine and vaginal secretions are acidic. Pathogens cannot grow in an acidic environment.

5. The stomach secretes hydrochloric acid, which helps in the process of digestion. This acid environment discourages the growth of pathogens entering the stomach.

Application of Medical Asepsis in the Medical Office

In the medical office, practices must be employed to reduce the number and hinder the transmission of pathogens. These practices are known as medical asepsis. *Medical asepsis* means that an object or area is clean and free from infection. There will still be nonpathogens present on a clean or medically aseptic substance or surface, but all the pathogens have been eliminated.

Handwashing is an important medical aseptic practice and is crucial in preventing the transmission of pathogens in the medical office. The medical assistant should wash the hands frequently, using the proper handwashing technique. Handwashing is particularly important as soon as one enters the medical office to begin the daily functions, before recording information in the patient's chart, before and after eating, after using a handkerchief, after using the rest room, after contact with grossly contaminated articles such as wastes, and before and after patient contact.

Other good aseptic practices in the medical office include the following:

1. Keeping the medical office free from dirt and dust, which can collect and carry microorganisms.

2. Making sure that the waiting room and examining rooms are well ventilated. Stuffy rooms encourage microorganisms to settle on objects.

3. Keeping the waiting and examining rooms bright and airy. Light discourages the growth of microorganisms.

4. Eliminating insects by the use of insecticides or window screens. Insects are a means of transmission of microorganisms.

5. Carefully disposing of wastes such as urine, feces, and respiratory secretions; all wastes should be handled as if they contained pathogens.

6. Wrapping grossly soiled items such as dressings, tissues, and cotton balls in waterproof bags before disposing of them. These items are a source of pathogens.

7. Not letting soiled items touch clothing.

8. Avoiding coughs and sneezes of patients. The water vapor expelled from the lungs with coughing and sneezing may contain pathogens.

9. Keeping equipment clean. Equipment that does not need to be sterilized should be cleaned thoroughly after patient use.

10. Using discretion in the amount of jewelry worn. Microorganisms can become lodged in the grooves and crevices of jewelry and serve as a means of transmission of pathogens.

PROCEDURE 1-1

HANDWASHING

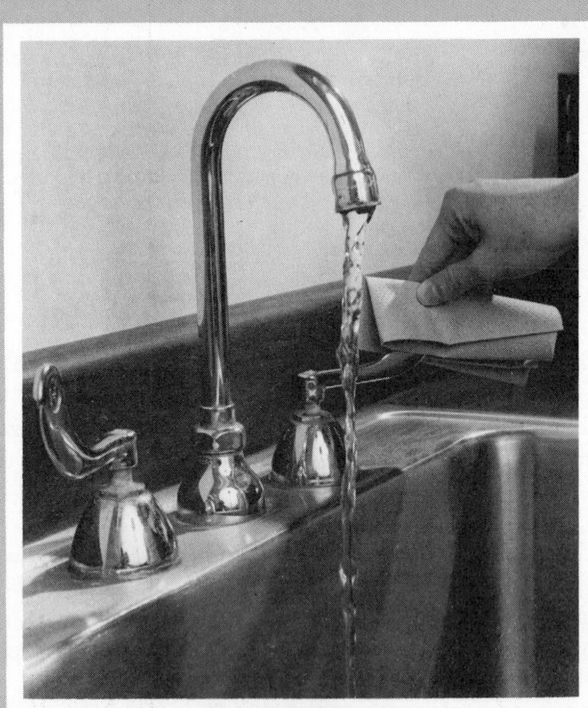

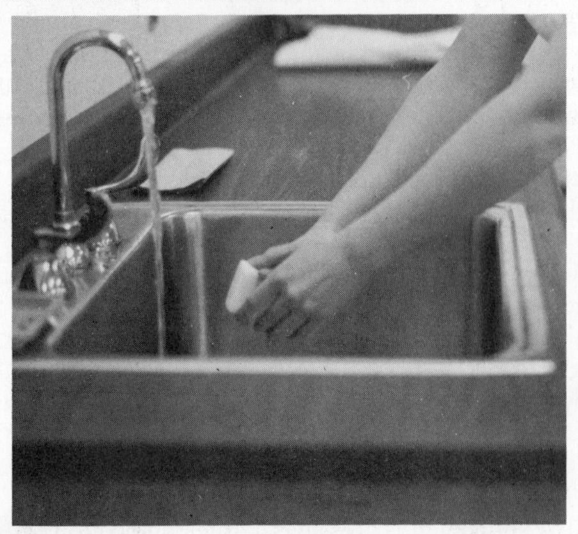

1. **PROCEDURAL STEP.** Remove all rings, except the plain wedding band.

PRINCIPLE. Microorganisms can lodge in the crevices and grooves of rings.

2. **PROCEDURAL STEP.** Stand at the sink, making sure clothing does not touch the sink.

PRINCIPLE. The sink is considered contaminated, and if the uniform touches the sink, it may pick up microorganisms and transfer them.

3. **PROCEDURAL STEP.** Turn on the faucets, using a paper towel.

PRINCIPLE. The faucets are considered contaminated because they harbor microorganisms.

4. **PROCEDURAL STEP.** Adjust the water temperature. The water should be warm to make the best suds.

PRINCIPLE. Water that is too hot or too cold tends to dry the skin, causing chapping and cracking and making it easy for pathogens to enter the body.

5. **PROCEDURAL STEP.** Discard the paper towel in the trash can.

PRINCIPLE. The paper towel is considered contaminated after touching the faucets.

6. **PROCEDURAL STEP.** Wet hands with water. The hands should be held lower than the elbows at all times. Be careful not to touch the inside of the sink, as it is also contaminated.

PRINCIPLE. By holding the hands lower than the elbows, bacteria and debris will be carried away from the arms and body and into the sink.

7. **PROCEDURAL STEP.** Apply soap to the hands. If liquid soap is used, apply approximately 1 teaspoon. If bar soap is used, it must be retained in the hands during sudsing up. (Note: If the bar soap is accidentally dropped on the floor or in the sink during the handwashing procedure, the medical assistant must repeat the procedure from the beginning.)

8. **PROCEDURAL STEP.** Rinse the bar soap before returning it to the soap dish. The soap dish should have drainage holes so that the soap can dry out — moisture encourages the growth of microorganisms.

PRINCIPLE. Microorganisms and debris accumulate on the soap during the handwashing procedure. Rinsing the soap helps to carry these away.

9. **PROCEDURAL STEP.** Wash the palms and backs of the hands with 10 circular motions. Use friction along with the circular motions to wash the palm and back of each hand.

PRINCIPLE. Friction helps to dislodge and remove microorganisms from the hands.

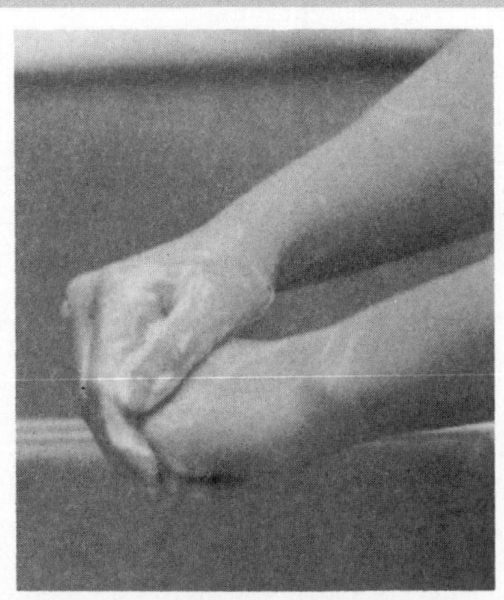

10. **PROCEDURAL STEP.** Wash the fingers with 10 circular motions. Interlace the fingers and thumbs and use friction and circular motions, while rubbing the fingers back and forth.

PRINCIPLE. This kind of movement helps to remove microorganisms and debris that have accumulated between the fingers.

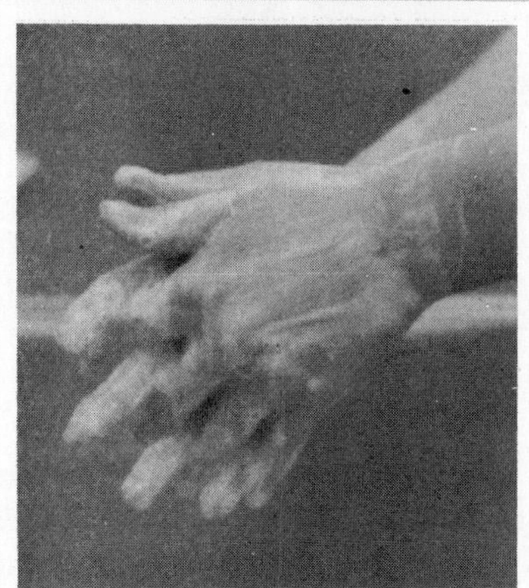

11. **PROCEDURAL STEP.** Rinse well, making sure to hold the hands lower than the elbows.

PRINCIPLE. Running water helps to rinse away dirt and microorganisms.

12. **PROCEDURAL STEP.** Wash wrists and forearms, using friction along with circular motions. (Note: The hands are washed first, as they are the most contaminated; thus organisms and dirt are washed away and not spread to the wrists and forearms.)

13. **PROCEDURAL STEP.** Rinse arms and hands.

PRINCIPLE. The running water rinses away the dirt and microorganisms.

14. **PROCEDURAL STEP.** Clean the fingernails with an orange stick. The fingernails should be cleaned at least once daily.

PRINCIPLE. Dirt and microorganisms collect underneath the fingernails.

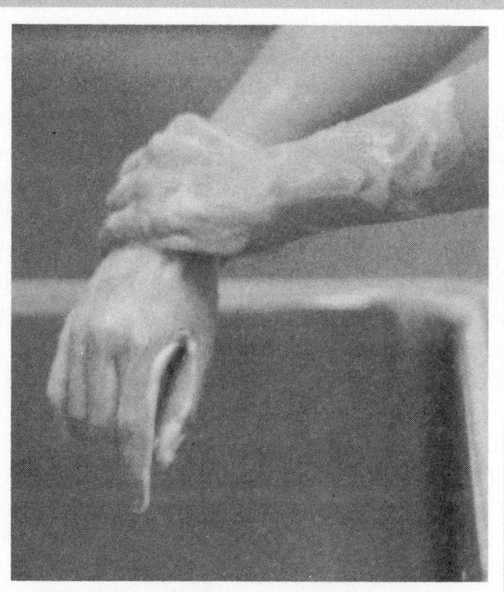

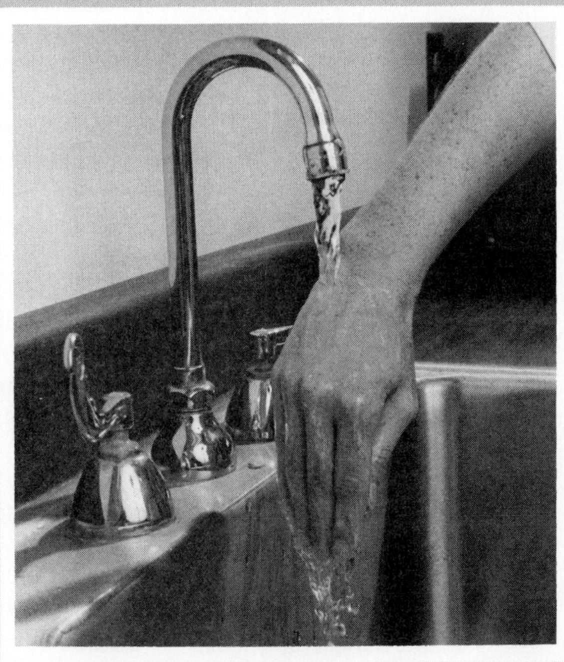

Continued

15. **PROCEDURAL STEP.** Repeat the handwashing procedure. For initial handwashing or when the hands are grossly contaminated, as when they come into contact with blood, pus, urine, or other contaminants, the handwashing procedure should be repeated. This is to ensure removal of all pathogens.

16. **PROCEDURAL STEP.** Dry the hands gently and thoroughly.
PRINCIPLE. Drying the hands gently prevents them from becoming chapped. Microorganisms can lodge in the crevices of chapped hands. Make sure the hands are dried completely, since wet skin may also cause chapping.

17. **PROCEDURAL STEP.** Turn off the water, using a paper towel.
PRINCIPLE. The faucet is considered contaminated, whereas the hands are medically aseptic or clean.

18. **PROCEDURAL STEP.** Wipe the area around the sink with a paper towel to remove water and debris that may have splashed onto the working area during the handwashing procedure.
PRINCIPLE. The water and dirt would result in sink contamination and encourage the growth of microorganisms.

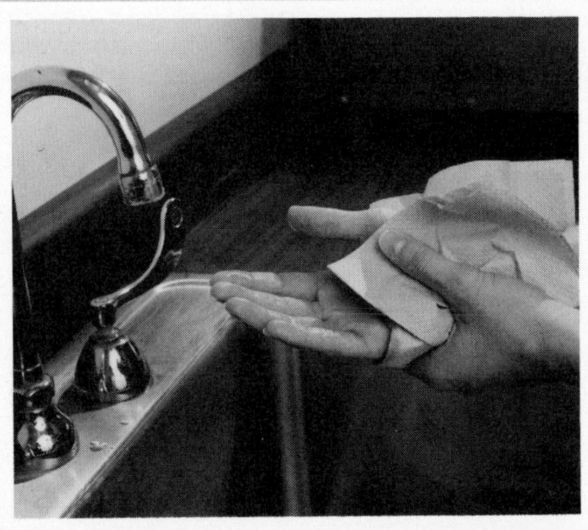

19. **PROCEDURAL STEP.** Do not touch the sink with the bare hands.
PRINCIPLE. The hands are now medically aseptic and the sink is considered contaminated.

Acquired Immunodeficiency Syndrome (AIDS)

Acquired immunodeficiency syndrome (AIDS) is a disorder of the immune system of the body and is characterized by the presence of opportunistic infections and unusual cancers that rarely afflict individuals with healthy immune systems. For example, a severe and rare type of pneumonia caused by the organism *Pneumocystis carinii* is frequently associated with AIDS patients, as is Kaposi's sarcoma, a type of cancer. AIDS is also known to damage the nervous system, which eventually results in varying degrees of dementia and other symptoms.

AIDS is caused by a retrovirus known as the *human immunodeficiency virus (HIV).* This virus is transmitted through contaminated body fluids, in particular, blood and semen. An individual infected with HIV may first experience a transient mononucleosis-like illness known as *acute HIV infection.* Symptoms of acute HIV infection include fever, pharyngitis, myalgia, arthralgia, and adenopathy. After these early symptoms have subsided (if they occur at all), the infected individual normally experiences a long incubation period, or years of latency, during which he or she is asymptomatic. At that time, the carrier may not realize the HIV infection is present, because the only evidence of HIV infection during the period of latency is the presence of an antibody to HIV that is detectable by blood tests.

Because of the length of time required by the body to develop HIV antibodies, however, these tests may fail to detect HIV for as long as 6 months after an individual has been infected. Because HIV may be transmitted with or without symptoms, it is during this period of latency that the danger of accidental transmission is greatest.

It is not yet known whether all HIV-infected individuals will develop AIDS. Current evidence suggests that 20 to 30 per cent of those infected with HIV will develop AIDS within the first 5 years. Some authorities project that 80 per cent of HIV carriers will develop AIDS within 10 years after infection. Furthermore, because there is no known cure for HIV infection at this time and the virus remains in the body for life, it may be that nearly all carriers will eventually develop the AIDS disease.

Before the development of full-blown AIDS (as identified by the presence of such disorders as *Pneumocystis carinii* pneumonia and Kaposi's sarcoma), many HIV–infected individuals experience a series of lesser symptoms. These include chronic enlargement of the lymph nodes, recurring fevers and sweats, persistent diarrhea, and a mononucleosis-like chronic fatigue. The combination of these symptoms is known as *AIDS–related complex (ARC).* Also characteristic of ARC are weight loss and ongoing dementia characterized by memory loss and other nervous disorders.

In summary, the AIDS virus infection cycle has four stages; however they may not all be experienced by every infected individual. They include:

1. Acute HIV infection.
2. A period of asymptomatic latency.
3. ARC.
4. The AIDS–defining disorders, such as *Pneumocystis carinii* pneumonia and Kaposi's sarcoma.

Transmission of AIDS

HIV has been isolated in blood, semen, saliva, tears, breast milk, cerebrospinal fluid, amniotic fluid, urine, and secretions of the female genital tract. However, the only documented transmission of the virus has occurred by exposure to contaminated blood and exchange of sexual and perinatal fluids. In the United States, AIDS has been concentrated primarily among the male homosexual population and intravenous drug users. The remaining cases are caused by the spread of HIV among recipients of contaminated blood transfusions, female sexual partners of other risk groups, and newborn babies of HIV–infected mothers.

The most common exposure to contaminated blood now occurs among needle-sharing intravenous drug users. Before 1985 there was some risk of becoming infected by way of contaminated blood transfusions. In March, 1985, the Food and Drug Administration approved the ELISA (enzyme-linked immunoabsorbent assay) for use in commercial blood banks, public health clinics, and plasma centers. Use of this test and the screening of potential donors for risk factors (e.g., homosexual contacts and drug use) have virtually eliminated the transmission of HIV through blood transfusions.

Studies have shown that HIV is not transmitted through casual contact, or even extensive contact such as occurs among family members of AIDS patients. Given that HIV is not easily transmitted, and, in fact, is apparently transmitted only during the exchange of contaminated body fluids, the risk to health-care workers is quite low. Still, parenteral exposure to HIV–contaminated blood or other body fluids should be considered a definite occupational risk, no matter how small. Studies by the United States Department of Health and Human Services Centers for Disease Control (CDC) have indicated that even when parenteral exposure to ***known*** HIV–contaminated blood has been documented, less than 1 per cent of health-care workers so exposed (and not at risk for other reasons) tested positive for HIV infection. These studies indicate that HIV is inefficiently transmitted, even during accidental needle-stick incidents or the exposure of mucous membrane or damaged skin to contaminated fluids.

AIDS Infection Precautions

Despite the low risk of infection, the serious nature of HIV infection and the likely subsequent development of AIDS warrant the use of precautionary measures by all health-care workers. Furthermore, because most HIV carriers are asymptomatic and may not be aware of their infection, precautions minimizing the risk of exposure to blood and body fluids should be taken with all patients at all times. The precautions are also recommended as a means of protection against other blood-borne pathogens such as hepatitis-B. The CDC has issued a recommended set of precautions for health-care workers, which are stated below.

Universal Precautions. Because medical history and examination cannot reliably identify all patients infected with HIV or other blood-borne pathogens, blood and body-fluid precautions should be consistently used for *all* patients. This approach, previously recommended by CDC and referred to as "universal blood and body-fluid precautions" or "universal precautions," should be used in the care of *all* patients, especially those in emergency-care settings, in which the risk of blood exposure is increased and the infection status of the patient is usually unknown.

1. All health-care workers should routinely use appropriate barrier precautions to prevent skin and mucous-membrane exposure, when contact with blood or other body fluids of any patient is anticipated. Gloves should be worn for touching blood and body fluids, mucous membranes, or nonintact skin of all patients, for handling items or surfaces soiled with blood or body fluids, and for performing venipuncture and other vascular access procedures. Gloves should be changed after contact with each patient. Masks and protective eye wear or face shields should be worn during procedures that are likely to generate droplets of blood or other body fluids to prevent exposure of mucous membranes of the mouth, nose, and eyes. Gowns or aprons should be worn during procedures that are likely to generate splashes of blood or other body fluids.
2. Hands and other skin surfaces should be washed immediately and thoroughly if contaminated with blood or other body fluids. Hands should be washed immediately after gloves are removed.
3. All health-care workers should take precautions to prevent injuries caused by needles, scalpels, and other sharp instruments or devices during procedures, when cleaning used instruments, during disposal of used needles, and when handling sharp instruments after procedures. To prevent needle-stick injuries, needles should not be recapped, purposely bent or broken by hand, removed from disposable syringes, or otherwise manipulated by hand. After they are used, disposable syringes and needles, scalpel blades, and other sharp items should be placed in puncture-resistant containers for disposal; the puncture-resistant containers should be located as close as is practical to the area in which they will be used. Large-bore reusable needles should be placed in a puncture-resistant container for transport to the reprocessing area.
4. Saliva has not been implicated in HIV transmission. However, to minimize the need for emergency mouth-to-mouth resuscitation, mouthpieces, resuscitation bags, or other ventilation devices should be available for use in areas in which the need for resuscitation is predictable.
5. Health-care workers who have exudative lesions or weeping dermatitis should refrain from all direct patient care and from handling patient-care equipment, until the condition resolves.
6. Health-care workers who are pregnant are not known to be at greater risk of contracting HIV infection than those who are not pregnant. However, if an individual develops HIV infection during pregnancy, the infant is at risk of infection resulting from perinatal transmission. Because of this risk, pregnant health-care workers should be especially familiar with and strictly adhere to precautions to minimize the risk of HIV infection.

Precautions for Laboratories. Blood and other body fluids from *all* patients should be considered infective. To supplement the universal blood and body-fluid precautions listed above, the following safeguards are recommended for health-care workers in clinical laboratories.

1. All specimens of blood and body fluids should be put in a well-constructed

container with a secure lid, to prevent leaking during transport. Care should be taken when collecting each specimen to avoid contaminating the outside of the container and the laboratory form accompanying the specimen.

2. All persons processing blood and body-fluid specimens (e.g., removing tops from vacuum tubes) should wear gloves. Masks and protective eye wear should be worn if mucous-membrane contact with blood or body fluids is anticipated. Gloves should be changed, and hands washed, after completion of specimen processing.

3. For routine procedures, such as histologic and pathologic studies or microbiologic culturing, a biologic safety cabinet is not necessary. However, biologic safety cabinets should be used whenever procedures are conducted that have a high potential for generating droplets. These include activities such as blending, sonicating, and vigorous mixing.

4. Mechanical pipetting devices should be used for manipulating all liquids in the laboratory. Mouth pipetting must not be done.

5. Use of needles and syringes should be limited to situations in which there is no alternative, and the recommendations for preventing injuries with needles outlined under Universal Precautions should be followed.

6. Laboratory work surfaces should be decontaminated with an appropriate chemical germicide after a spill of blood or other body fluids and when work activities are completed.

7. Contaminated materials used in laboratory tests should be decontaminated before reprocessing or should be placed in bags and disposed of in accordance with institutional policies for disposal of infective waste.

8. Scientific equipment that has been contaminated with blood or other body fluids should be decontaminated and cleaned before being repaired in the laboratory or transported to the manufacturer.

9. All persons should wash their hands after completing laboratory activities and should remove protective clothing before leaving the laboratory.

Sterilization and Disinfection. Standard sterilization and disinfection procedures for patient-care equipment currently recommended for use in a variety of health-care settings—including hospitals, medical and dental clinics and offices, hemodialysis centers, emergency care facilities, and long-term nursing-care facilities—are adequate to sterilize or disinfect instruments, devices, or other items contaminated with blood or other body fluids from persons infected with blood-borne pathogens, including HIV.

Instruments or devices that enter sterile tissue or the vascular system of any patient, or through which blood flows, should be sterilized before reuse. Devices or items that contact intact mucous membranes should be sterilized or receive high-level disinfection, a procedure that kills vegetative organisms and viruses but not necessarily large numbers of bacterial spores. Chemical germicides that are registered with the United States Environmental Protection Agency (EPA) as "sterilants" may be used either for sterilization or for high-level disinfection, depending on the contact time.

Medical devices or instruments that require sterilization or disinfection should be thoroughly cleaned before being exposed to the germicide, and the manufacturer's instructions for the use of the germicide should be followed. Further, it is important that the manufacturer's specifications for compatibility of the medical device with chemical germicides be closely followed. Information about the specific label claims of commercial germicides can be obtained by writing to the Disinfectants Branch, Office of Pesticides, Environmental Protection Agency, 401 M Street, SW, Washington, D. C. 20460.

Studies have shown that HIV is rapidly inactivated after being exposed to commonly used chemical germicides at concentrations much lower than those used in practice. Embalming fluids are similar to the types of chemical germicides that have been tested and found to completely inactivate HIV. In addition to commercially available chemical germicides, a solution of sodium hypochlorite (household bleach), prepared daily, is an inexpensive and effective germicide. Concentrations ranging from approximately 500 ppm (1 : 100 dilution of household bleach) sodium hypochlorite to 5000 ppm (1 : 10 dilution of household bleach) are effective, depending on the amount of organic material (e.g., blood, mucus) that is on the surface to be cleaned and disinfected. Commercially available chemical germicides may be more compatible with certain medical devices that might be corroded by repeated exposure to sodium hypochlorite, especially to the 1 : 10 dilution.

Cleaning and Decontaminating Spills of Blood or Other Body Fluids. Chemical germicides that are approved for use as "hospital disinfectants" and are turberculocidal when used at recommended dilutions can be used to decontaminate spills of blood and other body fluids. Strategies for decontaminating spills of blood and other body fluids in a patient-care setting are different than strategies for spills of cultures or other materials in clinical, public health, or research laboratories. In patient care areas, visible material should first be removed, and then the area should be decontaminated. With large spills of cultured or concentrated infectious agents in the laboratory, the contaminated area should be flooded with a liquid germicide before cleaning, then decontaminated with a fresh germicidal chemical. In both settings gloves should be worn during the cleaning and decontaminating procedures.

Infective Waste. No epidemiologic evidence is available to suggest that most medical waste is any more infective than residential waste. Moreover, there is no epidemiologic evidence that medical waste has caused disease in the community as a result of improper disposal. Therefore, identifying wastes for which special precautions are indicated is largely a matter of judgment about the relative risk of disease transmission. The most practical approach to the management of infective wastes is to identify those that have the potential for causing infection during handling and disposal and for which some special precautions appear prudent. Medical wastes that seem to warrant special precautions include microbiology laboratory waste, pathology waste, and blood specimens or blood products. Although any item that has had contact with blood exudates or secretions may be potentially infective, it is not usually considered practical or necessary to treat all such waste as infective. Infective waste, in general, should either be incinerated or should be autoclaved before disposal in a sanitary land fill. Bulk blood, suctioned fluids, excretions, and secretions may be carefully poured down a drain connected to a sanitary sewer. Sanitary sewers may also be used to dispose of other infectious wastes capable of being ground and flushed into the sewer.

Study Questions

1. What is a microorganism?
2. What are the basic requirements needed for growth and multiplication of microorganisms?
3. What is medical asepsis?
4. What are the six recommendations included in the universal precautions for infection control?

2 VITAL SIGNS

CHAPTER OUTLINE

BODY TEMPERATURE
- How Body Temperature is Maintained
- Methods for Taking Body Temperature
- Body Temperature Range
- Variations in Body Temperature
- Pyrexia
- Glass Thermometers
- Temperature Sheaths
- Cleaning Glass Thermometers
- Electronic Thermometer

PULSE
- Mechanism of the Pulse
- Sites for Taking the Pulse
- Pulse Rate
- Rhythm and Volume

RESPIRATION
- Mechanism of Respiration
- Control of Respiration
- Respiratory Rate
- Rhythm and Depth of Respiration
- Respiratory Abnormalities
- Color of the Patient

BLOOD PRESSURE
- Mechanism of Blood Pressure
- Normal Blood Pressure
- Equipment to Measure Blood Pressure
- Factors Affecting Blood Pressure
- Korotkoff Sounds

INTRODUCTION

Vital signs, also known as cardinal signs, indicate a patient's condition; they are objective guideposts, indicating that life is present. The four vital signs are temperature, pulse, and respiration (TPR), and blood pressure (BP).

The normal ranges of the vital signs are finely adjusted, and any deviation from normal may indicate disease. During the course of an illness, variations in the vital signs may take place. The medical assistant should be alert to any significant changes and report them to the physician, as they may indicate a change in the patient's condition. When patients visit the medical office vital signs are routinely checked to establish each patient's baseline measurements, within the normal range, against which future measurements can be compared. The medical assistant should have a thorough knowledge of the vital signs and attain proficiency in taking them.

This chapter is divided into four units, covering each of the vital signs. Each unit has separate objectives, vocabulary lists, procedures, and study questions. In addition, general objectives are provided for the chapter as a whole.

GENERAL OBJECTIVES

After completing this chapter, you should be able to do the following:

1. Define a vital sign.
2. List the four vital signs.
3. Explain the purpose for taking vital signs.

• VOCABULARY •

axilla (ak-sil' ah)—The armpit.
Centigrade or Celsius thermometer (sen' ti-grād or sel' se-us ther-mom' ĕ-ter)—A thermometer on which the freezing point of water is 0° and the boiling point of water is 100°.
conduction (kon-duk' shun)—The transfer of energy, such as heat, from one object to another.
convection (kon-vek' shun)—The transfer of energy, such as heat, in the form of currents.
crisis (kri' sis)—A sudden falling of an elevated body temperature to normal.
disinfectant (dis" in-fek' tant)—A substance that kills disease-producing organisms.
Fahrenheit thermometer (far' en-hīt ther-mom' ĕ-ter)—A thermometer on which the freezing point of water is 32° and the boiling point of water is 212°.
fever (fe' ver)—A body temperature that is above normal. Synonym for pyrexia.
frenulum linguae (fren' u-lum ling' gwe)—The midline fold that connects the undersurface of the tongue with the floor of the mouth.
hyperpyrexia (hi" per-pi-rek' se-ah)—An extremely high fever.
lysis (li' sis)—The gradual return of the body temperature to normal.
pyrexia (pi-rek' se-ah)—A body temperature that is above normal. Synonym for fever.
radiation (ra" de-a' shun)—The transfer of energy, such as heat, in the form of waves.
subnormal (sub-nor' mal)—A body temperature that is below normal.

COMPETENCIES

After completing this unit, you should be able to demonstrate the proper procedures to perform the following:

1. Apply and remove a temperature sheath.
2. Take and record oral body temperature.
3. Take and record rectal body temperature.
4. Take and record axillary body temperature.
5. Take and record body temperature with an electronic thermometer.
6. Clean glass thermometers.

LEARNING OBJECTIVES

After completing this unit, you should be able to do the following:

1. Define the terms listed in the vocabulary.
2. Define body temperature.
3. Give examples of four ways in which heat is produced in the body and four ways in which heat is lost from the body.
4. List the three sites for taking body temperature and explain why these sites are used.
5. List three instances in which the rectal method for taking body temperature would be preferred over the oral method.
6. Explain why the rectal method is considered the most accurate method for taking body temperature and why the axillary method is considered the least accurate method.
7. State the normal body temperature range and the average body temperature.
8. List and explain four factors that should be taken into consideration when evaluating body temperature.
9. List and explain the three stages included in the course of a fever.
10. List and explain the parts of a glass thermometer.
11. Explain the principles underlying each step in the oral, rectal, and axillary temperature procedures.

Body Temperature

How Body Temperature is Maintained

Body temperature represents a balance between the heat produced in the body and the heat lost from the body (Fig. 2–1). A constant temperature range must be maintained in order for the body to function properly.

Most of the heat produced in the body is through voluntary and involuntary muscle contractions. Voluntary muscle contractions involve the muscles over which the body has control, for example, the moving of legs or arms. Involuntary muscle contractions involve the muscles over which the body has no control; physiologic processes such as digestion, the beating of the heart, and shivering are examples of this.

Body heat is also produced by cell metabolism. Heat is produced when nutrients are broken down in the cells. Fever and strong emotional states increase heat production in the body.

Heat is lost from the body through the urine and feces and in water vapor from the lungs. Perspiration also contributes to heat loss. Perspiration is the excretion of moisture through the pores of the skin. When the moisture evaporates, heat is released and the body is cooled.

Conduction, convection, and radiation all cause loss of heat from the body. *Conduction* is the transfer of heat from one object to another; heat can be transferred by conduction from the body to a cooler object it touches. *Convection* is the transfer of heat through air currents; cool air currents can cause the body to lose heat. *Radiation* is the transfer of heat in the form of waves; body heat is continuously radiating into cooler surroundings.

Methods for Taking Body Temperature

There are three methods for taking body temperature: *oral* (by mouth), *rectal* (by rectum), and *axillary* (by axilla). The sites used for taking temperature must be located in a space as closed as possible to prevent air currents from interfering with the temperature reading. The sites should also have an abundant blood supply, so that the temperature of the entire body is obtained, and not just the temperature of only a part of the body.

The oral method is the most convenient and the most commonly used method for taking body temperature. When the medical assistant records a temperature,

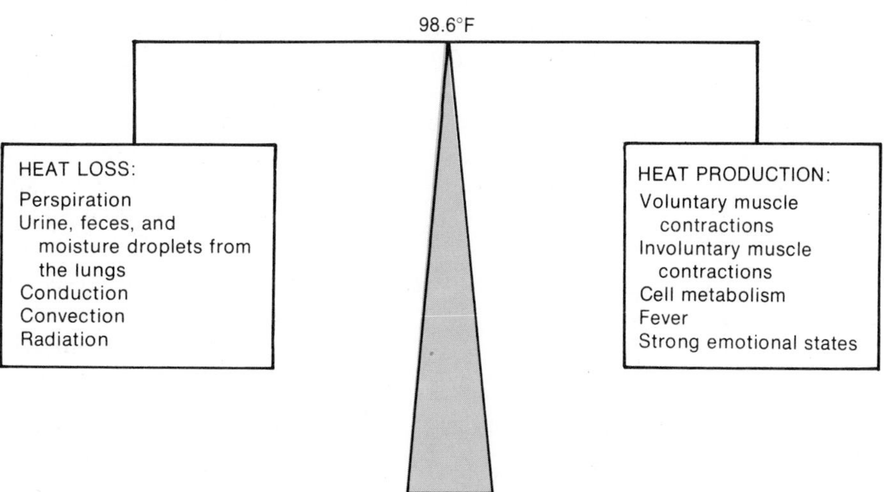

FIGURE 2–1. Body temperature represents a balance between the heat produced in the body and the heat lost from the body.

the physician assumes it has been taken through the oral route, unless it is otherwise noted. There is a rich blood supply under the tongue in the area located on either side of the frenulum linguae. This is the area in which the thermometer should be placed to receive the most accurate reading. The patient must keep his or her mouth closed during the procedure to provide a closed space for the thermometer.

The rectal temperature is the most accurate measurement of body temperature. The rectum is highly vascular and, of the three sites, provides the most closed cavity. The temperature obtained through the rectal route measures approximately 1°F higher than the same temperature taken through the oral route. The medical assistant should make a notation on the patient's chart if the temperature has been taken rectally. The rectal method is generally used for infants and young children, unconscious patients, and mouth-breathing patients and when greater accuracy in body temperature is desired.

The axillary method is the least accurate of the three methods, because the axilla is more open to air currents than the mouth or rectum. The axillary method is used when the medical assistant is unable to use the other two methods. It is often used with preschoolers who are not yet old enough to understand how to hold a thermometer in their mouths for mouth-breathing patients and for patients with oral inflammation or who have had oral surgery. The temperature obtained through the axillary method measures approximately 1°F lower than the same temperature taken through the oral route. As with the rectal method, the medical assistant should make a notation to tell the physician that the temperature was taken through the axillary route.

Body Temperature Range

The purpose of taking body temperature is to establish the patient's baseline recording and to monitor an abnormally high or low body temperature. The normal body temperature range is 97 to 99° Fahrenheit (F), the average temperature being 98.6°F, which is equal to 37° centigrade or Celsius (C). The body temperature can be taken by using a Fahrenheit or a Celsius (centigrade) thermometer. The Fahrenheit thermometer is most often employed in the medical office.

A body temperature below 97°F is classified as *subnormal.* This means that the heat being lost from the body is greater than the heat being produced. An individual usually cannot survive with a subnormal temperature of less than 93.2°F (34°C).

A body temperature above 99°F indicates a *fever,* or *pyrexia.* If the temperature exceeds 99°F, the heat being produced in the body is greater than the heat being lost. A temperature reading above 105.8°F (41°C) is known as *hyperpyrexia.* Hyperpyrexia is a serious condition, and a temperature above 109.4°F (43°C) is generally fatal.

Variations in Body Temperature

Normal variations may occur in the day-to-day activities of an individual, causing fluctuations in the body temperature. Rarely does the body temperature stay the same throughout the course of a day. The medical assistant should take the following points into consideration when evaluating a patient's temperature:

Emotional states — Strong emotions, such as crying or extreme anger, can increase the body temperature. This is important to consider when working with young children, who frequently cry during examination procedures or when they are ill.

Time of day — During sleep, body metabolism slows down, as do muscle contractions. The temperature of the body is lowest in the morning before metabolism and muscle contractions begin speeding up.

Patient's normal body temperature	Some patients normally run a low or high temperature. The medical assistant should review the patient's past vital sign recordings.
Environment	Cold weather tends to decrease the body temperature, whereas hot weather increases it.
Physical exercise	Vigorous physical exercise causes an increase in voluntary muscle contractions, which raises the body temperature.
Pregnancy	Cell metabolism increases during pregnancy, which in turn raises body temperature.
Age of patient	Infants and young children normally have a higher body temperature than adults because their heat-regulating mechanism is not yet fully established. Older people usually have a lower body temperature.

Pyrexia

Fever, or pyrexia, denotes that a patient's temperature has risen above 99°F. Fever is generally associated with the presence of disease. An individual with a fever feels hot to the touch and has a flushed appearance. The course of a fever can be divided into the following three stages:

1. The *onset* is when the temperature first begins to rise. The rise may be slow or sudden.
2. During the *stadium,* the temperature rises and falls in one of the following three patterns:
   a. For the patient with *continued fever,* the temperature is continuously elevated above normal, with less than 1°F of fluctuation in a 24-hour period.
   b. An *intermittent fever* is one in which the temperature alternately rises and falls and at times returns to normal or even subnormal.
   c. A *remittent fever* is characterized by a rising and falling of an elevated temperature. It does not return to normal until the patient has recovered.
3. The *subsiding* stage is when the temperature returns to normal. It can return to normal gradually (known as *lysis*) or suddenly (known as a *crisis*).

Glass Thermometers

The glass thermometer is the type most commonly used in the medical office (Fig. 2–2). It consists of two parts—the *bulb* and the *stem.* Mercury is contained in the bulb of the thermometer. Mercury is a metal that expands when exposed to heat and rises in a sealed column located in the center of the thermometer.

The bulb has a constriction that does not allow the mercury to fall back once it has risen in the sealed column. It is necessary to shake the thermometer with a snapping wrist motion to make the mercury return to the bulb. The mercury should be at a level of 96°F or below, before a patient's temperature is taken; otherwise, the reading may be inaccurate.

The stem of the thermometer contains calibrations, which are divided into two-tenths of a degree (0.2°) on the Fahrenheit thermometer and into one-tenth of a degree (0.1°) on the Celsius thermometer. The temperature range on the Fahrenheit thermometer is 94 to 108°, and on the Celsius thermometer it is 34 to 42° (Fig. 2–3). A body temperature above or below these ranges is rare.

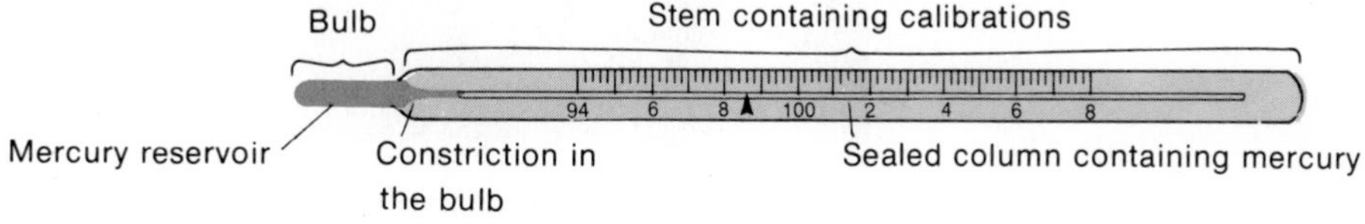

FIGURE 2–2. The parts of a mercury thermometer.

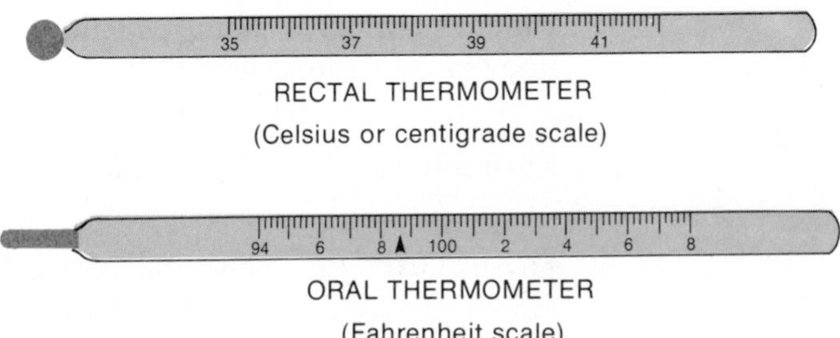

FIGURE 2–3. Glass mercury thermometers illustrating the difference in the shape of the bulb between the rectal and oral thermometers. The rectal thermometer exhibits the centigrade scale and the oral thermometer exhibits the Fahrenheit scale.

The bulb of an oral thermometer is long and slender to provide a greater surface area for contact with the vascular tissues of the mouth or axilla. The bulb of the rectal thermometer is short and blunt for easier insertion into the rectum (Fig. 2–3). An oral thermometer should not be used to take a rectal temperature, as the long, slender bulb may puncture the rectal mucosa. The medical assistant should store oral and rectal thermometers in separate containers. Thermometers are usually color coded at the stem end to facilitate identifying them; the oral thermometer has a blue tip, and the rectal thermometer has a red tip.

If the thermometer breaks, the medical assistant should take care to make sure the pieces are carefully disposed of, to avoid injury. Mercury is best picked up by brushing the beads onto a piece of paper, without allowing the mercury to touch the skin, and then properly disposing of it.

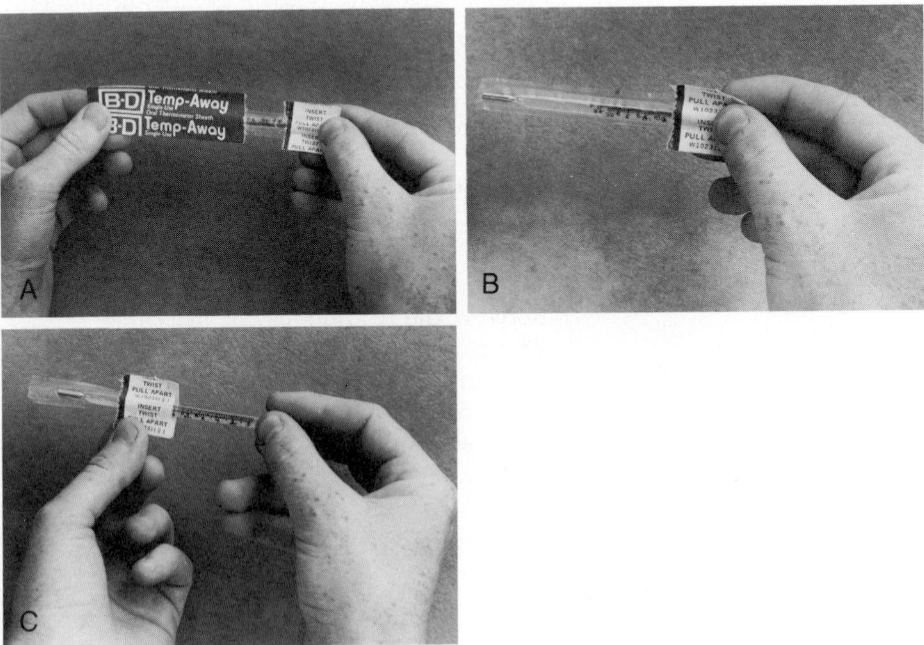

FIGURE 2–4. Application and removal of a temperature sheath. *A,* The sheath is applied according to the manufacturer's instructions. *B,* The sheath should completely encase the thermometer. *C,* As the sheath is pulled off the stem, it inverts, which encloses secretions and bacteria.

Temperature Sheaths

A temperature sheath is a clear, plastic disposable cover that fits over the bulb and stem of a thermometer (Fig. 2–4). Temperature sheaths can be used for the measurement of oral, rectal, and axillary temperature. The rectal sheaths are prelubricated for easier insertion. The thermometer must be shaken down before the sheath is applied so that the calibrations can be clearly read. The sheath is applied according to the manufacturer's instructions, which are usually listed on the label (Fig. 2–4*A*). The medical assistant should make sure that the sheath completely encases the thermometer and is not torn (Fig. 2–4*B*); if tearing occurs, a new sheath should be applied. The patient's temperature is measured according to the oral, rectal, or axillary body temperature procedures presented on the following pages. Once the temperature has been measured, the sheath is removed. As it is pulled off of the stem, the sheath inverts, thereby enclosing secretions and bacteria and reducing the transmission of microorganisms (Fig. 2–4*C*). To ensure an accurate temperature reading, the thermometer must be read after removing the plastic sheath, which should then be properly discarded following the medical office policy.

Cleaning Glass Thermometers

Hot water cannot be used to clean a glass thermometer, because it causes the mercury to expand too far in the sealed column, and the thermometer could break.

The following procedure is used to clean glass thermometers:

1. Wash the thermometer in cool sudsy water to remove surface dirt. Either soap or detergent can be used.
2. Rinse the thermometer under cold running water.
3. Thoroughly dry the thermometer. If the thermometer is wet when immersed in the chemical solution, the water decreases the strength of the chemical by diluting it.
4. Immerse the thermometer in a chemical disinfectant such as benzalkonium chloride (Zephiran Chloride) or alcohol. A period of at least 20 minutes is usually recommended for this step.
5. Rinse the thermometer again under cold running water to remove all traces of disinfectant.
6. Place the thermometer in its proper storage container.

PROCEDURE 2-1
TAKING BODY TEMPERATURE — ORAL

1. **PROCEDURAL STEP.** Wash the hands.

PRINCIPLE. The hands should be clean and free from contamination so that pathogens will not be transferred to the patient.

2. **PROCEDURAL STEP.** Assemble the equipment. The equipment includes an **oral thermometer** and **tissues.** If the thermometer has been stored in a chemical solution, rinse it off with cold water and wipe it dry with a clean soft tissue, using a firm rotating motion.

PRINCIPLE. Chemicals may irritate the mucosa of the mouth and have an unpleasant taste. Cold water must be used to rinse the thermometer, because hot water causes the mercury to expand too far, breaking the thermometer. Wiping the thermometer dry by using a rotating motion ensures that all sides are wiped.

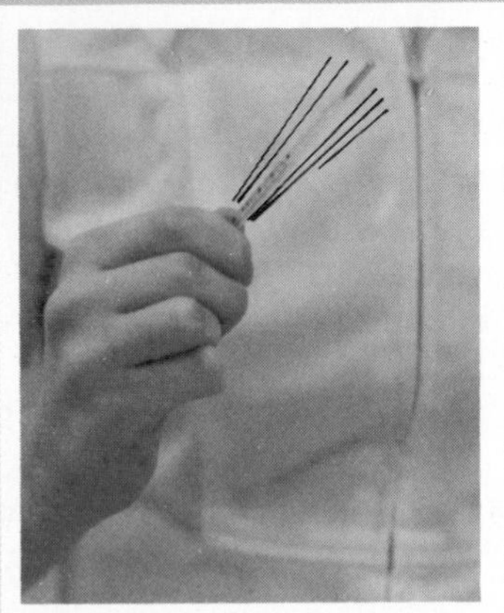

3. **PROCEDURAL STEP.** Check the level of the mercury in the thermometer. Hold the thermometer horizontally at eye level and rotate it slowly, to obtain the best reading.

4. **PROCEDURAL STEP.** If the level of mercury is above 96°F, it needs to be shaken down, in order to obtain an accurate temperature reading. Hold the thermometer firmly between the thumb and forefinger. Shake the thermometer downward with a snapping wrist movement. Repeat this motion until the mercury is below 96°F. Do not allow the thermometer to hit a hard object during this process, to prevent breaking the thermometer.

PRINCIPLE. The constriction in the bulb prevents the mercury from falling on its own.

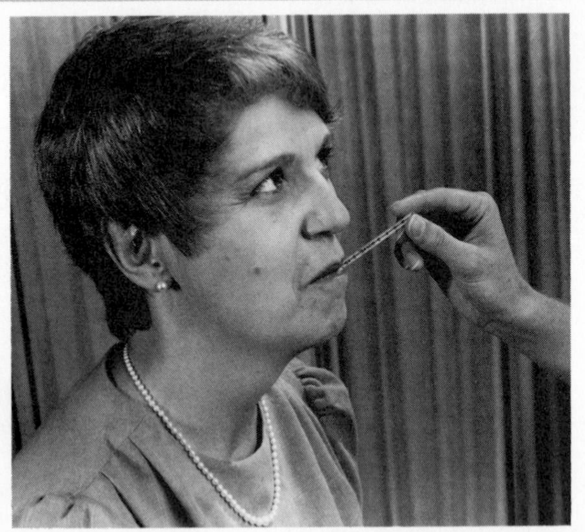

5. **PROCEDURAL STEP.** Identify the patient and explain the procedure.

PRINCIPLE. It is important to explain what you will be doing, since a fearful or apprehensive patient may register an increased body temperature. If the patient has been drinking a hot or cold beverage or has been smoking, the medical assistant must wait 15 to 30 minutes before taking the temperature. Otherwise, a temperature reading of the mouth, and not the body, will be obtained.

6. **PROCEDURAL STEP.** Place the bulb of the thermometer in the patient's mouth in the pocket located on either side of the frenulum linguae.

PRINCIPLE. The long slender bulb provides for good contact with the rich blood supply located in the tissue under the tongue.

7. **PROCEDURAL STEP.** Instruct the patient to keep the mouth closed and to hold the thermometer in place with the lips.

PRINCIPLE. If the mouth is not closed tightly, cooler air from the outside affects the temperature reading. The thermometer must be held in place with the lips — not the teeth — to prevent the patient from biting down on it and breaking it.

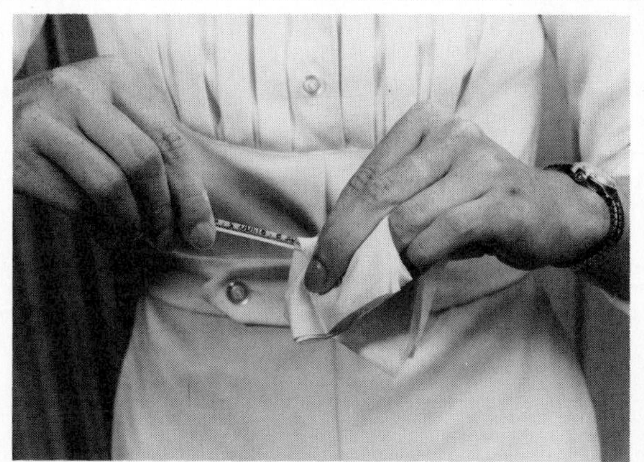

8. **PROCEDURAL STEP.** Leave the thermometer in place for 3 to 5 minutes. The medical assistant should remain in the room to reassure the patient and to remove the thermometer as soon as the body temperature has registered. The pulse and respiration may be taken during this time.
PRINCIPLE. The thermometer must remain in the mouth long enough for an accurate temperature reading to register.

9. **PROCEDURAL STEP.** Remove the thermometer and wipe it from stem to bulb with a clean soft tissue, using a firm rotating motion.
PRINCIPLE. The thermometer should be wiped from the stem toward the bulb end to carry microorganisms away from the medical assistant's fingers. Wiping it also helps to remove mouth secretions and makes it easier to read.

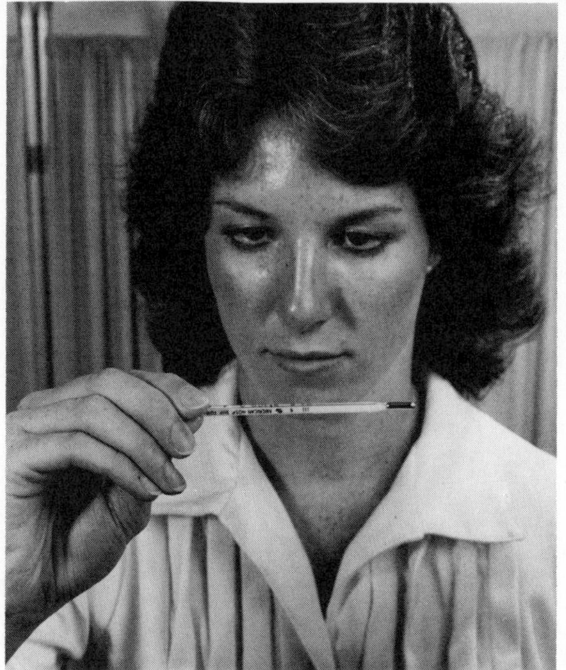

10. **PROCEDURAL STEP.** Read the thermometer. To obtain the best reading, hold the thermometer horizontally and rotate it slowly at eye level until the column of mercury is clearly visible. The temperature is read at the point at which the mercury level ends. Each long line represents 1° and each short line represents 0.2° on a Fahrenheit thermometer. Read to the nearest 0.2°. (The temperature indicated on this thermometer is 101.4°F.)

11. **PROCEDURAL STEP.** Shake down the mercury, and place the used thermometer in the designated container for cleansing and disinfecting. Oral and rectal thermometers should be stored in separate containers.

12. **PROCEDURAL STEP.** Wash the hands.
PRINCIPLE. Microorganisms from the patient may have been transferred to the medical assistant's hands.

13. **PROCEDURAL STEP.** Record the reading. Include the patient's name, the date and time, and the oral temperature reading. Place your initials next to the recording.
PRINCIPLE. Patient data should be properly recorded to aid the physician in the diagnosis and to provide future reference.

94 6 8 100 2 4 6 8

Record data below.

DATE	TIME	PATIENT'S NAME	TEMPERATURE

PROCEDURE 2-2

TAKING BODY TEMPERATURE—RECTAL

1. **PROCEDURAL STEP.** Wash the hands.

PRINCIPLE. The hands should be clean and free from contamination so that pathogens are not transferred to the patient.

2. **PROCEDURAL STEP.** Assemble the equipment. The equipment includes a **rectal thermometer, a lubricant,** and **tissues.** If the thermometer is stored in a chemical solution, rinse it off with cold water and wipe it dry with a clean soft tissue, using a firm rotating motion.

PRINCIPLE. Chemicals may irritate the mucosa of the rectum. Cold water must be used to rinse the thermometer, because hot water may cause breakage.

3. **PROCEDURAL STEP.** Check the level of the mercury in the thermometer. Hold the thermometer horizontally at eye level and rotate it slowly, to obtain the best reading.

4. **PROCEDURAL STEP.** If the level of mercury is above 96°F, it will need to be shaken down in order to obtain an accurate temperature reading. Hold the thermometer firmly between the thumb and forefinger. Shake the thermometer downward with a snapping wrist movement.

PRINCIPLE. The constriction in the bulb prevents the mercury from falling on its own.

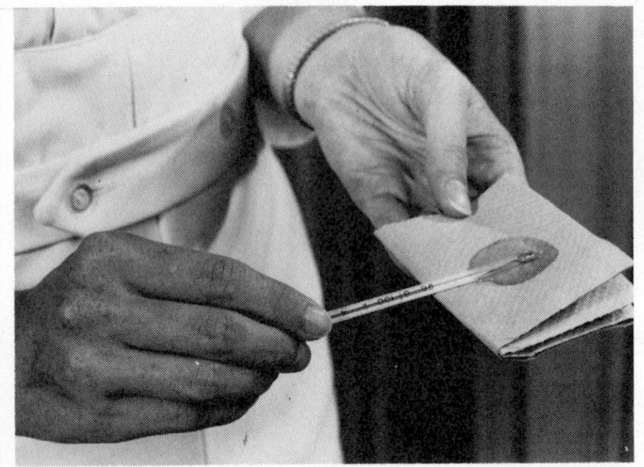

5. **PROCEDURAL STEP.** Identify the patient and explain the procedure.

PRINCIPLE. It is important to explain what you will be doing, since body temperature may be higher in a fearful or apprehensive patient.

6. **PROCEDURAL STEP.** Lubricate the thermometer for easier insertion into the rectum. Place some lubricant from a tube or jar on a paper wipe and lubricate the bulb end up to a level of 1 inch.

PRINCIPLE. A lubricated thermometer can be inserted more easily and does not irritate the delicate rectal mucosa. Placing the lubricant on a paper wipe prevents contamination of the remaining lubricant in the tube or jar.

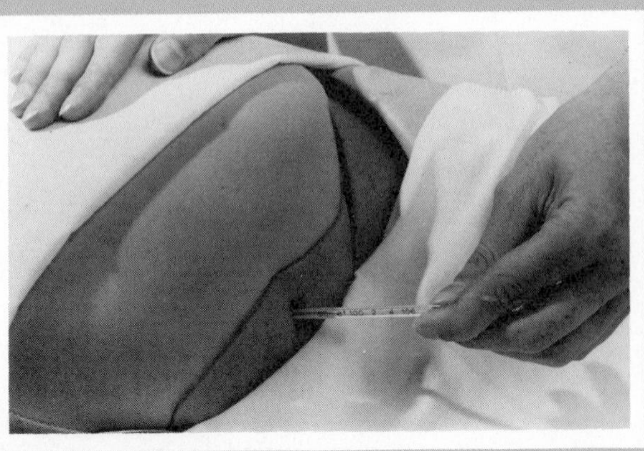

7. **PROCEDURAL STEP.** Position the patient. *Adults:* Position the patient on his or her abdomen or side, and drape the patient to expose only the anal area. *Infants:* Position the infant on his or her back, grasping the ankles and placing the index finger between the ankle bones.

PRINCIPLE. Correct positioning allows for clear viewing of the anal opening and provides for proper insertion of the thermometer. Draping reduces patient embarrassment and provides warmth.

8. **PROCEDURAL STEP.** Spread the buttocks to expose the anal opening and insert the lubricated bulb of the thermometer approximately 1½ inches into the rectum for adults and ½ inch for infants. Allow the buttocks to fall back in place. If the patient is an infant or if the adult is unconscious or confused, the thermometer should be held in place until the temperature registers. Other patients should be advised to remain still.
PRINCIPLE. The thermometer must be inserted correctly to prevent injury to the tissue of the anal opening. Patient movement could cause the thermometer to work itself further into the rectum, possibly damaging the rectal mucosa. Patient movement may also cause the thermometer to slip out of the rectum.

9. **PROCEDURAL STEP.** Leave the thermometer in place for 3 to 5 minutes. The medical assistant should remain in the room to reassure the patient and to remove the thermometer as soon as the body temperature has registered. Having the patient breathe through the mouth will help to relax the individual.
PRINCIPLE. The thermometer must remain in the rectum long enough for an accurate temperature reading to register.

10. **PROCEDURAL STEP.** Remove the thermometer in the same direction as that in which it was inserted, and wipe it from stem to bulb with a clean soft tissue, using a firm rotating motion. Wipe the anal area to remove excess lubricant.
PRINCIPLE. The lubricant and any fecal matter must be wiped away to provide for easier reading of the thermometer. The thermometer is wiped from the stem toward the bulb end to carry microorganisms away from the medical assistant's fingers.

11. **PROCEDURAL STEP.** Read the thermometer as you would when taking an oral temperature.

12. **PROCEDURAL STEP.** Shake down the mercury, and place the used thermometer in the designated container for cleansing and disinfecting. Oral and rectal thermometers should be stored in separate containers.

13. **PROCEDURAL STEP.** Wash the hands.
PRINCIPLE. Microorganisms from the patient may have been transferred to the hands of the medical assistant.

14. **PROCEDURAL STEP.** Record the reading. Include the patient's name, the date and time, and the rectal temperature. The symbol ® must be charted next to the temperature reading to tell the physician that a rectal reading was taken. (Example: 98.6°F ®.) Include your initials next to the recording.
PRINCIPLE. Patient data should be properly recorded to aid the physician in the diagnosis and to provide for future reference.

Record data below.

DATE	TIME	PATIENT'S NAME	TEMPERATURE

PROCEDURE 2-3

TAKING BODY TEMPERATURE—AXILLARY

Note: Many of the principles for taking temperature have already been stated and are not included in this procedure.

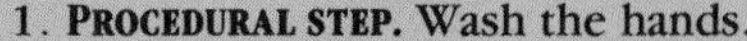

1. **PROCEDURAL STEP.** Wash the hands.

2. **PROCEDURAL STEP.** Assemble the equipment. The equipment includes a **thermometer** and **tissues.** If the thermometer is stored in a chemical solution, rinse it off with cold water and wipe it dry with a clean soft tissue, using a firm rotating motion.
   PRINCIPLE. Chemicals may irritate the skin of the axilla.

3. **PROCEDURAL STEP.** Check the level of the mercury in the thermometer.

4. **PROCEDURAL STEP.** Shake the mercury to a level of 96°F or below, if necessary.

5. **PROCEDURAL STEP.** Identify the patient and explain the procedure.

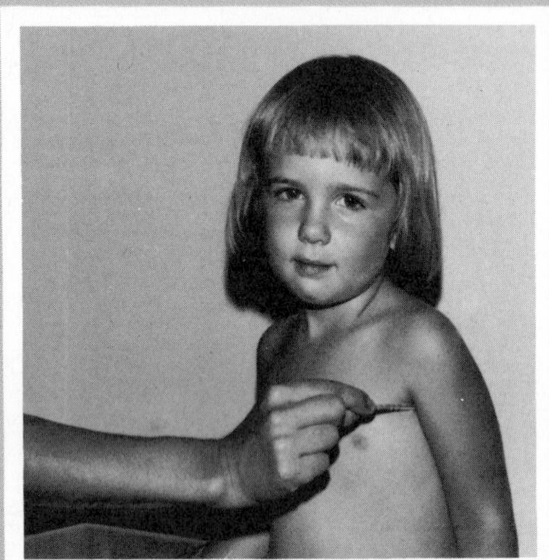

6. **PROCEDURAL STEP.** Make sure the axilla is dry. If it is wet, pat it dry with a clean cloth. Place the bulb of the thermometer in the center of the axilla, and instruct the patient to hold his or her arm tightly against the chest. The thermometer and arm should be held in place for small children and any other patients who cannot maintain the position themselves.
   PRINCIPLE. Rubbing the axilla causes an increase in the temperature in that area due to friction, resulting in an inaccurate temperature reading. Interference from outside air currents is reduced when the arm is held tightly against the chest; in addition, the thermometer is prevented from falling and breaking.

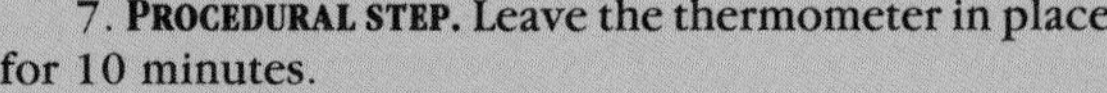

7. **PROCEDURAL STEP.** Leave the thermometer in place for 10 minutes.
   PRINCIPLE. The thermometer must remain in the axilla long enough for an accurate temperature reading to register. The axilla is not as closed a space as the mouth or rectum and therefore is more subject to the influence of air currents.

8. **PROCEDURAL STEP.** Remove the thermometer and wipe it from stem to bulb with a clean soft tissue, using a firm rotating motion.

9. **PROCEDURAL STEP.** Read the thermometer.

10. **PROCEDURAL STEP.** Shake down the mercury and place the used thermometer in the designated container for cleansing and disinfecting.

11. **PROCEDURAL STEP.** Wash the hands.

12. **PROCEDURAL STEP.** Record the reading. Include the patient's name, the date and time, and the axillary temperature reading. The symbol Ⓐ must be charted next to the temperature reading to tell the physician that an axillary reading was taken (example: 97.6° Ⓐ). Include your initials next to the recording.

Record data below.

DATE	TIME	PATIENT'S NAME	TEMPERATURE

Electronic Thermometer

An electronic thermometer is often used in the medical office to measure oral, rectal, and axillary body temperature. An electronic thermometer takes less time to measure temperature than does a glass thermometer; the time varies between 10 and 60 seconds, depending on the manufacturer. In addition, it is easier to read the results because the temperature measurement is digitally displayed on a screen. An electronic thermometer consists of interchangeable oral and rectal probes attached to a battery-operated portable unit that sits in a rechargeable base. A disposable soft plastic cover is placed over the probe to prevent the transmission of microorganisms between patients. Depending on the method of taking temperature, the probe is inserted in the mouth, rectum, or axilla and is left in place until a beep is emitted from the thermometer. When the beep sounds, the patient's temperature in degrees Fahrenheit is displayed on the screen. The plastic cover is then removed from the probe and properly disposed of, according to the medical office policy.

PROCEDURE 2-4

TAKING BODY TEMPERATURE WITH AN ELECTRONIC THERMOMETER

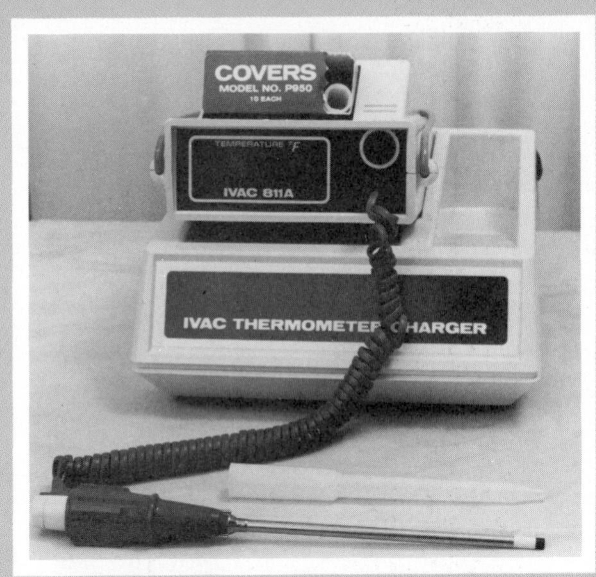

1. **PROCEDURAL STEP.** Wash the hands, and assemble the equipment. The equipment includes the **electronic thermometer**, the **appropriate probe (oral/axillary or rectal)**, and a **plastic probe cover.**

2. **PROCEDURAL STEP.** Attach the proper probe to the thermometer unit. Next, insert the probe into the face of the thermometer. The probe collars are color coded as follows: Oral and axillary—blue-collared probe; Rectal—red-collared probe.

   PRINCIPLE. The probe collars are color coded for ease in identifying them.

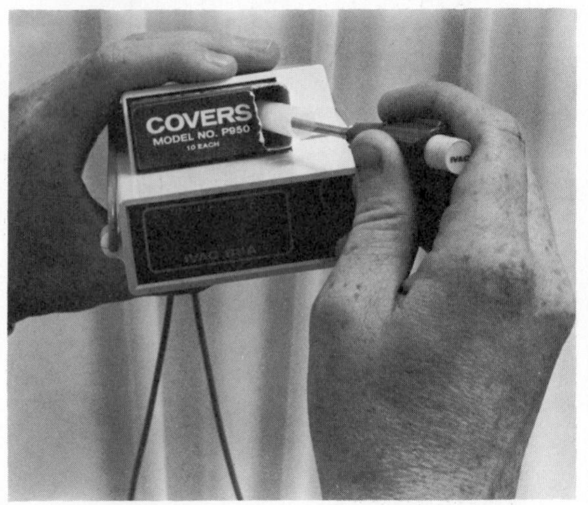

3. **PROCEDURAL STEP.** Remove the thermometer unit from its rechargeable base. Grasp the probe by the collar, and remove it from the face of the thermometer. Firmly attach a disposable plastic probe cover to the probe.

   PRINCIPLE. Removing the probe from the thermometer automatically turns on the thermometer. The probe cover prevents the transfer of microorganisms from one patient to another.

4. **PROCEDURAL STEP.** Identify the patient, and explain the procedure.

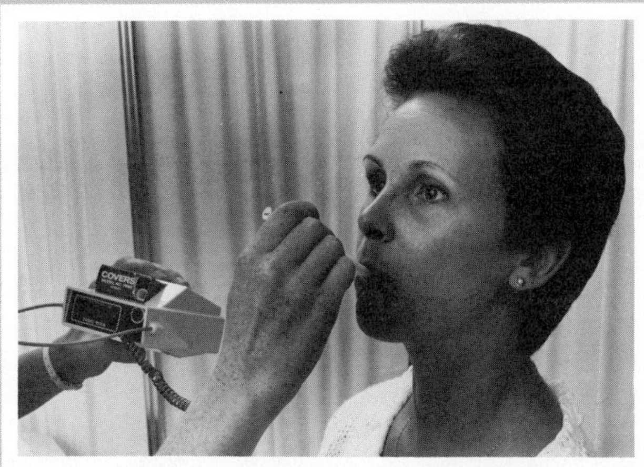

5. **PROCEDURAL STEP.** Take the patient's temperature by inserting the probe as follows:
Oral—Place the probe under the tongue in the pocket located on either side of the frenulum linguae.
Axillary—Place the probe in the center of the axilla, and instruct the patient to hold the arm tightly against the chest.
Rectal—Lubricate the end of the probe up to a level of 1 inch. Spread the buttocks and place the probe approximately 1½ inches into the rectum for adults and ½ inch for infants. (Note: Some rectal probes do not require lubrication. Check with the instruction manual for the manufacturer's recommendation).

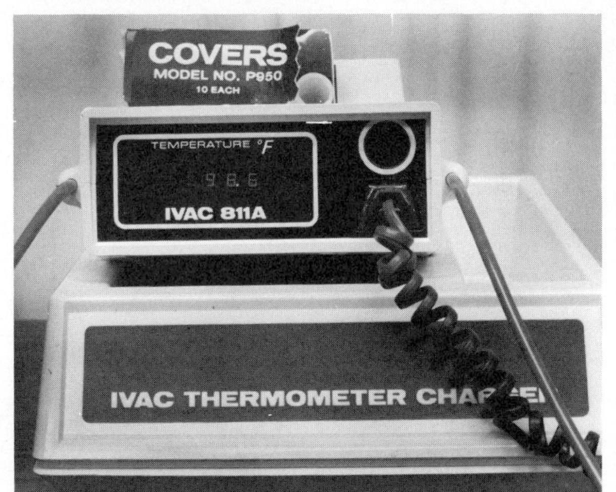

6. **PROCEDURAL STEP.** Hold the probe in place until the audible tone is heard. At that time, the patient's temperature appears as a digital display on the screen. (The temperature indicated on this thermometer is 98.6° F.)

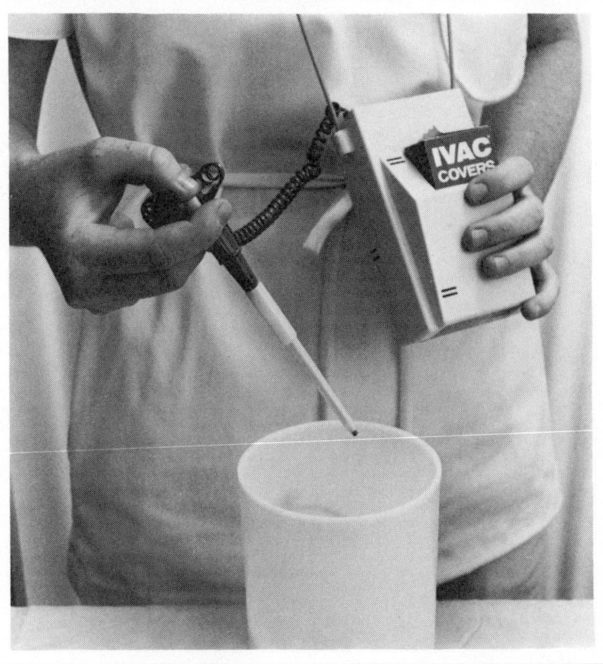

7. **PROCEDURAL STEP.** Remove the probe from the mouth, axilla, or rectum and discard the probe cover in the appropriate receptacle by pushing the ejection button. Do not allow your fingers to come in contact with the probe cover.
PRINCIPLE. The probe cover should not be touched, to prevent the transfer of microorganisms from the patient to the medical assistant.

8. **PROCEDURAL STEP.** Return the probe to its stored position in the thermometer unit.
PRINCIPLE. Returning the probe to the unit automatically turns off and resets the thermometer.

9. **PROCEDURAL STEP.** Wash the hands and record the results. Include the patient's name, the date and time, and the temperature reading. Place your initials next to the recording.
PRINCIPLE. Patient data should be properly recorded to aid the physician in the diagnosis and to provide future reference.

10. **PROCEDURAL STEP.** Store the thermometer unit in the base, which recharges the unit.

Continued

Record data below.

DATE	TIME	PATIENT'S NAME	TEMPERATURE

Study Questions

1. How is heat produced in the body? How is heat lost from the body?
2. What is the normal body temperature range and the average body temperature?
3. What factors should be taken into consideration when evaluating body temperature?

COMPETENCIES

After completing this unit, you should be able to demonstrate the proper procedures to perform the following:

1. Take and record the radial pulse.
2. Take and record the apical pulse.

LEARNING OBJECTIVES

After completing this unit, you should be able to do the following:

1. Define the terms listed in the vocabulary.
2. Explain what causes pulse to occur and the purpose of measuring the pulse rate.
3. List the conditions that must exist in order to use a particular part of the body as a site for taking the pulse.
4. List and be able to locate eight sites for taking the pulse.
5. Identify one use of each of the eight pulse sites.
6. State the normal range for pulse rate.
7. List and explain four factors that affect the pulse rate.
8. Explain the principles underlying each step in the radial and apical pulse procedures.

• VOCABULARY •

antecubital space (an″ te-ku′ bĭ-tal spās)—The space located at the front of the elbow.

aorta (a-or′ tah)—The major trunk of the arterial system of the body. The aorta arises from the upper surface of the left ventricle.

arrhythmia (ah-rith′ me-ah)—An irregular rhythm.

bounding pulse (bownd-ing puls)—A pulse with an increased volume that feels very strong and full.

bradycardia (brad″ e-kar′ de-ah)—An abnormally slow heart or pulse rate (below 60 beats per minute).

intercostal (in″ ter-kos′ tal)—Between the ribs.

tachycardia (tak″ e-kar′ de-ah)—An abnormally fast heart or pulse rate (over 100 beats per minute).

thready pulse (thrĕd′ ē puls)—A pulse with a decreased volume that feels weak and thin.

Pulse

Mechanism of the Pulse

When the left ventricle of the heart contracts, blood is forced from the heart into the aorta. The aorta is already filled with blood and must expand to accept the blood being pushed out of the left ventricle. The elastic tissue in the wall of the aorta allows it to expand to accommodate the new supply of blood. When the heart relaxes, the aorta recoils to its original size. The expansion and recoiling of the aorta send a wave of vibration from the aorta through the walls of the arterial system. This vibration, known as the *pulse,* can be felt as a light tap by an examiner. The pulse rate is measured by counting the number of beats per minute. The contraction and relaxation of the heart (or heart rate) can thus be determined by taking the pulse rate.

The purpose of taking pulse is to establish the patient's baseline recording and to assess the pulse rate following special procedures, medications, or disease processes that affect heart functioning.

Sites for Taking Pulse

The pulse is felt most strongly when a superficial artery is held against a firm tissue, such as bone. The most common site for taking the pulse is the radial artery, which is located on the inner aspect of the wrist just below the thumb. The radial pulse is easily accessible, and the pulse rate can be taken with no discomfort to the patient.

Other sites used for taking the pulse include those shown in Figure 5–2 and described on the following page.

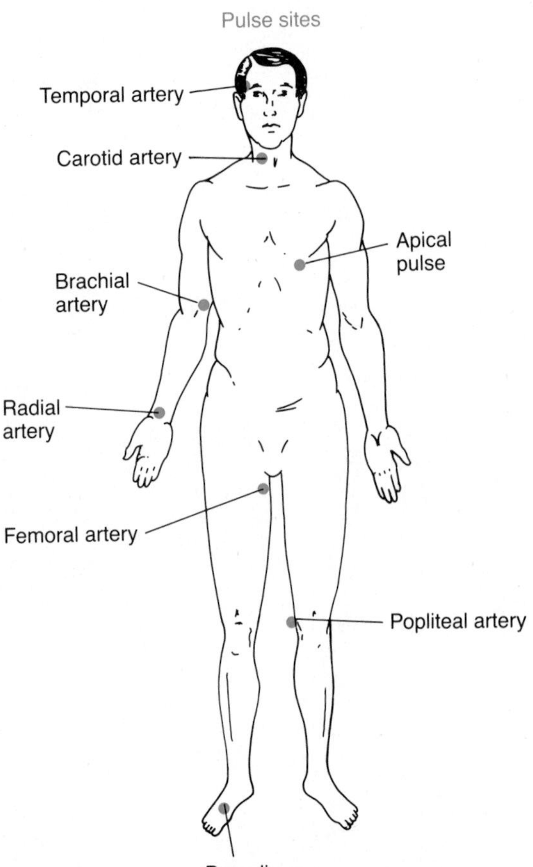

FIGURE 2–5. Common sites where the pulse can be felt.

Brachial artery	The brachial pulse is located in the antecubital space and is used when taking blood pressure. This site is also used to measure pulse in infants during cardiac arrest.
Temporal artery	The temporal pulse is located in front of the ear and just above eye level. This site is used to measure pulse when the radial pulse is not accessible.
Carotid artery	The carotid pulse is located on the anterior side of the neck slightly to one side of the midline. This site is used to measure pulse in infants, in adults undergoing cardiac arrest, and to assess circulation to the brain.
Femoral artery	The femoral pulse is located in the middle of the groin. This site is used to measure pulse in infants and children and in adults during cardiac arrest, as well as to assess circulation to a lower extremity.
Popliteal artery	The popliteal pulse is located at the back of the knee and is most easily detected when the knee is slightly flexed. This site is used to measure blood pressure when the brachial pulse is not accessible and to assess circulation to a lower extremity.
Dorsalis pedis artery	The pedal pulse is located on the upper surface of the foot, between the first and second metatarsal bones. This site is used to assess circulation to the foot.

If the medical assistant is having difficulty feeling the pulse at the sites mentioned, the *apical pulse* can be taken. In addition, this pulse site is often used to measure pulse in infants and in children up to 3 years of age. The apical pulse has a stronger beat and is more easily heard. The diaphragm of the stethoscope is lightly placed over the apex of the heart, which is located in the fifth intercostal space, approximately 1 to 3 inches to the left of the sternum. This position generally falls just below the left nipple.

Pulse Rate

The normal, resting pulse rate for a healthy adult ranges from 60 to 100 beats per minute, the average falling between 70 and 80 beats per minute.

Pulse rate can vary, depending on the following:

Age The pulse varies inversely with age. As the age increases, the pulse rate decreases. The pulse rates of the various age groups follow:

Infants	115 to 130 beats per minute
Children (ages 1 to 7)	80 to 120 beats per minute
Children (age 7 to adult)	72 to 90 beats per minute
Adults	70 to 80 beats per minute

Sex	Female adults tend to have a slightly faster pulse rate than male adults.
Physical exercise	Physical activity, such as running or swimming, will increase the pulse rate.
Emotional states	Strong emotional states, such as crying or anger, will increase the pulse rate.

Metabolism	Increased body metabolism, such as occurs during pregnancy, will increase the pulse rate.
Drugs	Certain drugs have a tendency to increase the pulse rate, whereas others will decrease it.

An abnormally fast heart or pulse rate (more than 100 beats per minute) is known as *tachycardia.* Tachycardia may indicate diseased states such as hemorrhaging or heart disease. However, an individual's pulse rate may normally exceed 100 beats per minute during vigorous exercise or in strong emotional states.

Bradycardia is an abnormally slow heart or pulse rate (below 60 beats per minute). Normally, a pulse rate below 60 may occur during sleep; trained athletes often have low pulse rates.

Rhythm and Volume

In addition to measuring the pulse rate, the medical assistant should also determine the rhythm and volume of the pulse.

The *rhythm* of a pulse denotes the time interval between heart beats, a normal rhythm having the same time interval between each two beats. Any irregularity in the heart's rhythm is known as an *arrhythmia* and is characterized by unequal or irregular intervals between the heart beats.

The *volume* of the pulse refers to the strength of the heart beat. The amount of blood pumped into the aorta by each contraction of the left ventricle should remain constant, making the pulse feel strong and full. If the blood volume decreases, the pulse feels weak and may be difficult to detect. This type of pulse is usually accompanied by a fast heart rate and is described as a *thready pulse.* An increase in the blood volume results in a pulse that feels extremely strong and full; this is known as a *bounding pulse.*

Any abnormalities occurring in the rhythm or volume of the pulse should be accurately recorded in the patient's chart by the medical assistant. A pulse that has a normal rhythm and volume is recorded as being regular and strong.

PROCEDURE 2-5
MEASURING RADIAL PULSE

1. **PROCEDURAL STEP.** Wash the hands, identify the patient, and explain the procedure. A **watch with a second hand** is needed to take the pulse rate.

Observe the patient for any signs that may result in an increase or decrease in the pulse rate.

PRINCIPLE. Pulse rate can vary, according to the factors listed on page 33.

2. **PROCEDURAL STEP.** Position the patient in a sitting or lying position. The patient's arm should be placed alongside the body in a comfortable position, with the wrist slightly flexed, in order to relax the muscles and tendons over the pulse site.

PRINCIPLE. Relaxed muscles and tendons over the pulse site make it easier to palpate the pulse.

3. **PROCEDURAL STEP.** Place the three middle fingertips over the radial pulse site while resting the thumb on the back of the patient's wrist.

PRINCIPLE. The medical assistant should not take the pulse with the thumb, because the thumb has a pulse of its own. The result may be measurement of the medical assistant's pulse and not the patient's pulse.

4. **PROCEDURAL STEP.** Apply moderate, gentle pressure directly over the site until the pulse can be felt.

PRINCIPLE. A normal pulse can be felt with moderate pressure. Too much pressure applied to the radial artery closes it off, and no pulse is felt.

5. **PROCEDURAL STEP.** Count the number of pulsations per minute. The rhythm and volume of the pulse should also be noted.

PRINCIPLE. The pulse rate may be counted for a full minute, or for half a minute and multiplied by two. A full minute is recommended if any abnormalities occur in the rhythm or volume.

6. **PROCEDURAL STEP.** Record the results. Include the patient's name, the date and time, and the pulse rate, rhythm, and volume. Indicate the site for taking the pulse (radial pulse). Include your initials next to the recording.

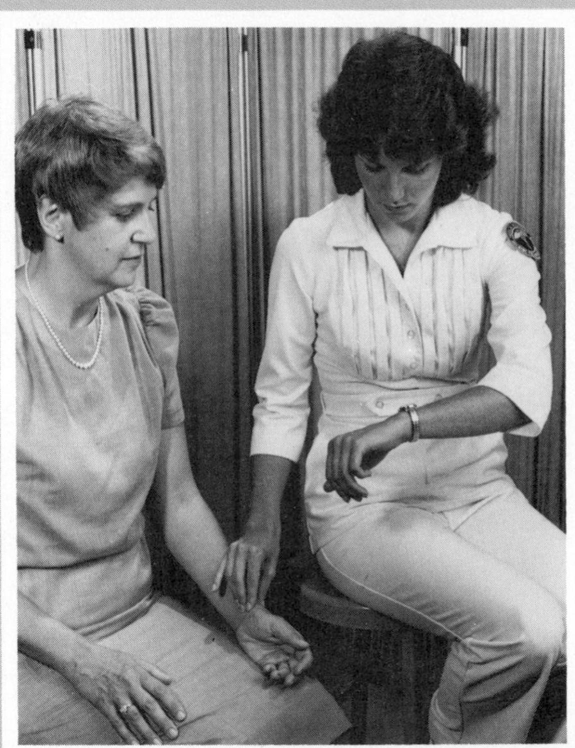

Record data below:

DATE	TIME	PATIENT'S NAME	PULSE

PROCEDURE 2-6
MEASURING APICAL PULSE

1. **PROCEDURAL STEP.** Wash the hands, identify the patient, and explain the procedure.

2. **PROCEDURAL STEP.** Assemble the equipment. A **watch with a second hand** and a **stethoscope** are needed to take the apical pulse. Clean the earpieces of the stethoscope with an antiseptic wipe.
PRINCIPLE. Cleaning the earpieces helps to prevent the transmission of microorganisms.

3. **PROCEDURAL STEP.** Position the patient in a lying (supine) or sitting position.
PRINCIPLE. A supine or sitting position allows for access to the apex of the heart.

4. **PROCEDURAL STEP.** Warm the diaphragm of the stethoscope with your hand. Insert the earpieces of the stethoscope into your ears, with the earpieces directed slightly forward, and place the diaphragm over the apex of the heart. The apex of the heart is located in the fifth intercostal space at the junction of the left midclavicular line.
PRINCIPLE. Warming the diaphragm helps to reduce the discomfort of having a cold object placed on the chest. In addition, a cold diaphragm could startle the patient, resulting in an increase in the pulse rate. The earpieces should be directed forward, permitting them to follow the direction of the ear canal, which facilitates hearing.

5. **PROCEDURAL STEP.** Listen for the heart beat and count the number of beats per minute. Also note the rhythm and volume of the heart beat. The medical assistant will hear a "lubb-dupp" sound through the stethoscope. This sound occurs as a result of the closing of the valves of the heart. Each "lubb-dupp" is counted as one beat.

6. **PROCEDURAL STEP.** Record the results. Include the patient's name, the date and time, and the apical pulse rate, rhythm, and volume. Indicate the site used for taking the pulse (apical pulse). Include your initials next to the recording.
PRINCIPLE. Good recording techniques provide for a more complete patient record.

7. **PROCEDURAL STEP.** Clean the earpieces of the stethoscope with an antiseptic wipe.

Record data below.

DATE	TIME	PATIENT'S NAME	PULSE

Study Questions

1. What causes pulse to occur?
2. What is the normal adult range for pulse rate?
3. What factors affect the pulse rate?

• VOCABULARY •

alveolus (pl. alveoli) (al-ve' o-lus; al-ve' o-li)—A thin-walled air sac of the lungs in which the exchange of oxygen and carbon dioxide takes place.
apnea (ap-ne' ah)—The temporary cessation of breathing.
cyanosis (si" ah-no' sis)—A bluish discoloration of the skin and mucous membranes.
dyspnea (disp' ne-ah)—Labored or difficult breathing.
eupnea (ūp-ne' ah)—Normal respiration.
exhalation (eks" hah-la' shun)—The act of breathing out.
hyperpnea (hi" perp-ne' ah)—An abnormal increase in the rate and depth of respiration.
hypopnea (hi-pop' ne-ah)—An abnormal decrease in the rate and depth of respiration.
hypoxia (hi-pok' se-ah)—A reduction in the oxygen supply to the tissues of the body.
inhalation (in" hah-la' shun)—The act of breathing in.
orthopnea (or" thop-ne' ah)—The condition in which breathing is easier when an individual is in a standing or sitting position.
stertorous respiration (ster' to-rus res" pi-ra' shun)—Noisy and snoring respiration.
tachypnea (tak" ip-ne' ah)—An abnormal increase in the respiratory rate.

COMPETENCY

After completing this unit, you should be able to demonstrate the proper procedure to perform the following:

Measure respiration and record results.

LEARNING OBJECTIVES

After completing this unit, you should be able to do the following:

1. Define the terms listed in the vocabulary.
2. Explain the purpose of respiration.
3. State what occurs during inhalation and exhalation.
4. Explain the difference between external and internal respiration.
5. Discuss how respiration can be controlled, involuntarily and voluntarily, in the body.
6. State the normal respiratory rate of an adult.
7. List and explain three factors that affect the respiratory rate.
8. Explain the principles underlying each step in the procedure for measuring respiration.

Respiration

Mechanism of Respiration

The purpose of respiration is to provide for the exchange of oxygen and carbon dioxide between the atmosphere and the blood. Oxygen is taken into the body to be used for vital body processes, and carbon dioxide is given off as a waste product.

Each respiration is divided into two phases: *inhalation* and *exhalation.* During inhalation or inspiration, the diaphragm descends and the lungs expand, causing air containing oxygen to move from the atmosphere into the lungs. Exhalation, or expiration, involves the removal of carbon dioxide from the body. The diaphragm ascends and the lungs return to their original state, so that air containing carbon dioxide is expelled. One complete respiration is composed of one inhalation and one exhalation.

Respiration may be classified as either *external* or *internal.* External respiration involves the exchange of oxygen and carbon dioxide between the alveoli of the lungs and the blood. The blood, located in small capillaries, comes in contact with the alveoli, picks up oxygen, and carries it to the cells of the body. At this point, the oxygen is given off to the cells and carbon dioxide is picked up by the blood to be transported as a waste product to the lungs. The exchange of oxygen and carbon dioxide between the body cells and the blood is known as internal respiration.

Control of Respiration

The medulla oblongata, located in the brain, is the control center for involuntary respiration. A build-up of carbon dioxide in the blood sends a message to the medulla, which then triggers respiration to occur automatically.

To a certain extent, respiration is also under voluntary control. An individual can control respiration during activities such as singing, laughing, talking, eating, and crying. Voluntary respiration is ultimately under the control of the medulla oblongata. The breath can be held for only a certain length of time, after which carbon dioxide begins to build up in the body, resulting in a stimulus to the medulla that causes respiration to occur involuntarily. Small children may voluntarily hold their breath during a temper tantrum. A parent who does not understand the principles of respiration may be concerned that the child will cease breathing. The medical assistant should be able to explain that involuntary respiration will eventually occur, and the child will resume breathing.

Since an individual can control his or her respiration, the medical assistant should measure respirations without the patient's knowledge. Patients may change their respiratory rate unintentionally if they are aware that they are being tested. An ideal time to measure respiration is before or after the pulse is taken.

Respiratory Rate

The respiratory rate of a normal healthy adult may range from 16 to 20 respirations per minute. With most adults, there is a ratio of one respiration for every four pulse beats. For example, if the respiratory rate is 18, the pulse rate would be approximately 72 beats per minute. An abnormal increase in the respiratory rate is referred to as *tachypnea.*

There are certain factors that the medical assistant should take into consideration when measuring the respiratory rate. These include age, physical activity, strong emotions, illness, and drugs. As age increases, the respiratory rate decreases. Therefore, we would expect the respiratory rate of a child to be faster than that of an adult. Physical activity and strong emotional states increase the respiratory rate. Also, a patient with a fever has an increased respiratory rate: one of the ways in which heat is lost from the body is through the lungs; therefore, a fever causes an increased respiratory rate as the body tries to rid itself of the excess heat.

Certain drugs may increase the respiratory rate, whereas others may decrease it. The medical assistant who is unsure of what effect a particular drug may have should consult a drug reference such as the *Physician's Desk Reference* (PDR).

Rhythm and Depth of Respiration

Both the *rhythm* and *depth* should be noted when measuring respiration. Normally, the rhythm should be even and regular, and the pauses between inhalation and exhalation should be equal.

The depth of respiration indicates the amount of air that is inhaled or exhaled during the process of breathing. Some illnesses result in an abnormal increase in the rate and depth of the respirations; this condition is known as *hyperpnea.* A patient with hyperpnea exhibits a very rapid and panting type of respiration. In contrast, a patient's respiration may show an abnormal decrease in the rate and depth; this condition is termed *hypopnea.* The depth is approximately one-half that of normal respiration. Normal respiration is referred to as *eupnea.* The rate is approximately 16 respirations per minute, the rhythm is even and regular, and the depth is normal.

Respiratory Abnormalities

A patient who is having labored or difficult breathing has a condition known as *dyspnea.* Asthma, emphysema, and vigorous physical exertion can result in dyspnea. The patient with dyspnea may find it easier to breathe while in a sitting or standing position. This state is called *orthopnea* and it is also a common symptom of congestive heart failure.

Apnea refers to a temporary absence of respiration. *Stertorous respirations* are unusually noisy, snoring respirations, which may be due to a partial obstruction of the upper airway.

Color of the Patient

The patient's color should also be observed while the respiration is being measured. A lack of oxygen (hypoxia) results in a condition known as *cyanosis,* which causes a bluish discoloration of the skin and mucous membranes. Cyanosis is first observed in the nail beds and lips because these are areas in which the blood vessels lie close to the surface of the skin.

PROCEDURE 2-7
MEASURING RESPIRATION

1. **PROCEDURAL STEP.** Make sure the patient is unaware that his respirations are being monitored. This can be accomplished in the following manner: After taking the pulse, the medical assistant should continue to hold three fingers on the patient's wrist with the same amount of pressure and measure his respirations.
   PRINCIPLE. If the patient is aware that respiration is being taken, his breathing may change.

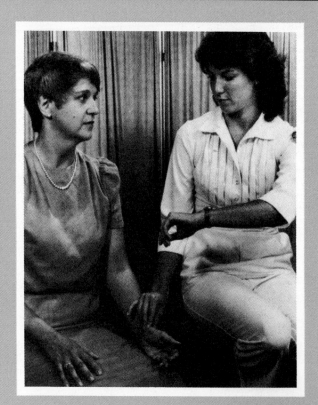

2. **PROCEDURAL STEP.** Observe the rise and fall of the patient's chest as the patient inhales and exhales.
   PRINCIPLE. One complete respiration includes one inhalation and one exhalation.

3. **PROCEDURAL STEP.** Count the number of respirations per minute. The respiratory rate should be counted for a full minute, or for one-half minute and multiplied by two. A full minute is recommended if any abnormalities occur in the rhythm or depth. Also note the rhythm and depth of the respiration. Observe the patient's color.

4. **PROCEDURAL STEP.** Record results. Include the patient's name, the date and time, and the respiratory rate, rhythm, and depth. Place your initials next to the recording.

Record data below.

DATE	TIME	PATIENT'S NAME	RESPIRATION

Study Questions

1. What is the purpose of respiration?
2. What is the difference between external and internal respiration?
3. What is the normal respiratory rate of an adult?
4. What factors affect the respiratory rate?

• VOCABULARY •

diastole (di-as' to-le)—The phase in the cardiac cycle in which the heart relaxes between contractions.

diastolic pressure (di" ah-stol' ik presh' ur)—The point of lesser pressure on the arterial walls, which is recorded during diastole.

hypertension (hi" per-ten' shun)—High blood pressure.

hypotension (hi" po-ten' shun)—Low blood pressure.

manometer (mah-nom' ĕ-ter)—An instrument for measuring pressure.

meniscus (mē-nis' kus)—The curved surface on a column of liquid in a tube.

sphygmomanometer (sfig" mo-mah-nom' ē-ter)—An instrument for measuring arterial blood pressure.

stethoscope (steth' o-skōp)—An instrument for amplifying and hearing sounds produced by the body.

systole (sis' to-le)—The phase in the cardiac cycle in which the ventricles contract, sending blood out of the heart and into the aorta and pulmonary aorta.

systolic pressure (sis-tol' ik presh' ur)—The point of maximum pressure on the arterial walls, which is recorded during systole.

COMPETENCY

After completing this unit, you should be able to demonstrate the proper procedure to perform the following:

Take and record blood pressure.

LEARNING OBJECTIVES

After completing this unit, you should be able to do the following:

1. Define the terms listed in the vocabulary.
2. Define blood pressure.
3. Explain why the diastolic pressure is lower than the systolic pressure.
4. State the normal range for blood pressure. Explain why age is an important consideration when taking blood pressure.
5. List three factors that affect the blood pressure.
6. Identify the different parts of a stethoscope and a sphygmomanometer.
7. List the three different cuff sizes and explain when each would be employed.
8. Identify the Korotkoff sounds.
9. Explain the principles underlying each step in the blood pressure procedure.

Blood Pressure

Mechanism of Blood Pressure

Blood pressure measures the pressure or force exerted on the walls of the arteries by the blood. Each time the ventricles contract, blood is pushed out of the heart and into the aorta and pulmonary aorta, exerting pressure on the walls of the arteries. This phase in the cardiac cycle is known as *systole,* and it represents the highest point of blood pressure in the body, or the *systolic pressure.* The phase of the cardiac cycle in which the heart relaxes between contractions is referred to as *diastole.* The *diastolic pressure* (recorded during diastole) is lower, owing to the relaxation of the heart. Thus, contraction and relaxation of the heart result in two different pressures, systolic and diastolic.

Normal Blood Pressure

The normal adult range for blood pressure is 110/60 to 140/90. The numbers to the left of the slash represent the systolic pressure, and the numbers to the right of the slash represent the diastolic pressure. Blood pressure is measured in millimeters of mercury. A blood-pressure reading of 120/80 means that there was enough force to raise a column of mercury 120 mm during systole and 80 mm during diastole.

Age is an important consideration when determining whether or not a patient's blood pressure is normal. As age increases, the blood pressure gradually increases: a 6-year-old child may normally have a reading of 90/60, whereas a young healthy adult will generally have a blood-pressure reading of approximately 120/80, and it would not be unusual for a 60-year-old man to have a reading of 140/90. Blood pressure should be taken during each office visit to allow the physician to compare the patient's readings over a period of time. This is a good preventive measure in guarding against serious illness. A single blood-pressure reading taken on one occasion does not accurately characterize an individual's blood pressure. Several blood-pressure readings, taken on different occasions, are needed to provide a good index of an individual's blood pressure.

Equipment to Measure Blood Pressure

The equipment needed to measure blood pressure includes a *stethoscope* and a *sphygmomanometer.* The stethoscope amplifies sounds produced by the body and allows the medical assistant to hear them (Fig. 2–6). Before using the stethoscope, the medical assistant should make sure that it is in proper working condition.

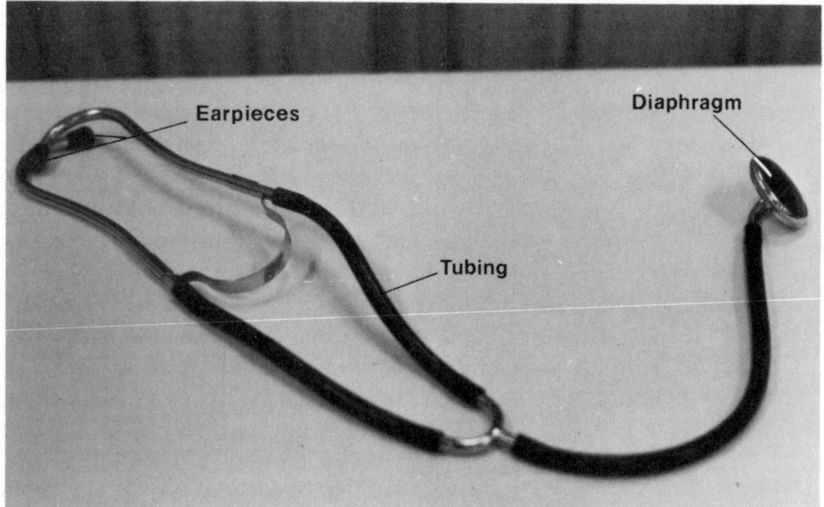

FIGURE 2–6. The parts of a stethoscope.

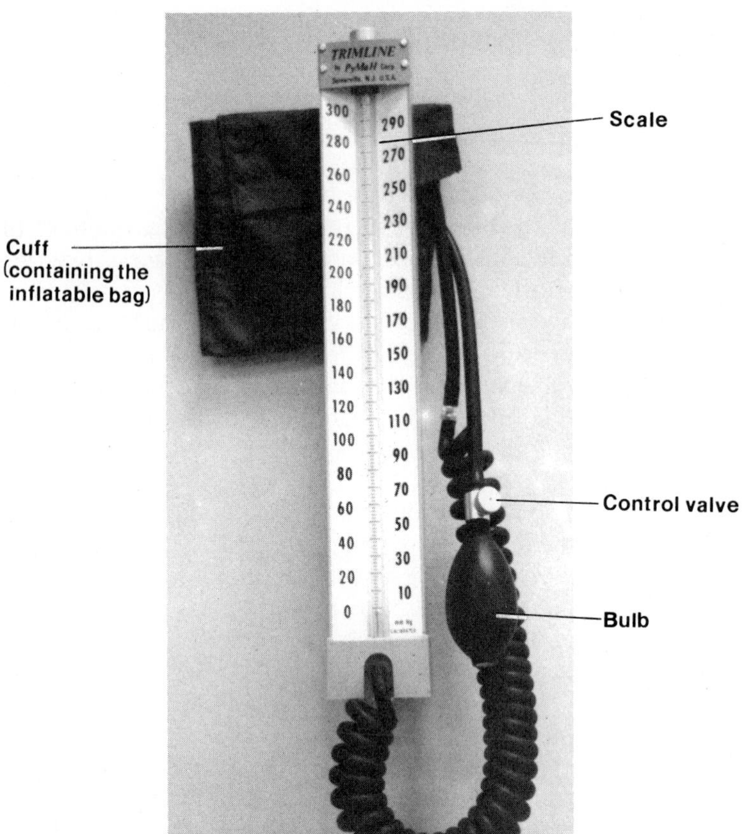

FIGURE 2–7. The parts of a mercury gravity sphygmomanometer (wall model).

The sphygmomanometer is an instrument that measures arterial blood pressure. It consists of an inflatable bag surrounded by a covering known as the cuff, an inflatable bulb, a control valve, and a manometer containing a scale for registering the pressure (Fig. 2–7).

The cuff is available in three different sizes: pediatric, adult, and thigh. The diameter of the limb determines the size of cuff to use; the width of the cuff should be 20 per cent greater than the diameter of the limb. Pediatric cuffs are used for children and for adults with small arms. The adult cuff is used for the average-sized adult arm, and the thigh cuff is used for taking blood pressure from the thigh or for adults with large arms. The cuff should fit snugly and should be applied so that the center of the inflatable bag is directly over the artery to be compressed. The cuff has an interlocking, self-sticking substance (Velcro) that allows for easy closure.

Two types of manometers are in common use: the *mercury gravity manometer* and the *aneroid manometer.* The mercury manometer is more reliable and accurate and does not require recalibration. The aneroid manometer is less bulky but requires regular calibration against a mercury gravity manometer. The manometer must be placed in the correct position for proper viewing. The medical assistant should be no farther than 3 feet from the scale of the manometer. The portable mercury manometer should be placed on a flat surface so that the mercury column is in a vertical position. The wall model mercury manometer is mounted securely against a wall, thereby placing the mercury column in a vertical position. The top portion of the mercury column curves slightly upward and is known as the *meniscus.* The blood pressure should be read at the top of the meniscus with the eye at the same level as the meniscus of the mercury column. The aneroid manometer is placed so that it may be viewed directly.

Factors Affecting Blood Pressure

Fluctuations in an individual's blood pressure are normal during the course of a day. When one awakens, the blood pressure is lower as a result of the decreased metabolism and physical activity that occur during sleep. As metabolism and activity increase during the day, the blood pressure rises. A patient who has been involved in vigorous physical activity should be given an opportunity to rest before a reading is taken. Strong emotional states, such as anger or fear, increase the blood pressure. If the medical assistant observes such a reaction, an attempt should be made to calm the patient before taking blood pressure. Other factors that may increase the blood pressure include pain, a recent meal, smoking, and bladder distention.

In some cases, the blood pressure of a patient who is in a lying or standing position may be different from that measured when the patient is in a sitting position. A notation should be made on the patient's chart if the reading was obtained in any position other than sitting, using the following abbreviations: *L* (lying) and *St* (standing).

Excessive pressure on the walls of the arteries, or high blood pressure, is known as *hypertension.* Reduced pressure on the arterial walls, or low blood pressure, is referred to as *hypotension.*

The Korotkoff Sounds

The Korotkoff sounds are used to determine the systolic and diastolic blood pressure readings. When the cuff is inflated, the brachial artery is compressed, so that no audible sounds are heard through the stethoscope. As the cuff is deflated, at a rate of 2 to 3 millimeters of mercury (mmHg) per heart beat, the sounds become audible.

Phase I is when the first faint but clear tapping sound is heard. The sound is recorded as the systolic pressure. It gradually increases in intensity. As the cuff continues to deflate, *Phase II* occurs, in which the sounds have a murmuring or swishing quality. Further deflation results in *Phase III,* when the sounds become crisper and increase in intensity. During *Phase IV,* the sounds become muffled. According to the American Heart Association, the onset of the muffled sounds is regarded as the best index of the diastolic pressure. *Phase V* is the point at which the sounds disappear. Some authorities believe that the diastolic pressure falls midway between Phases IV and V; therefore, some physicians may want the medical assistant to record both Phases IV and V as the diastolic pressures (e.g., 128/76/72).

The medical assistant should practice listening to these sounds and be able to identify the various phases.

PROCEDURE 2-8

MEASURING BLOOD PRESSURE

1. **PROCEDURAL STEP.** Wash the hands and assemble the equipment. The equipment needed includes a **stethoscope,** a **sphygmomanometer,** and an **alcohol wipe.** Be sure to select the proper patient cuff size. Clean the earpieces of the stethoscope with the alcohol wipe.

2. **PROCEDURAL STEP.** Identify the patient and explain the procedure. While explaining the procedure, observe the patient for any signs that would influence the reading, such as anger, fear, pain, recent physical activity, and others. If it is not possible to reduce or eliminate these influences, list them in the patient's chart.

3. **PROCEDURAL STEP.** Position the patient comfortably in a sitting position. The arm should be at heart level, well supported and well extended, with the palm facing upward. Roll up the patient's sleeve approximately 5 inches above the elbow. If the sleeve does not roll up or is too tight after being rolled up, remove the sleeve from the arm. Make a notation in the patient's chart if the lying or standing position was used to take blood pressure. Abbreviations that can be used are L (lying) and St (standing).

   PRINCIPLE. Placing the arm above heart level may cause the reading to be falsely low. The position of the arm allows easy access to the brachial artery. A tight sleeve causes partial compression of the brachial artery.

4. **PROCEDURAL STEP.** Place the cuff on the patient's arm so that the lower edge of the cuff is 1 to 2 inches above the bend in the elbow. The inflatable bag should be centered over the brachial artery.

   PRINCIPLE. The cuff should be up far enough to prevent the stethoscope from touching it; otherwise, extraneous sounds may be picked up. Centering the inflatable bag allows for complete compression of the brachial artery.

5. **PROCEDURAL STEP.** Wrap the cuff smoothly and snugly around the patient's arm and secure the end of it.

   PRINCIPLE. Applying the cuff properly prevents it from bulging or slipping. This permits application of an equal pressure over the brachial artery.

6. **PROCEDURAL STEP.** Position the manometer for direct viewing and at a distance of no more than 3 feet.

   PRINCIPLE. The medical assistant may have trouble seeing the scale on the manometer if it is placed more than 3 feet away.

7. **Procedural step.** Place the earpieces of the stethoscope in your ears, with the earpieces directed slightly forward. During the blood pressure measurement, the tubing of the stethoscope should hang freely and should not be permitted to rub against any object. Making sure the arm is well extended, palpate the brachial pulse with the fingertips and place the diaphragm gently but firmly over the artery. Hold the diaphragm with your thumb and place your fingers under the patient's elbow; there should be no gap between the skin and the diaphragm. Make sure the diaphragm is not touching the cuff.

Principle. The earpieces should be directed forward, permitting them to follow the direction of the ear canal, which facilitates hearing. If the stethoscope tubing rubs against an object, extraneous sounds may be picked up, which will interfere with an accurate measurement. Locating the brachial pulse allows for good positioning of the diaphragm over the brachial artery. A well-extended arm allows for easier palpation of the brachial pulse. Good contact of the diaphragm with the skin helps to transmit clear and audible Korotkoff sounds through the earpieces of the stethoscope.

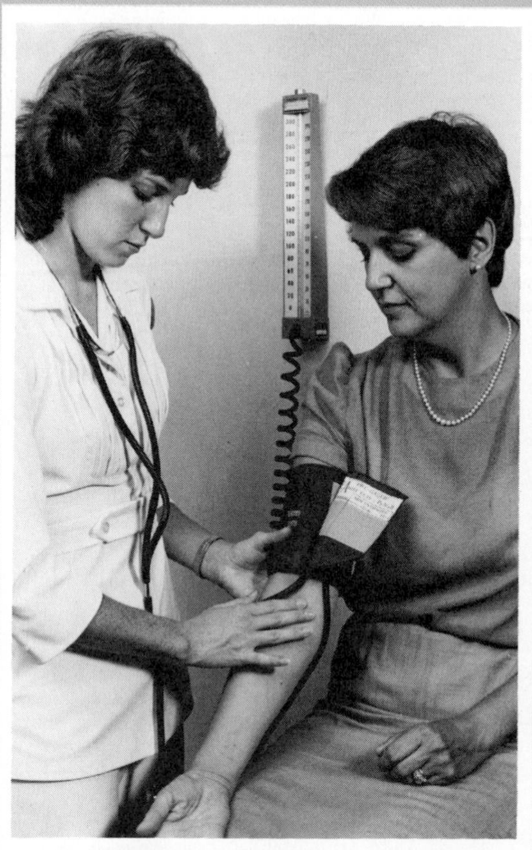

8. **Procedural step.** Close the valve on the bulb by turning the thumbscrew in a clockwise direction until it feels tight. Pump air into the inflatable bag as rapidly as possible up to a level of approximately 20 to 30 mmHg above the palpated or previously measured systolic pressure. Explain to the patient that this will cause a numbing and tingling sensation in the arm.

Principle. Inflation of the cuff compresses and closes off the brachial artery so that no blood flows through the artery. A preliminary determination of the systolic pressure, by palpation, allows the medical assistant to estimate how high to inflate the cuff. The procedure for palpating the systolic pressure is explained on page 49. If the patient has had the blood pressure measured previously at the medical office, the recorded systolic pressure can be used to determine how high to inflate the cuff.

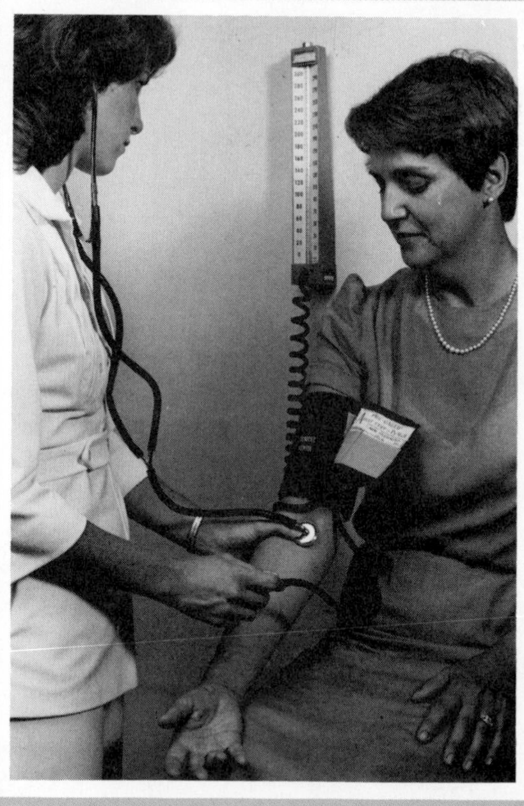

9. **Procedural step.** Release the pressure at a moderately steady rate of 2 to 3 mmHg per heart beat by slowly turning the thumbscrew in a counterclockwise direction. This opens the valve and allows the air in the cuff to slowly escape. Listen for the first clear tapping sound (Phase I of the Korotkoff sounds). This represents the systolic pressure. Note this point on the scale of the manometer.

Principle. The systolic pressure is the point at which the blood first begins to spurt through the artery as the cuff pressure begins to decrease; it represents the pressure that occurs on the walls of the arteries during systole.

10. **Procedural step.** Continue to deflate the cuff while listening to the Korotkoff sounds. Listen for the onset of the muffled sound that occurs during Phase IV and note this point on the scale of the manometer. If Phase V is to be recorded, continue to deflate the cuff and note the point on the scale at which the sounds cease.

Continued

PRINCIPLE. Phase IV marks the diastolic pressure (which represents the pressure that occurs on the walls of the arteries during diastole); the cuff pressure is reduced and blood is flowing freely through the brachial artery.

11. **PROCEDURAL STEP.** Quickly and completely deflate the cuff to zero. If you could not obtain an accurate blood-pressure reading, wait 15 to 30 seconds and repeat the blood pressure procedure outlined previously. Remove the earpieces of the stethoscope from your ears and carefully remove the cuff from the patient's arm.

PRINCIPLE. Venous congestion results when blood pressure is taken, which will alter a second reading if it is taken too soon.

12. **PROCEDURAL STEP.** Record the results. Include the patient's name, the date and time, and the blood pressure reading. Place your initials next to the recording.

13. **PROCEDURAL STEP.** Clean the earpieces with alcohol and properly replace the equipment.

Record data below.

DATE	TIME	PATIENT'S NAME	BLOOD PRESSURE

PROCEDURE 2-9
DETERMINING SYSTOLIC PRESSURE BY PALPATION

1. Locate the radial pulse with the fingertips.

2. Close the valve on the bulb and pump air into the bulb until the pulsation ceases.

3. Release the valve at a moderate rate of 2 to 3 mmHg per heart beat, while palpating the artery with the fingertips.

4. Record the point at which the pulsation reappears as the palpated systolic pressure.

5. Deflate the cuff completely and wait 15 to 30 seconds before checking the blood pressure.

Study Questions

1. What is blood pressure?
2. Why is the diastolic pressure lower than the systolic pressure?
3. What is the normal range for blood pressure?
4. What factors affect the blood pressure?

3

THE PATIENT EXAMINATION

CHAPTER OUTLINE

The Health History
Charting in the Medical Record
Symptoms
Weight and Height
Positioning and Draping
Preparation of the Examination Room
Preparation of the Patient
The Physical Examination

COMPETENCIES

After completing this chapter, you should be able to demonstrate the proper procedure to perform the following:

1. Complete a health history form.
2. Operate and care for equipment and instruments used during the physical examination, according to the manufacturer's instructions.
3. Prepare the examining room.
4. Take weight and height, and record the results.
5. Prepare a patient for a physical examination.
6. Position and drape a patient in the following positions: horizontal recumbent, dorsal recumbent, dorsal lithotomy, prone, knee-chest, and Sims.
7. Assist the physician during the physical examination.

LEARNING OBJECTIVES

After completing this chapter, you should be able to do the following:

1. Define the terms listed in the vocabulary.
2. Identify the three components of a complete patient examination.
3. List and describe the seven parts of the health history.
4. List the guidelines that should be followed in recording the chief complaint.
5. Explain the function of the medical record.
6. List and describe eight areas in which the medical assistant is responsible for recording information in the patient's chart.
7. List and describe six guidelines to follow to ensure accurate and concise charting.
8. List three examples each of subjective symptoms and objective symptoms.
9. Identify common symptoms and gather information related to them.
10. Identify equipment and instruments used during the physical examination.
11. List and define the four methods of examining the patient. State an example of the use of each during the physical examination.

• VOCABULARY •

audiometer (aw″de-om′ĕ-ter)—An instrument used to measure hearing.

auscultation (aw″skul-ta′shun)—The process of listening to the sounds produced within the body to detect any signs of disease.

charting (chart′ing)—The process of making written entries about a patient in the medical record.

clinical diagnosis (klin′e-k′l di″ag-no′sis)—A tentative diagnosis obtained through the evaluation of the health history and the physical examination, without the benefit of laboratory or diagnostic tests.

conjunctiva (kon″junk-ti′vah)—The mucous membrane that lines the eyelids and covers the eyeball, except for the cornea.

diagnosis (di″ag-no′sis)—The scientific method of determining and identifying a disease.

differential diagnosis (dif″er-en′shal di″ag-no′sis)—A determination of which of two or more diseases with similar symptoms is producing the patient's symptoms.

familial (fə-mil′yəl)—Occurring or affecting members of a family more frequently than would be expected by chance.

inspection (in-spek′shun)—The process of observing a patient to detect any signs of disease.

medical record (mĕd′i-k′l rĕk′erd)—A written record of the important aspects regarding a patient, his or her care, and the progress of his or her illness (also known as "the chart").

objective symptom (ob-jek′tiv simp′tom)—A symptom that can be observed by an examiner.

ophthalmoscope (of-thal′mo-skōp)—An instrument for examining the interior of the eye.

otoscope (o′to-skōp)—An instrument for examining the external ear canal and tympanic membrane.

palpation (pal-pa′shun)—The process of feeling with the hands to detect signs of disease.

percussion (per-kush′un)—The process of tapping the body to detect signs of disease.

percussion hammer (per-kush′un ham′er)—A hammer with a rubber head, used for testing reflexes.

retina (ret′i-nah)—The interior structure of the eye, which picks up and transmits light impulses to the optic nerve.

speculum (spek′u-lum)—An instrument for opening a body orifice or cavity for viewing.

subjective symptom (sub-jek′tiv simp′tom)—A symptom that is felt by the patient but is not observable by an examiner.

symptom (simp′tom)—Any change in the body or its functioning that indicates that a disease is present.

tonometer (to-nom′ĕ-ter)—An instrument for measuring pressure within the eye.

tympanic membrane (tim-pan′ik mem′brān)—A thin, semi-transparent membrane located between the external ear canal and middle ear that receives and transmits sound waves. Also known as the ear drum.

Introduction

An important and frequent responsibility of the medical assistant is to assist with patient examinations. People are becoming more aware of the need for a yearly physical examination to detect early signs of illness and to prevent serious health problems. Also, a physical examination is often a prerequisite for employment, for entering the military service and schools, and for obtaining an insurance policy.

A complete patient examination consists of three parts: the health history, the physical examination of each body system, and the laboratory and diagnostic tests. The results are used by the physician to determine the patient's general state of health, to arrive at a diagnosis and prescribe treatment, and to observe any change in a patient's illness after treatment has been instituted.

The term *diagnosis* refers to the scientific method of determining and identifying a disease through the evaluation of the health history, the patient's symptoms, and laboratory tests and diagnostic procedures. The importance of establishing a diagnosis is to provide a logical basis for treatment and prognosis. There are different kinds of diagnoses. The *clinical diagnosis* is obtained through the evaluation of the health history and the physical examination without the benefit of laboratory or diagnostic tests. Outside laboratories generally ask the physician to list the clinical diagnosis on the laboratory request form to assist the laboratory in correlating the clinical laboratory data with the needs of the physician. Two or more diseases may have similar symptoms; the *differential diagnosis* involves determining which of these diseases is producing the patient's symptoms.

The medical assistant is responsible for the preparation of the examining room, equipment, and supplies and for preparing the patient for examination. That individual is also responsible for assisting the patient, assisting the physician, collecting specimens, and performing certain aspects of laboratory and diagnostic testing.

The Health History

The health history is a collection of data obtained by interviewing the patient (Fig. 3-1). It aids the physician in making a complete diagnosis of the patient's condition. A thorough history is taken on a new patient and subsequent office visits provide additional information regarding changes in the patient's illness or treatment. A quiet, comfortable room that allows for privacy encourages the patient to communicate more honestly and openly. Showing genuine interest in and concern for the patient helps to reduce apprehension and facilitates the collection of data. The health history is usually taken before the physical examination, providing the physician the opportunity to compare findings. The health history consists of seven parts or sections, which are listed and described below.

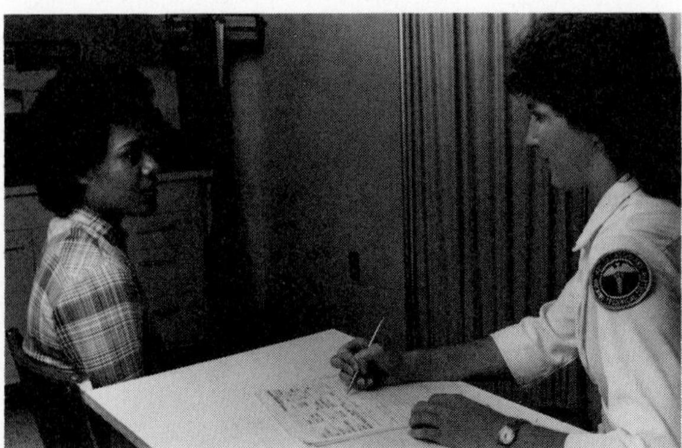

FIGURE 3-1. Collecting data from the patient for the health history.

Introductory Data

The introductory or identification data section is included at the beginning of the health history form to obtain basic data on all new patients (Fig. 3–2*A*). This information is used for a number of administrative procedures, such as preparing a new patient's chart, billing, and completing insurance forms. The introductory data section is completed by the patient and includes the following information:

Patient's name
Address
Telephone number (home)
Place of employment
Telephone number (work)
Responsible party
Age
Date of birth
Sex
Race
Marital status
Occupation
Insurance company and policy number
Social security number

Chief Complaint

The chief complaint (CC) identifies the patient's reason for seeking care, that is, the symptom causing the patient the most trouble. The chief complaint is used as a foundation for the more detailed information that will be obtained in the Present Illness and Review of Systems sections of the health history. The medical assistant is usually responsible for obtaining the chief complaint from the patient and recording it in the patient's chart. In most offices, this information is recorded on a preprinted lined form (Fig. 3–2*G*). Certain guidelines must be followed in obtaining and recording the chief complaint and are described as follows:

1. An open-ended question should be used to elicit the chief complaint from the patient. Examples include the following:
   a. What seems to be the problem?
   b. How can we help you today?
   c. What can we do for you today?
2. The chief complaint should be limited to one or two symptoms and should refer to a specific, rather than vague, symptom.
3. The chief complaint should be recorded concisely and briefly, using the patient's own words as much as possible.
4. The duration of the symptom (onset) should be included in the chief complaint.
5. The medical assistant should avoid using names of diseases or diagnostic terms to record the chief complaint.

The following are correct and incorrect examples of recording chief complaints:

1. Correct Examples
   a. Burning during urination that has lasted for 2 days.
   b. Pain in the shoulder that started 2 weeks ago.
   c. Shortness of breath for the past month.
2. Incorrect Examples
   a. Has not felt well for the past 2 weeks. (This statement refers to a vague, rather than a specific, complaint.)
   b. Ear pain and fever. (The duration of the symptom is not listed.)

c. Dysuria upon urination indicative of a urinary tract infection. (Names of diseases and diagnostic terms should not be used to record the chief complaint; the duration of the symptom is not listed.)

Present Illness

The present illness (PI) is an expansion of the chief complaint and includes a full description of the current status of the patient's illness, from the time of its onset. To complete this section of the health history, the patient is asked questions to obtain a detailed description of the symptom causing the patient the most problem. This information is recorded on the same preprinted lined form used to record the chief complaint (Fig. 3–2*G*), following the charting guidelines outlined on page 62. The medical assistant may be responsible for completing this section of the health history. Much skill and practice in asking the proper questions are required to obtain more detailed information. A general guide for obtaining further information on symptoms is presented on page 64, whereas a more thorough study for analyzing a symptom is included in the *Student Manual* (Supplemental Education for Chapter 3: Taking Patient Symptoms).

Past History

The past medical history is a review of the patient's past medical status (Fig. 3–2*C*). Obtaining information on past medical care assists the physician in providing optimal patient care for the current problem. Most medical offices ask the patient to complete this section of the health history through a checklist type of form. The medical assistant should assist the patient with this section, as necessary, by offering to answer any questions regarding the information required. The past history includes the following areas:

Major illnesses
Childhood diseases
Unusual infections
Injuries/accidents
Hospitalizations and operations
Previous medical tests
Immunizations
Allergies
Medications: past and present

Family History

The family history is a review of the health status of the patient's blood relatives (Fig. 3–2*B*). This section of the health history focuses on diseases that tend to be familial. A *familial* disease is one that occurs in or affects members of a family more frequently than would be expected by chance. Examples of familial diseases include hypertension, heart disease, allergies, and diabetes mellitus. The patient usually completes this section of the health history and is asked to provide the following information on each blood relative:

Age
State of health
Presence of any significant disease
If deceased, cause of death

Text continued on page 60

PATIENT HEALTH HISTORY

(A) IDENTIFICATION DATA Please print the following information.

Today's date ____/____/____ File no. ____________

Name ______________________________ ____ Male ____ Female ________ Race Date of birth ____/____/____

Address ______________________________ ____ Married ____ Separated ____ Divorced ____ Widowed ____ Single

______________________________ ________ Zip Code Insurance provider ______________________________

Telephone ______________ Home number ______________ Work number Policy number ______________________________

Social Security or Medicare No. ______________________________ Occupation ______________________________

(B) FAMILY HISTORY: For each member of your family, follow the grey or white line across the page and check the boxes for:

1. Their present state of health
2. Any illnesses they have had

PRINT NAMES BELOW	Good health	Poor health	Deceased	If deceased, write in age and cause of death. Include fatal accidents and suicides.	Allergies or asthma	Anemia	Bleed easily	Diabetes	Cancer or tumor	Epilepsy	Glaucoma	Genetic disease	Alcoholism	Kidney or bladder trouble	Stomach / duodenal ulcer	Nervous breakdown	Rheumatism or arthritis	High blood pressure	Heart trouble	Gout
Father:																				
Mother:																				
Brothers/Sisters:																				
Spouse:																				
Child:																				
Child:																				
Child:																				
Child:																				
Paternal relatives (in each box, write how many affected with) →																				
Maternal relatives (in each box, write how many affected with) →																				
(C) YOUR HEALTH HISTORY (begin here with illnesses) →																				

PAST HISTORY

Additional Illnesses or Problems: Mark an X in the box next to any of the following that you have now or have ever had

- ☐ eye infections
- ☐ thyroid disease
- ☐ eczema
- ☐ hives or rashes
- ☐ bronchitis
- ☐ emphysema
- ☐ pneumonia
- ☐ pancreatitis
- ☐ liver disease
- ☐ diverticulosis
- ☐ hernia
- ☐ hemorrhoids
- ☐ neuralgia or neuritis
- ☐ tension/anxiety
- ☐ depression
- ☐ childhood hyperactivity
- ☐ chicken pox
- ☐ German measles
- ☐ scarlet fever
- ☐ measles
- ☐ mumps
- ☐ polio
- ☐ rheumatic fever
- ☐ malaria
- ☐ mononucleosis
- ☐ venereal disease
- ☐ yellow jaundice
- ☐ tuberculosis
- ☐ ______________
- ☐ ______________

Have you ever been turned down for life insurance, military service or employment because of health problems? . . . . ____ Yes ____ No

Major Hospitalizations: If you have ever been hospitalized for any major medical illness or operation, write in your most recent hospitalizations below. Check this box ☐ if you have had more than four such hospitalizations. (Do not include normal pregnancies)

	Year	Operation or Illness	Name of Hospital	City and State
1st Hospitalization				
2nd Hospitalization				
3rd Hospitalization				
4th Hospitalization				

Tests and Immunizations: Mark an X next to those that you have had. Enter the year when you last were given the tests or "shots."

	Year			Year	
☐	19___	chest x-ray	☐	19___	smallpox "shots"
☐	19___	kidney x-ray	☐	19___	tetanus "shots"
☐	19___	G.I. series	☐	19___	polio series
☐	19___	colon x-ray	☐	19___	typhoid "shots"
☐	19___	gallbladder x-ray	☐	19___	flu injections
☐	19___	electrocardiogram	☐	19___	mumps "shots"
☐	19___	TB test	☐	19___	measles "shots"
☐	19___	sigmoidoscopy	☐	19___	______________

Medicines: Mark an X in the box next to any medicines that you are now taking, or that you are sensitive or allergic to.

taking	allergic to:		taking	allergic to:	
☐	☐	antibiotics	☐	☐	aspirin
☐	☐	penicillin	☐	☐	diet pills
☐	☐	sulfa	☐	☐	antacids
☐	☐	opiates/codeine	☐	☐	laxatives
☐	☐	diuretics/water pills	☐	☐	cold tablets
☐	☐	sedatives	☐	☐	______________
☐	☐	stimulants/caffeine	☐	☐	______________
☐	☐	Demerol	☐	☐	______________
☐	☐	blood pressure medicine			

Your Signature: ______________________________

CONTINUE TO NEXT PAGE

FIGURE 3–2. Example of a health history form. The health history consists of the following sections: *A*, Introductory Data, *B*, Family History, *C*, Past History.

Illustration continued on following page

(D) PERSONAL HISTORY

EDUCATION:

_____ Years elementary
_____ Years high school
_____ Years college, technical, business, etc.

OCCUPATIONAL HISTORY:

Occupation _______________________________ Years _____
Previous occupation _______________________ Years _____
Military service __________________________
Overseas? _______________________________

Have you been exposed to any of the following in your work environment?

_____ Excess dust (coal, lime, rock)	_____ Smoke or auto exhaust fumes
_____ Sand	_____ Radiation
_____ Chemicals	_____ Insecticides
_____ Cleaning fluids/solvents	_____ Paints
_____ Hair spray	_____ Other toxic materials

Please answer the following questions by writing an X on the line in front of the word Yes or No, except where you are asked for specific information.

If a question doesn't apply, skip it and go on to the next one.

This information is obviously highly confidential and will be released to other health professionals or insurance carriers only with your signed consent.

DIET HISTORY/EXERCISE

1. Do you eat a good breakfast?	1. _____ Yes _____ No
2. Do you snack between meals (soft drinks, chips, candy bars)?	2. _____ Yes _____ No
3. Do you eat fresh fruits and vegetables each day?	3. _____ Yes _____ No
4. Do you eat whole grain breads and cereals?	4. _____ Yes _____ No
5. Is your diet high in fat content?	5. _____ Yes _____ No
6. Is your diet high in cholesterol content?	6. _____ Yes _____ No
7. Is your diet high in salt content?	7. _____ Yes _____ No
8. Do you habitually use laxatives?	8. _____ Yes _____ No
9. Do you exercise on a regular basis?	9. _____ Yes _____ No
10. Does your job require strenuous, sustained physical work?	10. _____ Yes _____ No
11. Are you allergic to any foods?	11. _____ Yes _____ No
12. How many glasses of milk do you drink each day?	12. ______________
13. How many glasses of water do you drink each day?	13. ______________
14. How would you describe your overall eating habits?	14. _____ Excellent _____ Good _____ Fair _____ Poor

FIGURE 3-2 *Continued. D,* Personal History.

SOCIAL HISTORY/HABITS

15. Are you very nervous around strangers? .... 15. ____ Yes ____ No
16. Do you find it hard to make decisions? .... 16. ____ Yes ____ No
17. Do you find it hard to concentrate or remember? .... 17. ____ Yes ____ No
18. Do you usually feel lonely or depressed? .... 18. ____ Yes ____ No
19. Do you often cry? .... 19. ____ Yes ____ No
20. Would you say you have a hopeless outlook? .... 20. ____ Yes ____ No
21. Do you have difficulty relaxing? .... 21. ____ Yes ____ No
22. Do you have a tendency to worry a lot? .... 22. ____ Yes ____ No
23. Are you troubled by frightening dreams or thoughts? .... 23. ____ Yes ____ No
24. Do you have a tendency to be shy or sensitive? .... 24. ____ Yes ____ No
25. Do you have a strong dislike for criticism? .... 25. ____ Yes ____ No
26. Do you lose your temper often? .... 26. ____ Yes ____ No
27. Do little things often annoy you? .... 27. ____ Yes ____ No
28. Are you disturbed by any work or family problems? .... 28. ____ Yes ____ No
29. Are you having any sexual difficulties? .... 29. ____ Yes ____ No
30. Have you ever considered committing suicide? .... 30. ____ Yes ____ No
31. Have you ever desired or sought psychiatric help? .... 31. ____ Yes ____ No
32. Have you gained or lost much weight recently? .... 32. ____ Yes ____ No
33. Do you have a tendency to be too hot or too cold? .... 33. ____ Yes ____ No
34. Have you lost your interest in eating lately? .... 34. ____ Yes ____ No
35. Do you always seem to be hungry? .... 35. ____ Yes ____ No
36. Are you more thirsty than usual lately? .... 36. ____ Yes ____ No
37. Are there any swellings in your armpits or groin? .... 37. ____ Yes ____ No
38. Do you seem to feel exhausted or fatigued most of the time? .... 38. ____ Yes ____ No
39. Do you have difficulty either falling asleep or staying asleep? .... 39. ____ Yes ____ No
40. Do you participate in physical activity or exercise less than three times a week? .... 40. ____ Yes ____ No
41. How much do you smoke per day? .... 41. ____ cigarettes
    ____ cigars/pipes
    ____ don't smoke
42. Do you take two or more alcoholic drinks a day? .... 42. ____ Yes ____ No
43. Do you drink more than six cups of coffee or tea a day? .... 43. ____ Yes ____ No
44. Are you a regular user of sleeping pills, marijuana, tranquilizers, pain killers, etc.? .... 44. ____ Yes ____ No
45. Have you ever used heroin, cocaine, LSD, PCP, etc.? .... 45. ____ Yes ____ No
46. Do you drive a motor vehicle more than 25,000 miles a year? .... 46. ____ Yes ____ No
47. How often do you use seat belts when riding in cars? .... 47. ____ never
    ____ sometimes
    ____ always
48. List any country outside the United States you have visited in the past six months .... 48. ____________
49. Do you live in: (A) an apartment (B) a house (C) a trailer (D) other .... 49. ____________
50. When did you last have a physical examination? .... 50. ____________

FIGURE 3-2*D* *Continued.*

Illustration continued on following page

(E) Name____Date________________

Doctor's notes ____

____

____

REVIEW OF SYSTEMS

HEAD and NECK

92. ____ frequent headaches
93. ____ neck pains
94. ____ neck lumps or swelling

EYES

95. ____ wears glasses
96. ____ blurry vision
97. ____ eyesight worsening
98. ____ sees double
99. ____ sees halo
100. ____ eye pains or itching
101. ____ watering eyes
102. ____ eye trouble

EARS

103. ____ hearing difficulties
104. ____ earaches
105. ____ running ears
106. ____ buzzing in ears
107. ____ motion sickness

MOUTH

108. ____ dental problems
109. ____ swellings on gums or jaws
110. ____ sore tongue
111. ____ taste changes

NOSE and THROAT

112. ____ congested nose
113. ____ running nose
114. ____ sneezing spells
115. ____ headcolds
116. ____ nose bleeds
117. ____ sore throat
118. ____ enlarged tonsils
119. ____ hoarse voice

RESPIRATORY

120. ____ wheezes or gasps
121. ____ coughing spells
122. ____ coughs up phlegm
123. ____ coughed up blood
124. ____ chest colds
125. ____ excessive sweating, night sweats

CARDIOVASCULAR

126. ____ high blood pressure
127. ____ racing heart
128. ____ chest pains
129. ____ dizzy spells
130. ____ shortness of breath
131. ____ shortness of breath at night
132. ____ more pillows to breathe
133. ____ swollen feet or ankles
134. ____ leg cramps
135. ____ heart murmur

DIGESTIVE

heartburn ____ 49.
bloated stomach ____ 50.
belching ____ 51.
stomach pains ____ 52.
nausea ____ 53.
vomited blood ____ 54.
difficulty swallowing ____ 55.
constipation ____ 56.
loose bowels ____ 57.
black stools ____ 58.
grey stools ____ 59.
pain in rectum ____ 60.
rectal bleeding ____ 61.

URINARY

night frequency ____ 62.
day frequency ____ 63.
wets pants or bed ____ 64.
burning on urination ____ 65.
brown, black or bloody urine ____ 66.
difficulty starting urine ____ 67.
urgency ____ 68.

MALE GENITAL

weak urine stream ____ 69.
prostate trouble ____ 70.
burning or discharge ____ 71.
lumps on testicles ____ 72.
painful testicles ____ 73.

FEMALE GENITAL

last menstrual period ____/____/____ 74.
post-menopausal or hysterectomy ____ 75.
noticed vaginal bleeding ____ 76.

abnormal LMP ____ 77.
heavy bleeding during periods ____ 78.
bleeding between periods ____ 79.
bleeding after intercourse ____ 80.
recent vaginal itching/discharge ____ 81.
no monthly breast exam ____ 82.
lump or pain in breasts ____ 83.
complications with birth control ____ 84.
last Pap test ____/____ 85.

OBSTETRIC HISTORY

gravida ______ 86.
para ______ 87.
pre-term ______ 88.
miscarriages ______ 89.
still births ______ 90.
has had an abortion ____ 91.

MUSCULOSKELETAL

1. ____ aching muscles or joints
2. ____ swollen joints
3. ____ back or shoulder pains
4. ____ painful feet
5. ____ handicapped

SKIN

6. ____ skin problems
7. ____ itching or burning skin
8. ____ bleeds easily
9. ____ bruises easily

NEUROLOGICAL

10. ____ faintness
11. ____ numbness
12. ____ convulsions
13. ____ change in handwriting
14. ____ trembles

MOOD

15. ____ nervous with strangers
16. ____ difficulty in making decisions
17. ____ lack of concentration or memory
18. ____ lonely or depressed
19. ____ cries often
20. ____ hopeless outlook
21. ____ difficulty relaxing
22. ____ worries a lot
23. ____ frightening dreams or thoughts
24. ____ shy or sensitive
25. ____ dislikes criticism
26. ____ loses temper
27. ____ annoyed by little things
28. ____ work or family problems
29. ____ sexual difficulties
30. ____ considered suicide
31. ____ desired psychiatric help

GENERAL

32. ____ weight changes
33. ____ tends to be hot or cold
34. ____ loss of interest in eating
35. ____ always hungry
36. ____ more thirsty lately
37. ____ armpits or groin swelling
38. ____ fatigue
39. ____ sleeping difficulties
40. ____ exercises less than 3 times per week
41. ____ cigarettes ____ cigars/pipes ____ don't smoke
42. ____ two or more alcoholic drinks per day
43. ____ over 6 cups of coffee/tea per day
44. ____ uses sleeping pills, marijuana, tranquilizers
45. ____ has used hard drugs
46. ____ drives vehicle over 25,000 miles per year
47. ____ never ____ sometimes ____ always wears seat belts
48. ______________ visited in the last 6 months

Special problems or symptoms: ____

____

____

____

____

Patient's Signature: ______________________________

FIGURE 3–2 *Continued. E,* Review of Systems.

Ⓕ NAME AGE

OCCUPATION ______ SOC. SEC. # ______

<table>
<tr><td rowspan="2">Height ___
Weight ___
Build ___
(Sm. Med. Lg. Obese.)
Pulse ___
Resp. ___
Temp. ___</td><td rowspan="2">BLOOD PRESSURE
Sitting
R / : L /
Standing
R / : L /
Lying
R / : L /</td><td rowspan="2">VISION
Without Glasses
Far R 20/ L 20/
Near R / L /
With Glasses
Far R 20/ L 20/
Near R / L /
Tonometry R ___ L ___
Colorvision ___
(Ishihara plates missed)
Peripheral Fields R ___ L ___</td><td>Diagnostic Tests</td><td>Results</td></tr>
<tr><td></td><td></td></tr>
<tr><td>AUDIOMETRIC TESTING</td><td colspan="2">250 500 1000 2000 4000 8000
R ___ ___ ___ ___ ___ ___
L ___ ___ ___ ___ ___ ___
Gross Hearing ___</td><td></td><td></td></tr>
<tr><td colspan="3">PULMONARY FUNCTION</td><td colspan="2"></td></tr>
</table>

Ⓖ Initial Problem List

Employment status ______ Physician's signature ______

DATE ______

FIGURE 3-2 *Continued. F* and *G*, The Chief Complaint and Present Illness are recorded in the section labeled *G*, while the results of routine procedures are recorded in section *F*.

Personal History

This section of the health history includes information on the patient's personal life, including the daily routine, health habits, family situation, and living environment (Fig. 3–2*D*). The personal history is important because personal factors in a patient's life may have an impact on the condition of that individual as well as influence the course of treatment or therapy chosen by the physician. The personal history also provides the physician with information regarding the effect that the illness may have on the patient's daily living pattern. If it is necessary for the individual to make a major lifestyle adjustment (e.g., stop smoking, reduce working hours), the physician may recommend available support services to assist in this transition. This section of the history is usually completed by the patient and includes the following areas:

Education
Occupational history
Diet history
Exercise
Social history
Habits

Review of Systems

A review of systems (ROS) is a systematic review of each body system in order to detect any symptoms that have not yet been revealed. The importance of the review of systems is that it assists in identifying symptoms that might otherwise remain undetected. The physician usually completes the review of systems by asking a series of detailed and direct questions relating to each body system; the results of this section of the health history assist the physician in a preliminary assessment of the type and extent of physical examination required. Refer to Figure 3–2*E* for an example of a review of systems form.

Charting in the Medical Record

A *medical record* (often called "the chart") is a written record of the important information regarding a patient, including the care of that individual and the progress of the illness. *Charting* is the process of making written entries about a patient in the medical record and is performed by individuals in the medical office who are involved with the health care of the patient. The patient's record is considered a legal document; therefore, the information must be recorded as completely and as accurately as possible. The medical assistant must always keep in mind that the information contained within the patient's medical record is strictly confidential and must not be read by or discussed with anyone except the physician or medical staff involved with the care of the patient.

The patient's medical record serves several functions. It provides an efficient and effective method by which information can be shared among members of the medical office. For example, the charting of an ultrasound treatment that has been administered by the medical assistant informs the physician that the patient received the treatment that was ordered. The physician uses the information in the medical record as a basis for making decisions regarding the patient's care and treatment. In addition, the medical record serves to document the results of the treatment and the patient's progress. The patient's medical record also serves as a legal document. The law requires that a record be maintained to document the care and treatment being received by the patient. If something goes wrong, good charting works to legally protect the physician and the medical staff. On the other hand, incomplete records could be used as evidence in court to show that the patient did not receive the quality of care that meets generally accepted standards.

The specific information contained in the medical record may vary slightly from one medical office to another but generally includes the patient's health history, the results of the physical examination, laboratory reports, the results of diagnostic tests such as x-rays and electrocardiograms, progress notes relating to the patient's care and treatment, and the patient's diagnosis and prognosis. Most medical offices record the patient's health data on preprinted health forms, which are stored in a folder labeled with the patient's name (constituting the patient's medical record). A large variety of forms are available; the type of form utilized is based upon the specific needs of each medical office. (Fig. 3–2 is an example of a health history form, and Fig. 3–7 is an example of a form used to record the results of the physical examination.)

Types of Charting Entries

The medical assistant will be recording information in the patient's medical record, which is considered one of the most important responsibilities in the medical office. Areas in which the medical assistant is most apt to be making entries include the following.

Recording Patient Symptoms. The medical assistant may be responsible for recording symptoms obtained during office visits or telephone conversations in the patient's medical record. The medical assistant must be sure to record this information in a clear, complete, and concise manner so it is meaningful to the physician. Each symptom should be described completely. For example, if a patient complains about pain in the lower abdomen, additional information is needed to describe the pain, including the type, specific location, onset, intensity, precipitating factors, and duration of the pain. Complete and concise descriptions provide the physician with baseline data, against which a later improvement or worsening of the patient's condition can be compared. Refer to page 63 for a discussion of guidelines to follow for recording patient symptoms.

Recording Procedures Performed on the Patient. Procedures can be classified into two general categories. A *diagnostic procedure* is performed to assist in the diagnosis of a patient's condition; examples include electrocardiography, x-ray examination, and proctosigmoidoscopy. A *therapeutic procedure* is curative in nature and is performed to treat a patient's condition. Examples of therapeutic procedures include the administration of medication, ear and eye irrigations, and therapeutic ultrasound. Procedures should be recorded immediately after being performed; from a legal standpoint, a procedure that is not documented was not performed. Specific information to be recorded is included with each procedure presented in this text. In general, the following information must be included: the date and time, the type of procedure (e.g., ear irrigation), the outcome (e.g., cerumen removed from the ear canal), the patient's reaction, and the medical assistant's initials.

Medications Administered to the Patient. Recording information regarding medications is an important responsibility in the medical office. Included in the recording should be the date and time, the route of administration, the name of the medication, the dosage given, the injection site used (for parenteral medication), any significant observations or patient reactions, and the medical assistant's initials.

Specimens Collected from the Patient. Each time a specimen is collected from a patient, the medical assistant should chart the date and time the specimen was collected, the type of specimen, and the area of the body from which the specimen was obtained. If the specimen is to be sent to an outside laboratory for testing, this information should also be recorded, including the date the specimen was picked up or mailed. In this way, the physician will know that the specimen was sent to the laboratory, when test results are not back yet.

Laboratory Tests Ordered. Laboratory testing involves the analysis and study of materials, fluids, or tissues obtained from patients to assist in diagnosing and treating disease. Each time a laboratory test is ordered for a patient, this informtion should be recorded in the patient's chart, including the date and the type of test(s) ordered. If the patient does not undergo the test, documented proof exists that the test was ordered. Recording laboratory tests that were ordered protects the physician legally as well as refreshes the physician's memory of tests being run on the patient that are not yet back from the laboratory.

Results of Laboratory Tests. In most medical offices, the laboratory report (containing the laboratory test results) is placed in the patient's chart; therefore, it is not necessary to record the results. In some offices, however, the medical assistant may be required to transcribe the test results onto another form. In cases of a stat request or abnormal findings, the test results are telephoned to the medical office, thus requiring the medical assistant to record the results on a reporting form. Careful recording is essential to avoid errors, which in turn could affect the patient's diagnosis.

Progress Notes. Progress notes involve updating the medical record with new information each time the patient visits or telephones the medical office. Progress notes serve to document the patient's health status from one visit to the next and may include such areas as the results of treatment (e.g., drug or diet therapy, additional symptoms experienced by the patient, additional laboratory or diagnostic tests ordered). The medical assistant must make sure to include the date with each progress note entry.

Instructions Given to the Patient Regarding Medical Care. Many times it is necessary to relay instructions to a patient regarding medical care (e.g., wound care, cast care, care of sutures). The medical assistant should chart this information, making sure to include the date and the type of instructions relayed to the patient. A growing number of medical offices have printed instruction sheets that are given to the patient. The patient is asked to sign a form indicating that he or she has read and understands the instructions. The form is then signed by the medical assistant, who functions as a witness. This protects the physician legally in the event that the patient fails to follow the instructions and causes further harm or damage to a body part.

Other areas in which the medical assistant is responsible for making entries in the patient's medical record include missed or canceled appointments, telephone calls from patients, medication refills, and changes in medication or dosage by the physician.

Guidelines for Proper Charting

In order to ensure accurate and concise charting, specific guidelines must be followed. These are listed and described as follows:

1. *Check the name on the chart before making an entry to be sure you have the correct chart.* If the medical assistant records in the wrong patient's chart by mistake, information such as a procedure that was performed on a patient may be excluded from that individual's record. As previously stated, from a legal standpoint, a procedure not documented was not performed.
2. *Use dark ink (black or dark blue) to make entries in the patient's chart.* Dark ink must be used to provide a permanent record. In addition, entries made in dark

ink are easier to reproduce, should the record be duplicated for insurance company purposes, patient referral, microfilming, and so on.

3. *Write in legible hand-printed or written handwriting.* In order for the medical record to be meaningful to others, the medical assistant must be sure to record information legibly. If the medical assistant's handwriting is not legible, the information should be printed.

4. *Record information accurately, using phrases or sentences.* Information should be recorded precisely and accurately, using phrases or sentences. The medical assistant should be brief but complete and should avoid vagueness and duplication of information. It is not necessary to include the patient's name in the entry, because the entire chart centers on one patient; it is therefore assumed the information refers to that patient. (Because this text is designed to be used by a student performing procedures in a classroom setting, each text procedure requires the student to record the patient's name for the sake of clarity. In a medical office setting the name is found on the patient's chart and does not need to be included in the entry.) Each phrase or sentence should begin with a capital letter and end with a period. Each new topic should begin on a separate line and be dated with the month, day, and year. Standard abbreviations, medical terms, and symbols should be used to help save time and space. It is important, however, that the medical assistant first check the medical office policy to determine those abbreviations, medical terms, and symbols that are commonly used in that office to avoid confusing others reading the chart. In addition, correct spelling is essential for accuracy in charting. If in doubt about the spelling of a word, check a dictionary.

5. *Chart immediately after performing each procedure.* Once a procedure has been performed, it should be charted without delay. If a time lapse occurs between performing the procedure and charting it, the medical assistant may not remember certain aspects of the procedure such as the results of the treatment or the patient's reaction. Procedures should never be charted in advance. The individual performing the procedure should be the one to chart it; in other words, never chart for someone else.

6. *Never erase or obliterate a recording.* If an error is made in charting, the medical assistant must never erase or obliterate the recording. Should the physician or medical staff be involved in litigation, erased or obliterated entries tend to reduce credibility. If incorrect information is charted, the medical assistant should draw a single line through the incorrect information, thus permitting the incorrect information to remain legible. The word "error" is then written above the incorrect data, including the date and the medical assistant's initials. Some medical offices may request that the reason for the change also be recorded. The correct information is then inserted immediately following the error (Fig. 3–3).

The medical assistant should always take the time to record properly in the patient's medical record. Good charting helps to coordinate efforts in the medical office and leads to high-quality patient care.

Symptoms

A *symptom* is any change in the body or its functioning that indicates the presence of disease. Symptoms can be classified as *subjective* or *objective.* A subjective symptom is one that is felt by the patient and cannot be observed by another

error 12/7/8 - JB
12/7/8– OPV, 0.5ml, ~~IM~~ JB
P.O.

FIGURE 3–3. Proper method for correcting an error in the patient's medical record.

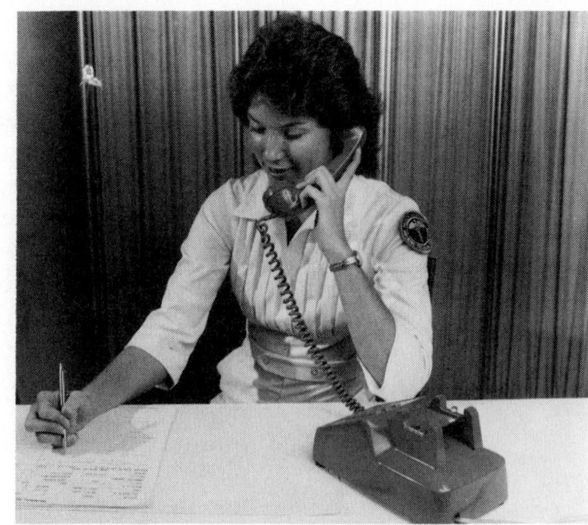

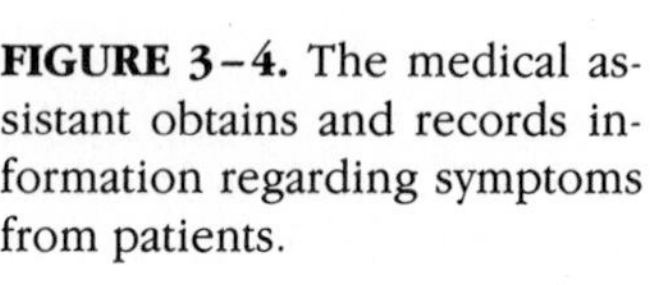

FIGURE 3–4. The medical assistant obtains and records information regarding symptoms from patients.

person. Pain, pruritus, vertigo, and nausea are examples of subjective symptoms. An objective symptom is one that can be observed by another person as well as by the patient. Rash, coughing, and cyanosis are objective symptoms.

When patients relate information regarding their symptoms to the medical assistant during office visits and telephone conversations, the medical assistant should obtain as much detailed information as possible. Information conveyed during a telephone conversation helps determine whether the patient needs to be seen and the immediacy of the situation (Fig. 3–4).

The following is a general guide the medical assistant can follow to gather additional information on symptoms:

1. ***What?*** What exactly is experienced by the patient? Does the symptom occur suddenly or gradually? Does anything make it worse?
2. ***Where?*** Where is the symptom located?
3. ***When?*** When did the symptom first occur? How long does it last after occurring? Does anything precipitate it?

The medical assistant should have a thorough knowledge of common symptoms and be able to recognize them. The following is a list of common symptoms:

Integumentary System

Diaphoresis	Excessive perspiration.
Flushing	A red appearance to the skin, which generally affects the face and neck. A flushed appearance is commonly present with a fever.
Jaundice	A yellow appearance to the skin, first evident in the whites of the eyes.
Rash	An eruption on the skin.

Circulatory System

Bradycardia	An abnormally slow pulse rate.
Dehydration	A decrease in the amount of water in the body. The patient will have a flushed appearance, dry skin, and a decreased output of urine.

Edema	The retention of fluid in the tissues, resulting in swelling. The skin over the area is tight. Edema is most easily observed in the extremities.
Tachycardia	An abnormally fast pulse rate.

Gastrointestinal System

Anorexia	The patient has a loss of appetite and a lack of interest in food.
Constipation	A condition in which the stool becomes hard and dry, resulting in difficult passage from the rectum. The consistency of the stool, rather than the frequency of defecation, is used as a guide in determining the presence of constipation. (Frequency of bowel movements varies with the individual. Some people have a bowel movement only every 2 to 3 days but are not constipated.) Other symptoms of constipation include headache, nausea, and general malaise.
Diarrhea	The passage of an increased number of loose, watery stools. The fecal material moves rapidly through the intestinal tract, resulting in decreased absorption by the body of water, electrolytes, and nutrients. Other symptoms usually associated with diarrhea are intestinal cramping and general weakness.
Flatulence	The presence of excessive gas in the stomach or intestines.
Nausea and vomiting	Nausea is a sensation of discomfort in the stomach with a feeling that vomiting may occur. Vomiting is the ejection of the stomach contents through the mouth, also known as *emesis.* The ejected content is known as *vomitus.*

Respiratory System

Cough	An involuntary and forceful exhalation of air followed by a deep inhalation. A cough may be productive (meaning a discharge is produced) or nonproductive (when no discharge is present).
Cyanosis	A bluish discoloration of the skin due to a lack of oxygen.
Dyspnea	Labored or difficult breathing.
Epistaxis	Hemorrhaging from the nose or a nosebleed.

Nervous System

Chill	A feeling of coldness accompanied by shivering. Chills are generally present with a fever.
Convulsion	Involuntary contractions of the muscles.
Fever or pyrexia	A body temperature that is higher than normal.

Headache	A feeling of pain or aching in the head. It is a common symptom that accompanies many illnesses. Tension, fatigue, and eye strain can result in a headache.
Pain	Irritation of pain receptors, resulting in a feeling of distress or suffering. Pain is an important indication that a part of the body is not working properly.
Pruritus	Severe itching.
Vertigo	A feeling of dizziness or lightheadedness.

Weight and Height

The medical assistant routinely takes weight and height measurements on many different types of patients. A change in weight may be significant in the diagnosis of a patient's condition and in evaluating the course of treatment. Underweight and overweight patients who follow a diet therapy program should be weighed at intervals to determine their progress. Maternity patients are weighed during each prenatal visit. A sudden gain in weight may indicate edema. Children are weighed and measured during each office visit to observe their pattern of growth.

The weight can be compared against a chart that serves as a general guide to determine if the patient's weight falls within normal limits (see Table 3–1).

Positioning and Draping

Correct positioning of the patient facilitates the examination by permitting better access to the part being examined or treated. The basic positions commonly used in the medical office are the horizontal recumbent, dorsal recumbent, dorsal lithotomy, prone, knee-chest, and Sims (Fig. 3–5). The position utilized depends upon the type of examination or procedure to be performed. The medical assistant is responsible for knowing the correct position for each examination or treatment.

The patient is draped during positioning to provide for modesty, comfort, and warmth. The part to be examined is the only part that should be exposed. Patient gowns and drapes are made of cloth or disposable paper.

The *horizontal recumbent* or *supine position* is used during the physical examination of the head, chest, abdomen, and extremities and to test reflexes. The patient lies flat on the back and is covered with a drape. As the physician examines the patient, the drape is moved accordingly to expose the parts being examined.

The *dorsal recumbent position* is used for vaginal or rectal examinations. The patient is positioned on the back with the thighs rotated outward and the knees sharply flexed. A drape is positioned diagonally over the patient with one corner of the drape over the patient's chest, one corner wrapped around each leg, and the remaining corner over the pubic area. When the physician is ready to examine the patient, the center corner is folded back over the abdomen, exposing the genital area.

The *dorsal lithotomy position* is also used for vaginal or rectal examinations. It is the same as the dorsal recumbent position except that the patient's feet are placed in stirrups. The stirrups are positioned so that they are level with the examining table and pulled out approximately one foot from the edge of the table. The patient's knees are bent and the feet moved into the stirrups. The medical assistant then instructs the patient to slide the buttocks to the edge of the examining table and to rotate the thighs outward as far as is comfortable. The patient is draped in the same way as for the dorsal recumbent position. When the medical assistant is helping the patient out of the stirrups, both the patient's legs should be lifted at the same time to avoid strain on the back and abdominal muscles.

The *prone position* is used for examination of the back. The patient is positioned on the abdomen with the head turned to one side. The arms can be placed above the head or alongside the body. The patient is covered with a drape.

PROCEDURE 3-1
MEASURING WEIGHT AND HEIGHT

WEIGHT

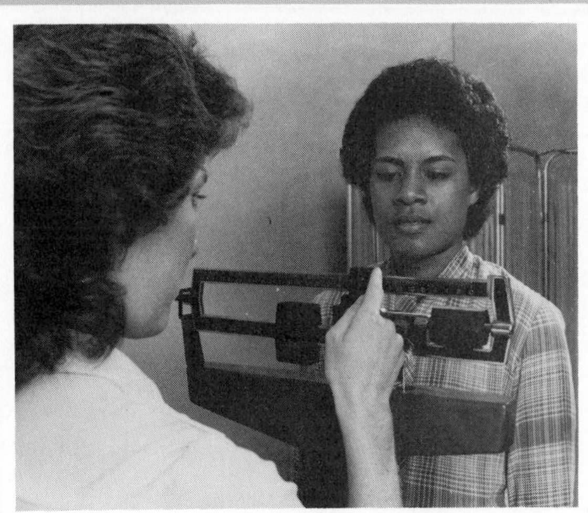

1. Wash the hands.

2. Check the balance scale for accuracy.

3. Instruct the patient to remove his or her shoes for a more accurate reading. A good medical aseptic practice is to place a paper towel on the scale to protect the patient's feet.

4. Assist the patient onto the scale.

5. Instruct the patient not to move.

6. Balance the scale and read results.

7. Return the balance to the resting position.

HEIGHT

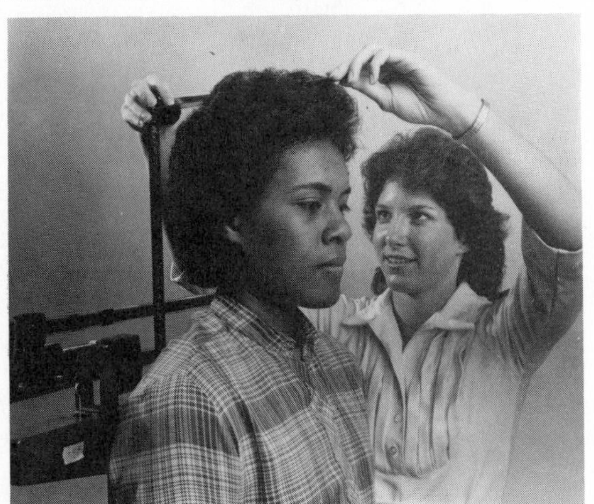

1. Instruct the patient to stand erect and look straight ahead, with his or her back to the scale.

2. Keeping the bar of the measuring scale in a vertical position, lift the bar above the patient's head.

3. Open the bar out into a horizontal position and move it down until it just touches the top of the patient's head.

4. Instruct the patient to step down and put on his or her shoes.

5. Read the marking.

6. Return the bar to the resting position.

7. Record the weight and height correctly.

DATE	TIME	PATIENT'S NAME	WEIGHT	HEIGHT

TABLE 3-1. 1983 Metropolitan Height and Weight Tables*

MEN

Height Feet	Height Inches	Small Frame	Medium Frame	Large Frame
5	2	128–134	131–141	138–150
5	3	130–136	133–143	140–153
5	4	132–138	135–145	142–156
5	5	134–140	137–148	144–160
5	6	136–142	139–151	146–164
5	7	138–145	142–154	149–168
5	8	140–148	145–157	152–172
5	9	142–151	148–160	155–176
5	10	144–154	151–163	158–180
5	11	146–157	154–166	161–184
6	0	149–160	157–170	164–188
6	1	152–164	160–174	168–192
6	2	155–168	164–178	172–197
6	3	158–172	167–182	176–202
6	4	162–176	171–187	181–207

WOMEN

Height Feet	Height Inches	Small Frame	Medium Frame	Large Frame
4	10	102–111	109–121	118–131
4	11	103–113	111–123	120–134
5	0	104–115	113–126	122–137
5	1	106–118	115–129	125–140
5	2	108–121	118–132	128–143
5	3	111–124	121–135	131–147
5	4	114–127	124–138	134–151
5	5	117–130	127–141	137–155
5	6	120–133	130–144	140–159
5	7	123–136	133–147	143–163
5	8	126–139	136–150	146–167
5	9	129–142	139–153	149–170
5	10	132–145	142–156	152–173
5	11	135–148	145–159	155–176
6	0	138–151	148–162	158–179

* Courtesy of Metropolitan Life Insurance Company.

Source of basic data: 1979 Build Study. Society of Actuaries and Association of Life Insurance Medical Directors of America, 1980.

Notes:

1. Weight at ages 25–29 based on lowest mortality. Weight in pounds according to frame (in indoor clothing weighing 5 pounds for men and 3 pounds for women; shoes with 1-inch heels).
2. To make an approximation of your frame size: Extend your arm and bend the forearm upward at a 90-degree angle. Keep fingers straight and turn the inside of your wrist toward your body. If you have a caliper, use it to measure the space between the two prominent bones on *either side* of your elbow. Without a caliper, place the thumb and index finger of your other hand on these two bones. Measure the space between your fingers against a ruler or tape measure. Compare it with the tables below that list elbow measurements for *medium-framed* men and women. Measurements lower than those listed indicate that you have a small frame. Higher measurements indicate a large frame.

Height in 1″ Heels Men	*Elbow Breadth Men*	*Height in 1″ Heels Women*	*Elbow Breadth Women*
5′2″–5′3″	2½″–2⅞″	4′10″–4′11″	2¼″–2½″
5′4″–5′7″	2⅝″–2⅞″	5′0″–5′3″	2¼″–2½″
5′8″–5′11″	2¾″–3″	5′4″–5′7″	2⅜″–2⅝″
6′0″–6′3″	2¾″–3⅛″	5′8″–5′11″	2⅜″–2⅝″
6′4″	2⅞″–3¼″	6′0″	2½″–2¾″

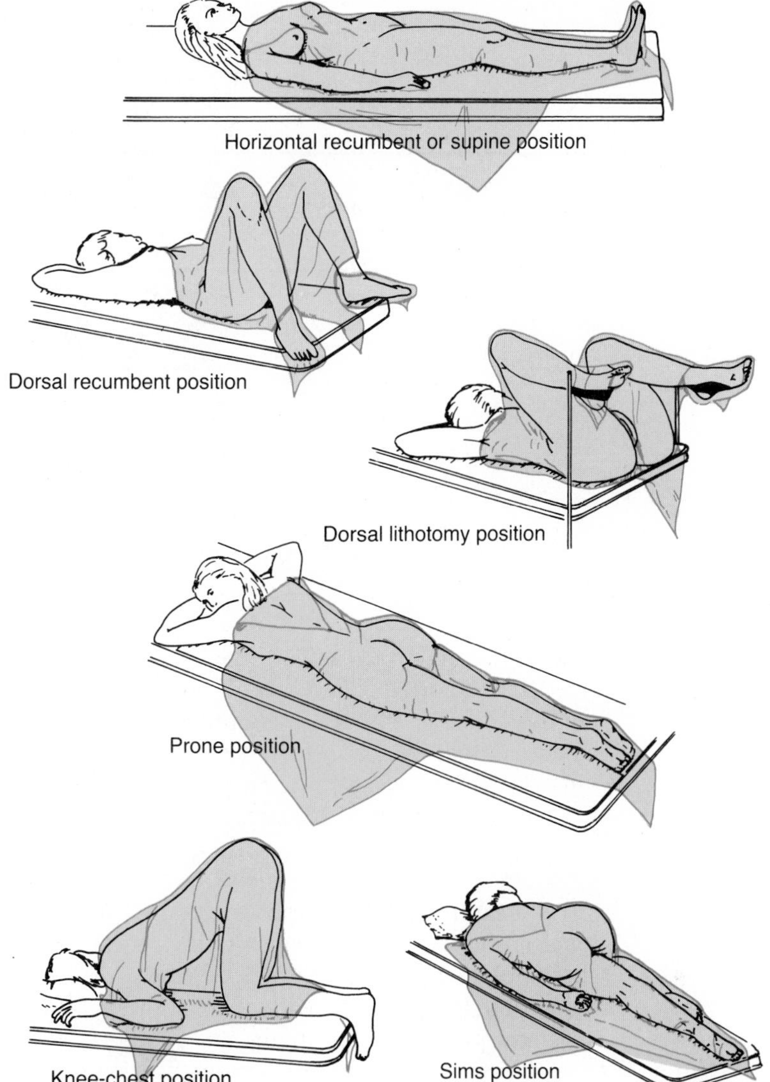

FIGURE 3–5. Positioning and draping the patient.

The *knee-chest position* is commonly used to examine the rectum or to perform a sigmoidoscopy. The patient kneels with the chest resting on the examining table. The buttocks are elevated while the back is kept straight. The patient's head, chest, and arms should be supported on the table. The head is turned to one side, and the elbows can rest on the table or the arms can be positioned above the head. A pillow can be used under the chest for support and to promote relaxation. The knees and lower legs are separated about a foot apart. The patient is draped using the diamond-shaped arrangement or with the use of two draw sheets, one across the legs and the other across the back. This is a difficult position to maintain, and the patient should not be put into this position until just before the examination. Specially constructed tables are available that offer support and that can be tilted to place the patient in the knee-chest position.

Sims position can be used for examination of the vagina or rectum or for colon treatments such as an enema. The patient is positioned on the left side with the left arm behind the body and the right arm forward with the elbow bent. Both legs are flexed, with the right leg flexed sharply and the left leg flexed slightly. The patient is draped, with a small portion of the drape folded back to expose the anal area.

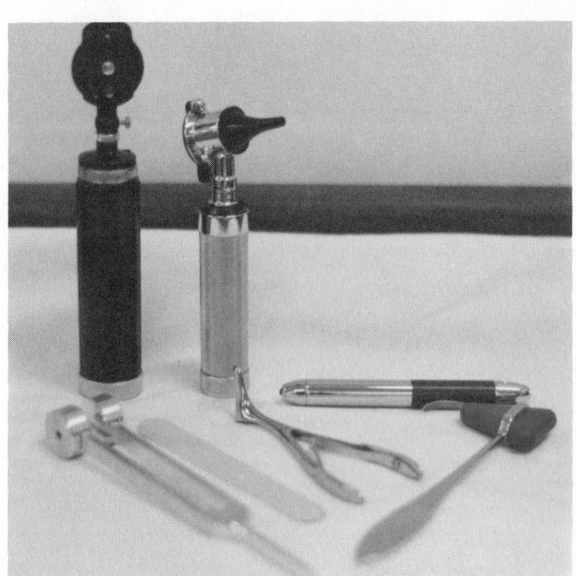

FIGURE 3-6. Examples of common instruments used for the physical examination. Starting at the far lefthand corner and going in a clockwise direction, these instruments are the ophthalmoscope, otoscope, pen flashlight, percussion hammer, nasal speculum, tongue blade, and tuning fork.

Preparation of the Examining Room

The examining room should be clean, free of clutter, and well lit. Waste baskets should be emptied frequently, especially if they contain articles that may harbor microorganisms. The room should be well ventilated, and air freshener kept on hand to help eliminate odors. A proper temperature should be maintained, keeping in mind that a temperature that is comfortable for a fully clothed patient may be too cold for one who has disrobed.

Countertops and faucets should be cleaned frequently, and dust removed from furniture and towel dispensers.

The examining table paper is changed after each patient by unrolling a fresh length. The medical assistant should check to make sure that there is an ample supply of clean gowns and drapes ready for use. Some physicians prefer to use disposable linens, and an adequate supply of these must be kept at all times.

Patient privacy is important. The medical assistant is responsible for making sure that the door is closed during examinations.

Equipment, instruments, and supplies used for patient examination should be cleaned accordingly and prepared, ready for use by the physician. Equipment and instruments must be checked on a regular basis for proper working condition. This protects the patient from harm due to faulty equipment and also protects the physician and the medical assistant.

The equipment, instruments, and supplies needed for the physical examination vary according to the physician's preference, method, and specialty (Fig. 3-6). The medical assistant is responsible for knowing how to operate and care for each piece of equipment and each instrument. The manufacturer includes an instruction manual, which should be read carefully and thoroughly.

The following is a list of articles, along with their uses, that may be employed during the physical examination:

Patient examination gown	A gown made of cloth or disposable paper and used to provide patient modesty, comfort, and warmth
Drapes	Drapes are made of cloth or disposable paper and are used to reduce patient exposure
Sphygmomanometer	An instrument used to measure blood pressure
Stethoscope	An instrument used to measure blood pressure and to auscultate various parts of the body such as the heart and lungs

Thermometer	An instrument used to measure body temperature
Balance-beam scale	A device used to measure weight and height
Tape measure	A device used to measure a part of the body such as the circumference of the head
Otoscope	A lighted instrument with a lens, used to examine the external ear canal and tympanic membrane
Tuning fork	A small metal instrument consisting of a stem and two prongs, used to test hearing acuity
Ophthalmoscope	A lighted instrument with a lens, for examining the interior of the eye
Tonometer	An instrument for measuring pressure within the eye
Tongue blade	A flat wooden blade used to examine the patient's mouth and pharynx
Percussion hammer	A hammer with a rubber head, used for testing reflexes
Speculum	An instrument used for opening a body orifice or cavity for viewing (e.g., an ear speculum or a vaginal speculum)
Clean gloves	Used by the physician to examine the rectum and vagina
Lubricant	An agent that is applied to the physician's gloved hand or to a speculum that reduces friction between parts and provides for easier insertion
Specimen bottle	Container in which a body specimen is placed for transport to the laboratory
Tissues	Used for wiping instruments such as a thermometer and for wiping body secretions
Cotton-tipped applicator	A small piece of cotton wrapped around the end of a slender wooden stick, for the collection of a specimen from the body
Gooseneck lamp	A light mounted on a flexible movable stand used to focus light on an area for good visibility
Penlight flashlight	A small flashlight used to provide better visibility of the mouth and pharynx and to check pupillary reflexes
Kidney basin	A kidney-shaped container in which used instruments are deposited
Waste container	A container used for depositing soiled disposable articles

Preparation of the Patient

After the physician completes the health history, the medical assistant prepares the patient for the physical examination. At this time, the medical assistant generally takes vital signs and measurements of weight and height. The physician may also request that the medical assistant perform a visual acuity test. The results of these routine procedures are recorded in the patient's chart, usually on a preprinted form (Fig. 3–2*F*).

The medical assistant first explains the purpose of the examination and offers to answer any questions. Patient apprehension and embarrassment can be reduced by addressing the patient by name, by adopting a friendly and supportive attitude, and by speaking clearly, distinctly, and slowly. This also facilitates the examination.

The patient should be asked if he or she needs to empty the bladder before the examination. An empty bladder makes the examination easier and is more comfortable for the patient. If a urine specimen is needed, the patient is requested to void.

Instructions to the patient should be specific, so that he or she understands what items of clothing to remove and where to place the clothing. The disrobing facility should be comfortable and provide privacy. It is helpful to have hooks or hangers for patients' clothing. Instructions for putting on the examination gown and for locating the gown opening help to reduce patient confusion. If the medical assistant senses that the patient will have trouble undressing, assistance should be offered.

The medical assistant is responsible for making the patient's chart available for review and use by the physician. It is suggested that the chart be placed outside the examining room; the chart contains medical terms, which, if seen by the patient, could cause confusion and apprehension. The physician will explain the contents of the chart, using terms that the patient can understand.

The physical examination is performed with the patient positioned on an examination table, which is specially constructed to facilitate the examination. For safety purposes, it is advisable to help the patient on and off the table, using the foot stool.

The collection and testing of specimens is discussed in later chapters.

The Physical Examination

There are four methods used to gather information during the examination: inspection, palpation, percussion, and auscultation.

Inspection involves observation of the patient for any signs of disease. The patient's color, speech, deformities, skin condition (rashes, scars, warts), body contours, orientation to the surroundings, body movements, and anxiety level all can supply clues to his or her condition. The medical assistant should develop a high level of observational skills to assist the physician in noting any significant physical characteristics.

Palpation involves the physician feeling with the fingers or hands to determine the placement and size of organs, the presence of any lumps, or the existence of pain, swelling, or tenderness. Examining the breasts and taking the pulse are performed by palpation. Palpation often helps to verify data obtained during inspection.

Percussion involves tapping the patient with the fingers and listening to the sounds produced to determine the size, density, and location of underlying organs. This method is often used to examine the chest, back, and abdomen.

Auscultation is listening to the sounds of the body with the aid of a stethoscope. This method is used when listening to the heart and lungs or when taking blood pressure.

The patient is usually in a sitting position on the examination table when the physician enters the examining room. This makes it convenient for the physician to begin with an examination of the hands and arms. The patient is next instructed to assume the horizontal recumbent position. The physician examines the patient's head and proceeds systematically toward the feet, which facilitates the examination process and requires the fewest number of position changes by the patient. The results of the physical examination are recorded by the physician in the patient's chart. Figure 3–7 is an example of a preprinted form used for this purpose.

Data Base System PHYSICAL EXAMINATION

INSTRUCTIONS:
(WNL) Within Normal Limits
(POS) Positive findings (X) Omitted

1. GENERAL
a. Posture ____
b. Gait ____
c. Speech ____
d. Appearance ____
e. Emotion ____

2. HEAD
a. Hair ____
b. Masses ____
c. Shape ____
d. Bruits ____
e. Tenderness ____
f. Sinus ____
g. Articulations ____

3. EYES
a. Lids R ___ L ___
b. Sclera R ___ L ___
c. Conjunctiva R ___ L ___
d. Muscles R ___ L ___
e. Cornea R ___ L ___
f. Pupils R ___ L ___
g. Fundi R ___ L ___
h. Light R ___ L ___
i. Bruit R ___ L ___
j. Accommodation R ___ L ___

4. EARS
a. Pinna R ___ L ___
b. Canal R ___ L ___
c. Drum R ___ L ___
d. Weber ____
e. Rinne ____

5. NOSE
a. Septum ____
b. Mucosa R ___ L ___
c. Obstruction ____

6. MOUTH/THROAT
a. Lips ____
b. Breath ____
c. Tongue ____
d. Pharynx ____
e. Tonsils ____
f. Teeth ____
g. Dentures ____
h. Caries ____
i. Larynx ____
j. Floor ____

7. NECK
a. Thyroid ____
b. Trachea ____
c. Veins ____
d. Nodes R ___ L ___
e. Bruits R ___ L ___
f. Carotid R ___ L ___

8. LUNGS
a. Chest ____
b. Symmetry ____
c. Diaphragm ____
d. Rubs ____
e. Bruit ____
f. Sounds ____
g. Fremitus ____

9. HEART
a. PMI ____
b. Rate ____
c. Rhythm ____
d. Thrill ____
e. Rub ____
f. Murmur ____
g. Palpation ____

10. BREASTS
a. Nodes R ___ L ___
b. Nipple R ___ L ___
c. Areolar R ___ L ___
d. Symmetry ____
e. Discharge ____

11. ABDOMEN
a. Sounds ____
b. Masses ____
c. Tenderness ____
d. Organs ____
e. Hernia R ___ L ___
f. Bruit R ___ L ___
g. Femoral R ___ L ___
h. Ing. Nodes R ___ L ___

12. MUSCULOSKELETAL
a. Cervical ____
b. Thoracic ____
c. Lumbar ____
d. Sacral ____
e. Pelvic ____
f. Rib Cage ____

13. FEMALE GENITALS
a. Labia ____
b. Bartholin gland ____
c. Urethra ____
d. Vagina ____
e. Cervix ____
f. Uterus ____
g. Adnexa R ___ L ___
h. Pap smear done ____

14. MALE GENITALS
a. Penis ____
b. Scrotum ____
c. Testicles ____
d. Discharge ____
e. Scars ____
f. Meatus ____
g. Epididymis ____

15. RECTAL
a. Masses ____
b. Anus ____
c. Sphincter ____
d. Prostate ____
e. Pilonidal ____
f. Fissure ____
g. Hemorrhoids ____
h. Sigmoid ____ ___cm.
i. Mucosa ____
j. Other ____

16. SKIN
a. Scars ____
b. Marks ____
c. Texture ____
d. Sweat ____
e. Color ____
f. Ulcers ____

17. NEUROLOGICAL

	Strength*	Reflex**
a. Biceps	R ___ L ___	R ___ L ___
b. Triceps	R ___ L ___	R ___ L ___
c. Knee	R ___ L ___	R ___ L ___
d. Ankle	R ___ L ___	R ___ L ___

e. Romberg ____
f. Babinsky ____
g. Cranial N ____
h. Sensory ____
i. Coordination ____
j. Tremor ____
k. Vibratory ____

*When testing strength use grades: Weak (W); Normal (N); Strong (S)
**When testing reflexes use: Absent (A); Present (P); Brisk (B)

18. EXTREMITIES
a. Range of Motion
Shoulder ____ Knee ____
Elbow ____ Ankle ____
Wrist ____ Hand ____
Hip ____ Foot ____
Phalanges ____

b. General	UR ___	UL ___	LR ___	LL ___
c. Muscular	UR ___	UL ___	LR ___	LL ___
d. Bruits	UR ___	UL ___	LR ___	LL ___
e. Edema	UR ___	UL ___	LR ___	LL ___
f. Varicosities	UR ___	UL ___	LR ___	LL ___

Signature ____

FIGURE 3-7. An example of a preprinted form for recording results of the physical examination.

An outline of the specific examinations included in a complete physical examination is presented below.

I. Examination of the arms and hands
- A. Inspection of the hands for general appearance
- B. Inspection of the fingernails
- C. Inspection of the skin condition of the arms
- D. Palpation of the forearm and upper arm for tenderness and lumps

II. Examination of the head and neck
- A. Inspection of the size and shape of the head
- B. Inspection of the hair and scalp
- C. Palpation of the head and neck for lumps or swelling
- D. Palpation of the trachea

III. Examination of the eyes, ears, and nose
- **A. Eyes**
  1. Inspection of the eyelids and eyeballs
  2. Inspection of the conjunctiva for irritation
  3. Inspection of eye movements
  4. Test for pupillary reaction by shining a light into each pupil
  5. Inspection of the retina using an ophthalmoscope
  6. Test for measuring pressure within the eye, using a tonometer
- **B. Ears**
  1. Inspection of the size and shape of the ears
  2. Inspection of the external ear canal and tympanic membrane, using an otoscope
  3. Test for hearing, using a tuning fork or audiometer
- **C. Nose**
  1. Inspection for patency or signs of irritation, using a nasal speculum
  2. Test for the sense of smell

IV. Examination of the lips, mouth, and throat
- A. Inspection of the lips for color, moisture, lumps, and cracking
- B. Inspection of the mouth, gums, teeth, tongue, and pharynx

V. Examination of the chest
- **A. Chest and lungs**
  1. Inspection of the size and shape of the chest
  2. Inspection of the respiratory movements
  3. Percussion of the chest sounds
  4. Auscultation of the lungs, while the patient breathes through the mouth, to listen to breath sounds
  5. Palpation of the ribs for tenderness
- **B. Breasts (female patient)**
  1. Inspection for redness or inflammation
  2. Inspection of the nipple for bleeding, discharge, or inversion
  3. Palpation of the breasts for lumps
  4. Palpation of axillary lymph nodes for lumps
- **C. Heart**
  1. Inspection, palpation, and percussion of the area over the heart
  2. Auscultation of heart sounds
  3. Electrocardiogram to assess heart function

VI. Examination of the abdomen
- A. Inspection for contour, symmetry, skin condition, and nutritional state
- B. Auscultation for bowel sounds
- C. Percussion to assess underlying organs
- D. Palpation for underlying organs, tenderness, and lumps

VII. Examination of the genitalia and rectum

A. Male patient

1. Observation of the penis and urethra for ulceration or discharge
2. Observation of the scrotum and palpation of the testes for lumps or tenderness
3. Palpation of the rectum and prostate gland for lumps or tenderness
4. Stool specimen to test for occult blood

B. Female patient

1. Inspection of the external genitalia for ulceration or redness
2. Inspection of the vagina and cervix using a vaginal speculum to detect color, lacerations, tenderness, and discharge
3. Specimen collection from the vagina and cervix for the Papanicolaou test
4. Bimanual pelvic examination to palpate the uterus and ovaries to assess for size, shape, tenderness, and lumps
5. Palpation of the rectum for lumps or tenderness
6. Stool specimen to test for occult blood

VIII. Examination of the lower extremities

A. Inspection of the conditions of the skin
B. Palpation of the leg muscles
C. Inspection for tenderness or lumps
D. Inspection of the toenails

IX. Neurologic examination

A. Determination of the sense of pain and touch
B. Use of a percussion hammer to test reflexes
C. Observation of the patient for incoordination, tremors, or speech defects

PROCEDURE 3-2

ASSISTING WITH THE PHYSICAL EXAMINATION

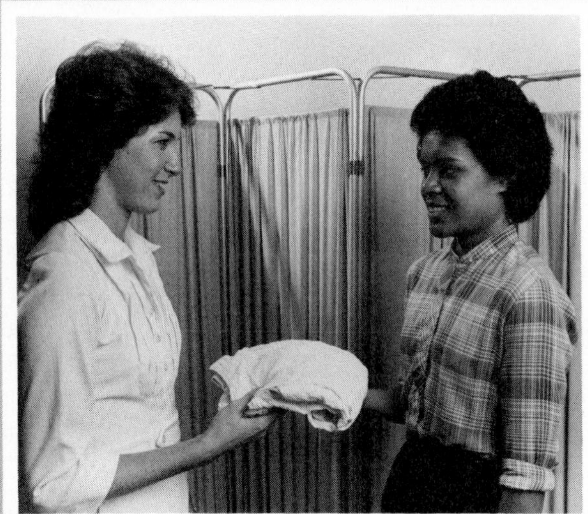

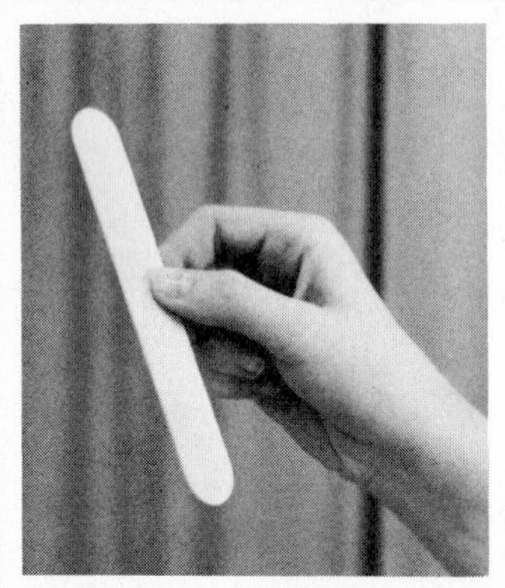

1. Prepare the examining room. Make sure the room is clean, free of clutter, and well lit, and the room temperature is comfortable for the patient. Unroll a fresh length of paper on the examining table, and check to make sure there is an ample supply of clean gowns and drapes.

2. Wash the hands.

3. Assemble the **equipment according to physician preference and the type of examination to be performed.** Arrange the instruments and supplies in a neat and orderly manner on a table or tray. Do not allow one article to lie on top of another.

4. Identify the patient and explain the procedure.

5. Measure the vital signs and record them accurately.

6. Measure visual acuity and record results.

7. Measure the weight and height, and record the results.

8. Instruct and prepare the patient for the examination. Include having the patient void, collecting urine specimen (if required), and instructing the patient on disrobing and putting on the examination gown.

9. Check to make sure everything is prepared for the physical examination, inform the physician that the patient is ready, and make the chart available to the physician.

10. Assist the physician with the examination of the body systems. The patient is generally placed in a sitting position for examination of the eyes, ears, nose, and throat. Assist the physician by handing the ophthalmoscope, otoscope, and tongue blade. Dim the lights when the physician is ready to use the ophthalmoscope. The dim light will help to dilate the patient's pupils, thus providing the physician with better visualization of the interior of the eye. The tongue blade should be transferred by holding it at the center to prevent contact with the patient's secretions, which may contain pathogens. Offer reassurance to the patient to help reduce apprehension.

11. Position the patient as required for examination of the remaining body systems. The medical assistant should be able to place and drape the patient in the proper position for examination of a particular part of the body.

12. Wash the hands.

13. Record results as necessary and as indicated by the physician. Proper charting techniques provide for a complete patient record.

14. Assist and instruct the patient. Assist the patient off the examining table to prevent falls. Elderly patients frequently become dizzy after being positioned on the examining table. Give the patient instructions on dressing and on further discussion with the physician regarding prescriptions, medication, and a return visit. Instructions given by the medical assistant involving medical care should be explained in terms the patient can understand. In most cases, the use of medical terms should be avoided. Chart any instructions given to the patient in his or her medical record.

15. Clean the examining room in preparation for the next patient.

Study Questions

1. What are the three components of a complete patient examination?
2. What is the function of the medical record?
3. What is the difference between a subjective symptom and an objective symptom?
4. What are the four methods used in examining the patient?

4

THE EYE AND EAR

CHAPTER OUTLINE

THE EYE
- **Structure of the Eye**
- **Visual Acuity**
- **Assessment of Color Vision**
- **Eye Irrigation**
- **Eye Instillation**

THE EAR
- **Structure of the Ear**
- **Ear Instillation**
- **Ear Irrigation**

INTRODUCTION

The medical assistant is responsible for performing a variety of procedures involving the eye and the ear. An understanding of the structure and function of the eye and the ear is essential in mastering skill in these areas.

A distance and near visual acuity test is usually included as part of the routine physical examination. This test is used as a screening device to detect deficiencies in vision.

The medical assistant may be responsible for testing color vision with the use of specially prepared colored plates. As a result of this testing, color blindness can be detected. Color blindness is an inability to distinguish certain colors; the most common confusion is between the colors red and green. This is particularly significant if the patient is involved in activities or employment that relies upon the ability to distinguish colors, such as interior decorating, flying a plane, and art.

Hearing tests may also be included as part of the routine physical examination. During contact with the patient, the medical assistant should be alert to any signs that may indicate the patient is having difficulty hearing what is being said. A watch held next to the patient's ear can be used as a screening test for hearing acuity. The use of tuning forks or an audiometer provides for a more accurate determination of hearing acuity. An ***audiometer*** is an instrument that emits sound waves at various frequencies. The patient is instructed to indicate when a sound at a given frequency can be heard.

Performing or teaching the patient to perform eye and ear irrigations and instillations is a frequent responsibility of the medical assistant. ***Irrigation*** is washing a body canal with a flowing solution. ***Instillation*** is dropping a liquid into a body cavity. Eye and ear irrigations and instillations should be performed, using the important principles of medical asepsis outlined in Chapter 1.

GENERAL OBJECTIVES

After completing this chapter, you should be able to do the following:

1. List four tests or procedures that are performed on the eye and ear in the medical office.
2. Define the terms irrigation and instillation.

• VOCABULARY •

canthus (kan' thus)—The junction of the eyelids at either corner of the eye.
hyperopia (hi" per-o' pe-ah)—Farsightedness.
instillation (in" stĭ-la-shun)—The dropping of a liquid into a body cavity.
irrigation (ir" ĭ-ga' shun)—The washing of a body canal by a flowing solution.
myopia (mi-o' pe-ah)—Nearsightedness.
ophthalmologist (of" thal-mol' o-jist)—A medical doctor who specializes in diagnosing and treating disorders of the eye.
optician (op-tish' an)—A professional who grinds lenses and places them in frames.
optometrist (op-tom' ĕ-trist)—A licensed practitioner who is skilled in measuring visual acuity and is qualified to prescribe corrective lenses.
presbyopia (pres" be-o' pe-ah)—A decrease in the elasticity of the lens due to aging, resulting in a decreased ability to focus on close objects.
refraction (re-frak' shun)—The deflection or bending of light rays by a lens.

COMPETENCIES

After completing this unit, you should be able to demonstrate the proper procedure to perform the following:

1. Measure distance visual acuity, and record the results.
2. Measure near visual acuity, and record the results.
3. Assess color vision, and record the results.
4. Perform an eye irrigation, and record the procedure.
5. Perform an eye instillation, and record the procedure.

LEARNING OBJECTIVES

After completing this unit, you should be able to do the following:

1. Define the terms listed in the vocabulary.
2. Identify the structures that constitute the eye, and explain the function of each.
3. Define visual acuity.
4. State the causes of myopia, hyperopia, and presbyopia, and indicate what visual difficulty is present with each.
5. Explain the difference between an ophthalmologist, an optometrist, and an optician.
6. Explain the significance of the top and bottom numbers next to each line of letters on the Snellen eye chart.
7. Explain the difference between congenital and acquired color vision defects.
8. State three reasons for performing an eye irrigation and an eye instillation.
9. Explain the principles underlying the steps in each eye procedure.

The Eye

Structure of the Eye

Three different layers make up the eye (Fig. 4–1). The outer layer is the *sclera,* which is composed of tough, white, fibrous connective tissue. The front part of the sclera is modified to form a transparent covering over the colored part of the eye; this covering is known as the *cornea.*

The middle layer of the eye is the *choroid.* It is composed of many blood vessels and is highly pigmented. The blood vessels nourish the other layers of the eye, whereas the pigment works to absorb stray light rays.The front part of the choroid is specialized into the ciliary body, the suspensory ligaments, and the iris. The *ciliary body* contains muscles that control the shape of the lens. The function of the *suspensory ligaments* is to suspend the lens in place. The *lens* itself is responsible for focusing the light rays on the retina. The colored part of the eye is the *iris,* which controls the size of the pupil. The *pupil* is the opening in the eye that permits the entrance of light rays.

The third and innermost layer of the eye is the *retina.* Light rays come to a focus on the retina and are subsequently transmitted to the brain, by way of the optic nerve, to be interpreted.

The *anterior chamber* is the area between the cornea and iris, and the *posterior chamber* is the area between the iris and lens. Both chambers are filled with a substance known as the *aqueous humor.* Between the lens and the retina is a transparent jelly-like material filling the eyeball, known as the *vitreous humor.* Its function is to help maintain the shape of the eyeball.

The *conjunctiva* is a membrane that lines the eyelids and covers the front of the eye, except for the cornea. The conjunctiva covering the sclera is transparent, except for some capillaries, which allows the white sclera to show through.

Visual Acuity

Visual acuity refers to acuteness or sharpness of vision. A person with normal visual acuity can see clearly and is able to distinguish fine details both close up and at some distance.

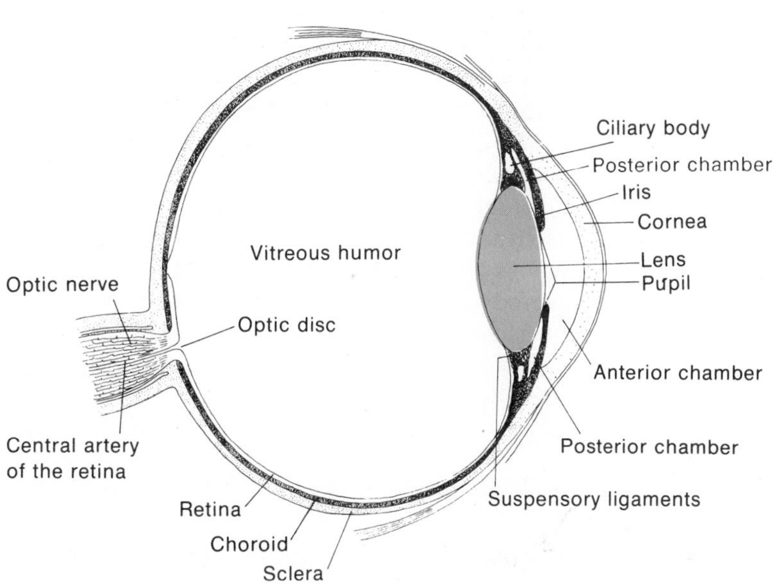

FIGURE 4–1. The internal structure of the eye.

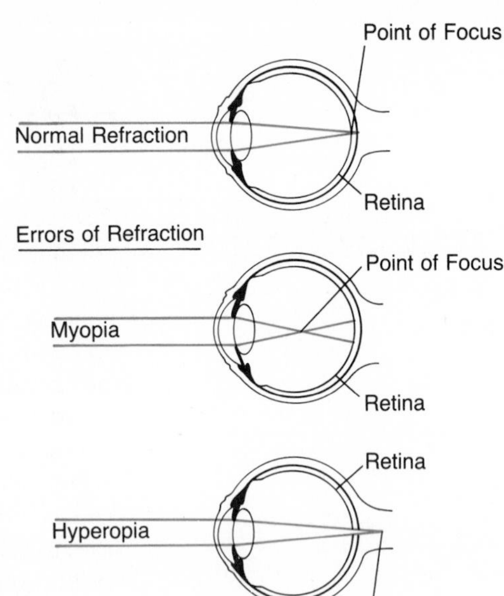

FIGURE 4-2. Diagram of normal refraction as compared with myopia (nearsightedness) and hyperopia (farsightedness), which are errors of refraction that cause visual defects.

Errors of refraction are the most common causes of defects in visual acuity. *Refraction* refers to the ability of the eye to bend the parallel light rays coming into it so they can be focused on the retina. An error of refraction means that the light rays are not being refracted or bent properly and therefore are not adequately focused on the retina. A defect in the shape of the eyeball can cause a refractive error. Errors of refraction can be improved with the use of corrective lenses.

A person who is nearsighted has a condition termed *myopia.* The eyeball is too long from front to back, causing the light rays to be brought to a focus in front of the retina. The myopic person has difficulty seeing objects at a distance and may squint and have headaches as a result of eye strain (Fig. 4-2). A concave lens is used to correct this condition by causing the light rays to come to a focus on the retina.

A person who is farsighted has a condition known as *hyperopia.* The eyeball is too short from front to back, resulting in a different type of refractive error, in which the light rays are brought to a focus behind the retina. This person has difficulty viewing objects at a reading or working distance (Fig. 4-2). A convex lens is used to correct this condition by causing the light rays to come to a focus on the retina.

In most people, a decrease in the elasticity of the lens of the eye begins to occur after age 40. This condition is known as *presbyopia,* and it results in a decreased ability to focus clearly on objects close up.

There are several types of professionals involved in the care of the eyes. An *ophthalmologist* is a medical doctor who specializes in diagnosing and treating disorders of the eye. An ophthalmologist is qualified to prescribe drugs and corrective lenses and to perform eye surgery. An *optometrist* is a licensed practitioner who is skilled in measuring visual acuity. The optometrist is qualified to prescribe corrective lenses for the treatment of refractive errors. This professional is not a physician and therefore is not permitted to diagnose or treat other eye disorders or to perform eye surgery. An *optician* is a professional who grinds lenses and places them in frames.

Measuring Distance Visual Acuity

Myopia can be diagnosed (in combination with other tests) by a distance visual acuity test. In the medical office, the Snellen eye chart is most often used. There are two types of charts (Figs. 4-3 and 4-4): one type, used for school-aged

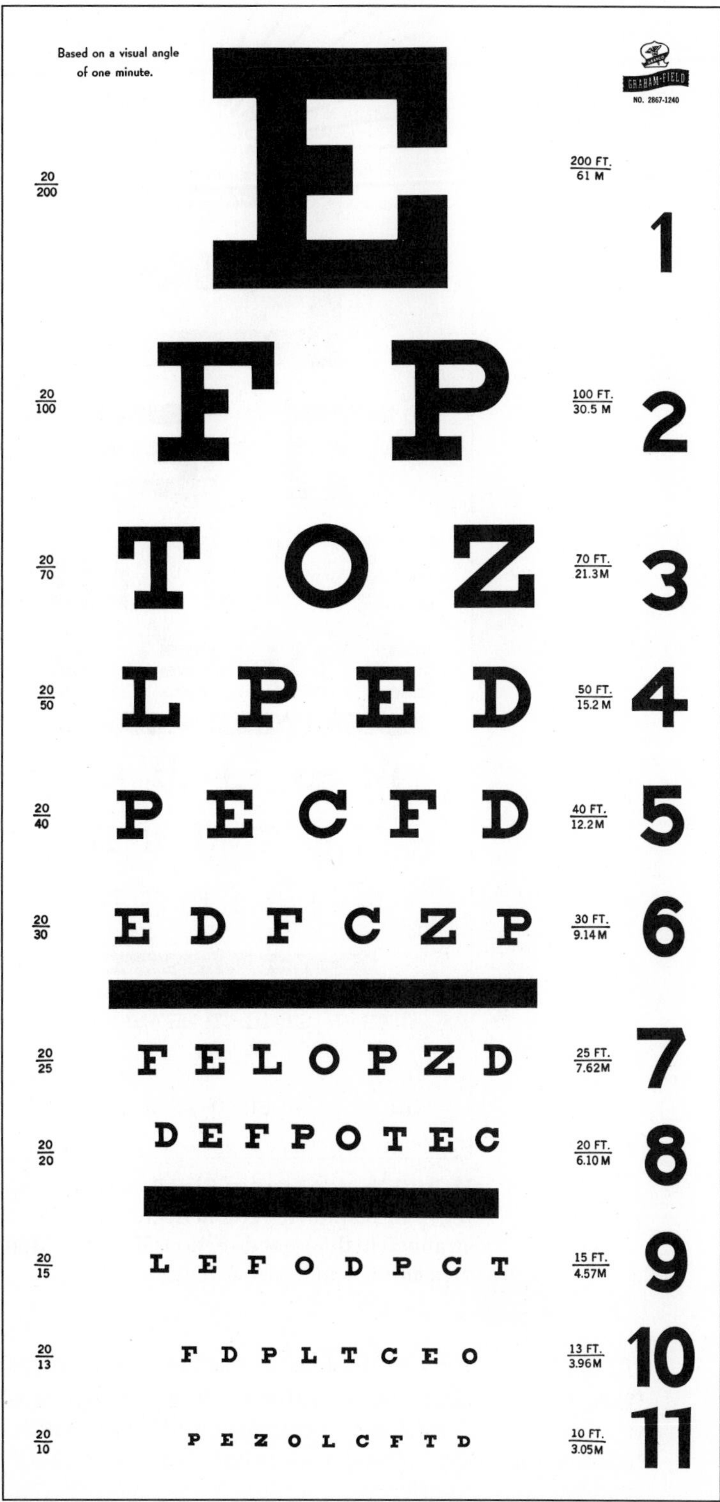

FIGURE 4–3. A Snellen eye chart consisting of letters in decreasing sizes, which is used to measure distance visual acuity.

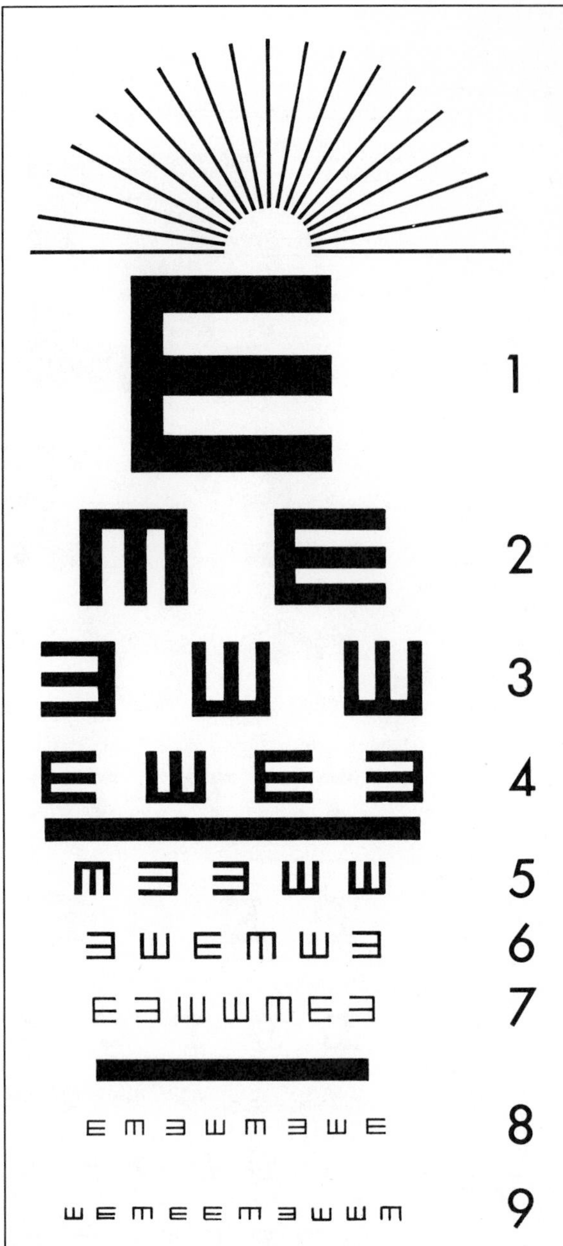

FIGURE 4–4. A Snellen Big E eye chart consisting of the capital letter E in decreasing sizes and arranged in different directions, which is used to measure distance visual acuity.

children and adults, consists of a chart of letters in decreasing sizes. The other type, used for preschool children, non–English-speaking people, and nonreaders, is composed of the capital letter E in decreasing sizes and arranged in different directions. Visual acuity charts with pictures of common objects are also available for use with preschoolers. These charts tend to be less accurate than the Snellen charts. Some children are unable to identify the objects because of lack of recognition rather than a defect in visual acuity. It is suggested that the Snellen Big E chart be used with preschoolers.

Snellen eye charts are available with the letters printed on a cardboard poster or as a self-illuminating unit mounted on a portable stand. The latter has the advantage of being easier to adjust to each patient's eye level.

The visual acuity test should be performed in a well-lit room, free from distractions. The test is usually performed at a distance of 20 feet; this can be conveniently marked off in the medical office with paint or a piece of tape so that it does not have to be remeasured each time the test is given.

At the side of each row of letters on the chart are two numbers, separated by a line. The number above the line represents the distance (in feet) at which the test is conducted. It is usually 20, as most eye tests are conducted at this distance. The number below the line represents the distance from which a person with normal visual acuity can read the row of letters. The line marked 20/20 indicates normal distance visual acuity, or 20/20 vision. This means a person could read what he or she was supposed to read at a distance of 20 feet.

A visual acuity reading of 20/30 means this was the smallest line that the individual could read at a distance of 20 feet. People with normal acuity would be able to read this line at a distance of 30 feet.

A visual acuity reading of 20/15 means this was the smallest line that the individual could read at a distance of 20 feet. It indicates above-average acuity for distance vision. People with normal acuity would be able to read this line at 15 feet.

The acuity should be measured in each eye separately, traditionally beginning with the right eye. Most physicians prefer that the patient keep contact lenses or glasses on during the test, except for reading glasses; the medical assistant should record in the patient's chart the type of corrective lenses worn by the patient during the test. An opaque object such as a paper cup or eye occluder should be held over the eye not being tested. The patient's hands should not be used to cover the eye, as this may encourage peeking through the fingers, especially in the case of children. The patient should be instructed to leave open the eye not being tested, since closing it causes squinting of the eye that is being tested.

PROCEDURE 4-1

MEASURING DISTANCE VISUAL ACUITY

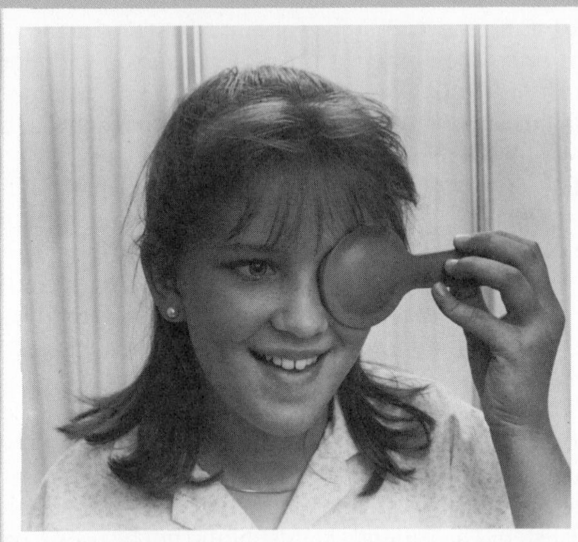

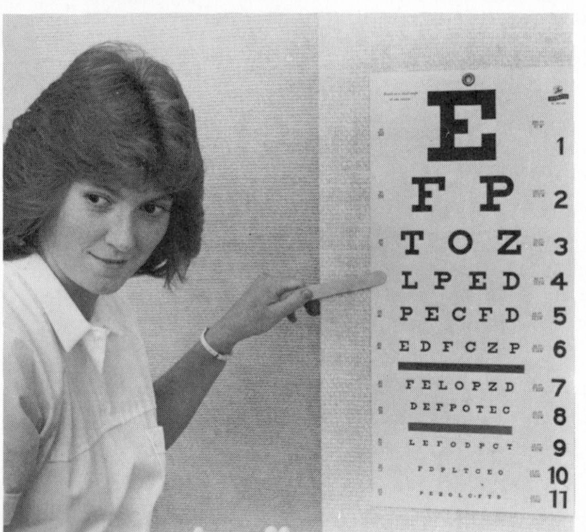

1. **PROCEDURAL STEP.** Wash the hands.

2. **PROCEDURAL STEP.** Assemble the equipment. The equipment needed includes a **Snellen eye chart** and **a paper cup or an eye occluder.** An occluder may be desired to expose one line of the chart at a time.

3. **PROCEDURAL STEP.** Identify the patient and explain the procedure. The patient should be told that he or she will be asked to read several lines of letters. The patient should not have an opportunity to study or memorize the letters before beginning the test. The patient should be instructed not to squint during the test, as squinting temporarily improves vision.

4. **PROCEDURAL STEP.** Place the patient in a comfortable position 20 feet from the chart. The patient may sit or stand. (It is helpful to have the distance permanently marked off to prevent having to measure each time the test is performed.)

5. **PROCEDURAL STEP.** Position the center of the Snellen chart at the patient's eye level. The medical assistant stands next to the chart during the test to indicate to the patient the line to be identified.
PRINCIPLE. Make sure the chart is at the patient's eye level rather than your eye level, to provide the most accurate results.

6. **PROCEDURAL STEP.** Ask the patient to cover the left eye with the paper cup or occluder. Instruct the patient to keep the left eye open. During the test, the medical assistant should check to make sure the patient is keeping the left eye open.
PRINCIPLE. Keeping the left eye open prevents squinting of the right eye.

7. **PROCEDURAL STEP.** Measure the visual acuity of the right eye first. Ask the patient to orally identify one line at a time on the Snellen chart, starting with the 20/70 line (or a line that is several lines above the 20/20 line). An occluder can be used to expose only the line to be identified.
PRINCIPLE. It is best to start at a line that is above the 20/20 line to give the patient a chance to gain confidence and to become familiar with the test procedure. The medical assistant should establish a pattern of beginning with the same eye each time the test is performed (traditionally the right eye). This helps to reduce errors during the recording of results.

8. **PROCEDURAL STEP.** If the patient is able to read the 20/70 line, proceed down the chart until the smallest line of letters the patient can read is reached. If the patient is unable to read the 20/70 line, proceed up the chart until the smallest line of letters the patient can read is reached.

9. **PROCEDURAL STEP.** Observe the patient for any unusual symptoms while he or she is reading the letters, such as squinting, tilting of the head, or watering of the eyes.

PRINCIPLE. These symptoms may indicate that the patient is having difficulty identifying the letters.

10. **PROCEDURAL STEP.** Ask the patient to cover the right eye with a paper cup or occluder and to keep the right eye open. Measure the visual acuity in the left eye as described in Steps 7 and 8.

During the test the medical assistant should check to make sure the patient is keeping the right eye open.

PRINCIPLE. Keeping the right eye open prevents squinting of the left eye.

11. **PROCEDURAL STEP.** Record the results. Observe the numbers to the side of the smallest line of letters that the patient was able to read. If one or two letters were missed, the visual acuity is recorded with a minus sign next to the bottom number, along with the number of letters missed. Latin abbreviations are used to record the visual acuity in each eye. The abbreviation for the right eye is OD (oculus dexter) and the abbreviation for the left eye is OS (oculus sinister). For example, if a patient reads the line marked 20/20 with the right eye and misses one letter, the visual acuity would be recorded as follows: OD 20/20 – 1. If the patient wears corrective lenses, record this information in the patient's chart.

Record any unusual symptoms that the patient may have exhibited during the test. Include the patient's name, the date and time, and your initials next to the recording.

Record data below.

DATE	TIME	PATIENT'S NAME	RESULTS OF VISUAL ACUITY TESTING

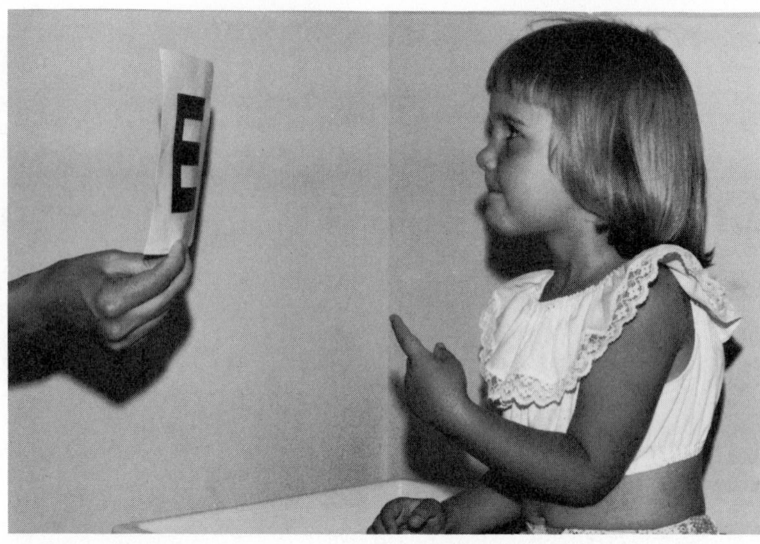

FIGURE 4-5. Teaching a preschooler to point in the direction of the open part of the capital letter E.

Measuring Distance Visual Acuity in Preschoolers

With minor variations, Procedure 4-1: Measuring Distance Visual Acuity can be used to test distance visual acuity in preschoolers. The Snellen Big E chart is utilized for this purpose.

A child needs a complete and thorough explanation of what is expected of him or her before beginning the test. Tell the child you will be playing a pointing game. Do not force the child to play the game, because the results would then tend to be inaccurate. Draw the capital letter E on an index card, and teach the child to point in the direction of the open part of the E by turning the card in different directions (up, down, to the right, and to the left). Using such phrases as the "fingers" or the "legs of the table" to describe the open part of the E helps the child understand what is expected (Fig. 4-5). Allow the child to practice the pointing game with the index card until you are sure this level of skill has been mastered. Be sure to praise the child when the correct response is given.

The child may need help in holding the paper cup or occluder in place. The aid of another person would then be required.

Measuring Near Visual Acuity

Near visual acuity testing assesses a patient's ability to read objects close up (i.e., at a reading or working distance); the test results are used to detect patients with hyperopia or presbyopia.

The test is conducted with a card similar to the Snellen eye chart, except for the size of the type, which ranges from the size of newspaper headlines down to considerably smaller print such as would be found in a telephone directory (Fig. 4-6). The test card is available in a variety of forms such as printed paragraphs, printed words, pictures, and Es.

The test should be performed in a well-lit room free from distractions. It is conducted with the patient holding the test card at a distance between 14 and 16 inches. The acuity should be measured in each eye separately, traditionally beginning with the right eye. The eye not being tested should be kept closed. If the patient wears reading glasses, they should be worn during the test.

No. 1.
.37M

In the second century of the Christian era, the empire of Rome comprehended the fairest part of the earth, and the most civilized portion of mankind. The frontiers of that extensive monarchy were guarded by ancient renown and disciplined valor. The gentle but powerful influence of laws and manners had gradually cemented the union of the provinces. Their peaceful inhabitants enjoyed and abused the advantages of wealth.

No. 2.
.50M

fourscore years, the public administration was conducted by the virtue and abilities of Nerva, Trajan, Hadrian, and the two Antonines. It is the design of this, and of the two succeeding chapters, to describe the prosperous condition of their empire; and afterwards, from the death of Marcus Antoninus, to deduce the most important circumstances of its decline and fall; a revolution which will ever be remembered, and is still felt by

No. 3.
.62M

the nations of the earth. The principal conquests of the Romans were achieved under the republic; and the emperors, for the most part, were satisfied with preserving those dominions which had been acquired by the policy of the senate, the active emulations of the consuls, and the martial enthusiasm of the people. The seven first centuries were filled with a rapid succession of triumphs; but it was

No. 4.
.75M

reserved for Augustus to relinquish the ambitious design of subduing the whole earth, and to introduce a spirit of moderation into the public councils. Inclined to peace by his temper and situation, it was very easy for him to discover that Rome, in her present exalted situation, had much less to hope than to fear from the chance of arms; and that, in the prosecution of

No. 5.
1.00M

the undertaking became every day more difficult, the event more doubtful, and the possession more precarious, and less beneficial. The experience of Augustus added weight to these salutary reflections, and effectually convinced him that, by the prudent vigor of

No. 6.
1.25M

his counsels, it would be easy to secure every concession which the safety or the dignity of Rome might require from the most formidable barbarians. Instead of exposing his person or his legions to the arrows of the Parthinians, he obtained, by an honor-

No. 7.
1.50M

able treaty, the restitution of the standards and prisoners which had been taken in the defeat of Crassus. His generals, in the early part of his reign, attempted the reduction of Ethiopia and Arabia Felix. They marched near a thou-

No. 8.
1.75M

sand miles to the south of the tropic; but the heat of the climate soon repelled the invaders, and protected the unwarlike natives of those sequestered regions

No. 9.
2.00M

The northern countries of Europe scarcely deserved the expense and labor of conquest. The forests and morasses of Germany were

No. 10.
2.25M

filled with a hardy race of barbarians who despised life when it was separated from freedom; and though, on the first

No. 11.
2.50M

attack, they seemed to yield to the weight of the Roman power, they soon, by a signal

FIGURE 4–6. Example of a near visual acuity card.

The patient is asked to orally identify each line or paragraph of type. During the test, the patient should be observed for any unusual symptoms such as squinting, tilting the head, or watering of the eyes, which may indicate that the patient is having difficulty reading the card. The patient continues until reaching the smallest type that can be read.

The results are recorded as the smallest type that the patient could comfortably read with each eye at the distance at which the card is held (i.e., 14 to 16 inches). The recording will be based upon the type of test card used to conduct the test. For example, one type of card utilizes a recording method similar to that used with the Snellen eye test. For this type of near visual acuity card, the results would be recorded as 14/14 for a patient with normal near visual acuity. This means the patient read what was supposed to be read at a distance of 14 inches. Using the Jaeger system, a recording for a patient with normal visual acuity would be J2. Also included in the recording should be the patient's name, the date and time, corrective lenses worn, any unusual symptoms exhibited by the patient, and the medical assistant's initials.

Assessment of Color Vision

Defects in color vision may be classified as congenital or acquired. Congenital defects are the most common type and refer to a color vision deficiency that is inherited and therefore is present at birth. Congenital color vision deficiencies most often affect males. Acquired defects refer to a color vision deficiency that is acquired after birth, resulting from such factors as an eye injury, disease, or certain drugs. Color vision tests, such as the Ishihara test, detect color vision disturbances of congenital origin and are commonly performed as a screening measure in the medical office.

The Ishihara test for color blindness is a convenient and accurate method used to detect total color blindness and red-green blindness of congenital origin by assessing an individual's ability to perceive primary colors and shades of color. The Ishihara book contains a series of polychromatic plates consisting of primary colored dots arranged to form a numeral against a background of similar dots of contrasting colors (see inside back cover). Patients with normal color vision are able to read the appropriate numeral; however, patients with color vision defects read the dots as either not forming a number at all or as forming a completely different number than the one identified by the individual with normal color vision. The first plate in the book is designed to be read correctly by all individuals (those with normal vision and those exhibiting color vision deficiencies) and should be used to explain the procedure to the patient. Plates are also included in the book with winding colored lines for patients who are unable to read numbers, such as preschoolers and non–English-speaking individuals. The patient is asked to trace the line formed by the colored dots.

The Ishihara test should be conducted in a quiet room illuminated by natural daylight. If this is not possible, a room lit with artificial electric light may be used; however, the light should be adjusted to resemble the effect of natural daylight as much as possible. Using light other than that just described, such as bright sunlight, may change the appearance of the shades of color on the plates, leading to inaccurate test results. The medical assistant is responsible for performing the color vision test and recording results in the patient's chart. The physician will assess the results to determine if the patient has a deficiency in color vision. The Ishihara test consists of 14 color plates. Plates 1 through 11 are used to conduct the basic test, whereas Plates 12, 13, and 14 are used to further assess patients exhibiting a red-green color deficiency. Therefore, it is not necessary to include these plates (12, 13, and 14) in the test for those patients exhibiting normal color vision. In interpreting the results, if 10 or more plates are read normally, the patient's color vision is considered normal. If only 7 (or less than 7) out of the 11 Ishihara plates are read correctly, the patient is identified as having a color vision deficiency. (Note: It would be unusual for the medical assistant to obtain results in which the patient read 8 or 9 plates correctly. The test is structured so that a patient with a color vision defect generally does not read 8 or 9 plates correctly and the rest incorrectly. If this occurs, the patient requires additional assessment of color vision, using other color vision tests.) The procedure for assessing color vision using the Ishihara color plates is outlined on the following pages.

PROCEDURE 4-2
ASSESSING COLOR VISION

1. **PROCEDURAL STEP.** Assemble the equipment. The equipment needed includes the **Ishihara book of color plates.**

2. **PROCEDURAL STEP.** Conduct the test in a quiet room illuminated by natural daylight.
PRINCIPLE. Using unnatural light may change the appearance of the shades of color on the plates, leading to inaccurate test results.

3. **PROCEDURAL STEP.** Identify the patient and explain the procedure. Using the first (practice) plate as an example, the patient should be instructed to identify orally numbers formed by colored dots. The patient should be told that 3 seconds will be given to identify each plate.
PRINCIPLE. The first plate is designed to be read correctly by all individuals and is used to explain the procedure to the patient.

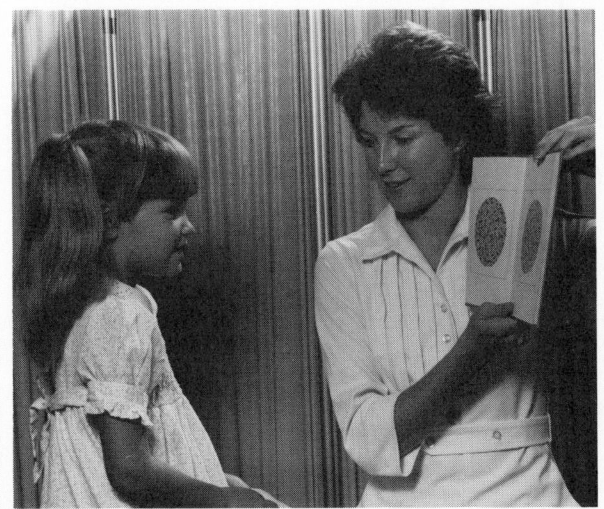

4. **PROCEDURAL STEP.** Hold the first plate 30 inches (75 cm) from the patient. The plate should be held at a right angle to the patient's line of vision. Both eyes should be kept open during the test.

5. **PROCEDURAL STEP.** Ask the patient to identify the number on the plate. Record results after each plate. Continue until the patient has viewed all of the plates.

6. **PROCEDURAL STEP.** Record results as follows: Record the plate identification number and the number indicated by the patient. If the patient is unable to identify a number, the mark X should be recorded to indicate the plate could not be read by the patient. An example is as follows:

Plate 5: 21 (This means the patient read the number 21 on Plate 5.)
Plate 6: X (This means the patient could not identify a number on Plate 6.)

Record any unusual symptoms that the patient may have exhibited during the test, such as squinting or rubbing the eyes. Include the patient's name, the date and time, and your initials next to the recording.

7. **PROCEDURAL STEP.** Return the Ishihara book to its proper place. The book of color plates must be stored in a closed position to protect it from light.
PRINCIPLE. Exposing the plates to excessive and unnecessary light results in fading of the color.

Continued

Record data below.

DATE	TIME	PATIENT'S NAME	RESULTS OF COLOR VISION TESTING

PROCEDURE 4-3
EYE IRRIGATION

Eye irrigations are performed for the following purposes: to cleanse the eye by washing away foreign particles, ocular discharges, or harmful chemicals; to relieve inflammation through the application of heat; or to apply an antiseptic solution.

1. **Procedural step.** Wash the hands.

2. **Procedural step.** Assemble the equipment. The equipment needed includes a **towel, a basin to catch the solution, a rubber bulb syringe, a container to hold the solution, cotton balls,** and the **sterile solution ordered by the physician;** normal saline is generally used to irrigate the eye. Check the irrigating solution carefully with the physician's instructions to make sure you have obtained the correct solution. Check the expiration date of the solution. Check the solution label three times: while removing the solution from the shelf, while pouring the solution, and before returning it to its proper place.
Principle. The solution should be carefully compared with the physician's instructions to prevent an error. If the solution is outdated, consult the physician; it may produce undesirable effects, and the medical assistant could be held responsible.

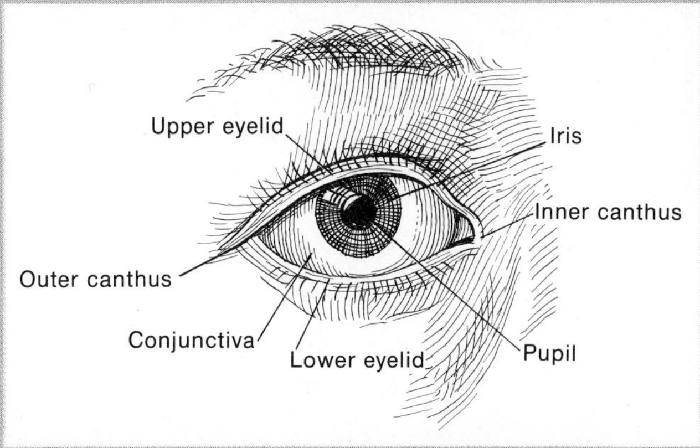

FIGURE 4-7. The external structure of the eye.

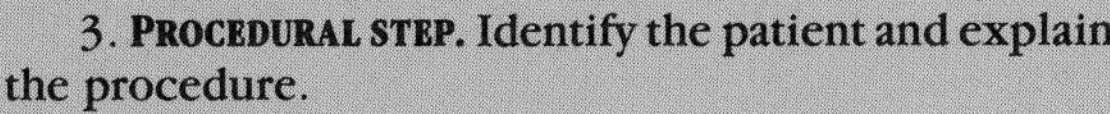

3. **Procedural step.** Identify the patient and explain the procedure.
Principle. Explain the purpose of the irrigation to the patient.

4. **Procedural step.** Position the patient. The patient may be placed in a sitting or lying position with the head turned in the direction of the affected eye. A basin should be positioned tightly against the patient's cheek under the affected eye to catch the irrigating solution. A towel should be placed on the patient's shoulder to protect the patient's clothing. If both eyes are to be irrigated, two separate sets of equipment must be used to prevent cross infection from one eye to the other.
Principle. The patient is positioned so the solution will flow away from the unaffected eye to prevent cross infection.

5. **Procedural step.** Cleanse the eyelids from inner to outer canthus with moistened cotton balls to remove any discharge or debris on the lids. The inner canthus is the inner junction of the eyelids next to the nose. The outer canthus is the junction of the eyelids farthest from the nose (Fig. 4-7). Normal saline or the solution ordered for the irrigation may be used.
Principle. The eyelids should be clean to prevent any foreign particles from entering the eye during the irrigation. Cleansing from inner to outer canthus prevents cross infection.

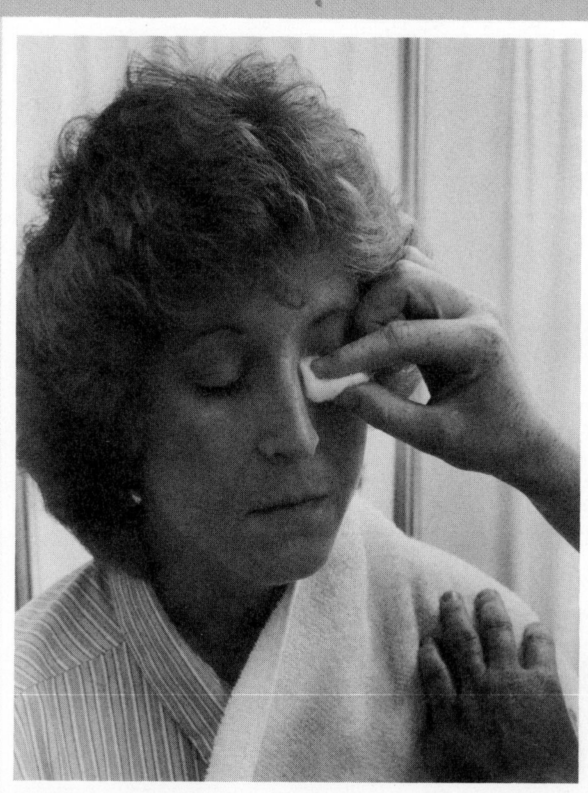

6. **Procedural step.** Fill the irrigating syringe with the solution by squeezing the bulb and slowly releasing it until the desired amount of solution enters the bulb.

Continued

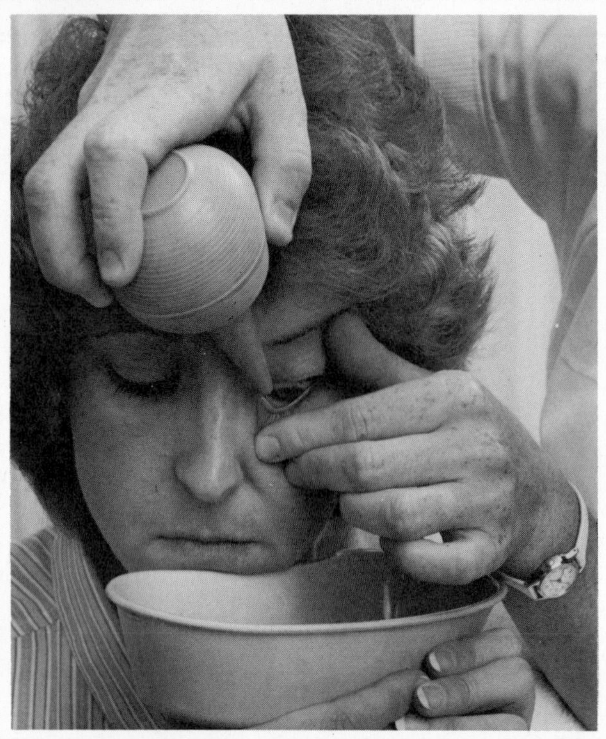

7. **PROCEDURAL STEP.** Separate the eyelids with the index finger and thumb to expose the lower conjunctiva and to hold the upper eyelid open.

PRINCIPLE. The medical assistant must hold the eye open during the procedure, since the patient will have a tendency to want to close it.

8. **PROCEDURAL STEP.** Hold the tip of the syringe approximately 1 inch above the eye. Gently release the solution onto the eye at the inner canthus. This allows the solution to flow over the eye at a moderate rate from the inner to the outer canthus. Direct the solution to the lower conjunctiva. To prevent injury, do not allow the syringe to touch the eye.

PRINCIPLE. The solution flows away from the unaffected eye to prevent cross infection. The cornea is sensitive and can be harmed easily. Therefore, the irrigating solution must be directed to the lower conjunctiva to prevent injury to the cornea.

9. **PROCEDURAL STEP.** Continue irrigating for the prescribed period of time or until the desired results have been obtained.

10. **PROCEDURAL STEP.** Dry the eyelids from inner to outer canthus with a dry cotton ball.

11. **PROCEDURAL STEP.** Wash the hands.

12. **PROCEDURAL STEP.** Record the procedure. Include the following: the patient's name; the date and time; the type, strength, and amount of solution used; which eye was irrigated; and any significant observations such as the presence of injury, discharge, swelling, unusual color, or patient reaction. Use the abbreviations listed in the next column to indicate which eye was irrigated:

OU Both eyes
OD Right eye
OS Left eye

Be sure to include your initials next to the recording.

13. **PROCEDURAL STEP.** Return the equipment.

Record data below.

DATE	TIME	PATIENT'S NAME	RECORDING

Eye Instillation

Eye instillations are performed to treat eye infections (with medication), to soothe an irritated eye, or to dilate the pupil or anesthetize the eye during an eye examination or treatment. Medication to be instilled in the eye may come in a liquid form, as eye (ophthalmic) drops, or as an eye (ophthalmic) ointment. The eye drops may be dispensed in a bottle with an eye dropper (screw-on) or in a flexible plastic container with an attached tip for administering the eye drops. Eye ointment is dispensed in a small metal tube with a very small nozzle for discharging the medication.

PROCEDURE 4-4
EYE INSTILLATION

1. **PROCEDURAL STEP.** Wash the hands.

2. **PROCEDURAL STEP.** Assemble the equipment. The equipment needed includes the eye medication in the form of **eye drops or eye ointment as ordered by the physician,** a **sterile eye dropper** for use with the eye drops (if one is not provided with the eye drops), and **cotton balls or tissues.** Check the medication carefully against the physician's instructions to make sure you have obtained the correct medication. The medication should bear the word *ophthalmic.* Check the expiration date. Check the drug label three times: while removing the medication from the shelf, before withdrawing the medication into the dropper, and before instilling the medication.
   PRINCIPLE. The medication should be carefully compared with the physician's instructions to prevent a drug error. Medication not bearing the word ophthalmic should never be placed in the eye because it could result in an injury to the eye. If the medication is outdated, consult the physician; it may produce undesirable effects, and the medical assistant could be held responsible.

3. **PROCEDURAL STEP.** Identify the patient and explain the procedure.
   PRINCIPLE. Explain the purpose of the instillation to the patient.

4. **PROCEDURAL STEP.** Place the patient in a sitting or supine position.

5. **PROCEDURAL STEP.** Prepare the medication. *Eye Drops:* Withdraw the medication into the dropper. *Eye Ointment:* Remove the cap from the nozzle of the tube.

6. **PROCEDURAL STEP.** Ask the patient to look up, and expose the lower conjunctival sac by using the fingers placed over a tissue. The fingers should be placed on the patient's cheekbone just below the eye, and the skin of the cheek should gently be drawn downward.
   PRINCIPLE. Looking up helps to keep the dropper from touching the cornea. It also helps to keep the patient from moving when the drops are instilled. The tissue is used to protect the fingers and to prevent the fingers from slipping.

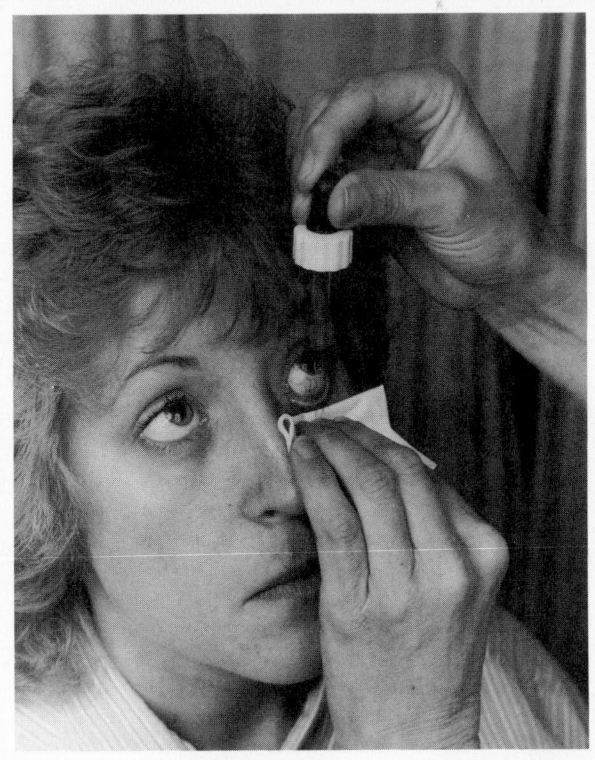

Continued

7. **PROCEDURAL STEP.** Insert the medication. *Eye Drops:* Place the correct number of eye drops in the center of the lower conjunctival sac. The tip of the dropper should be held approximately ½ inch above the sac. *Eye Ointment:* Place a thin ribbon of ointment along the length of the lower conjunctival sac from inner to outer canthus. Be careful not to touch the dropper or the tip of the ointment tube to the eye, because this could cause contamination of the dropper and tube. Discontinue the ribbon by twisting the tube.
PRINCIPLE. The medication must be placed in the conjunctival sac, rather than directly on the eyeball itself, as the medication may harm the cornea.

8. **PROCEDURAL STEP.** Discard any unused solution from the eye dropper. Do not touch the dropper to the outside of the bottle when returning it to the bottle.
PRINCIPLE. Touching the dropper to the outside of the bottle contaminates the dropper. Unused solution should not be returned to the bottle because it will contaminate the medication remaining in the bottle.

9. **PROCEDURAL STEP.** Ask the patient to close his or her eyes gently and move the eyeballs. Tell the patient that the instillation may temporarily blur the vision.
PRINCIPLE. Moving the eyeballs helps to distribute the medication over the entire eye. If the eyes are shut tightly, the drops or ointment is pushed out.

Record data below.

10. **PROCEDURAL STEP.** Dry the eyelid from inner to outer canthus with a dry cotton ball to remove any excess medication.

11. **PROCEDURAL STEP.** Wash the hands.

12. **PROCEDURAL STEP.** Record the procedure. Include the patient's name, the date and time, the type of eye medication, dosage and strength, which eye received the instillation, any observations made by the medical assistant (e.g., small amount of eye discharge present), and the patient's reactions. Include your initials next to the recording.

13. **PROCEDURAL STEP.** Replace the equipment.

DATE	TIME	PATIENT'S NAME	RECORDING

Study Questions

1. What is visual acuity?
2. What visual difficulty is present with each of the following: myopia, hyperopia, and presbyopia?
3. What is the purpose of performing an eye irrigation?
4. What is the purpose of performing an eye instillation?

COMPETENCIES

After completing this unit, you should be able to demonstrate the proper procedure to perform the following:

1. Perform an ear irrigation and record the procedure.
2. Perform an ear instillation and record the procedure.

LEARNING OBJECTIVES

After completing this unit, you should be able to do the following:

1. Define the terms listed in the vocabulary.
2. Identify the structures making up the ear and explain the function of each.
3. List two ways in which hearing acuity may be tested.
4. State three reasons each for performing an ear irrigation and an ear instillation.
5. Explain the principles underlying the steps in each ear procedure.

• VOCABULARY •

audiometer (aw″ de-om′ ĕ-ter)—An instrument used to measure hearing acuity.

cerumen (sĕ-roo′ men)—Ear wax.

impacted (im-pak′ ted)—Being wedged firmly together so as to be immovable.

otoscope (o′ to-skōp)—An instrument for examining the external ear canal and tympanic membrane.

tympanic membrane (tim-pan′ ik mem′ brān)—A thin, semitransparent membrane located between the external ear canal and middle ear that receives and transmits sound waves. Also known as the ear drum.

The Ear

Structure of the Ear

The ear has functions in hearing and in maintaining equilibrium. It consists of three divisions: the *external ear,* the *middle ear,* and the *inner ear.* The structures in the ear are illustrated in Figure 4–8. The functions of the structures in the external ear are discussed in this chapter because of their relationship to the ear procedures. The functions of the structures located in the middle and inner ears are omitted.

The external ear is composed of the auricle (or pinna) and the external auditory canal, also known as the external ear canal. The opening into this canal is the *external auditory meatus.*

The *auricle* is a flap of cartilage covered with skin that projects from the side of the head. Its function is to receive and collect sound waves and to direct them toward the external auditory canal.

The *external auditory canal* is approximately 1½ inches long and extends from the auricle to the tympanic membrane. The canal has an S-shaped curve as it leads inward. During either an examination with the otoscope or an ear instillation or irrigation, the canal must be straightened.

The *tympanic membrane* is at the end of the external auditory canal. It functions in receiving and transmitting sound waves.

Ear Irrigation

Ear irrigations are performed for the following purposes: to cleanse the external auditory canal to remove cerumen, discharge, or a foreign body; to relieve inflammation by applying an antiseptic solution; or to apply heat to the ear. Impacted cerumen must first be softened by instilling warm mineral oil or hydrogen peroxide for 10 to 15 minutes before irrigating.

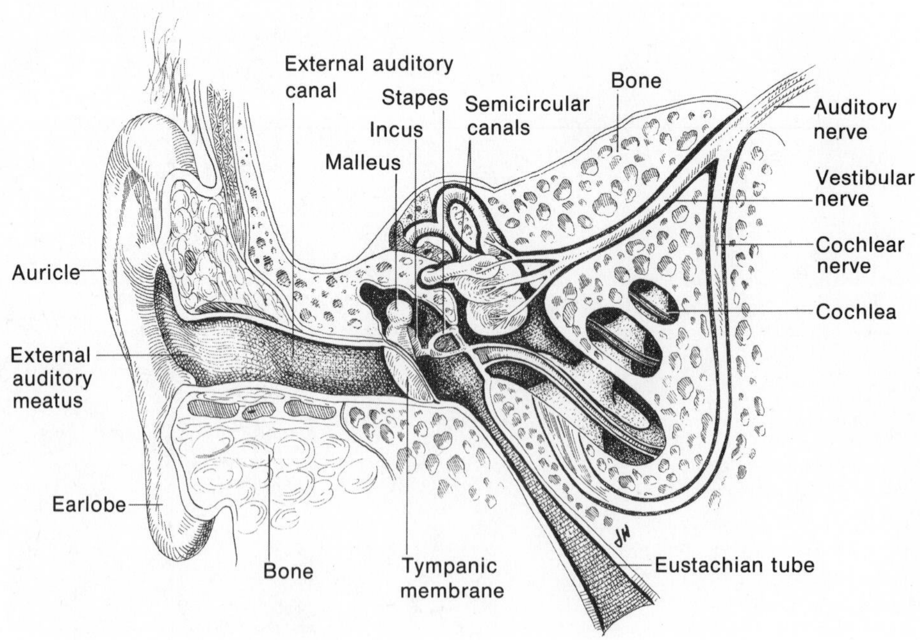

FIGURE 4–8. Structure of the ear.

The medical assistant should examine the external auditory canal with an otoscope before the irrigation to observe the area to be irrigated. If the irrigation is performed to cleanse the ear canal, the canal should be examined after the procedure to make sure it is clean. The ear canal must be straightened for proper viewing by pulling the ear upward and backward for adults, and downward and backward for children 3 years of age and younger. After 3 years of age, the canal is straightened using the technique described for adults. An ear irrigation should not be performed if the tympanic membrane is perforated, because this could result in a severe irritation or infection of the middle ear.

PROCEDURE 4-5
EAR IRRIGATION

1. **PROCEDURAL STEP.** Wash the hands.

2. **PROCEDURAL STEP.** Assemble the equipment. The equipment needed includes a **towel,** an **ear basin to catch the solution, a Pomeroy syringe or a soft rubber bulb syringe, a container to hold the solution, cotton balls,** and the **warmed irrigating solution (warmed to 100 to 105°F),** as ordered by the physician. Check the irrigating solution carefully against the physician's instructions to make sure you have obtained the correct solution. Check the expiration date of the solution. Check the label of the irrigating solution three times: while removing the solution from the shelf, while pouring the solution, and before returning it to its proper place.

Note: The Pomeroy syringe is made of metal. The medical assistant must be careful to avoid introducing the solution into the ear with too much pressure. This could result in rupture of the tympanic membrane. The rubber bulb syringe allows the solution to flow into the ear with less pressure. This type of syringe must be refilled several times during the procedure.

PRINCIPLE. The solution should be carefully compared with the physician's instructions to prevent an error. If the solution is outdated, consult the physician; it may produce undesirable effects, and the medical assistant could be held responsible.

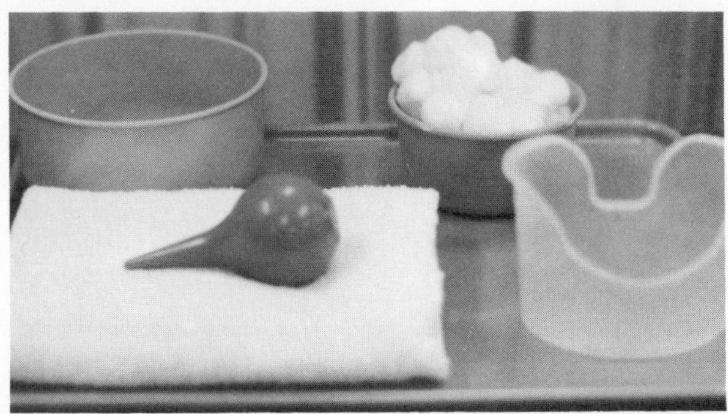

3. **PROCEDURAL STEP.** Identify the patient and explain the procedure.

PRINCIPLE. Explain the purpose of performing the irrigation—for example, to remove cerumen. Tell the patient the procedure is not painful; however, he or she may feel a minimal amount of discomfort and occasional dizziness as the ear solution comes in contact with the tympanic membrane.

4. **PROCEDURAL STEP.** Place the patient in a sitting position with the head tilted toward the affected ear. A towel should be placed on the patient's shoulders to protect clothing and to prevent water from running down the neck. Instruct the patient to hold the ear basin against the head under the affected ear to catch the irrigating solution.

PRINCIPLE. The patient is positioned so gravity aids the flow of the solution out of the ear and into the basin.

Continued

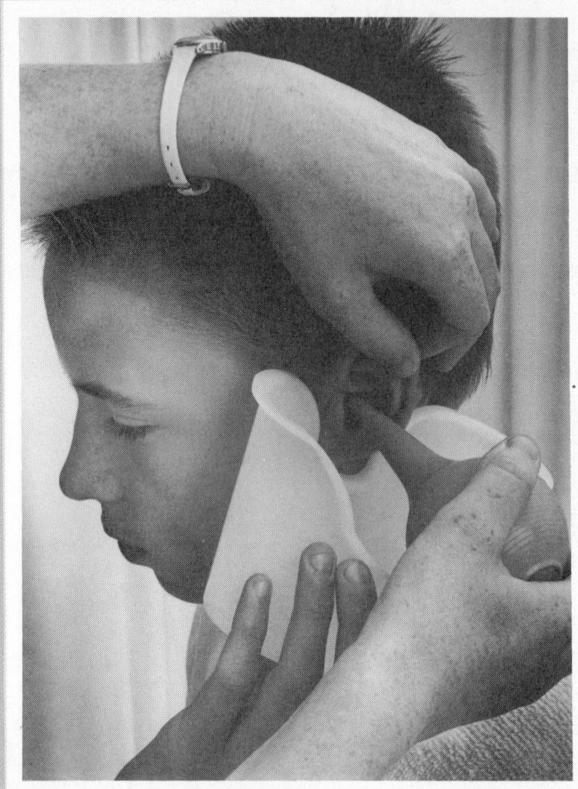

5. **PROCEDURAL STEP.** Cleanse the outer ear with a moistened cotton ball to remove any discharge or debris present. Normal saline or the solution ordered for the irrigation may be used.

PRINCIPLE. The outer ear should be clean to prevent any foreign particles from entering the ear canal during the irrigation.

6. **PROCEDURAL STEP.** Fill the syringe with the prescribed irrigating solution. Expel air from the syringe.

PRINCIPLE. Air forced into the ear is uncomfortable for the patient.

7. **PROCEDURAL STEP.** Straighten the external auditory canal. The canal is straightened by pulling the ear upward and backward for adults and downward and backward for children three years of age and younger.

PRINCIPLE. Straightening the canal permits the irrigating solution to reach all areas of the canal.

8. **PROCEDURAL STEP.** Insert the syringe tip into the ear and inject the irrigating solution toward the roof of the ear canal. It is important that the solution be injected toward the roof of the canal to prevent it from being injected directly onto the tympanic membrane. Do not insert the tip of the syringe too deeply.

PRINCIPLE. The tip of the syringe should be directed at the roof of the canal to prevent injury to the tympanic membrane and to aid in the removal of foreign particles by allowing the solution to flow down the length of the canal and out of the bottom. In addition, severe patient discomfort and dizziness may occur from the solution being injected directly onto the tympanic membrane. Inserting the tip of the syringe too deeply causes discomfort for the patient.

9. **PROCEDURAL STEP.** Continue irrigating for the prescribed period of time or until the desired results have been obtained. Make sure the tip of the syringe does not obstruct the canal opening so that the solution can flow freely out of the canal.

PRINCIPLE. Observe the returning solution to note the material present (e.g., cerumen, discharge, or a foreign object).

10. **PROCEDURAL STEP.** Dry the outside of the ear with a cotton ball. Have the patient lie on the affected side on the treatment table. Tell the patient that the ear will feel sensitive for a short period of time. Place a cotton wick in the ear canal if instructed to do so by the physician.

PRINCIPLE. Any remaining solution in the ear canal should be allowed to drain out. A cotton wick will help to make the patient's ear feel less sensitive after the irrigation.

11. **PROCEDURAL STEP.** Wash the hands.

12. **PROCEDURAL STEP.** Record the procedure. Include the following: the patient's name; the date and time; which ear was irrigated; the type, strength, and amount of solution used; any significant observations such as the presence of injury or the material returned in the irrigating solution; and patient reactions. Place your initials next to the recording.

13. **PROCEDURAL STEP.** Return the equipment.

Record data below.

DATE	TIME	PATIENT'S NAME	RECORDING

PROCEDURE 4-6
EAR INSTILLATION

Ear instillations are performed to soften impacted cerumen, to combat infection with the use of antibiotic ear drops, or to relieve pain.

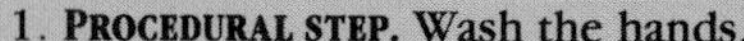

1. **PROCEDURAL STEP.** Wash the hands.

2. **PROCEDURAL STEP.** Assemble the equipment. The equipment needed includes **cotton balls,** the **medication as ordered by the physician,** and a **sterile ear dropper** for use with the ear drops (if one is not provided with the ear drops). Check the medication carefully against the physician's instructions to make sure you have obtained the correct medication. The medication should bear the word *otic.* Check the expiration date. Check the drug label three times: while removing the medication from the shelf, before withdrawing the medication into the dropper, and before instilling the medication.
PRINCIPLE. The medication should be carefully compared with the physician's instructions to prevent a drug error. Medication not bearing the word *otic* should not be placed in the ear because it could result in an injury to the ear. If the medication is outdated, consult the physician; it may produce undesirable effects, and the medical assistant could be held responsible.

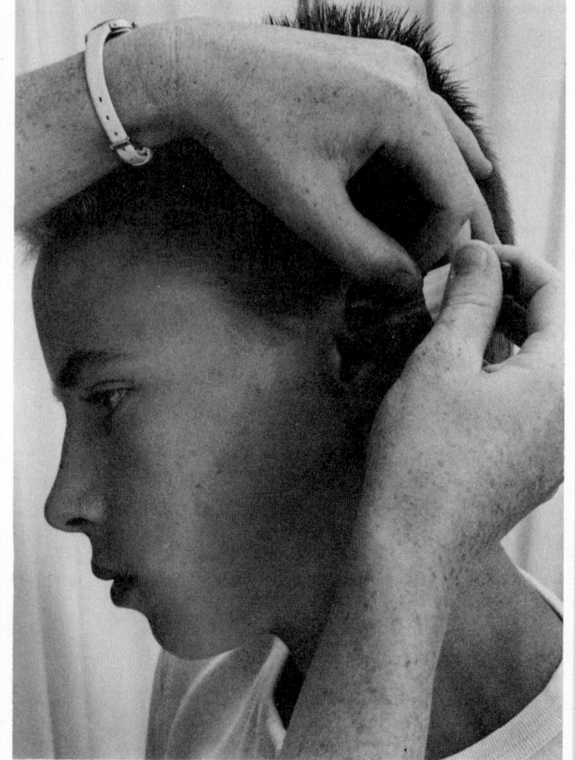

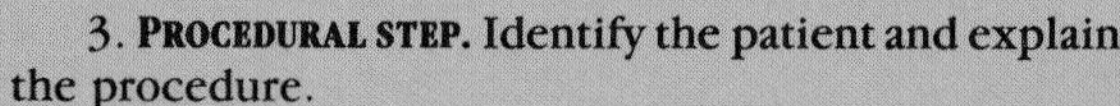

3. **PROCEDURAL STEP.** Identify the patient and explain the procedure.
PRINCIPLE. Explain the purpose of the instillation to the patient.

4. **PROCEDURAL STEP.** Place the patient in a sitting position with the head tilted in the direction of the unaffected ear.
PRINCIPLE. Gravity aids in the flow of the medication into the ear canal.

5. **PROCEDURAL STEP.** Withdraw the medication into the dropper.

6. **PROCEDURAL STEP.** Straighten the external auditory canal. The canal is straightened by pulling the ear upward and backward for adults, and downward and backward for children 3 years of age and younger.
PRINCIPLE. Straightening the canal permits the medication to reach all areas of the canal.

7. **PROCEDURAL STEP.** Place the tip of the dropper in the ear canal, and insert the proper amount of medication by squeezing the rubber bulb and instilling the correct number of drops along the side of the canal.

8. **PROCEDURAL STEP.** Instruct the patient to lie on the unaffected side.
PRINCIPLE. Lying on the unaffected side prevents the medication from running out.

9. **PROCEDURAL STEP.** Place a moistened cotton wick loosely in the ear canal if instructed to do so by the physician.

PRINCIPLE. The cotton ball prevents the medication from running out. Moistening the wick will prevent the medication from being absorbed by the cotton.

10. **PROCEDURAL STEP.** Wash the hands.

11. **PROCEDURAL STEP.** Record the procedure. Include the patient's name, the date and time, the type of ear medication, dosage and strength, which ear(s) received the instillation, any significant observations, and the patient's reaction. Place your initials next to the recording.

12. **PROCEDURAL STEP.** Replace the equipment.

Record data below.

DATE	TIME	PATIENT'S NAME	RECORDING

Study Questions

1. What is the purpose of performing an ear irrigation?
2. What is the purpose of performing an ear instillation?

5

PROMOTING TISSUE HEALING THROUGH PHYSICAL THERAPY

CHAPTER OUTLINE

Heat (Local Effects of Heat; Purpose of Applying Heat)
Cold (Local Effects of Cold; Purpose of Applying Cold)
Factors Affecting the Application of Heat and Cold
Ultrasound
Crutches
Axillary Crutch Measurement
Crutch Guidelines
Crutch Gaits
Canes
Walkers

COMPETENCIES

After completing this chapter, you should be able to demonstrate the proper procedure to perform the following:

1. Apply the following heat treatments, and record the results: hot water bag, heating pad, hot soak, and hot compress.
2. Apply the following cold treatments, and record the results: ice bag, cold compress, and chemical cold pack.
3. Administer an ultrasound treatment, and record the results.
4. Measure an individual for axillary crutches.
5. Instruct an individual in the proper procedure for each of the following crutch gaits: four-point, two-point, three-point, swing-to, and swing-through.
6. Instruct an individual in the proper procedure for using a cane.
7. Instruct an individual in the proper procedure for using a walker.

LEARNING OBJECTIVES

After completing this chapter, you should be able to do the following:

1. Define the terms listed in the vocabulary.
2. Give examples of moist and dry applications of heat and cold.
3. List the effects that occur from the local application of heat, and state three reasons for applying heat.
4. List the effects that occur from the local application of cold, and state three reasons for applying cold.
5. State three factors that should be taken into consideration when applying heat and cold.
6. Describe the general use of therapeutic ultrasound.
7. Explain the purpose of the ultrasound coupling agent.
8. Explain the principles underlying each step in the physical therapy procedures.
9. List four factors taken into consideration in determining the type of ambulatory assistive device prescribed for patient use.
10. Explain the difference between an axillary crutch and a Lofstrand crutch.
11. State three conditions that may result when axillary crutches are not fitted properly.
12. List the guidelines that should be followed by the patient to ensure safety during crutch use.
13. State the use of each of the following crutch gaits: four-point gait, two-point gait, three-point gait, swing-to gait, and swing-through gait.
14. List and describe the three types of canes.
15. Identify the patient conditions that would warrant the use of a cane and walker.

• VOCABULARY •

ambulation (am" bu-la' shun)—The ability to walk as opposed to being confined to bed.

compress (kom' pres)—A soft, moist, absorbent cloth that is folded in several layers and applied to a part of the body in the local application of heat or cold.

edema (ĕ-de' mah)—The retention of fluid in the tissues, resulting in swelling.

erythema (er" ĭ-the' mah)—Redness of the skin caused by congestion of capillaries in the lower layers of skin.

exudate (eks' u-dāt)—A discharge produced by the body tissues.

inflammation (in" flah-ma' shun)—The protective response of the tissues to injury or destruction. Local symptoms occurring at the site of the inflammation include pain, swelling, redness, and warmth.

soak (sōk)—The direct immersion of a body part in water or a medicated solution.

sprain (sprān)—Trauma to a joint, which causes injury to the ligaments.

strain (strān)—An overstretching of a muscle due to trauma.

suppuration (sup" u-ra' shun)—The process of pus formation.

toxin (tok' sin)—A poisonous or noxious substance.

Introduction

The application of heat and cold is used therapeutically to treat pathologic conditions such as infection and trauma. The medical assistant may be responsible for applying various forms of heat and cold at the medical office or for instructing patients in the proper procedure for applying heat or cold at home. Therefore, the medical assistant should have a basic understanding of the physiologic effects of heat and cold on the body and any adverse reactions that may occur if they are not administered correctly.

Heat and cold can be applied in either moist or dry forms. Examples of moist and dry applications of heat and cold commonly used are

1. Dry heat; hot water bag, heating pad
2. Moist heat: hot soak, hot compress
3. Dry cold: ice bag, chemical cold pack
4. Moist cold: cold compress

Heat and cold are applied for short periods of time (generally 15 to 30 minutes) to produce desired therapeutic results. The application may be repeated at time intervals specified by the physician. Prolonged application of heat or cold is not recommended, as it can result in adverse secondary effects. The type of heat or cold application utilized for a particular condition depends upon the purpose of the application, the location and condition of the affected area, and the age and general health of the patient. The physician will instruct the medical assistant to apply a heat or cold treatment based upon these factors.

Heat and cold receptors located in the skin readily adapt to changes in temperature, eventually resulting in diminished heat or cold sensations. The temperature actually remains the same and is providing the intended therapeutic effects. However, the patient, not perceiving the same degree of temperature, may want to increase the intensity of the application without realizing the inherent dangers involved. Excessive heat or cold could result in tissue damage. The medical assistant should fully explain to the patient the necessity of maintaining a safe temperature range during the application.

Heat

Local Effects of Heat

The local effects of applying moderate heat to the body for a short period of time (approximately 15 to 30 minutes) include dilatation or an increase in diameter of the blood vessels in the area as the body tries to rid itself of excess heat from the blood to the environment (Fig. 5–1). This results in an increased blood supply to the area, and tissue metabolism increases. Nutrients and oxygen are provided to the cells at a faster rate, and wastes and toxins are carried away faster. The skin in the area becomes warm and exhibits erythema. *Erythema* is the redness of the skin caused by congestion of capillaries in the lower layers of the skin. These physiologic effects of moderate heat applied to a localized area promote healing. However, prolonged application of heat (more than 1 hour) produces secondary effects that reverse this healing process. Blood vessels constrict, and blood supply to the area decreases. The medical assistant must be careful to apply heat for a length of time specified by the physician.

Purpose of Applying Heat

Heat functions in relieving pain, congestion, muscle spasms, and inflammation. Heat promotes muscle relaxation and therefore is often used for the relief of pain due to the excessive contraction of muscle fibers. Edema or swelling already present in the tissues can be reduced through the application of heat, because the increased blood supply functions to increase the absorption of fluid from the tissues through the lymphatic system. Heat, usually in the form of a moist compress, can be used to soften exudates. An *exudate* is a discharge produced by the body's tissues. At times, exudates may form a hard crust over an area and require removal. Heat also increases *suppuration,* or the process of pus formation to help in the relief of inflammation by breaking down infected tissues. However, heat is not recommended for the initial treatment of acute inflammation or trauma.

Cold

Local Effects of Cold

The application of moderate cold to a localized area produces constriction or a decrease in diameter of blood vessels in the area as the body attempts to prevent heat loss from the blood to the environment (see Fig. 5–1). This leads to decreased blood supply to the area. Tissue metabolism decreases, less oxygen is utilized, and fewer wastes accumulate. The skin becomes cool and pale. Prolonged application of cold (more than 1 hour) has a reverse secondary effect. Blood vessels dilate and there is an increase in tissue metabolism. The medical assistant must apply cold for the recommended length of time only, to prevent secondary effects.

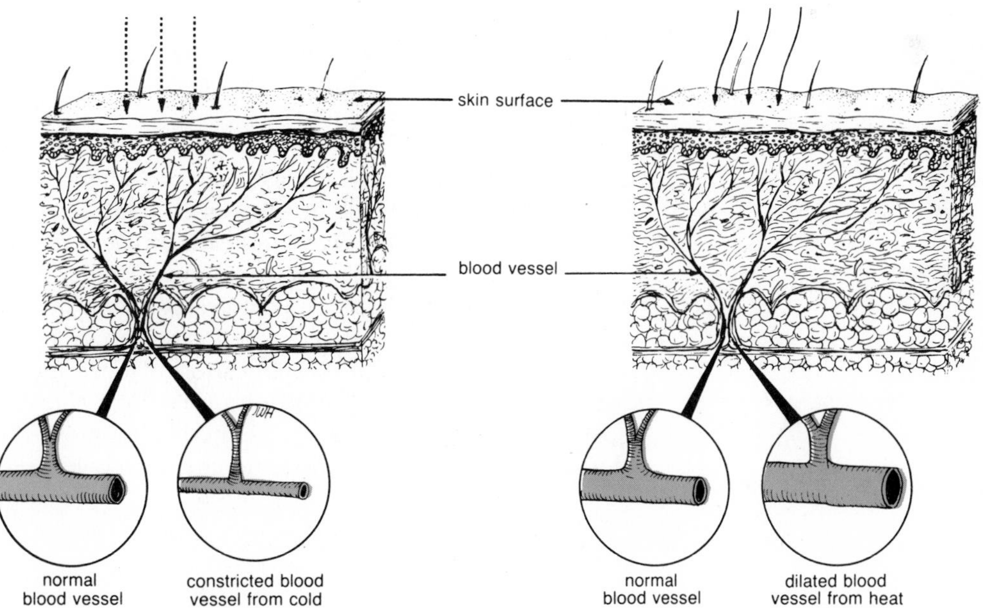

FIGURE 5–1. Effects of the local application of heat and cold. (From Wood, L. A., and Rambo, B. J.: *Nursing Skills for Allied Health Services.* Philadelphia, W.B. Saunders Company, Volume 2, 1980.)

Purpose of Applying Cold

The application of moderate cold for a short period of time is used to prevent edema or swelling. Cold may be applied immediately after an individual has suffered direct trauma such as a bruise, sprain, muscle strain, or fracture. The cold limits the accumulation of fluid in the body tissues by constricting blood vessels and reducing the leakage of fluid into the tissues. Through the constriction of peripheral blood vessels, cold can be used to control bleeding. Cold temporarily relieves pain because of its anesthetic, or numbing, effect, which reduces stimulation of the nerve receptors. Cold also slows the movement of blood and tissue fluids in the affected area, resulting in less pressure against nerve receptors, and therefore less pain. In the early stages of an infection, the local application of cold will function to inhibit the activity of microorganisms. In this way, suppuration is decreased and inflammation is reduced. Cold applications should always be placed in a protective covering, because applying cold directly to the skin could result in a skin burn.

Factors Affecting the Application of Heat and Cold

Before applying heat or cold, certain factors must be taken into consideration to prevent unfavorable reactions such as tissue necrosis. The temperature may need to be adjusted based upon the following conditions:

1. *The age of the patient.* Young children and elderly patients tend to be more sensitive to the application of heat or cold.
2. *Location of the application.* Certain areas of the body are more sensitive to the application of heat or cold, especially thin areas of the skin and areas that are usually covered by clothing, such as the chest, back, and abdomen. The skin of the hands and face is not as sensitive and is better able to tolerate temperature change. Broken skin, such as is found with an open wound, is more sensitive to heat and cold as well as being more prone to tissue damage.
3. *Impaired circulation.* Patients with impaired circulation tend to be more sensitive to heat or cold. This impairment may be at the site of the application or a system problem involving the entire body.
4. *Impaired sensation.* Patients with impaired sensation must be watched very carefully, since tissue damage may occur from the application of heat or cold without the patient's awareness.
5. *Individual tolerance to change in temperature.* Some individuals cannot tolerate temperature change as easily as others. The medical assistant should observe the area to which the heat or cold has been applied before, during, and after the treatment for signs indicating that a modification in temperature is needed. Prolonged erythema or paleness, pain, swelling, or blisters should be reported to the physician. The medical assistant should also ask the patient if the application feels comfortable or if it is too hot or too cold.

Procedures for the local application of heat and cold are presented on the following pages; heat application procedures (hot water bag, heating pad, hot soak, and hot compress) are presented first, followed by cold application procedures (ice bag, cold compress and chemical cold pack).

PROCEDURE 5-1
APPLYING A HOT WATER BAG

1. **PROCEDURAL STEP.** Wash the hands.

2. **PROCEDURAL STEP.** Assemble the equipment. The equipment needed includes the **hot water bag,** a **protective covering for the bag,** a **graduated pitcher for water,** and **a bath thermometer.**

3. **PROCEDURAL STEP.** Identify the patient and explain the procedure. Explain the purpose of applying the hot water bag—for example, to relieve pain.

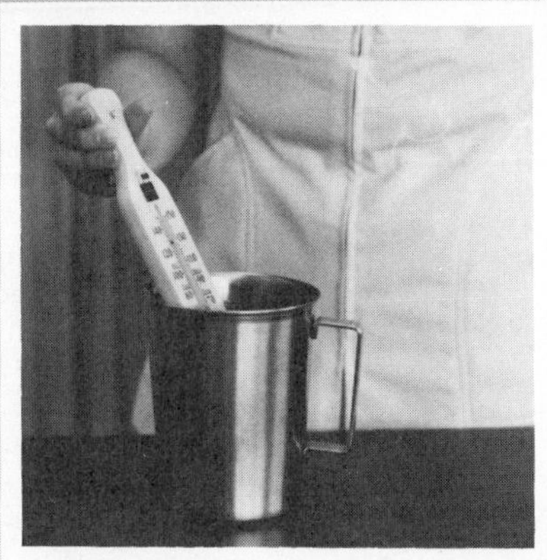

4. **PROCEDURAL STEP.** Fill the graduated pitcher with hot tap water. Test the temperature of the water with a bath thermometer. It should range between 115 and 125°F (46 and 52°C) for adults and older children and between 105 and 115°F (41 and 46°C) for infants, children under 2 years old, and elderly patients.
PRINCIPLE. The temperature should never exceed 125°F, to avoid burning the patient.

5. **PROCEDURAL STEP.** Fill the hot water bag one-third to one-half full of water.
PRINCIPLE. A hot water bag that is not completely full is lighter in weight and easier to mold to the body area.

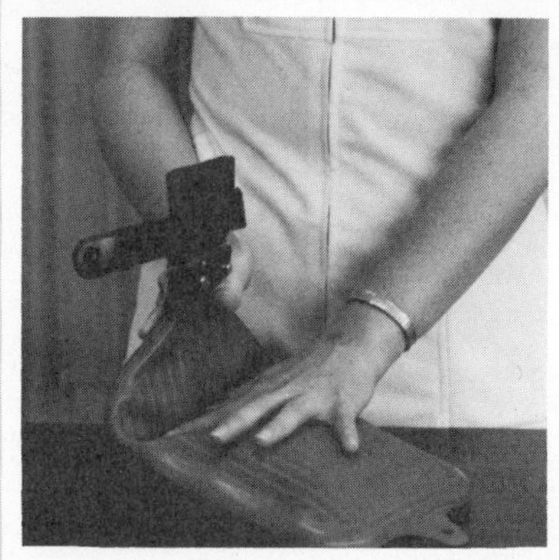

6. **PROCEDURAL STEP.** Expel the excess air from the bag by resting the bag on the table and flattening it, while holding the neck upright until the water reaches the neck. Air can also be expelled by holding the bag upright and squeezing the unfilled part until the water reaches the neck. Screw in the stopper or fasten the top with special closure tabs.
PRINCIPLE. Air is a poor conductor of heat and also makes it difficult to mold the hot water bag to the body area.

7. **PROCEDURAL STEP.** Dry the outside of the bag and test for leakage by holding the bag upside down.
PRINCIPLE. Leaking water will get the patient wet and may burn the patient.

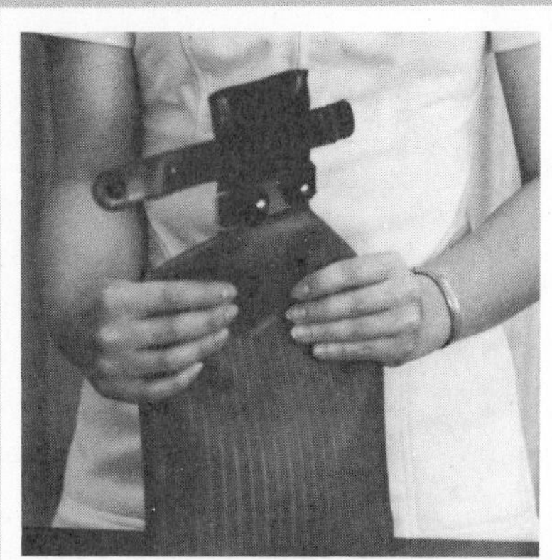

8. **PROCEDURAL STEP.** Place the bag in the protective covering.
PRINCIPLE. The cover helps to absorb perspiration and lessens the danger of burning the patient.

9. **PROCEDURAL STEP.** Place the bag on the patient's affected body area. Ask the patient how the temperature feels. The hot water bag should feel warm but not uncomfortable.
PRINCIPLE. Individuals vary in their ability to tolerate heat.

Continued

10. **PROCEDURAL STEP.** Administer the treatment for the proper length of time as designated by the physician. Check the patient's skin periodically for signs of an increase or decrease in redness or swelling, and ask the patient whether the site is painful.

11. **PROCEDURAL STEP.** Refill the bag with hot water as needed to maintain the proper temperature, making sure to remove an equal amount of the cooler water.

12. **PROCEDURAL STEP.** Wash the hands and record the procedure. Include the patient's name, date and time, method of heat application (hot water bag), temperature of the hot water bag, location and duration of the application and appearance of the application site. Place your initials next to the recording.

13. **PROCEDURAL STEP.** Properly care for the hot water bag. Dispose of or launder the protective covering. Cleanse the hot water with a warm detergent solution, rinse thoroughly, and dry by hanging the bag upside down with the top removed. Store the bag by screwing on the stopper, leaving air inside to prevent the sides from sticking.

Record data below.

DATE	TIME	PATIENT'S NAME	RECORDING

PROCEDURE 5-2
APPLYING A HEATING PAD

The electric heating pad consists of a network of wires that function to convert electric energy into heat to provide a constant and even heat application. The wires must not be bent or crushed. This could damage the pad, resulting in overheating of parts of the pad and leading to burns or fire. Pins must not be inserted in the pad as a means of securing it, because if a pin comes in contact with a wire, an electric shock could result. To prevent electric hazards, heating pads should not be used over areas containing moisture, such as wet dressings.

1. **PROCEDURAL STEP.** Wash the hands.

2. **PROCEDURAL STEP.** Assemble the equipment. The equipment needed includes the **heating pad** and a **protective covering.**

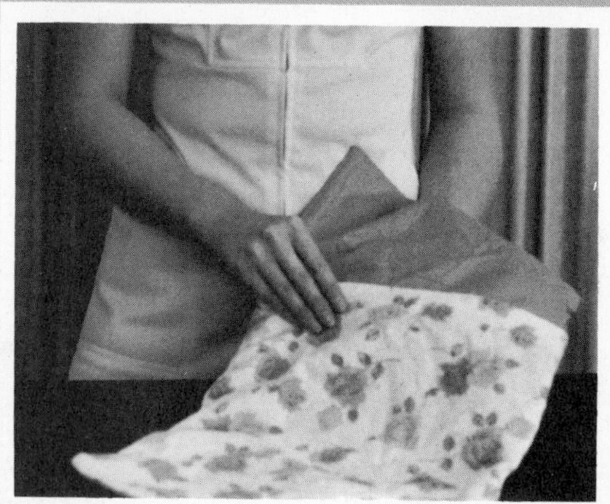

3. **PROCEDURAL STEP.** Identify the patient and explain the procedure. Patients should be instructed not to lie on the heating pad.
PRINCIPLE. Lying on the pad causes heat to accumulate and burn the patient.

4. **PROCEDURAL STEP.** Place the heating pad in the protective covering.
PRINCIPLE. The protective covering provides more comfort for the patient and functions to absorb perspiration.

5. **PROCEDURAL STEP.** Connect the plug to an electric outlet. Set the selector switch at the proper setting, as designated by the physician (usually low or medium).

6. **PROCEDURAL STEP.** Place the heating pad on the patient's affected body area. Ask the patient how the temperature feels. The heating pad should feel warm but not uncomfortable.

7. **PROCEDURAL STEP.** Instruct the patient not to turn the control higher, so as to prevent a burn that may be caused by excessive heat.
PRINCIPLE. The patient's heat receptors eventually become adjusted to the temperature change, resulting in a decreased heat sensation, and the patient may be tempted to increase the temperature.

8. **PROCEDURAL STEP.** Administer the treatment for the proper length of time as designated by the physician. Check the patient periodically for signs of an increase or decrease in redness or swelling and ask the patient if the site is painful.

9. **PROCEDURAL STEP.** Wash hands and record the procedure. Include the patient's name, date and time, method of heat application (heating pad), temperature setting of the pad, location and duration of the application, and appearance of the application site. Place your initials next to the recording.

10. **PROCEDURAL STEP.** Return equipment.

Continued

Record data below.

DATE	TIME	PATIENT'S NAME	RECORDING

PROCEDURE 5-3
APPLYING A HOT SOAK

A *soak* is the direct immersion of a body part in water or a medicated solution. A soak can be applied to an extremity or a part of the torso. Hot soaks function to cleanse open wounds, to increase suppuration, to increase the blood supply to an area to hasten the healing process, or to apply a medicated solution to an area. Applying a soak to an open wound requires the use of sterile technique.

1. **PROCEDURAL STEP.** Wash the hands.

2. **PROCEDURAL STEP.** Assemble the equipment. The equipment needed includes the **soaking solution** (as ordered by the physician), a **bath thermometer,** a **basin for immersion,** and **bath towels.**

3. **PROCEDURAL STEP.** Identify the patient and explain the procedure.

4. **PROCEDURAL STEP.** Fill the basin half full with the soaking solution.

5. **PROCEDURAL STEP.** Check the temperature of the solution with a bath thermometer. The temperature for an adult should range between 105 and 110°F (41 and 44°C).

6. **PROCEDURAL STEP.** Place the patient in a comfortable position to avoid fatigue and muscle strain. Pad the side of the basin with a towel to provide for patient comfort.

7. **PROCEDURAL STEP.** Slowly and gradually immerse the patient's affected body part in the solution. Ask the patient how the temperature feels.
PRINCIPLE. The affected body part should be allowed to become accustomed to the change in temperature gradually.

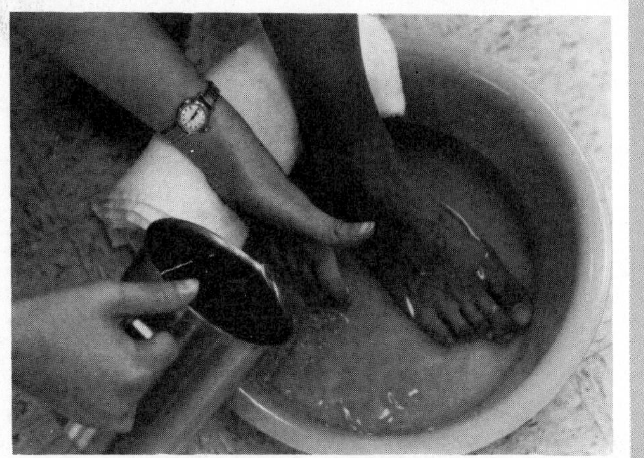

8. **PROCEDURAL STEP.** Test the temperature of the solution frequently. Remove cooler fluid every 5 minutes to keep the solution at a constant temperature. Pour the hot water in near the edge of the basin by placing your hand between the patient and water. Stir the water as you pour.
PRINCIPLE. Water should be added away from the patient's body part to prevent burning the patient. Stirring in the water helps to distribute the heat and to keep the temperature constant.

9. **PROCEDURAL STEP.** Apply the hot soak for the proper length of time, as designated by the physician (usually 15 to 20 minutes). Check the patient's skin periodically for signs of an increase or decrease in redness or swelling, and ask the patient whether the site is painful.

10. **PROCEDURAL STEP.** Completely dry the affected part.

11. **PROCEDURAL STEP.** Wash the hands and record the procedure. Include the patient's name, date and time, method of heat application (hot soak), the temperature of the soak, location and duration of the application, and the appearance of the application site. Place your initials next to the recording.

12. **PROCEDURAL STEP.** Return and properly care for the equipment.

Record data below.

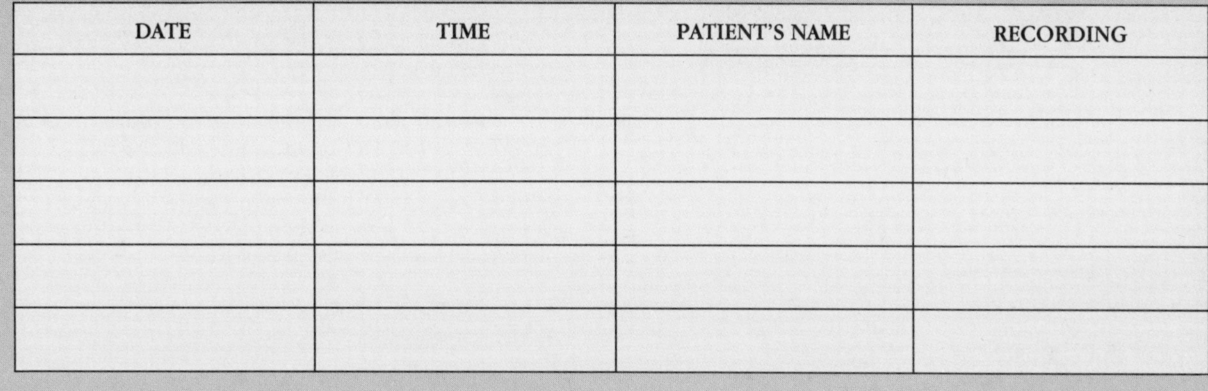

DATE	TIME	PATIENT'S NAME	RECORDING

PROCEDURE 5-4
APPLYING A HOT COMPRESS

A *compress* is a soft, moist, absorbent cloth, such as a gauze dressing or washcloth that is folded into several layers and applied to a body part. Hot compresses are used to increase suppuration, to improve circulation to a body part to aid in healing, and to promote drainage from infection. Applying a hot compress to an open wound requires the use of sterile technique.

1. **PROCEDURAL STEP.** Wash the hands.

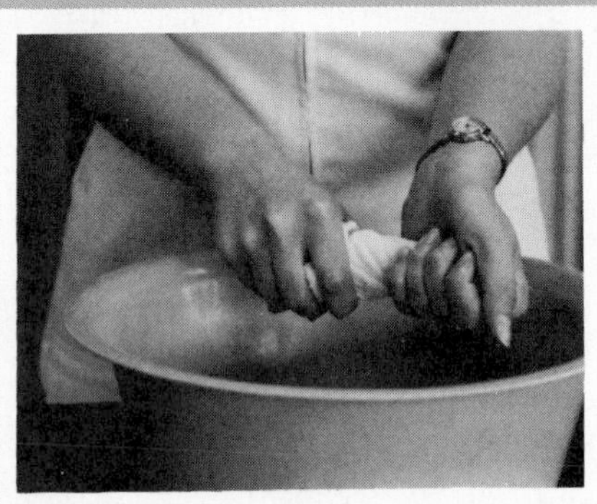

2. **PROCEDURAL STEP.** Assemble the equipment. The equipment needed includes the **solution** (as ordered by the physician), a **bath thermometer, gauze squares or washcloths,** and a **basin to hold the solution.**

3. **PROCEDURAL STEP.** Identify the patient and explain the procedure.

4. **PROCEDURAL STEP.** Check the temperature of the solution with the bath thermometer. The temperature for an adult should range between 105 and 110°F (41 and 44°C).

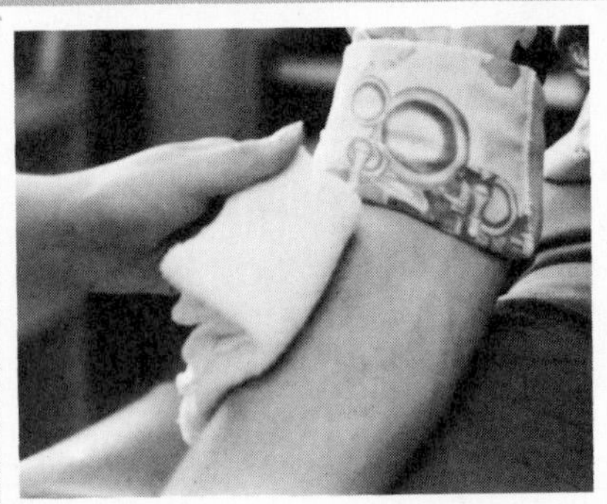

5. **PROCEDURAL STEP.** Wring out the compress to rid it of excess moisture. The compress should be wet but not dripping. Apply it lightly at first to the affected site to allow the patient gradually to become used to the heat. The medical assistant may want to cover the compress with a waterproof cover to help hold the heat in. Ask the patient how the temperature feels. The compress should be applied as hot as the patient can comfortably tolerate.

   PRINCIPLE. The waterproof cover prevents cool air currents from coming in contact with the compress and reduces the number of times the compress needs to be changed.

6. **PROCEDURAL STEP.** Place additional compresses in the solution so they are ready for use.

7. **PROCEDURAL STEP.** Repeat the application of the compress every 2 to 3 minutes for the duration of time specified by the physician (usually 15 to 20 minutes). Check the patient's skin periodically for signs of an increase or decrease in redness or swelling and ask the patient whether the site is painful.

8. **PROCEDURAL STEP.** Check the temperature of the water periodically. Add more hot water if needed.

9. **PROCEDURAL STEP.** Thoroughly dry the affected part.

10. **PROCEDURAL STEP.** Wash hands and record the procedure. Include the patient's name, date and time, method of heat application (hot compress), temperature of the solution, location and duration of the application, and appearance of the application site. Place your initials next to the recording.

11. **PROCEDURAL STEP.** Return and properly care for the equipment.

Record data below.

DATE	TIME	PATIENT'S NAME	RECORDING

PROCEDURE 5-5
APPLYING AN ICE BAG

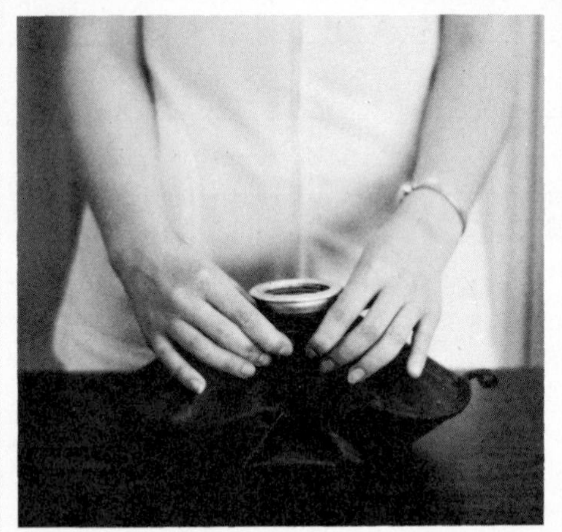

1. **PROCEDURAL STEP.** Wash the hands.

2. **PROCEDURAL STEP.** Assemble the equipment. The equipment needed includes the **ice bag, a protective covering,** and **small pieces of ice (ice chips or crushed ice).**

3. **PROCEDURAL STEP.** Identify the patient and explain the procedure. Explain the purpose of applying the ice bag—for example, to prevent swelling.

4. **PROCEDURAL STEP.** Check the ice bag for leakage.
PRINCIPLE. A leaking bag will get the patient wet and cause chilling.

5. **PROCEDURAL STEP.** Fill the bag one-half to two-thirds full with small pieces of ice.
PRINCIPLE. Small pieces of ice work better than larger pieces because they reduce the amount of air spaces in the bag, resulting in better conduction of cold. In addition, small pieces of ice allow the bag to mold better to the body area.

6. **PROCEDURAL STEP.** Expel air from the bag by squeezing the empty top half of the bag together and screwing on the stopper.
PRINCIPLE. Air is a poor conductor of cold and also makes it difficult to mold the ice bag to the body area.

7. **PROCEDURAL STEP.** Thoroughly dry the bag and place it in the protective covering.
PRINCIPLE. The protective covering provides for patient comfort and absorbs the moisture that condenses on the outside of the bag.

8. **PROCEDURAL STEP.** Place the bag on the patient's affected body area. Ask the patient how the temperature feels. The application of ice is usually uncomfortable, but most patients tolerate it if they know how much benefit may be derived from it.
PRINCIPLE. Individuals vary in their ability to tolerate cold.

9. **PROCEDURAL STEP.** Administer the treatment for the proper length of time, as designated by the physician (*usually until the area feels numb,* approximately 20 to 30 minutes). Check the patient's skin periodically for signs of an increase or decrease in redness or swelling, and ask the patient whether the site is painful. If extreme paleness and numbness or a mottled blue appearance occurs at the application site, remove the bag and notify the physician.

10. **PROCEDURAL STEP.** Refill the bag with ice and change the protective covering if needed.

11. **PROCEDURAL STEP.** Wash the hands and record the procedure. Include the patient's name, date and time, method of cold application (ice bag), location and duration of the application, and appearance of the application site. Place your initials next to the recording.

12. **PROCEDURAL STEP.** Properly care for the ice bag. Dispose of or launder the protective covering as required. Cleanse the ice bag with a warm detergent solution, rinse thoroughly, and dry by hanging the bag upside down with the top removed. Store the bag by screwing on the stopper, leaving air inside to prevent the sides from sticking.

Record data below.

DATE	TIME	PATIENT'S NAME	RECORDING

PROCEDURE 5-6
APPLYING A COLD COMPRESS

Cold compresses are used to relieve pain and inflammation and to treat conditions such as headaches, injured eyes, and tooth extractions.

1. **PROCEDURAL STEP.** Wash the hands.

2. **PROCEDURAL STEP.** Assemble the equipment. The equipment needed includes **gauze squares or washcloths, ice cubes,** and a **basin to hold the water.**

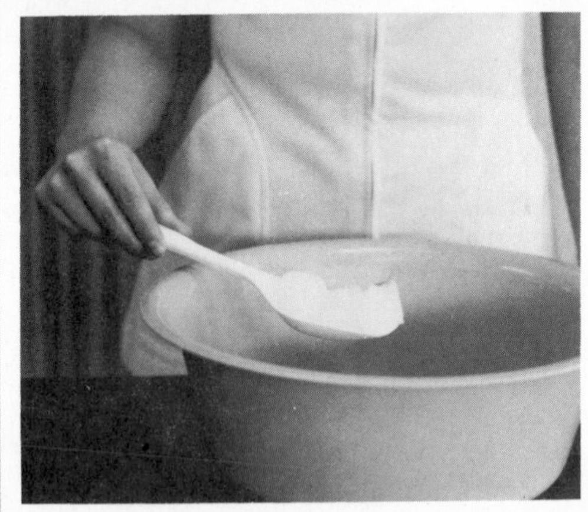

3. **PROCEDURAL STEP.** Identify the patient and explain the procedure.

4. **PROCEDURAL STEP.** Prepare the water by placing large ice cubes in the basin and adding a small amount of water.
PRINCIPLE. Using larger pieces of ice prevents them from sticking to the compress and slows the rate at which they melt in the water.

5. **PROCEDURAL STEP.** Wring out the compress to rid it of excess moisture. The compress should be wet but not dripping. Apply it lightly at first to the affected site to allow the patient gradually to become used to the cold. The medical assistant may want to cover the compress with an ice bag to help keep it cold and to reduce the number of times it needs to be changed. Ask the patient how the temperature feels.

6. **PROCEDURAL STEP.** Place additional compresses in the solution to be ready for use.

7. **PROCEDURAL STEP.** Repeat the application of the compress every 2 to 3 minutes for the duration of time specified by the physician (usually 15 to 20 minutes). Check the patient's skin periodically for signs of an increase or decrease in redness or swelling, and ask the patient whether the site is painful.

8. **PROCEDURAL STEP.** Add ice if needed to keep the water cold.

9. **PROCEDURAL STEP.** Thoroughly dry the affected part.

10. **PROCEDURAL STEP.** Wash hands and record the procedure. Include the patient's name, date and time, method of cold application (cold compress), location and duration of the application, and the appearance of the application site. Place your initials next to the recording.

11. **PROCEDURAL STEP.** Return and properly care for the equipment.

Record data below.

DATE	TIME	PATIENT'S NAME	RECORDING

PROCEDURE 5-7
APPLYING A CHEMICAL COLD PACK

Chemical cold packs are available in a variety of sizes and shapes (Fig. 5–2). Once activated, they provide a specific degree of coldness for a specific period of time (usually 30 to 60 minutes), as indicated on the package label. Most cold packs consist of a vinyl bag containing ammonium nitrate crystals. Enclosed within this bag is a smaller vinyl bag containing water. The cold pack is activated by applying pressure until the inner bag ruptures. This releases the water into the larger bag, and a chemical reaction occurs between the crystals and water, producing coldness. These packs are disposable, and, once the coldness diminishes, they should be discarded in an appropriate receptacle. Chemical cold packs should be stored at room temperature and are used as a replacement for ice bags for the local application of cold.

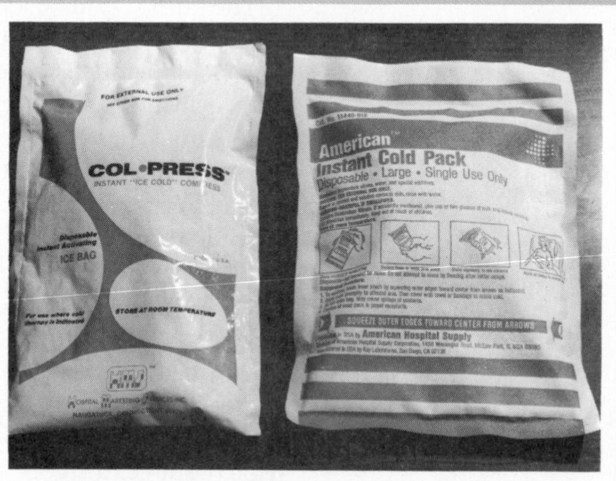

FIGURE 5–2. Disposable chemical cold packs.

The procedure for applying the pack is as follows:

1. Shake the crystals to the bottom of the bag.
2. Squeeze the bag firmly to break the inner water bag.
3. Shake the bag vigorously to mix the contents.
4. Apply the bag to the affected area.
5. Administer the treatment for the proper length of time.
6. Discard the bag in an appropriate receptacle.

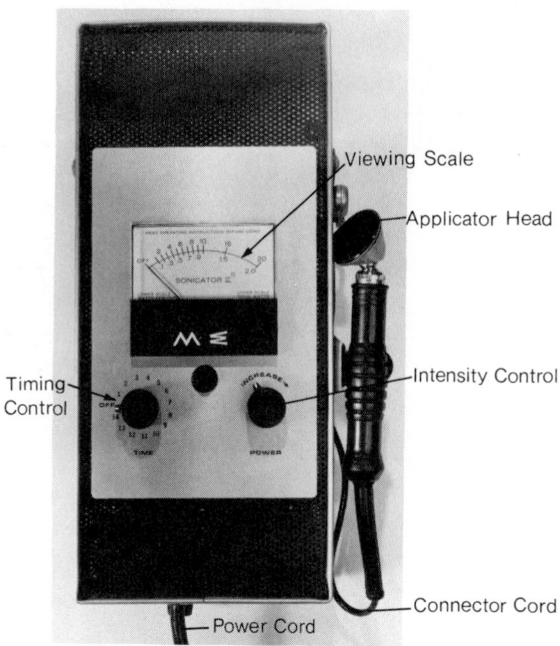

FIGURE 5-3. The parts of an ultrasound machine.

Ultrasound

Ultrasound operates on the basis of high-frequency sound waves that can be used therapeutically as a penetrating deep-heating agent for the soft tissues of the body, such as tendons and muscles. Many physicians utilize ultrasound in the medical office for the local application of heat to treat musculoskeletal disorders. The beneficial physiologic effects of ultrasound are primarily due to the deep heat produced in the tissues and include reduction of edema, breakup of exudates and precipitates, increased cellular metabolism, relief of pain, and micromassage. The physician may order ultrasound to treat such musculoskeletal conditions as sprains, strains, joint contractures, neuritis, arthritis, edema, synovitis, scar tissue, bursitis, fibrositis, osteoarthritis, dislocations, and pulled muscles and tendons. Therapeutic ultrasound must *not* be used over the eyeball, over malignant tumors, directly over the spinal cord, over the heart or brain, over reproductive organs or a pregnant uterus, or over areas of impaired sensation or inadequate circulation. The medical assistant is responsible for performing the ultrasound treatment, which includes preparing the patient, operating the machine, and administering the treatment.

The ultrasound machine consists of two main parts: the generator and the transducer. The generator is located within the main unit of the machine, which also contains the controls to operate the machine. The transducer consists of a crystal inserted between two electrodes and is located in a device termed the applicator head or sound head. The applicator head is a lightweight, hand-held device attached to the ultrasound machine by a connector cord (Fig. 5-3). The generator produces a high-frequency electric current that causes the crystal (located in the transducer) to vibrate and generate sound waves. The frequency of the sound waves produced by the transducer is above the frequency of sound waves audible by the human ear; therefore, no sound is heard when the machine is in operation. The applicator head is firmly placed on the patient's skin surface and is slowly and steadily moved over the treatment area, which allows the sound waves to penetrate the patient's soft tissues. As the sound waves travel through the tissues, part of the waves are absorbed by the tissues and transformed into heat. This produces a vigorous deep heating in the soft tissues of the body. A micromassage effect is also produced due to the mechanical vibration of the sound waves as they pass through the tissues, massaging them.

Air is a poor conductor of sound; therefore, a coupling agent must be used with ultrasound treatments to increase conductivity, thereby providing a good transmission of the sound waves to the patient's tissues. The coupling agent produces an air-free contact between the applicator head and the patient's skin and is available in the form of an oil, lotion, or gel. Examples of coupling agents include mineral oil and (commercially available) Soni-Gel and Lectro-Sonic. The coupling agent must be at room temperature and must be applied liberally to the treatment area of the patient's skin. Water may also be used as a coupling agent because it is a good conductor of sound. In this method, both the patient's skin surface to be treated and the applicator head are completely submerged under water. The applicator head is held ½ to 1 inch away from the patient's skin and is slowly and steadily moved, using a circular motion. The underwater method is advocated when the patient's skin is sensitive and cannot tolerate the direct pressure of the applicator head or when the body surface to be treated is uneven, as are the hands or feet, where it would be difficult to obtain a good contact between the patient's skin and the applicator head.

The applicator head must be moved continuously during the treatment in either a back-and-forth stroking motion or in a circular motion at a rate of 1 to 2 inches per second. The method used depends in large part on the area of the body to which the treatment is being applied. It is usually easier to use the stroking motion over larger body areas such as the back, and the circular motion over smaller areas such as the ankle. Moving the applicator head ensures a uniform distribution of heat in the tissues and prevents the occurrence of hot spots. A hot spot is a very small area in which the temperature rises rapidly if the applicator head is allowed to remain stationary. This could cause burns to the patient's tissues.

Ultrasound dosage is expressed in watt-minutes. Watt refers to the intensity of the sound waves ordered by the physician and minutes refers to the duration of the treatment. The dosage ordered by the physician depends on the area of the body that is receiving the treatment and the patient's condition. An acute condition requires a lower intensity treatment, whereas a chronic condition warrants a higher intensity. The underwater method also requires a higher intensity because some of the sound waves are absorbed and reflected by the water.

Ultrasound therapy is generally administered in a series of 6 to 12 treatments; the frequency of the treatment varies from once daily to three times per week. The duration of administration of the treatment usually progresses from 5 minutes at the beginning of the series to 8 to 10 minutes near the end of the treatments. An ultrasound treatment should never exceed 20 minutes.

The controls on the ultrasound machine include a timing control and an intensity control; additional controls may be present, depending on the type of machine in use. The timing control measures time in minutes; the time limit of most machines ranges from 0 to 15 minutes, which is sufficient because the majority of treatments rarely exceed 10 minutes. The intensity or power control governs the intensity of the sound waves, which are measured in watts; therapeutic ultrasound dosage usually ranges from 1 to 4 watts. A viewing scale indicates the intensity at which the machine has been set. The medical assistant must be able to operate each control; for example, if the physician orders an ultrasound treatment at 4 watts for a duration of 5 minutes, the medical assistant would first set the timing control at 5 (minutes) and then turn the intensity control until the viewing scale indicates that the intensity is at 4 watts.

During the treatment, the patient normally should not feel the ultrasound waves. If the patient indicates a feeling of burning or pain, the medical assistant should stop the treatment immediately and inform the physician. Any pain or discomfort usually indicates that the treatment dosage is too intense. Other causes of pain or discomfort include an insufficient amount of coupling medium applied to the treatment area and keeping the applicator head on one area too long.

PROCEDURE 5-8
ADMINISTERING AN ULTRASOUND TREATMENT

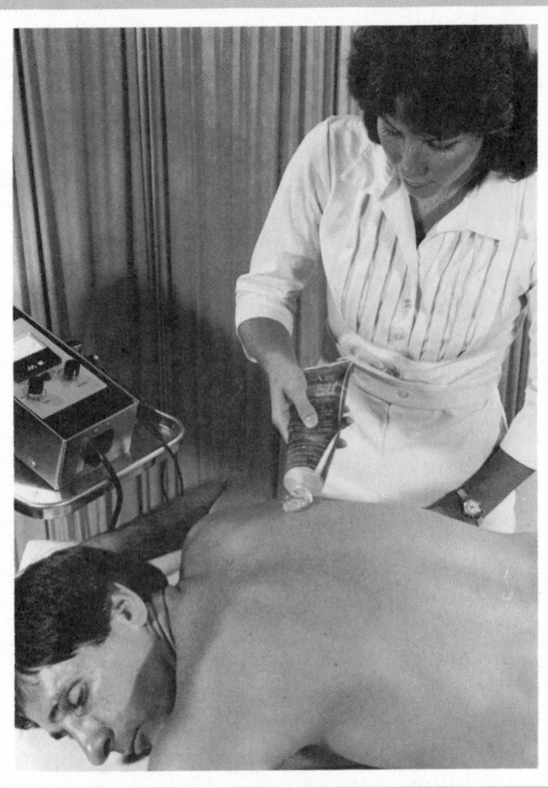

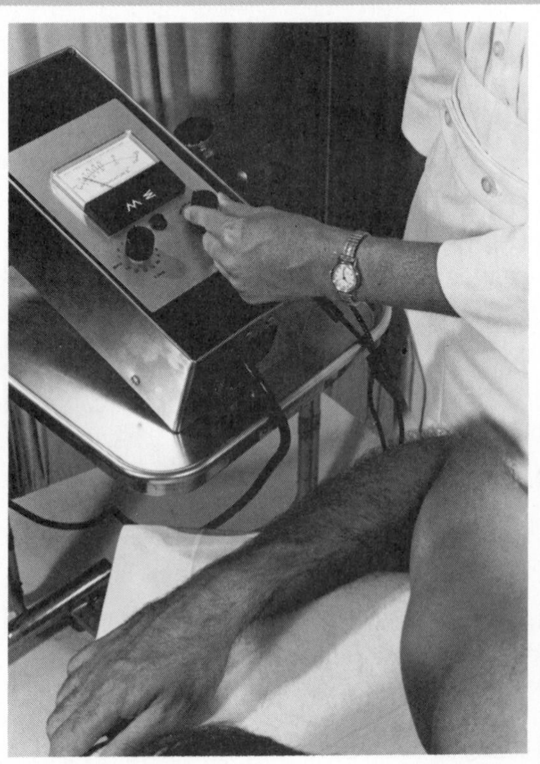

1. **Procedural step.** Wash the hands.

2. **Procedural step.** Assemble the equipment. The equpment needed includes the **ultrasound machine,** a **coupling agent,** and **paper towels.**

3. **Procedural step.** Identify the patient and explain the procedure. Tell the patient that the treatment will not take long and that any pain or discomfort experienced during the treatment should be reported immediately.

Principle. Pain or discomfort during the treatment may indicate that the intensity of the treatment dosage is too high.

4. **Procedural step.** Position the patient and prepare the skin. Ask the patient to remove appropriate clothing to expose the treatment area. Make sure the coupling medium is at room temperature and apply it liberally to the treatment area. Tell the patient that the coupling medium will feel cold. Use the applicator head to spread the coupling medium evenly over the treatment area. The coupling medium should completely cover, but should not flood, the area. Do not place the coupling medium on the ultrasound machine.

Principle. The coupling medium permits a good transmission of the sound waves to the patient's tissues. The coupling medium should be applied at room temperature so as not to be too uncomfortable for the patient.

5. **Procedural step.** Place the intensity control at the minimum position and set the timer to the amount of time stipulated for the ultrasound treatment as specified by the physician. Once the timer has activated the machine, check to make sure the intensity is at 0 watts.

6. **Procedural step.** Advance the intensity control to the treatment level (measured in watts) specified by the physician. Tell the patient that the applicator head will feel cold. Hold the applicator at a right angle to the patient's skin and, using a firm pressure, place the applicator head into the coupling medium in the treatment area.

7. **PROCEDURAL STEP.** Move the applicator head in a back-and-forth stroking motion or in a circular motion. If the stroking method is employed, use short strokes (approximately 1 inch in length), and gradually move the applicator head so that each stroke overlaps the previous stroke by one-half. Move the applicator head continuously at a rate of 1 to 2 inches per second.

PRINCIPLE. Moving the applicator head continuously ensures a uniform distribution of heat in the tissues and prevents overheating of the tissue in a small area (hot spot).

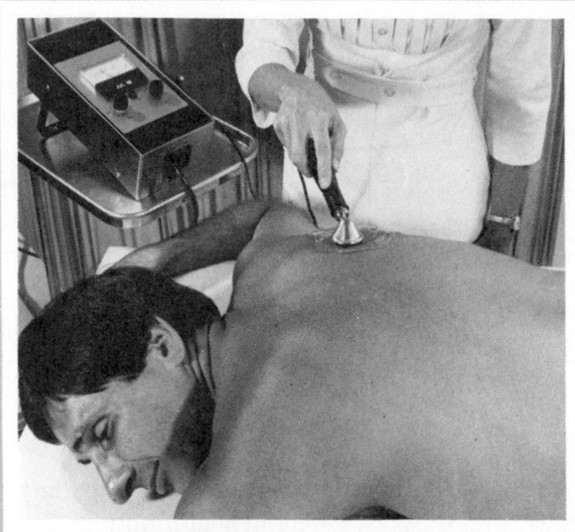

8. **PROCEDURAL STEP.** Continue the ultrasound treatment until the timer goes off. During the treatment, perform the following:
   a. Move the applicator head continuously.
   b. Do not remove the applicator head from the patient's skin and hold it up in the air.
   c. Stop the treatment immediately and notify the physician, if the patient complains of any pain or discomfort.

PRINCIPLE. Holding the applicator head in the air causes it to become hot, and it may burn the patient when it is placed back on the skin. It may also damage the crystal in the applicator head.

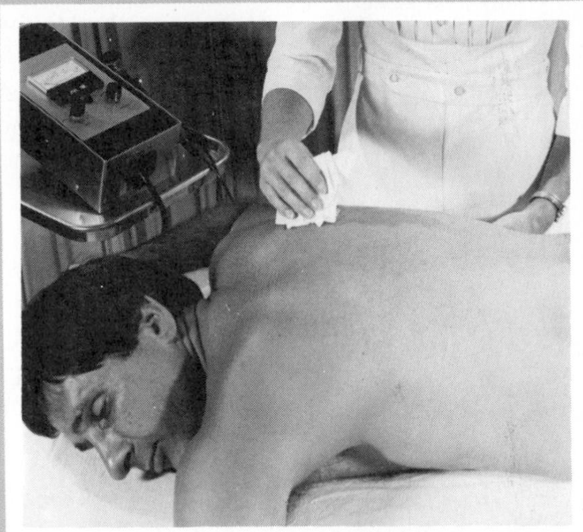

9. **PROCEDURAL STEP.** When the treatment time is completed, the timer automatically shuts off the machine. Remove the applicator head from the patient's skin and turn the intensity control to the minimum position.

10. **PROCEDURAL STEP.** Wipe the excess coupling medium from the patient's skin and applicator head with a paper towel. Instruct the patient to get dressed.

11. **PROCEDURAL STEP.** Wash the hands and record the procedure in the patient's chart. Include the patient's name, date and time, the location of the treatment, the duration of the treatment (in minutes) and the intensity used (in watts) and any unusual patient reaction.

Record data below.

DATE	TIME	PATIENT'S NAME	RECORDING

Assistive Devices for Ambulation

Mechanical assistive devices are used by individuals requiring aid in ambulation. The term *ambulation* refers to the ability to walk, as opposed to being confined to bed. Examples of assistive devices include crutches, canes, and walkers. The type of device used depends upon factors such as the type and severity of the disability, the amount of support required, and the patient's age and degree of muscular coordination. The assistive device may be prescribed for a temporary condition, such as a fracture or sprain to a lower extremity or disability following orthopedic surgery. It may also be prescribed for a more permanent condition, such as paralysis, deformity, or permanent weakness of the lower extremities.

Crutches

Crutches are artificial supports consisting of wood or tubular aluminum. They are used for patients requiring assistance in walking, as a result of disease, injury, or birth defects of the lower extremities. Crutches function by removing weight from the legs and transferring it to the arms.

The two main types of crutches are the *axillary crutch* and the *Lofstrand crutch* (Fig. 5–4). The axillary crutch is used most frequently and is made of wood or tubular aluminum. This type of crutch has a shoulder rest and handgrips and extends from the ground almost to the patient's axilla. The Lofstrand crutch consists of a single adjustable tube of aluminum that extends only to the forearm. A metal cuff, attached to the crutch, fits securely around the patient's forearm, while a handgrip covered with rubber extends from the crutch for means of weight bearing. The metal cuff and the handgrip function in stabilizing the patient's wrists to make walking safer and easier. One advantage of the Lofstrand crutch is that the individual can release the handgrip, enabling use of the hand, while the metal cuff

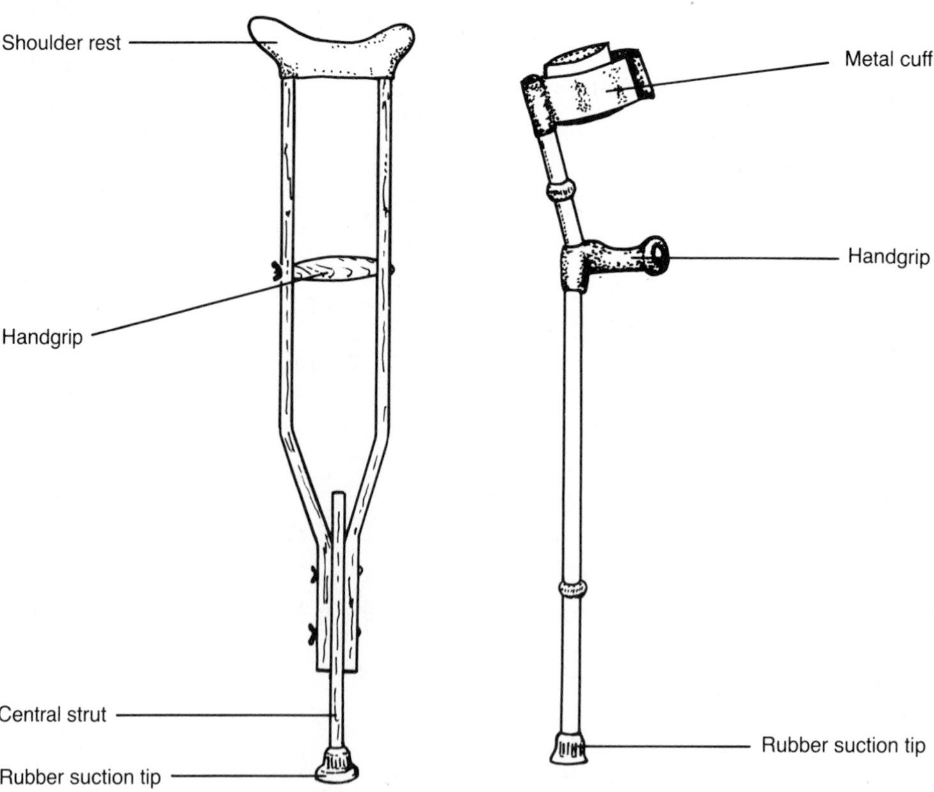

FIGURE 5–4. Types of crutches.

holds the crutch in place. The Lofstrand crutch is most often used by paraplegic individuals. Both the axillary and Lofstrand crutch require suction tips, which are generally made of rubber. The tips increase the surface tension to help prevent the crutches from slipping on a floor surface.

Axillary Crutch Measurement

The patient must be measured for axillary crutches to ensure the correct crutch length and the proper placement of the handgrip. Incorrectly fitted crutches increase the patient risk of developing back pain, nerve damage, and injuries to the axilla and palms of the hands, as follows: If the crutch is too long, the shoulder rest exerts pressure on the patient's axilla. This can injure the radial nerve in the brachial plexus, which eventually may lead to *crutch palsy,* a condition of muscular weakness in the forearm, wrist, and hand. In addition, crutches that are too long cause the patient's shoulders to be forced forward, preventing the patient from pushing his or her body off the ground. Crutches that are too short force the patient to be bent over and uncomfortable, also making the crutches awkward to use. If the handgrips are too low, pressure results on the patient's axilla, whereas handgrips that are too high are awkward. Crutches are designed using bolts and wing nuts, which allow for proper adjustment of both the length and handgrip level.

PROCEDURE 5-9
MEASURING FOR AXILLARY CRUTCHES

To correctly determine crutch length, the patient must wear shoes while being measured. The measurement can be taken with the patient in a standing position as outlined below.

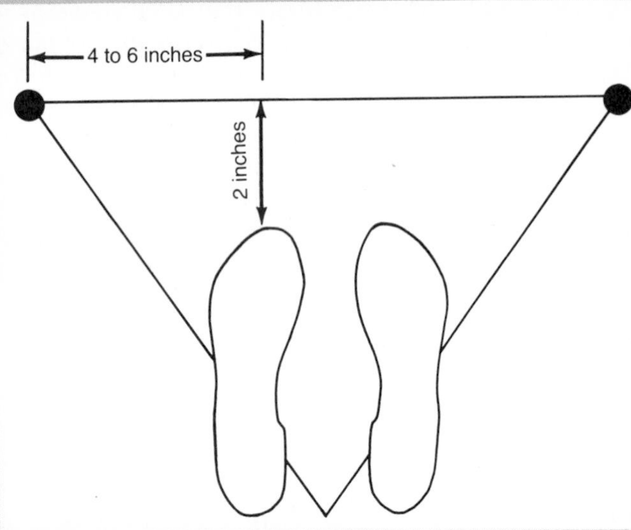

FIGURE 5-5. To measure the patient for axillary crutches, position the crutches with the tips at a distance of 2 inches in front of and 4 to 6 inches to the side of each foot. (Large dots represent crutch tips.)

1. Ask the patient to stand erect.

2. Position the crutches with the crutch tips at a distance of 2 inches (5 cm) in front of and 4 to 6 inches (15 cm) to the side of each foot (Fig. 5-5).

3. Adjust the crutch length so that the shoulder rests are approximately 1½ to 2 inches below the axilla. The length of the crutch is adjusted by removing the bolt and wing and sliding the central strut (support piece) at the bottom either upward or downward, as necessary, to attain the proper length. The strut is then secured by replacing the bolt and securely fastening the wing nut.

Once the crutch length measurement procedure has been completed, the correct placement of the handgrips must be determined. This is accomplished as follows:

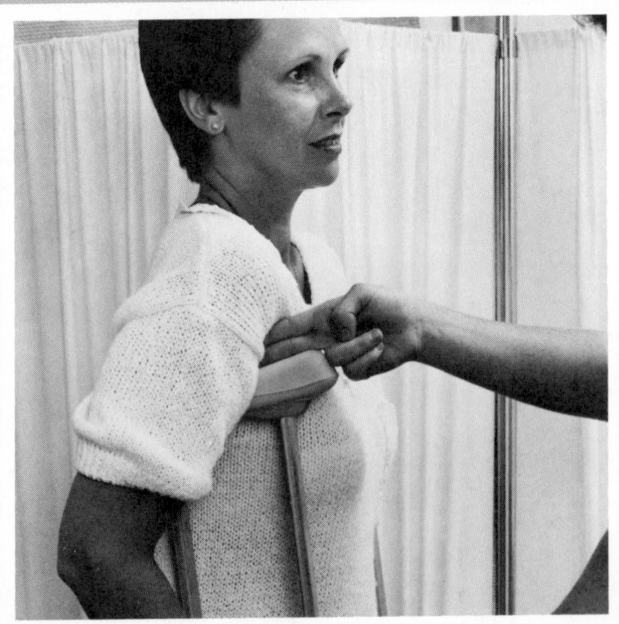

FIGURE 5-6. Checking the fit of axillary crutches.

1. Ask the patient to stand erect with a crutch under each arm and to support his or her weight by the handgrips.

2. Adjust the handgrips on the crutches so that the elbow is flexed to an angle of approximately 30 degrees. The handgrip level is adjusted by removing the bolt and wing nut and sliding the handgrip upward or downward, as required. The handgrip is then secured by replacing the bolt and tightly fastening the wing nut. The angle of elbow flexion can be verified using a measuring device known as a *goniometer*.

3. Check the fit of the crutches. If the crutches are measured correctly, the medical assistant should be able to insert two fingers between the top of the crutch and the axilla, when the patient is standing erect with the crutches under his or her arms (Fig. 5-6).

Crutch Guidelines

It is important that the patient be provided with specific guidelines to ensure safety while using crutches, to prevent injuries or falls. The medical assistant is responsible for instructing the patient in these guidelines as outlined below.

1. The weight of the body should be supported by the hands on the handgrips and the axillary pads pressing against the sides of the rib cage. The body weight should not be supported by the axilla, because pressure on the axilla may result in crutch palsy.
2. Tingling or numbness in the upper body should be reported to the physician. It may indicate the crutches are being used incorrectly or that the crutches are the wrong size.
3. The patient should practice correct posture to prevent strain on muscles and joints and to maintain proper body balance.
4. The shoulder rests of axillary crutches can be slightly padded for comfort, but the padding must not press against the axilla but rather the lateral rib cage. The handgrips can also be padded for increased patient comfort.
5. The crutches should be moved forward to the side, to prevent obstruction of the pathway for the feet.
6. Each step taken with crutches should be at a safe and comfortable distance. When first learning to use the crutches, the patient should take small steps, rather than large ones. The crutches should not be moved forward more than 12 to 15 inches with each step. A distance greater than this may cause the crutches to slide forward.
7. The crutch tips should be securely attached and inspected on a regular basis. If the crutch tips are worn down, they should be replaced with tips of the proper size.
8. Crutch tips should be kept dry to maintain their surface friction. If they become wet, the patient should dry them well before use.
9. The wing nuts holding the central strut and handgrips in place periodically should be checked for tightness.
10. Well-fitting flat shoes with firm, nonskid soles should be worn.
11. The patient should look ahead when walking rather than down at his or her feet.
12. The surface the patient is walking on must be clean, flat, dry, and well lighted. Throw rugs and objects serving as obstacles should temporarily be removed from the patient's environment.

Crutch Gaits

The type of crutch gait used depends upon the amount of weight the patient is able to support with one or both legs, the patient's physical condition, and muscular coordination. The patient should learn both a fast and a slow gait. The faster gait is used for making speed in open areas, and the slower one is used in crowded places. In addition, learning more than one gait reduces patient fatigue, because a different combination of muscles is used for each gait.

PROCEDURE 5-10

INSTRUCTING THE PATIENT IN CRUTCH GAITS

TRIPOD POSITION

The tripod position is the basic crutch stance used before crutch walking. It provides a wide base of support and enhances stability and balance (Fig. 5-7).

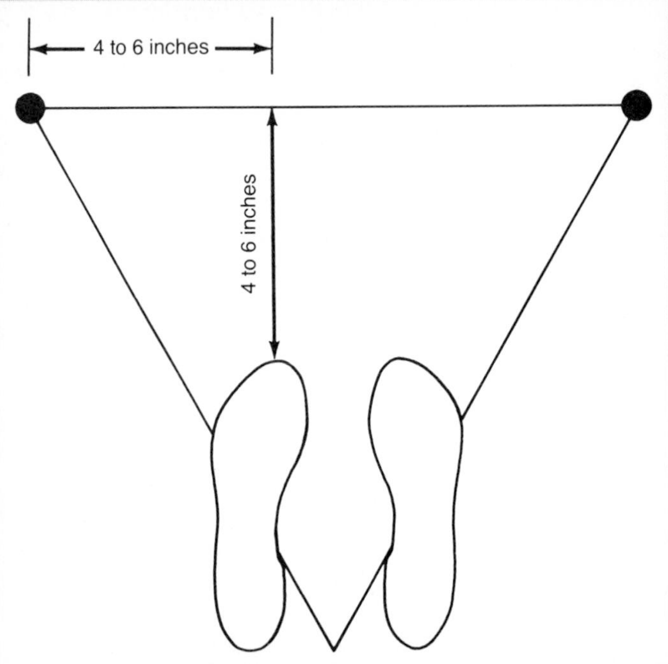

FIGURE 5-7. The tripod position is the basic crutch stance used before crutch walking. The crutch tips are placed 4 to 6 inches in front of the feet and 4 to 6 inches to the side of each foot. (Large dots represent crutch tips.)

Instruct the patient in the tripod position as outlined below.

1. Stand erect, and face straight ahead.

2. Place the tips of the crutches 4 to 6 inches (15 cm) in front of the feet and 4 to 6 inches (15 cm) to the side of each foot.

FOUR-POINT GAIT

The four-point gait is a very basic and slow gait. In order to use this gait, the patient must be able to bear considerable weight on both legs. The four-point gait is the most stable and safest of the crutch gaits, because it provides at least three points of support at all times. It is most often used with patients who have leg muscle weakness or spasticity, poor muscular coordination or balance, or degenerative leg joint disease. Instruct the patient in the procedure for the four-point gait following the steps in Figure 5–8.

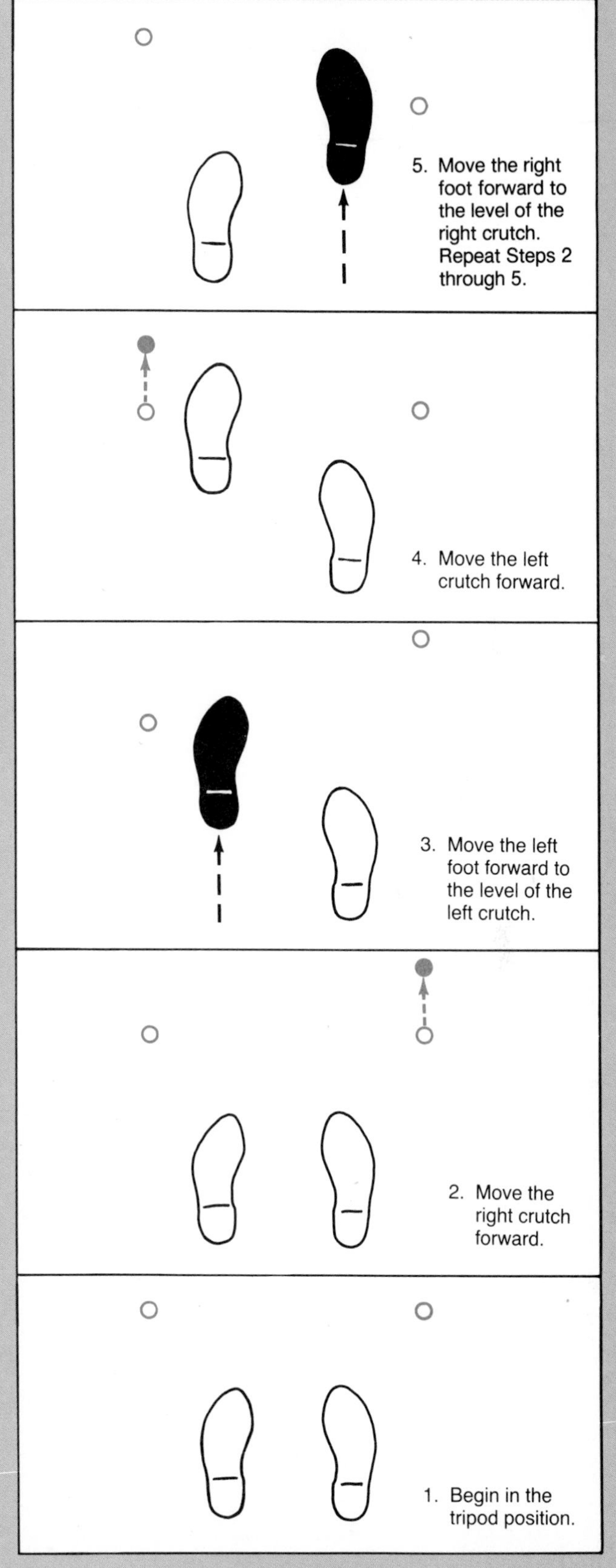

5. Move the right foot forward to the level of the right crutch. Repeat Steps 2 through 5.
4. Move the left crutch forward.
3. Move the left foot forward to the level of the left crutch.
2. Move the right crutch forward.
1. Begin in the tripod position.

FIGURE 5–8. Four-point crutch gait.

Continued

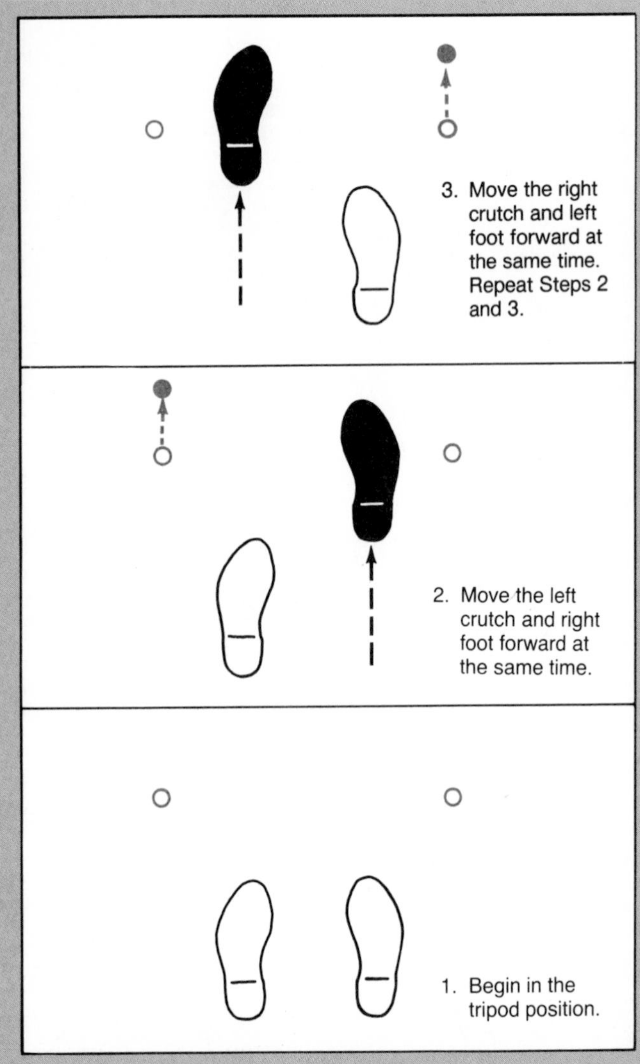

3. Move the right crutch and left foot forward at the same time. Repeat Steps 2 and 3.
2. Move the left crutch and right foot forward at the same time.
1. Begin in the tripod position.

FIGURE 5–9. Two-point crutch gait.

TWO-POINT GAIT

The two-point gait is similar to, but faster than, the four-point gait. This gait requires more balance because only two points support the body at one time. The two-point gait is used when the patient has partial weight bearing on each foot and good muscular coordination. Instruct the patient in the procedure for the two-point gait following the steps in Figure 5–9.

THREE-POINT GAIT

The three-point gait is used for the patient who cannot bear weight on one leg. The patient must be able to support his or her full weight on the unaffected leg. With this gait, the crutches and the unaffected leg alternately bear the patient's weight. This gait is used most often for amputees without a prosthesis, patients with musculoskeletal or soft-tissue trauma to a lower extremity (e.g., fracture, sprain), patients with acute leg inflammation, or patients who have had recent leg surgery. To use this gait, the patient must have good muscular coordination and arm strength. Instruct the patient in the procedure for the three-point gait following the steps in Figure 5–10.

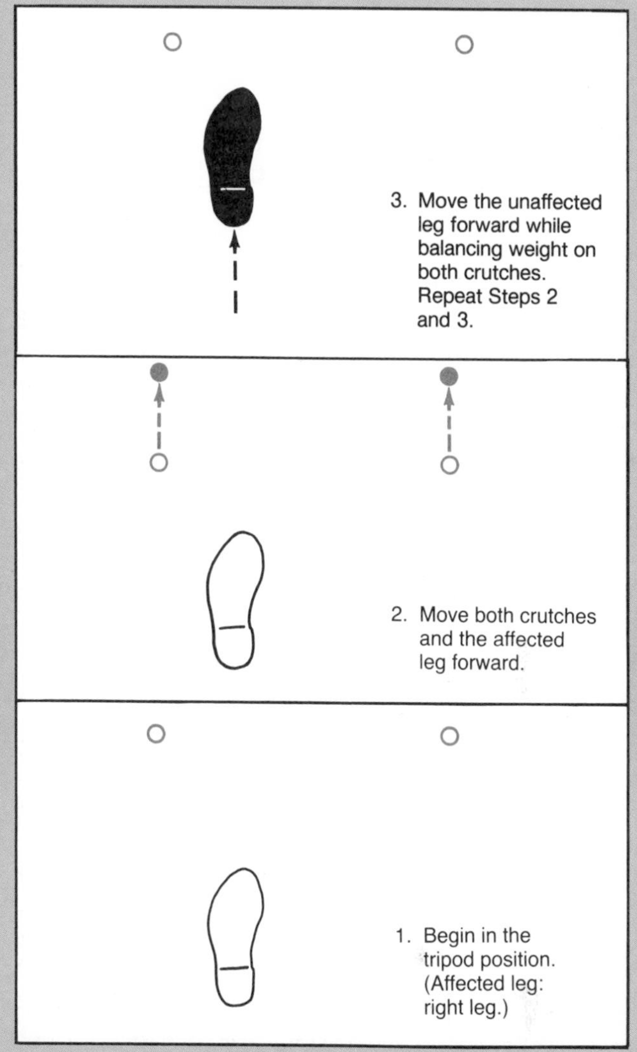

3. Move the unaffected leg forward while balancing weight on both crutches. Repeat Steps 2 and 3.
2. Move both crutches and the affected leg forward.
1. Begin in the tripod position. (Affected leg: right leg.)

FIGURE 5–10. Three-point crutch gait.

Continued

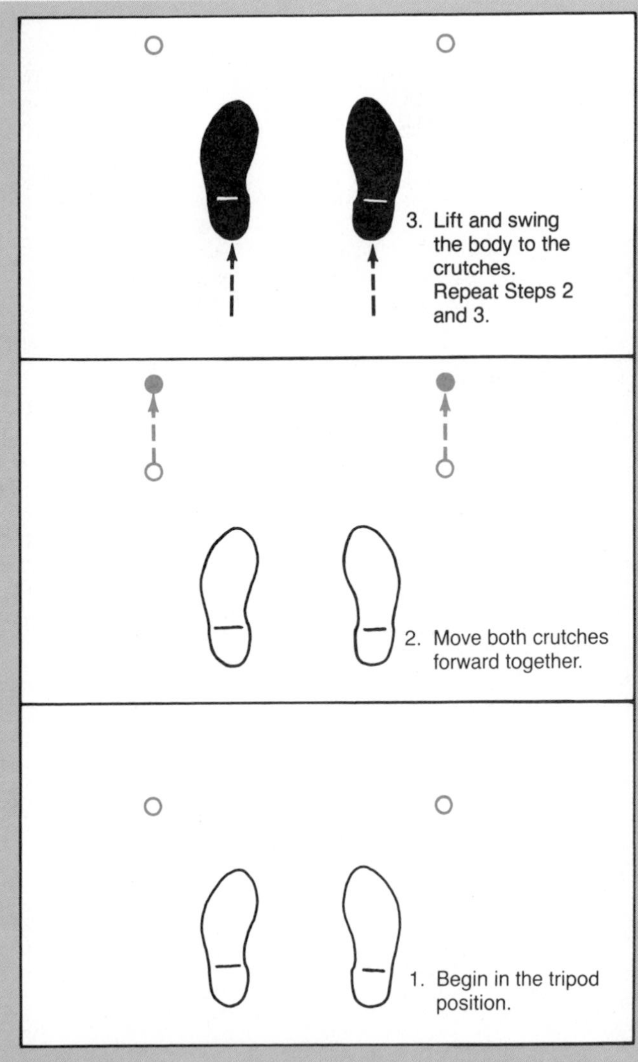
3. Lift and swing the body to the crutches. Repeat Steps 2 and 3.
2. Move both crutches forward together.
1. Begin in the tripod position.

FIGURE 5–11. Swing-to crutch gait.

SWING GAITS

The swing gaits include the swing-to gait and the swing-through gait and are used by patients with severe lower-extremity disabilities such as paralysis and by patients wearing supporting braces on their legs. Instruct the patient in the procedure for the swing-to-crutch gait, following the steps in Figure 5–11.

Instruct the patient in the procedure for the swing-through crutch gait following the steps in Figure 5–12.

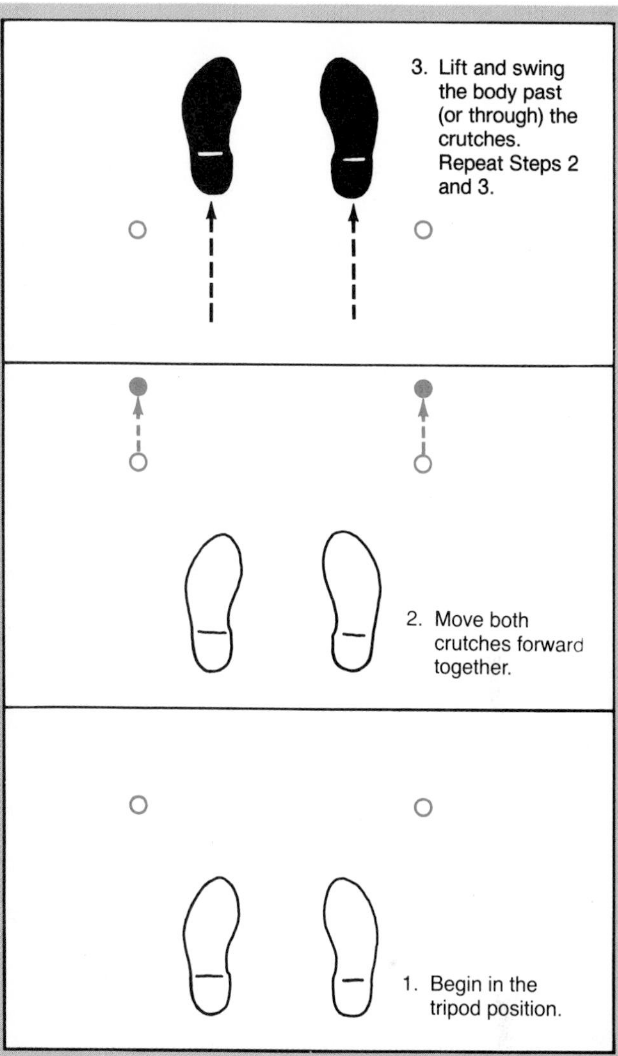

3. Lift and swing the body past (or through) the crutches. Repeat Steps 2 and 3.

2. Move both crutches forward together.

1. Begin in the tripod position.

FIGURE 5–12. Swing-through crutch gait.

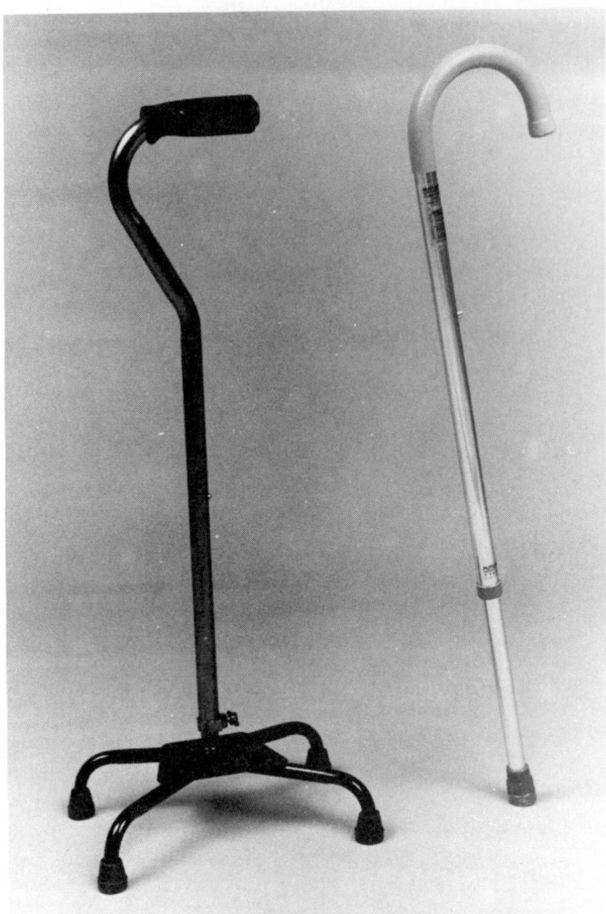

FIGURE 5–13. An example of a standard cane (right) and a tripod cane (left).

Canes

A cane is a lightweight, easily moveable device made of wood or aluminum with rubber suction tips used to help provide balance and support. Canes are generally used by patients who have weakness on one side of the body, such as those with hemiparesis, joint disabilities, and defects of the neuromuscular system. The three main types of canes are the *standard cane,* the *tripod cane,* and the *quad cane* (Fig. 5–13). The standard cane provides the least amount of support and is used by patients requiring only slight assistance in walking. The tripod and quad canes have three and four legs, respectively, a bent shaft, and a T-shaped handle with grips. They are easier to hold and provide greater stability than the standard cane because of the wider base of support. The disadvantage of the multi-legged cane is that it is bulkier and therefore more difficult to move. The cane length must be properly adjusted to ensure optimum stability. The cane handle should be approximately level with the greater trochanter, and the elbow should be flexed at a 25- to 30-degree angle. The patient should be instructed to stand erect and not lean on the cane to ensure good balance.

PROCEDURE 5-11
INSTRUCTING THE PATIENT IN USE OF A CANE

Instruct the patient in the use of a cane as outlined below.

1. Hold the cane on the strong side of the body (i.e., in the hand opposite the affected extremity).

2. The tip of the cane should be placed 4 to 6 inches to the side of the foot.

3. Move the cane forward approximately 12 inches (1 foot).

4. Move the affected leg forward to the level of the cane.

5. Move the strong leg forward and ahead of the cane and weak leg.

6. Repeat Steps 3 through 5.

Note: The cane and affected leg can be moved forward simultaneously (Steps 3 and 4); however the patient has less support with this method.

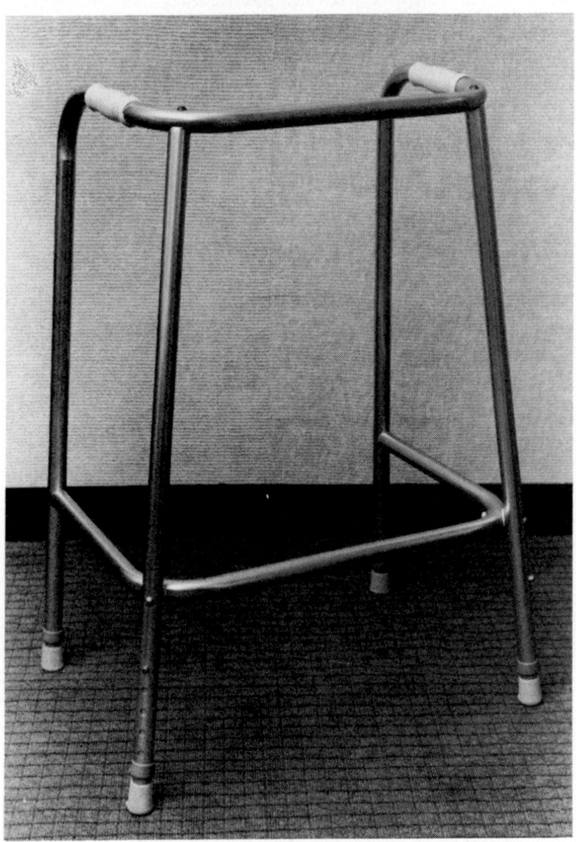

FIGURE 5–14. Example of a walker.

Walkers

A walker is an assistive device consisting of an aluminum frame with handgrips and four widely placed legs with rubber suction tips and one open side (Fig. 5–14). A walker is light and, therefore, easily moveable. For proper ambulation, the walker should extend from the ground to approximately the level of the patient's hip joint. Walkers are most often used by geriatric patients with weakness or balance problems. Because of its wide-base support, a walker provides the patient with a great amount of stability and security.

PROCEDURE 5-12
INSTRUCTING THE PATIENT IN USE OF A WALKER

Instruct the patient in the use of a walker as outlined below:

1. Pick up the walker, and move it forward approximately 6 inches.
2. Move the right foot and then the left foot up to the walker.
3. Repeat Steps 1 and 2.

Study Questions

1. What effects occur from the local application of heat?
2. What effects occur from the local application of cold?
3. What factors should be taken into consideration when applying heat or cold?
4. What is the general use of therapeutic ultrasound?
5. What factors are taken into consideration in determining the type of ambulatory assistive device to prescribe for patient use?
6. What guidelines should be followed by the patient to ensure safety during crutch use?

6

STERILIZATION AND DISINFECTION

CHAPTER OUTLINE

The General Sanitization Procedure
Physical Agents Used to Control Microorganisms (Boiling; Autoclave; Incineration; Dry Heat Oven)
Chemical Agents Used to Control Microorganisms (Disinfectants; Antiseptics)

COMPETENCIES

After completing this chapter, you should be able to demonstrate the proper procedure to perform the following:

1. Sanitize instruments, reusable needles and syringes, and rubber goods.
2. Wrap articles to be autoclaved.
3. Load the autoclave, operate the autoclave, and dry, remove, and store the load.
4. Care for and maintain the autoclave.
5. Chemically disinfect articles.

LEARNING OBJECTIVES

After completing this chapter, you should be able to do the following:

1. Define the terms listed in the vocabulary.
2. State the purpose of sanitization.
3. Explain why boiling cannot be used as a form of sterilization.
4. Explain the principle involved in sterilizing materials in the autoclave, and explain why the length of time necessary for autoclaving varies according to the type of article being sterilized.
5. State the qualities of a good wrapper for use in the autoclaving process.
6. List three principles that should be followed when loading the autoclave.
7. Explain the function of sterilization indicators, and list two types of indicators that may be used.
8. Explain how incomplete sterilization can occur when the autoclave is used, and list three causes.
9. List the materials that are best sterilized in a dry heat oven, and explain why a longer exposure period is needed for dry heat sterilization than for moist heat sterilization.
10. Identify four guidelines for operating the dry heat oven.
11. List the types of articles that are best disinfected with chemicals, and explain the basic guidelines for using a chemical disinfectant.

• VOCABULARY •

antiseptic (an" ti-sep' tik)—A substance that inhibits the growth of, or kills, disease-producing microorganisms but not their spores. An antiseptic is usually applied to living tissue.

autoclave (aw' to-klāv)—An apparatus for the sterilization of materials, using steam under pressure.

contaminate (kon-tam' i-nāt)—To soil, stain, or pollute; to make impure.

detergent (det-ter' jent)—An agent that purifies or cleanses.

disinfectant (dis" in-fek' tant)—A substance used to destroy disease-producing microorganisms but not necessarily their spores. Disinfectants are usually applied to inanimate objects.

incubate (in' ku-bāt)—To provide proper conditions for growth and development.

load (lōd)—The articles that are being sterilized.

sanitization (san" i-ti-za' shun)—A cleaning process to reduce the number of microorganisms to a safe level as determined by public health requirements.

spore (spōr)—A hard thick-walled capsule formed by some bacteria that contains only the essential parts of the protoplasm of the bacterial cell.

sterilization (ster" ll-i-za' shun)—The process of destroying all forms of microbial life.

thermolabile (ther" mo-la' bil)—Easily affected or changed by heat.

Introduction

The air and all objects around us contain microorganisms. The medical assistant is responsible for helping to reduce and eliminate micoorganisms to prevent the spread of disease. This can be accomplished by practicing good techniques of medical and surgical asepsis (refer to Chapters 1 and 7).

Physical and chemical agents can be used to destroy microorganisms found in the medical office or to inhibit their growth. The agent to be used depends on the number and type of microorganisms and the nature of the article on which they are found. Examples of physical agents commonly used in the medical office are moist heat and dry heat; examples of chemical agents are chemical disinfectants and antiseptics. Terms that will aid in understanding this chapter are listed below.

A *spore* is a hard, thick-walled capsule that some bacteria form by losing moisture and condensing their contents to contain only the essential parts of the protoplasm of the cell. Spores represent a resting and protective stage of the bacterial cell and are more resistant to drying, sunlight, heat, and disinfectants than is the vegetative form of the bacterium. Favorable conditions cause the spore to germinate into a vegetative bacterium, capable of reproducing again. Two examples of species of bacteria that are capable of forming spores are *Clostridium botulinum,* which causes botulism, and *Clostridium tetani,* which causes tetanus.

Sterilization is the process of destroying all forms of microbial life. An object that is *sterile* is free of all living microorganisms and spores. There can be no relative degrees of sterility—an object is classified as either sterile or not sterile. Agents commonly used to sterilize articles in the medical office include steam under pressure (the autoclave) and the dry heat oven.

Disinfection is the process of destroying disease-producing microorganisms; however, it does not necessarily kill the resistant spores. A disinfectant is usually a chemical, although there are other means of disinfecting, such as boiling; thus, disinfectants are generally applied to inanimate objects.

An *antiseptic* is a substance that also works by inhibiting the growth of, or killing, disease-producing microorganisms. Antiseptics are less toxic than disinfectants and can be applied to living tissue, such as the skin and mucous membranes. An antiseptic, like a disinfectant, is unable to kill spores.

The General Sanitization Procedure

Sanitization is a cleansing process that lowers the number of microorganisms to a safe level, as determined by public health requirements. In order for materials that are used in examinations, treatments, or office surgery to be properly sterilized or disinfected, they should first be cleansed, or sanitized.

The contaminated articles should be removed to a separate work area, away from contact with patients, to avoid the transfer of disease from pathogens that the articles may contain. If the articles cannot be sanitized immediately, they should be rinsed and/or placed in a soaking solution so that blood or any other organic matter does not dry and harden on them (this would be difficult to remove later on). The soaking solution must be rinsed off before the articles are sanitized. Most articles are best sanitized in a low-sudsing detergent that contains a rust inhibitor. After sanitization, the articles must be thoroughly rinsed to remove all traces of the detergent. The articles are then either sterilized or disinfected, depending upon what they are made of, what they are used for, and the medical office policy. The procedures for sanitizing instruments, reusable needles and syringes, and rubber goods are described on the following pages.

PROCEDURE 6-1
SANITIZING INSTRUMENTS

Instruments should be sanitized as soon as possible after use; otherwise, they should be rinsed with tap water and soaked in a detergent solution. Medical assistants must be careful not to cut themselves when handling sharp instruments, because this is another way in which infection can be spread. The procedure for sanitizing instruments is described as follows:

1. First rinse the instrument and then sanitize it in a low-sudsing detergent. The detergent should contain a blood solvent, if necessary.

2. Open hinged instruments and, using a small stiff brush, cleanse the grooves, crevices, or serrations, where contaminants such as blood, feces, or lubricants may collect. Otherwise, microorganisms can hide under these contaminants and therefore not be destroyed by the sterilization or disinfection process.

3. Check the instrument for proper working condition.

4. Rinse the instrument thoroughly with hot water; the hot water will precipitate the drying process.

5. Dry the instrument completely to prevent rusting. Instruments should not be lubricated or oiled, and all hinged instruments must be opened before they are sterilized or disinfected. This allows steam, heat, or chemicals to penetrate to all surfaces of the instrument.

6. Sterilize or disinfect the instrument according to the medical office policy.

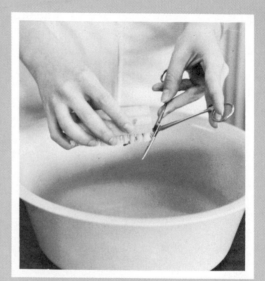

PROCEDURE 6-2
SANITIZING REUSABLE SYRINGES

Most medical offices use disposable needles and syringes to administer injections; however, reusable needles and syringes are commonly used in minor office surgery because they offer the advantage of being able to undergo the sterilization process. Because of this, reusable needles and syringes can be placed in a minor office surgery pack, which will also contain other instruments and supplies required for the surgery. The pack is then sterilized in the autoclave. In this way, the needle and syringe are already present in the surgical pack and do not have to be added before the physician performs the minor surgery.

Syringes must be sanitized as soon as possible after use to prevent the plunger from sticking to the barrel of the syringe. The procedure for sanitizing reusable needles and syringes follows.

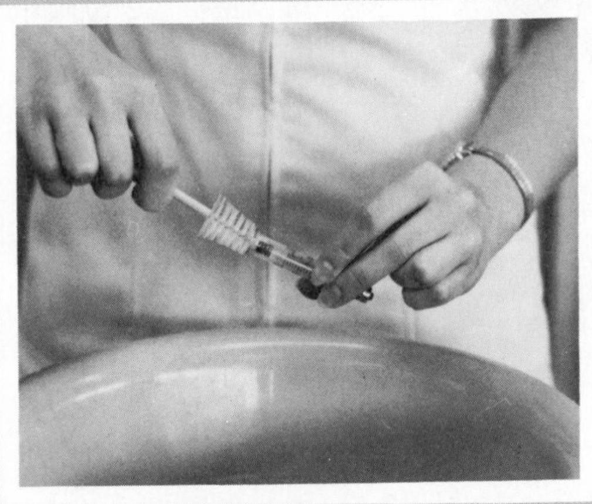

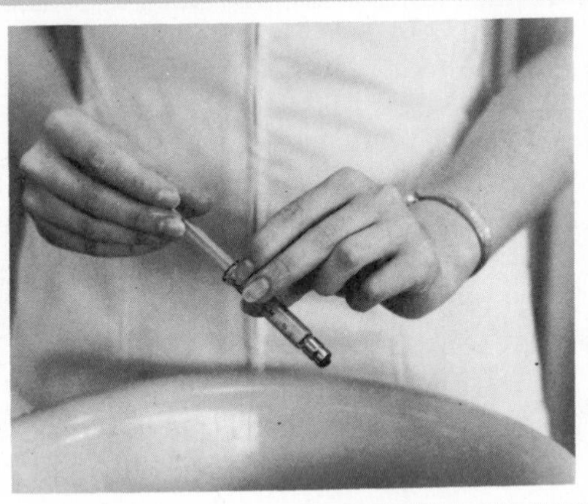

1. Separate the barrel and plunger, and rinse these parts with cold tap water immediately after use. This prevents contaminants, such as blood and medication, from drying and sticking to the surface of the syringe.

2. Wash the barrel and plunger with a low-sudsing, nonetching detergent. A nonetching detergent will not erode the ground glass surface of the syringe. Use a test tube brush to scrub the inside of the barrel of the syringe.

3. Thoroughly brush the outside of the syringe barrel and plunger. Force detergent through the tip of the syringe with the plunger.

4. Rinse thoroughly three times to make sure all the detergent is removed; for the first two rinses use tap water, and for the last rinse, use distilled water.

5. Wrap and sterilize the syringe according to the medical office policy.

PROCEDURE 6-3
SANITIZING REUSABLE NEEDLES

Protecting oneself is necessary when handling reusable needles to prevent accidental penetration of the skin and the transfer of infection.

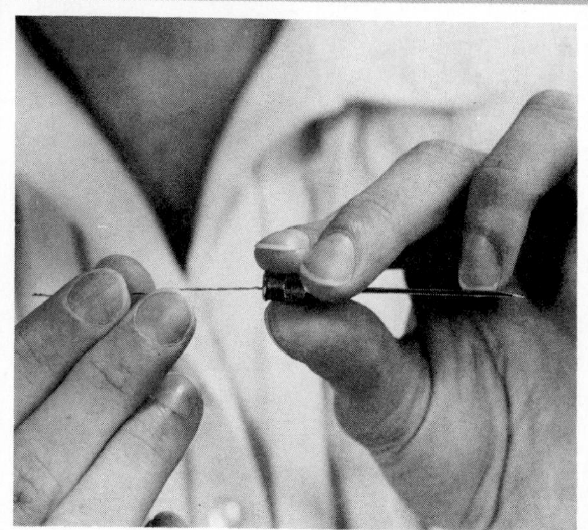

1. The needles should first be sterilized in the autoclave at 250°F for 30 minutes to remove contaminants such as harmful pathogens and thereby make the needles safe for handling by the medical assistant.

2. Insert a stylet through the lumen of the needle at the hub end to remove any contaminated matter present there; this prevents clogging of the lumen.

3. Place the needles in a hot solution of detergent that contains a blood solvent.

4. Clean the inside of the hub of the needle with a cotton applicator dipped in the detergent solution.

5. Wash the needles thoroughly, using a syringe to force the detergent solution through the lumen of the needle.

6. Inspect the point of the needle to determine if it needs to be sharpened. If the needle is dull or damaged, it must be resanitized after it has been sharpened.

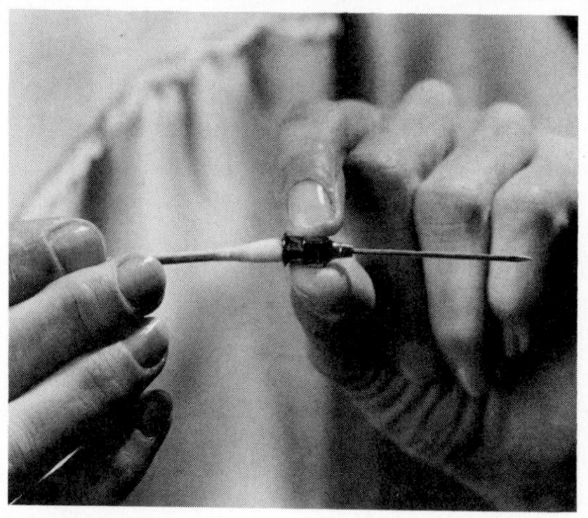

7. Rinse the hub and exterior of the needle with tap water. Rinse the lumen of the needle by forcing tap water through it twice with a syringe.

8. Wrap and sterilize according to the medical office policy.

PROCEDURE 6-4
SANITIZING RUBBER GOODS

Rubber goods are easily harmed by heat, light, and chemicals. Therefore, the medical assistant must try to protect them from excessive exposure to these agents. Examples of rubber goods used in the medical office include catheters, tubing, and gloves. The procedure for sanitizing rubber goods follows.

1. After use, rinse the rubber goods in cold water to remove organic matter.

2. Sanitize in a low-sudsing detergent.

3. Rinse thoroughly in fresh tap water.

SPECIAL INSTRUCTIONS FOR SANITIZING RUBBER GLOVES

1. During the sanitization process, cleanse the outside of the rubber gloves; then turn them inside out and repeat the cleansing process.

2. Rinse thoroughly. Fill the gloves with water and inspect them for any punctures and for organic matter that has not been removed.

3. Dry the gloves thoroughly and wrap them. The wrapping procedure is diagrammed in Figure 6-1.

When the dried rubber gloves are ready to be wrapped, they should first be powdered with a nonirritating starch preparation.

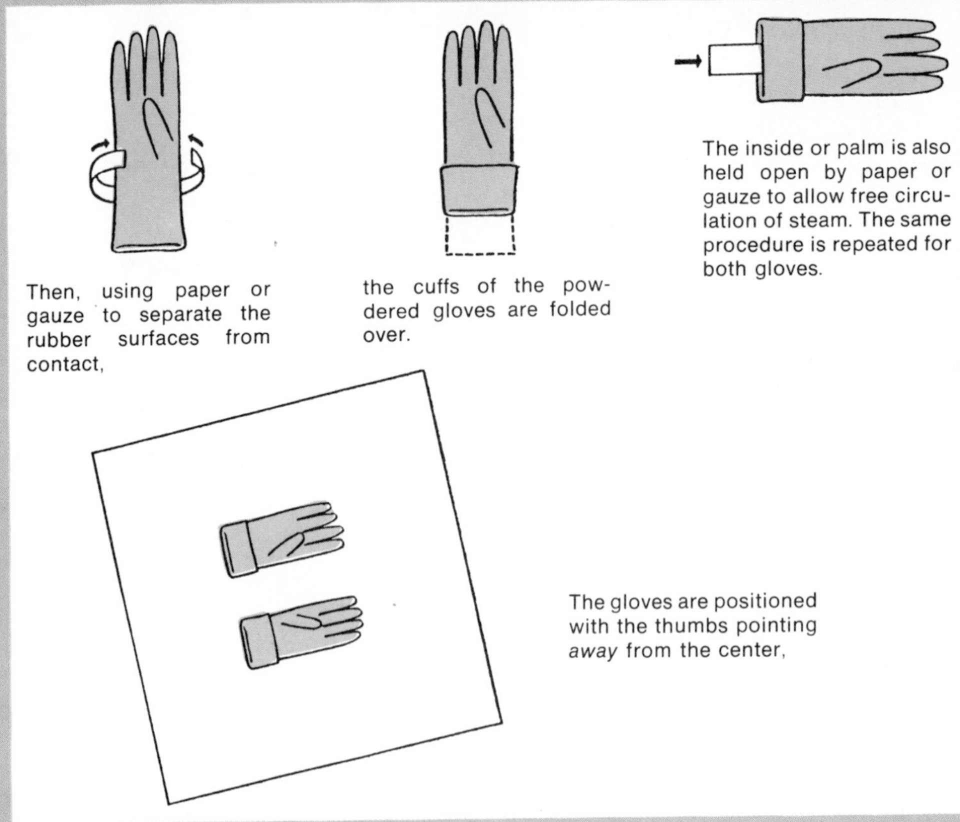

Then, using paper or gauze to separate the rubber surfaces from contact,
the cuffs of the powdered gloves are folded over.
The inside or palm is also held open by paper or gauze to allow free circulation of steam. The same procedure is repeated for both gloves.
The gloves are positioned with the thumbs pointing *away* from the center,

FIGURE 6-1. *See legend on opposite page*

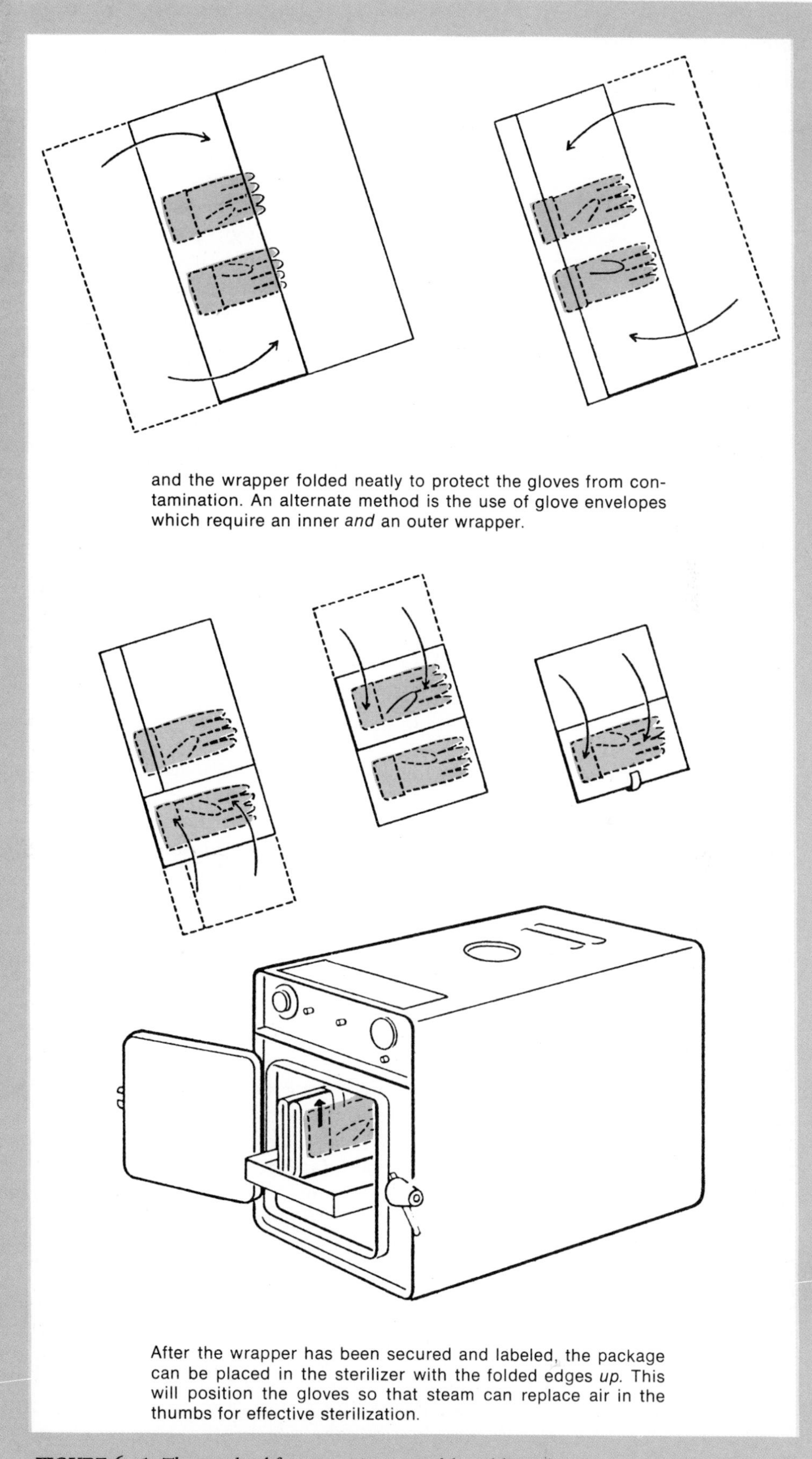

and the wrapper folded neatly to protect the gloves from contamination. An alternate method is the use of glove envelopes which require an inner *and* an outer wrapper.
After the wrapper has been secured and labeled, the package can be placed in the sterilizer with the folded edges *up*. This will position the gloves so that steam can replace air in the thumbs for effective sterilization.

FIGURE 6-1. The method for wrapping reusable rubber gloves.

Physical Agents Used to Control Microorganisms

Moist Heat

Boiling

Boiling functions as a disinfectant to kill most vegetative forms of microorganisms. However, this method cannot be used as a form of sterilization, because the maximum temperature that can be reached through boiling is 212°F (100°C). This temperature is not high enough to kill spores and the virus that causes hepatitis. Boiling can be used to disinfect instruments and supplies that do not penetrate body tissues; these instruments, such as nasal or aural specula, only come into contact with the outer skin or are shallowly inserted into body orifices.

The objects should first be thoroughly sanitized and then completely immersed in the water. Timing should not start until the water reaches a rolling boil, which is when the water boils slowly with the formation of only a few bubbles and liberates very little steam. A vigorous boil need not be maintained, because this will only reduce the water content through evaporation and the same temperature (212°F) can be obtained with a mild rolling boil. An object should be boiled for at least 15 minutes. Adding a 2 per cent solution of sodium carbonate will increase the disinfecting power of the boiling water and decrease corrosive action on metal instruments.

Steam Under Pressure—The Autoclave

The most commonly used method for sterilizing materials in the medical office is the autoclave. It is both dependable and efficient and can be used to sterilize objects that are not harmed by moisture or high temperature. Most autoclaves consist of an outer jacket surrounding an inner sterilizing chamber (Fig. 6–2). Water contained in a water reservoir is converted to steam under pressure. The steam is first allowed to enter the outer jacket and then, when the temperature builds up, it is permitted to enter the inner sterilizing chamber. The pressure plays no direct part in killing microorganisms; rather, it functions to attain a higher temperature than could be reached by the steam from boiling water (212°F). The cooler, drier air already present in the chamber is forced out through the air exhaust valve, which is located in the lower front area of the autoclave. It is important that all of the air in the chamber be replaced by steam. When air is present, the temperature in the autoclave is reduced and a temperature that is adequate for sterilization is not reached. When all of the air has been removed, the air exhaust valve seals off the inner chamber. The temperature, indicated on the gauge on the front of the autoclave, begins to rise.

The medical assistant should not set the timer on the autoclave until the gauge reaches the desired temperature. Generally, the autoclave is operated at approximately 15 pounds of pressure per square inch with a temperature of 250 to 254°F. The time varies according to what is being sterilized (Table 6–1). For example, steam can easily reach the surfaces of hard, nonporous goods such as glassware to kill microorganisms, requiring less sterilization time. On the other hand, porous items such as dressings require a longer sterilization time. Steam must penetrate to the center of the dressing fibers to assure sterilization. Rubber goods, however, may be damaged by exposure to excessive heat. To prevent this, the medical assistant should make sure to sterilize them for only the prescribed amount of time.

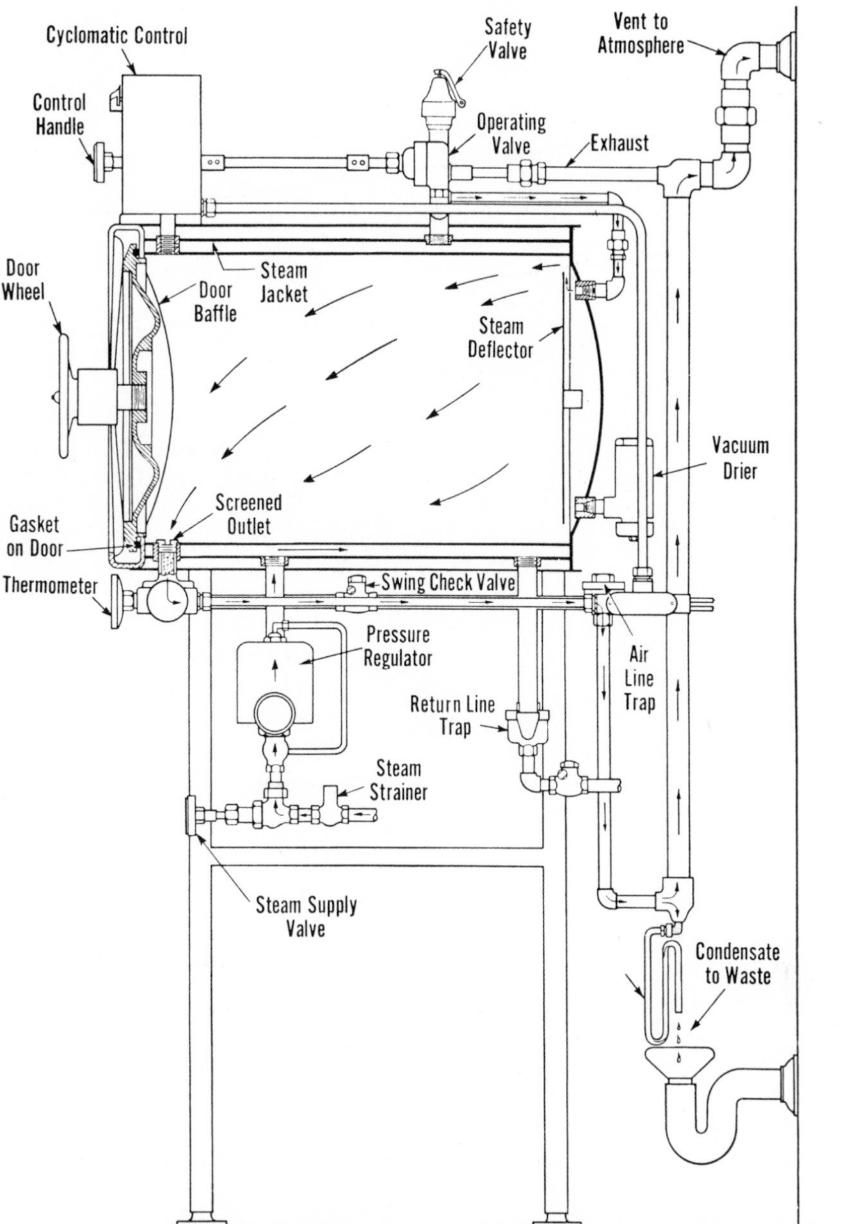

FIGURE 6–2. Diagrammatic illustration of steam-jacketed autoclave. Steam enters the *jacket*, a double-walled shell, at *source of steam* beneath the cylinder. It passes out the top through a pipe to which are attached a wheel valve admitting the steam to the inner *chamber*, a *safety valve*, and a gauge showing *pressure in the jacket*. The steam enters the inner chamber at the right of the diagram, filling the upper portion. Its pressure registers on the *chamber gauge*. It may be allowed to escape rapidly by the *exhaust valve*. If this is closed, steam pushes the cooler air in the lower portion out at the bottom (left), where the *thermometer* registers proper temperature only when the air is gone and is followed by the hot steam. The escaping steam may be allowed to flow out without building up any pressure if the *by-pass valve* is fully opened. If the by-pass valve is closed and the *shut-off valve* is opened, steam passes through the *thermostatic trap*, where the heat shuts off all but a pinhole opening. This causes pressure to build up in the chamber, yet prevents stagnation by permitting a constant minute flow of steam through the apparatus. (Courtesy of AMSCO/American Sterilizer Company, Erie, Pennsylvania 16512.)

TABLE 6-1. Minimum Sterilization Times

ARTICLES	TIME 250 TO 254°F (121 TO 123°C)
Glassware, empty, inverted Instruments, metal in covered or open tray, padded or unpadded Needles, unwrapped Syringes, unassembled, unwrapped	15 minutes
Flasked solutions, 75 to 250 ml Instruments, metal combined with other materials in covered and/or padded tray Instruments wrapped in double-thickness muslin Rubber gloves, catheters, drains, tubing, etc., unwrapped or wrapped in muslin or paper	20 minutes
Dressings, wrapped in paper or muslin—small packs only Flasked solutions, 500 to 1000 ml Needles, individually packaged in glass tubes or paper Syringes, unassembled, individually packed in muslin or paper Sutures, silk, cotton, or nylon, wrapped in paper or muslin Treatment trays, wrapped in muslin or paper	30 minutes

During the sterilization process, the steam penetrates the materials in the sterilizing chamber. The materials are cooler, so the steam condenses into moisture on them, giving up its heat. This heat serves to kill all microorganisms and their spores.

When the sterilization process is completed, the medical assistant must vent the chamber of steam to permit the pressure in the autoclave to drop and the chamber to cool. Some autoclaves will vent automatically, which eliminates having to vent them manually. The sterilized materials are moist and must be allowed to dry before they are removed from the autoclave, because microorganisms can move very quickly through moisture, resulting in contamination. The heat from the steam still present in the jacket aids in drying the articles. In addition, the door of the autoclave should be opened a crack to allow the moisture on the articles to change from a liquid to a vapor and thus to escape through the crack. The load should be allowed to dry for between 5 and 20 minutes, depending upon the manufacturer of the autoclave. The medical assistant must make sure her or his hands are clean and dry before removing the sterilized articles.

In order for the autoclave to work efficiently, it must be properly maintained. The instruction manual that accompanies it will contain specific information for the care and maintenance of that particular type of autoclave. In general, the interior of the autoclave should be washed every day with a mild detergent such as Calgonite; the chamber must be cool before the cleaning process is begun. A soft cloth or a soft brush can be used to clean the chamber, which should be rinsed thoroughly with clean, soft water. The chamber must be dried thoroughly and the door left open overnight. The metal shelves should be washed with Calgonite by the same method.

Preparing and Wrapping Articles. Articles to be sterilized in the autoclave must first be thoroughly sanitized according to the procedure described on pages 140 to 145. According to the medical office policy, the articles may then be wrapped. The purpose of wrapping articles is to protect them from recontamination during handling and storage after they have been sterilized. The wrapping material used should be made of a substance that is not affected by the sterilization process and should allow steam to penetrate, while preventing contaminants such as dust, insects, and microorganisms from entering during handling and storage. It should not tear or puncture easily and should allow the sterilized package to be

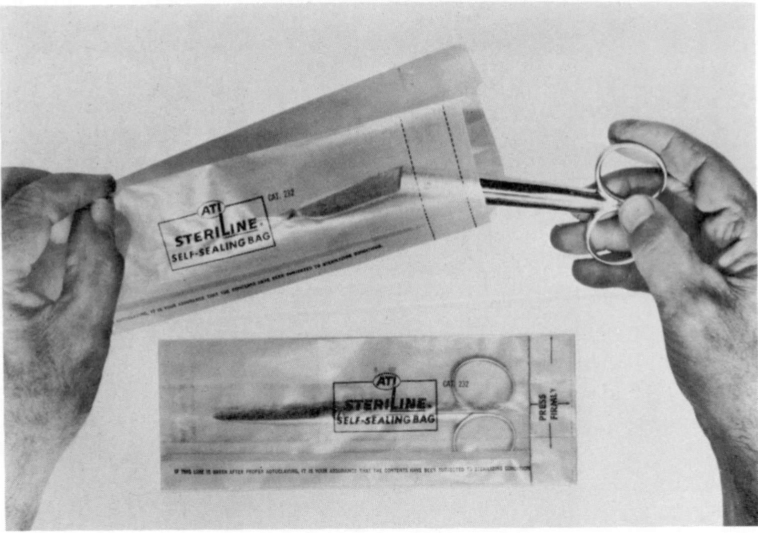

FIGURE 6–3. Disposable paper bags are available for sterilization of individual instruments and supplies in the autoclave. (Courtesy of Aseptic-Thermo Indicator, Parke, Davis & Company, North Hollywood, California 91609.)

opened without the contents being contaminated. A wrapper should not be used if it is torn or has a hole. Clean muslin and disposable paper are examples of wrapping material used for autoclaving (Fig. 6–3).

Articles must be wrapped in such a way that they do not become contaminated when the pack is opened. The proper method for wrapping instruments and supplies is diagrammed in Figure 6–4. First, the wrapper is placed on a clean, flat surface. The sanitized article is placed in the center of the wrapper. If the article has a movable part, such as a hinge joint, it must be left open to allow steam to penetrate all parts of the instrument. Next, the bottom edge of the wrapper is folded up over the article. The bottom corner of the wrapper is then folded back.

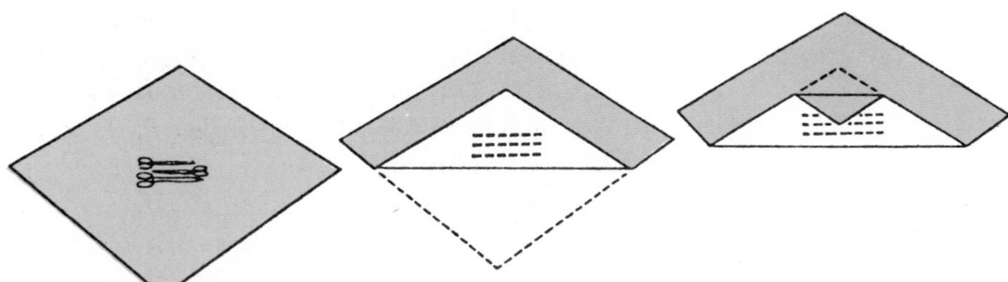

All items are placed in the center and the material folded up from the bottom, doubling back a small corner.

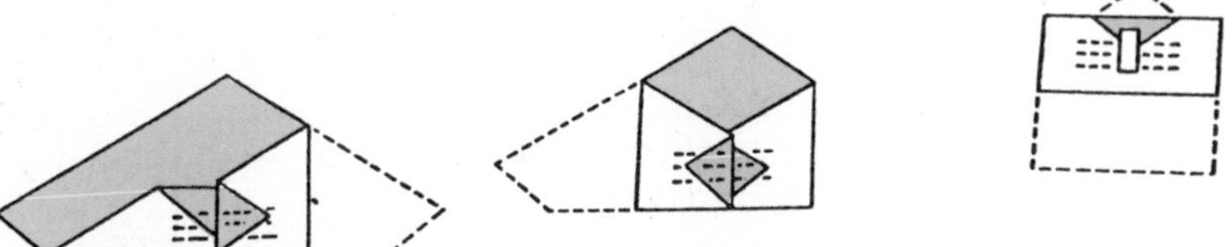

The right, then left, edges are folded over, again leaving corners doubled back. The pack is folded up from the bottom and secured with pressure-sensitive tape, then dated and labeled according to its contents. The pack should be firm enough for handling, but loose enough to permit proper circulation of steam. The materials included in each pack can be varied to suit the needs of each office, but the same wrapping pattern should be followed for all packs.

FIGURE 6–4. The method for wrapping instruments.

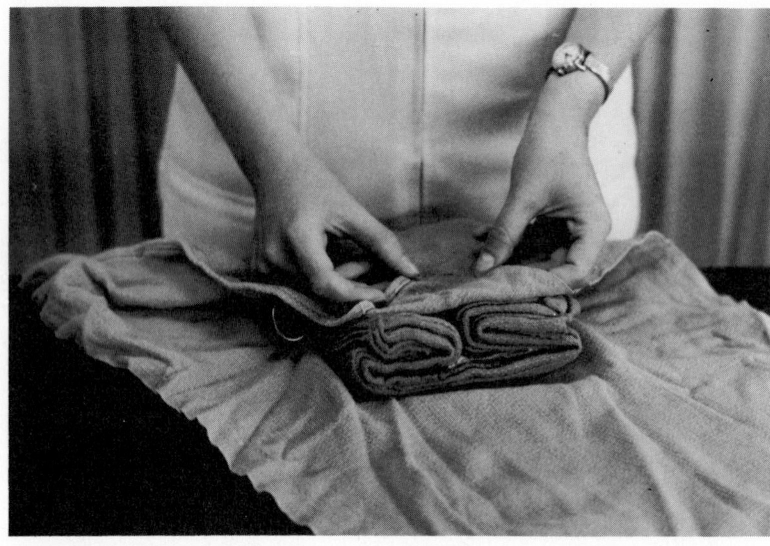

FIGURE 6–5. The medical assistant is preparing a prepackaged minor office surgery tray set-up. A sanitized fenestrated drape and surgical instruments have been placed in the center of the muslin wrapper. The bottom edge of the wrapper has been folded up over the articles and the medical assistant is in the process of folding back the bottom corner of the wrapper.

The right and then the left edges of the wrapper are folded over the article and both the right and left corners are folded back. Next, the pack is folded up from the bottom and secured with tape. The wrapped article is dated and labeled according to its contents (e.g., Dissecting Scissors, cvd 4/28/8_). This method of wrapping can be used for all types of instruments and supplies.

The medical assistant may be wrapping one or more articles in each pack; the number and type of articles placed in each pack is based on the needs of each medical office. If the medical office prepares prepackaged minor office surgery tray set-ups, there will be a variety of instruments and supplies that must be assembled in the pack (Fig. 6–5). The medical office usually maintains a list of the articles required for each minor office surgery pack, to be used as a guide in preparing it. The medical assistant must make sure to include all the required articles and label the pack according to its use (e.g., suture pack, cyst removal pack) (Fig. 6–6).

FIGURE 6–6. The wrapped minor office surgery pack is dated and labeled according to its use.

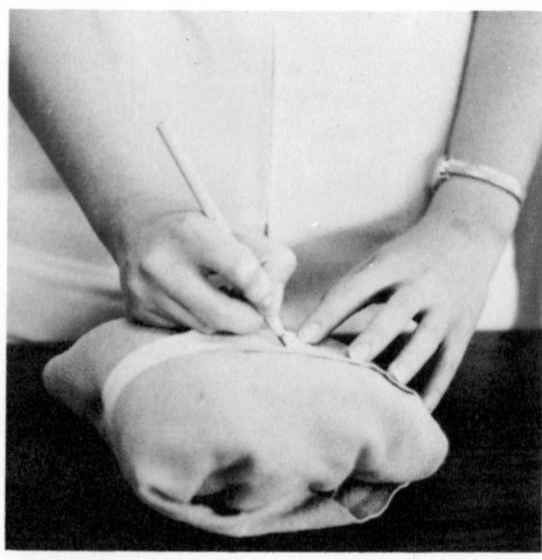

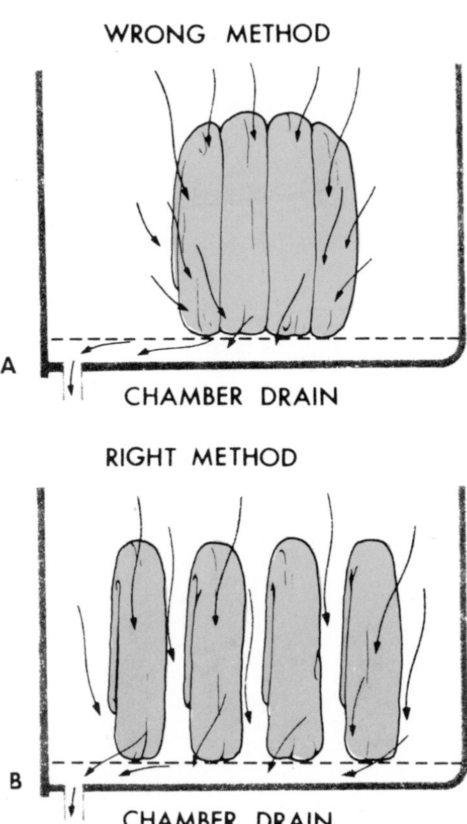

FIGURE 6–7. *A,* Improper arrangement of packs in autoclave. A large pack (here consisting of four smaller packs held closely together) prevents adequate penetration of steam, resulting in failure to sterilize the portions in the center of the mass. *B,* The large pack has been broken down into four small packs, and these are slightly separated from each other in the sterilizer. Steam will now permeate the entire mass quickly, and in the much shorter period of exposure needed there will be no oversterilized outer portions. (Courtesy of AMSCO/American Sterilizer Company, Erie, Pennsylvania 16512.)

Loading the Autoclave. The method by which the autoclave is loaded determines, to some extent, the effectiveness of the sterilization process. Small packs are best, because steam penetrates them more easily; it takes longer for steam to reach the center of a large pack to ensure sterilization. A pack should be no larger than 12 × 12 × 20 inches.

The materials should be packed as loosely as possible inside the autoclave, with approximately 1 to 3 inches separating all articles from each other and from the surrounding walls to allow for adequate steam penetration. Placing the articles too close together retards the flow of steam (Fig. 6–7). Jars and glassware should be placed on their sides in the autoclave with their lids removed. If they are placed upright, air might be trapped in them and they would not be properly sterilized. Trapped air should flow out and be replaced by steam during the sterilization process (Fig. 6–8).

Packs containing layers of fabric, such as dressings, should be placed in a vertical position. Steam flows from top to bottom, and this method allows the steam to penetrate the layers of fabric.

When fabrics, such as gauze dressings, and hard goods, such as jars, utensils, and treatment trays, are autoclaved together, the hard goods should be placed on the lowest shelves. This prevents the fabrics from becoming wet from the condensation that drips from the surface of the hard goods.

Sterilization Indicators. Materials that are being sterilized must be exposed to steam at a sufficient temperature and for a proper length of time. Sterilization indicators are available to determine the effectiveness of the procedure and to check against improper wrapping of articles, improper loading of the autoclave, or faulty operation of the autoclave. An article is not considered sterile unless the steam has penetrated to the center of it; therefore, many sterilization indicators are designed to be placed in the center of the article. The medical assistant should

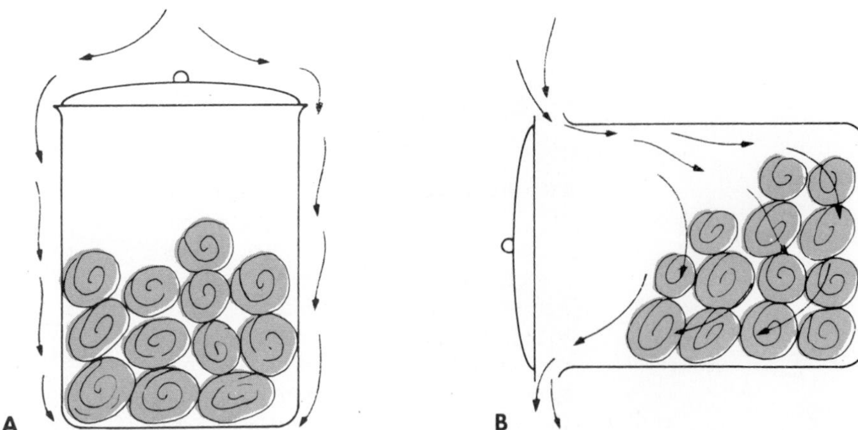

FIGURE 6–8. These line drawings show the correct and the incorrect way to place jars of dressings in the sterilizer. *A,* Right side up, even with the cover removed, all air is trapped within the jar. *B,* Resting on its side, with the cover held loosely in place, air will drain out and steam will promptly take its place, as indicated by the arrows. (Courtesy of AMSCO/American Sterilizer Company, Erie, Pennsylvania 16512.)

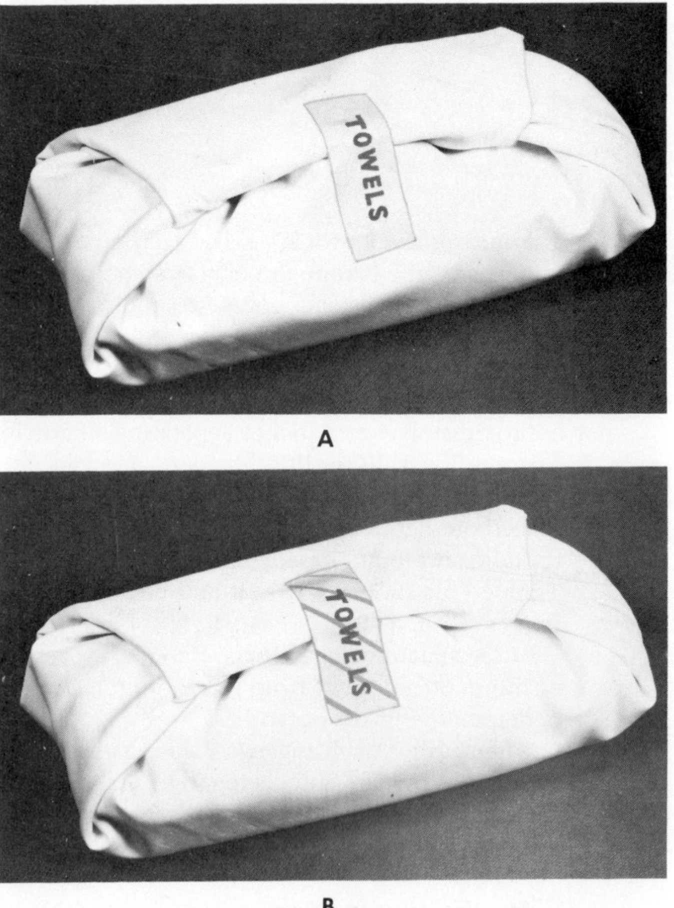

FIGURE 6–9. *A,* Before autoclaving: Autoclave tape easily and securely seals the wrapped articles in addition to identifying the contents. *B,* After autoclaving: Diagonal lines that appear on the tape during autoclaving indicate that the wrapped article has been autoclaved. (Courtesy of Aseptic-Thermo Indicator, Parke, Davis & Company, North Hollywood, California 91609.)

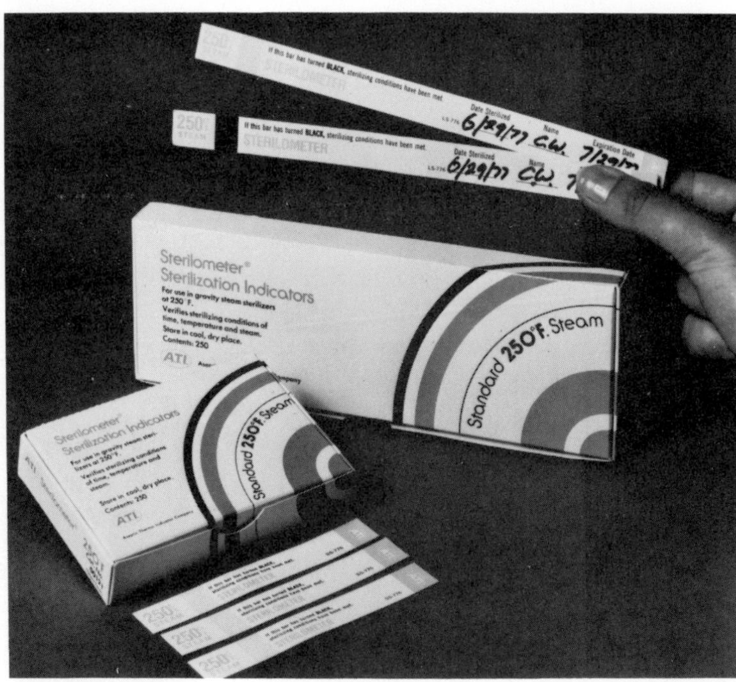

FIGURE 6–10. Sterilometer Sterilization Strips contain a thermolabile dye that changes from white to black when the correct combination of time, temperature, and steam has been attained. (Courtesy of Aseptic-Thermo Indicator, Parke, Davis & Company, North Hollywood, California 91609.)

thoroughly read the instructions that come with the sterilization indicators. The most reliable indicators check for the attainment of the proper temperature and also indicate the duration of that temperature.

Autoclave tape contains a chemical that changes color if it has been exposed to steam. The tape is available in a variety of colors, can be written on, and is useful for both closing and identifying the wrapped article (Fig. 6–9). However, autoclave tape is not intended to be a sterilization indicator. It does not assure that the proper sterilization time and temperature have been attained; it merely indicates that an article has been in the autoclave and that a high temperature has been attained.

Commercially prepared sterilization indicators containing a thermolabile dye change color when the correct combination of time, temperature, and steam has been reached. The indicator is usually placed in the center of each article to assure complete steam penetration and sterilization. Examples of this type of indicator include Sterilometer Sterilization Strips and Steam-Clox indicators (Figs. 6–10 and 6–11). Sealed glass tubes containing a wax pellet that melts when the necessary temperature has been reached are also available.

Culture tests are the best means available for determining the effectiveness of the sterilization procedure. These tests consist of strips of paper containing heat-resistant spores. A strip is placed in the center of two different wrapped articles. The articles are placed in areas of the autoclave that are the least accessible to steam penetration, such as the bottom shelf of the autoclave near the front (in close proximity to the air exhaust valve). After the strips have been exposed to sterilization conditions, they are removed from their wrappers and dropped into culture tubes containing a broth and are incubated for the period prescribed by the manufacturer (it may range from 24 hours to 7 days, depending upon the type of test used). If the proper sterilization conditions of time, temperature, and steam have been met, no growth should occur in the broth cultures. This would indicate that all the spores have been killed. Growth is evidenced by a clouding of the broth

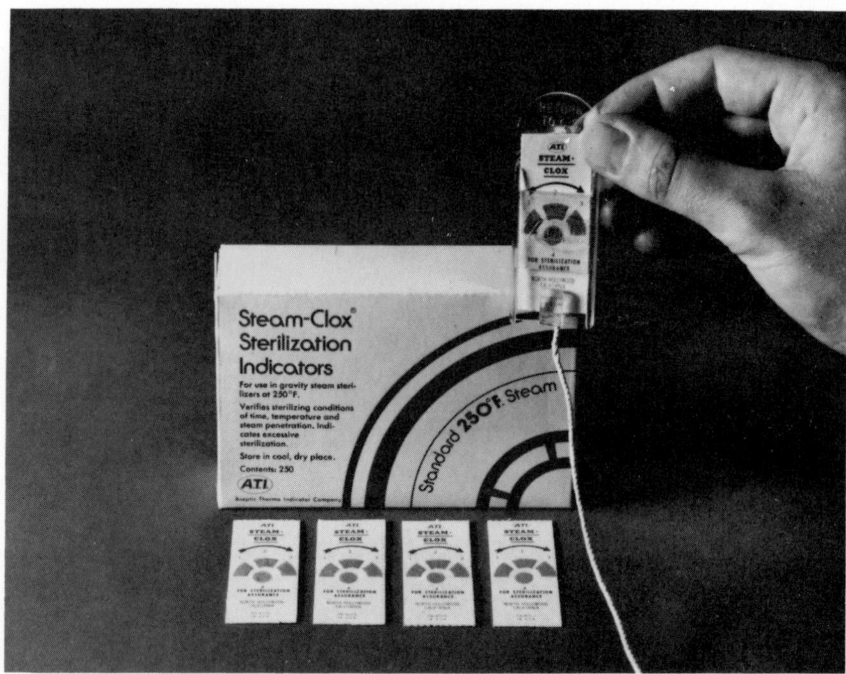

How to Use
1. ***Insert indicator into reusable holder.**
2. Place holder in center of each pack or package to be steam sterilized. Allow cord to extend from package.
3. Indicator changes color from purple to green as follows:

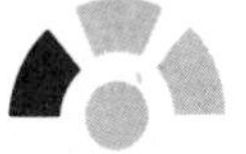
A. Insufficient steam penetration.

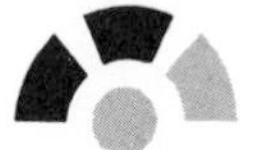
B. Partial steam penetration, but insufficient for complete sterilization.

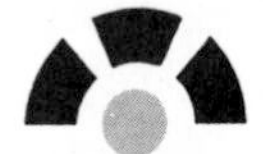
C. Sterilization conditions of time, temperature and steam have been achieved.

D. Excessive exposure time.

4. If indicator areas do not change color as described above, check sterilizing procedures and report to supervisor.

FIGURE 6–11. Steam-Clox sterilization indicators and how to use them and interpret results. (Courtesy of Aseptic-Thermo Indicator, Parke, Davis & Company, North Hollywood, California 91609.)

culture, whereas a clear culture indicates that no growth has occurred. A positive spore strip is generally used as a control to provide a comparison and to ensure that the broth contains the proper nutrients to encourage and support bacterial growth. The control is not exposed to sterilizing conditions and is dropped in a separate broth culture at the same time as the sterilized spore strips. The control should grow in the broth culture, causing the broth to become cloudy.

If an indicator does not change properly, a defect may be present in the sterilization technique or in the working condition of the autoclave. The article should be resterilized according to the proper procedure. If a defect in the working condition of the autoclave is suspected, the medical assistant should notify the physician, so that repairs can be arranged. Some of the causes of incomplete sterilization follow.

Causes of Improper Sterilization. Items may be improperly sterilized for a number of reasons, which are listed below along with some ways to avoid the problems.

Improper Preparation of Materials. The materials to be sterilized should be thoroughly sanitized first. Organic matter prevents adequate steam penetration to all surfaces of the article. Materials that are wrapped should be wrapped and sealed properly.

Incorrect Loading of the Autoclave. The materials should be packed loosely inside the autoclave to allow for adequate steam penetration. Packs containing layers of fabric should be placed in a vertical position to allow for good steam penetration. Lids should be removed from jars and glassware, which should be laid on their sides to prevent air from becoming trapped in them.

Faulty Operation of the Autoclave. The medical assistant should not start timing the autoclave until the correct sterilizing temperature is reached. This temperature must be maintained throughout the entire cycle.

Air in the Autoclave. Air in the autoclave takes up space that should be occupied by steam. Air is a poor conductor of heat and reduces the temperature in the autoclave, thus inhibiting complete sterilization.

Inadequate Drying of the Load. The load should be completely dry before it is removed from the autoclave. Microorganisms can easily move through moisture and contaminate the sterilized articles.

Storage. Sterilized articles should be stored in clean, dustproof areas that are free from insects and sources of contamination. Articles wrapped in muslin or disposable paper are considered sterile for 4 weeks. After this time, they should be resterilized. The medical assistant should check the date on each wrapped article before using it to make sure it is still considered sterile. If the package is torn or opened or if it becomes wet, it is no longer sterile and must be rewrapped and resterilized.

PROCEDURE 6-5
STERILIZING ARTICLES IN THE AUTOCLAVE

Sterilization procedures using the autoclave vary, depending on the type of autoclave and the medical office policy. However, a general procedure is outlined below to serve as a guideline for the medical assistant.

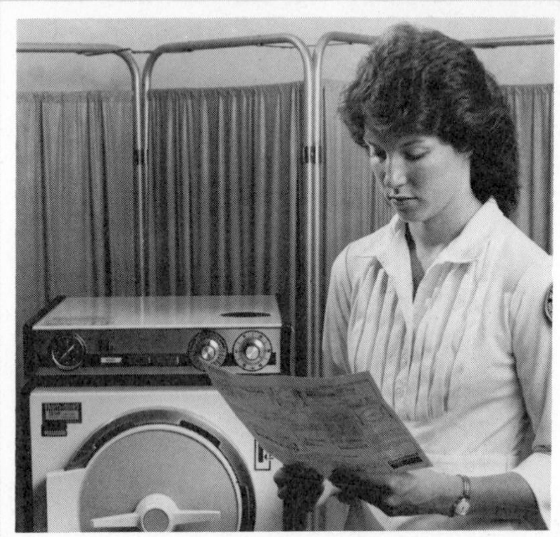

The medical assistant operates the autoclave according to the manufacturer's instructions.

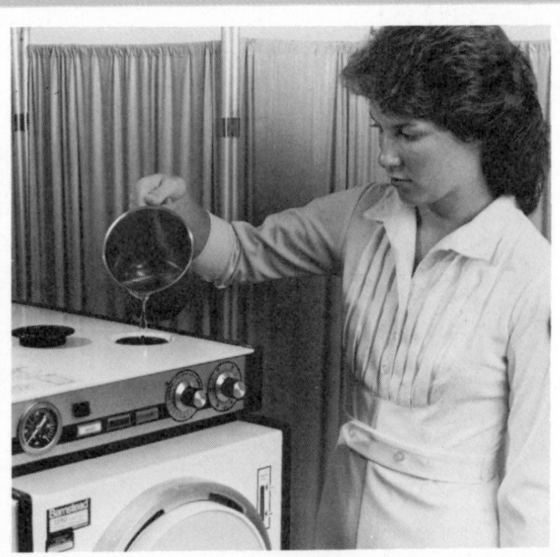

The water reservoir of the autoclave is filled with distilled water.

1. Remove the contaminated articles to a separate work area away from contact with patients. Refer to The General Sanitization Procedure, page 140.

2. Thoroughly sanitize the articles. Refer to the Sanitization Procedures, pages 141 to 145.

3. Wrap the articles, if required. Refer to Preparing and Wrapping Articles, pages 148 to 150.

4. Correctly position the sterilization indicators. Refer to Sterilization Indicators, pages 151 to 154.

5. Load the autoclave. Refer to Loading the Autoclave, page 151.

6. Operate the autoclave according to the procedure contained in the instruction manual. Also, refer to Steam Under Pressure — The Autoclave, page 146.

7. Dry the load according to the procedure contained in the instruction manual. Also, refer to Steam Under Pressure — The Autoclave, page 148.

8. Remove the load with clean dry hands.

9. Check the sterilization indicator to make sure the proper indicator response has taken place, pages 151 to 154.

10. Store the articles in a clean, dustproof area. Refer to Storage, page 155.

11. Maintain appropriate daily care of the autoclave according to the procedure contained in the instruction manual. Also, refer to Steam Under Pressure — The Autoclave, page 148.

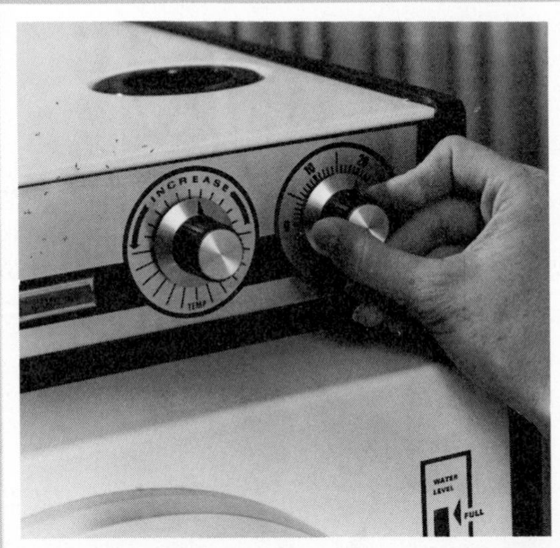

The medical assistant sets the timer on the autoclave when the temperature gauge reaches the desired temperature.

Dry Heat

Incineration

Incineration is a form of dry heat that destroys microorganisms immediately by direct flame. Incineration is commonly used to destroy contaminated disposable items such as tissues, dressings, and sputum cups. If the disposable item is grossly contaminated and likely to contain pathogens, it should first be wrapped in newspaper or a plastic bag to protect other patients and the trash collectors. Disposable plastic liners should be used in the trash cans to protect the person emptying the trash and to make sure no materials escape during transport to the incinerator. Burning must be complete to destroy all microorganisms and to prevent the spread of disease.

Dry Heat Oven

Dry heat ovens are used to sterilize articles that either cannot be penetrated by steam or may be damaged by it. For example, dry heat is less corrosive than moist heat for needles and instruments with sharp cutting edges; it does not dull their sharp points or edges. Oil, petroleum jelly, and powder cannot be penetrated by steam and must be sterilized in a dry heat oven. Moist heat sterilization tends to erode the ground glass surfaces of syringes, whereas dry heat does not.

A longer exposure period is needed with dry heat because microorganisms and spores are more resistant to dry heat than to moist heat and also because dry heat penetrates more slowly and unevenly than moist heat. The most commonly used temperature for dry heat sterilization is 320°F (160°C) for a duration of 1 to 2 hours, depending on the article being sterilized. Dry heat should not be used to sterilize rubber goods, because the long exposure period damages the rubber.

Muslin may be used to wrap articles for dry heat sterilization; however, high temperature of long duration may cause damage to the muslin fibers and shorten the life span of the muslin. A temperature over 320°F may cause charring or burning of the muslin. The recommended wrapping material is aluminum foil, because it is a good conductor of heat and also protects against recontamination during handling and storage. Dry heat sterilization indicators are available (Fig. 6–12) to determine the effectiveness of the sterilization process.

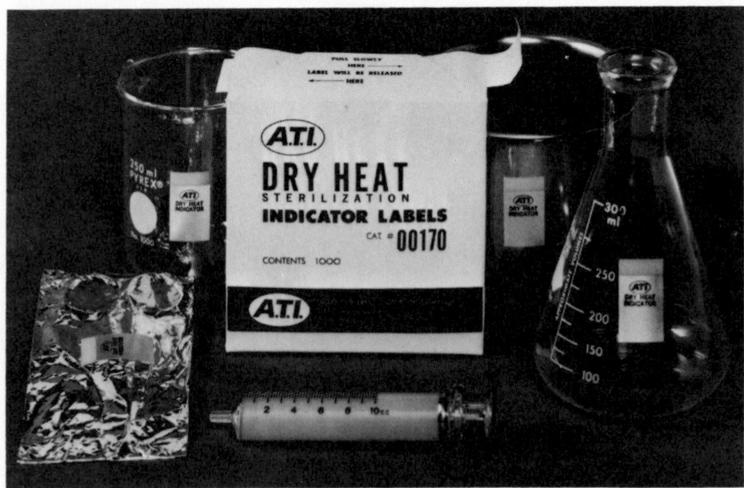

FIGURE 6–12. Dry heat sterilization indicators. (Courtesy of Aseptic-Thermo Indicator, Parke, Davis & Company, North Hollywood, California 91609.)

The guidelines for sterilizing materials in the dry heat oven are as follows:

1. Thoroughly sanitize the articles before sterilizing them.
2. Load the dry heat oven when it is cool to avoid burn injuries. Similarly, the dry heat oven should be unloaded when it is cool.
3. Do not overload the oven, but allow sufficient space between articles for adequate heat penetration to take place.
4. Remove lids from jars to prevent static air from being trapped inside them.
5. Do not start timing the load until the proper sterilization temperature has been reached.
6. Sterilize each article for the appropriate length of time and at the correct temperature.
7. Do not open the door during the sterilizing procedure. This may cool the temperature inside the oven, resulting in incomplete sterilization. In addition, the cool air rushing in from the outside may cause glassware to crack.
8. Allow the oven to cool before unloading it to prevent any glassware from cracking as cool air rushes in.

Chemical Agents Used to Control Microorganisms

Chemical Disinfectants and Antiseptics

Certain chemicals can be used as disinfectants and antiseptics to kill pathogens, but not necessarily their spores. Antiseptics are generally applied to living tissue such as the skin and mucosa of the throat, whereas chemical disinfectants are generally used on inanimate objects (Fig. 6–13). Disinfectants are too strong to be used on living tissue, because they may cause skin irritation. Chemicals are used to disinfect materials that may be damaged by heat, such as clinical thermometers. Since sterilization cannot be achieved with chemical disinfectants, they can only be used on those instruments and supplies that come into contact with the skin or are shallowly inserted into a body orifice. They cannot be used on instruments or supplies that penetrate the tissues of the body, since these articles must be sterile.

The article to be disinfected must first be thoroughly sanitized to remove organic matter such as dirt, blood, and feces. Organic matter may absorb the chemical disinfectant and inactivate it, and it also prevents the chemical from reaching the surface of the article; therefore, harmful pathogens may not be killed. After sanitization, the article should be thoroughly rinsed to remove all of the detergent, which may interfere with the disinfectant process. The article must be dried

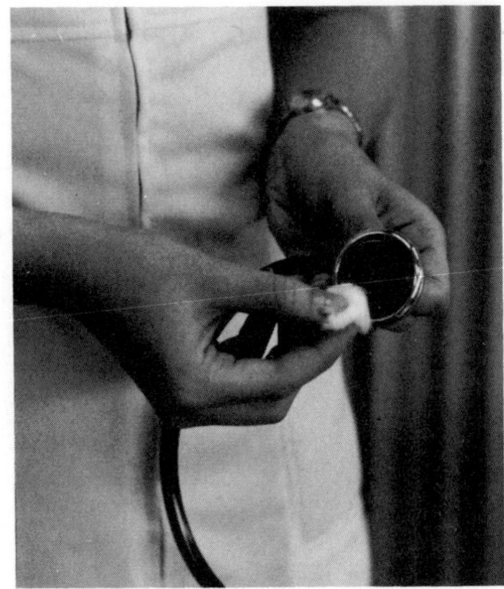

FIGURE 6–13. Cleaning the diaphragm of the stethoscope with alcohol, a chemical disinfectant.

completely because water dilutes the chemical and decreases its effectiveness. The medical assistant should read the instructions that come with each chemical before using it, for specific directions regarding its use. For instance, it may require dilution and will probably have to be applied for a certain length of time in order to kill all the pathogens that may be present. The instructions also state which microorganisms will not be killed. The article to be disinfected must be completely immersed in the chemical so that all parts are exposed to it. In addition, hinged instruments must be left open to allow the chemical to reach all parts of the instrument. The container holding the chemical must be kept covered and airtight to prevent evaporation of the chemical, which would change its potency. Some examples of chemical disinfectants utilized in the medical office follow.

Soap

Household soap is a good cleansing agent, but it is only a mild disinfectant. Most of its beneficial effects come from the mechanical scrubbing action associated with its use. In order to remove microorganisms effectively, scrubbing with soap should be followed by use of a suitable disinfectant. All the soap must be completely rinsed off before the article is immersed in the disinfectant.

Benzalkonium Chloride (Zephiran Chloride)

Benzalkonium chloride is a commonly used disinfectant. In a 1:1000 aqueous solution, it can be used for disinfecting instruments. It kills all vegetative bacteria, except tubercle bacilli and spores, in 30 minutes. Soap interferes with its action and should be removed by thorough rinsing, preferably with 70 per cent alcohol, because tap water may not remove all of the soap. Tincture of benzalkonium (1:750) is a colored solution that is used as a skin antiseptic for minor cuts and abrasions.

Alcohol

Alcohol is one of the most effective and widely used disinfectants and antiseptics. It kills all vegetative bacteria, including tubercle bacilli. Alcohol is commonly used to disinfect clinical thermometers, stethoscopes, and percussion hammers in the medical office. A disadvantage of alcohol is that it tends to rust instruments and dissolves the cement from around the lenses of instruments. The two types that are most commonly used are ethyl (grain) and isopropyl (rubbing) alcohol. The disinfecting action of ethyl alcohol is increased by the presence of water; therefore, a 70 per cent solution of ethyl alcohol is recommended. Stronger concentrations (95 or 100 per cent) are not as effective. Isopropyl alcohol is slightly more effective than ethyl alcohol, and its disinfecting action is increased in dilutions stronger than 70 per cent.

Phenol

Phenol is used mainly to disinfect walls, furniture, floors, and so forth. It is a corrosive poison and tends to be irritating to living tissue. It is expensive, and, because other disinfectants work as well, it is seldom used in the pure form. There are many derivatives of phenol that are more commonly used, including cresol, Lysol, and hexachlorophene (an example of a substance containing hexachlorophene is pHisoHex).

Iodine

Iodine is a well-known and commonly used disinfectant, but it does stain tissues and fabrics. It may be used to disinfect clinical thermometers. Tincture of iodine (containing 2 per cent iodine in an alcoholic solution) is used as an antiseptic for cuts and abrasions. Povidone-iodine (e.g., Betadine, Isodine) is an antiseptic consisting of povidone and iodine; unlike iodine, however, it does not stain skin and clothing. Povidone-iodine is frequently used in office procedures, including preoperative prepping of an operative site, postoperative application to prevent infection, and the treatment of minor wounds.

Other disinfectants include chlorine, formaldehyde (formalin), glutaraldehyde (Cidex), and several compounds of mercury: merbromin (Mercurochrome), nitromersol (Metaphen), and thimerosal (Merthiolate).

Study Questions

1. What is the purpose of sanitization?
2. What principles should be followed when loading the autoclave?
3. What is the function of sterilization indicators?
4. How can incomplete sterilization occur with the autoclave?

7

MINOR OFFICE SURGERY

CHAPTER OUTLINE

Surgical Asepsis
Instruments Used in Minor Office Surgery
Sterile Transfer Forceps
Wounds
The Healing Process
Insertion of Sutures
Suture Removal
Assisting with Minor Office Surgery
Medical Office Surgical Procedures

COMPETENCIES

After completing this chapter, you should be able to demonstrate the proper procedure to perform the following:

1. Apply and remove sterile gloves.
2. Open a sterile package.
3. Add a sterile article to a sterile field using a peel-apart package.
4. Use sterile transfer forceps.
5. Pour a sterile solution.
6. Change a sterile dressing and record results.
7. Remove sutures and record the procedure.
8. Set up a tray for each of the following surgical procedures: suture insertion, sebaceous cyst removal, incision and drainage of a localized infection, needle biopsy, ingrown toenail removal, colposcopy, cervical punch biopsy, and cryosurgery.
9. Assist the physician with minor office surgery.
10. Apply the following bandage turns: circular, spiral, spiral-reverse, figure-eight, and recurrent.
11. Apply a sling and make a cravat using a triangular bandage.
12. Apply a tubular gauze bandage and record the procedure.

LEARNING OBJECTIVES

After completing this chapter, you should be able to do the following:

1. Define the terms listed in the vocabulary.
2. Identify four types of procedures that require the use of surgical asepsis.
3. Describe the medical assistant's responsibilities during a minor surgical procedure.
4. List five guidelines that should be observed during a sterile procedure in order to maintain surgical asepsis.
5. Identify and explain the use and care of instruments commonly used for minor office surgery.
6. State the function of sterile transfer forceps, and list four guidelines to observe when using them.
7. Explain the difference between a closed and an open wound, and give an example of one type of closed wound and four types of open wounds.
8. List and explain the three phases involved in the healing process.
9. List two functions of a dressing.
10. Explain the method used to measure the diameter of suturing material.
11. Describe the two different types of sutures (absorbable and nonabsorbable), and give examples of uses for each.
12. Categorize suturing needles according to their type of point and their shape.
13. Explain the purpose of and procedure for each of the following minor surgical operations: sebaceous cyst removal, incision and drainage of a localized infection, needle biopsy, ingrown toenail removal, colposcopy, cervical punch biopsy, and cryosurgery.
14. State three functions of a bandage, and list four guidelines that should be observed when applying a bandage.
15. Identify the common types of bandages utilized in the medical office.

Continued

• VOCABULARY •

abrasion (ah-bra' zhun)—A wound in which the outer layers of the skin are damaged; a scrape.

abscess (ab' ses)—A collection of pus in a cavity surrounded by inflamed tissue.

absorbable suture (ab-sor' ba-b'l soo' cher)—Suture material that is gradually digested by tissue enzymes and absorbed by the body.

approximation (ah-prok' si-ma-shun)—The process of bringing two parts, such as tissue, together, through the use of sutures or other means.

bandage (ban' dij)—A strip of woven material used to wrap or cover a part of the body.

biopsy (bi' op-se)—The surgical removal and examination of tissue from the living body. Biopsies are generally done to determine if a tumor is benign or malignant.

capillary action (kap' i-ler" e ak' shun)—That action which causes liquid to rise along a wick, a tube, or a gauze dressing.

colposcope (kol' po-skōp)—A lighted instrument with a binocular magnifying lens used for the examination of the vagina and cervix.

colposcopy (kol-pos' ko-pe)—The visual examination of the vagina and cervix using a colposcope.

contaminate (kon-tam' i-nāt)—As it relates to sterile technique, to cause a sterile object or surface to become unsterile.

contusion (kon-too' zhun)—An injury to the tissues under the skin causing blood vessels to rupture, allowing blood to seep into the tissues; a bruise.

cryosurgery (kri" o-ser' jer-e)—The therapeutic use of freezing temperatures to treat chronic cervicitis and cervical erosion; also known as cryotherapy.

fibroblast (fi' -bro-blast)—An immature cell from which connective tissue can develop.

forceps (fōr' seps)—A two-pronged instrument for grasping and squeezing.

furuncle (fu' rung-k'l)—A localized staphylococcal infection that originates deep within a hair follicle; also known as a boil.

hemostasis (he" mo-sta' sis)—The arrest of bleeding by natural or artificial means.

incision (in-sizh' un)—A clean cut caused by a cutting instrument.

infection (in-fek' shun)—The condition in which the body or part of it is invaded by a pathogen.

infiltration (in" fil-tra' shun)—The process by which a substance passes into and is deposited within the substance of a cell, tissue, or an organ.

inflammation (in" flah-ma' shun)—A protective response of the body to trauma and the entrance of foreign matter. The purpose of inflammation is to destroy invading microorganisms and to repair injured tissue.

IUD (intrauterine device)—A mechanical device inserted into the uterine cavity for the purpose of contraception.

laceration (las" ĕ-ra' shun)—A wound in which the tissues are torn apart, leaving ragged and irregular edges.

ligate (li' gāt)—To tie off and close a structure such as a severed blood vessel.

local anesthetic (lo' kal an" es-thet' ik)—A drug that produces a loss of feeling and an inability to perceive pain in only a specific part of the body.

Mayo tray (ma' o tra)—A broad, flat metal tray placed on a stand and used to hold sterile instruments and supplies once it has been covered with a sterile towel.

needle biopsy (ne' d'l bi-op-se)—A type of biopsy in which tissue from deep within the body is obtained by the insertion of a biopsy needle through the skin.

nonabsorbable suture (non-ab-sor' ba-b'l soo' cher)—Suture material that is not absorbed by the body and either remains permanently in the body tissue and becomes encapsulated by fibrous tissue or is removed.

Continued

postoperative (pōst-op' er-ah-tiv)—After a surgical operation.

preoperative (pre-op' er-ah-tiv)—Preceding a surgical operation.

puncture (pungk' tur)—A wound made by a sharp pointed object piercing the skin.

scalpel (skal' pel)—A surgical knife used to divide tissues.

scissors (siz' erz)—A cutting instrument.

sebaceous cyst (se-ba' shus sist)—A thin closed sac or capsule containing fatty secretions from a sebaceous gland.

serum (se' rum)—The clear, straw-colored part of the blood that remains after the solid elements have been separated out of it.

sponge (spunj)—A porous, absorbent pad, such as a 4-inch gauze pad or cotton surrounded by gauze, used to absorb fluids, to apply medication, or to cleanse an area.

sterile (ster' il)—Free from all living microorganisms.

surgical asepsis (ser' je-kal a-sep' sis)—Those practices that keep objects and areas sterile or free from microorganisms.

sutures (soo' cherz)—Material used to approximate tissues with surgical stitches.

swaged needle (swājd ne' d'l)—A needle with suturing material permanently attached to the end of the needle.

wound (wo͞ond)—A break in the continuity of an external or internal surface caused by physical means.

16. Explain the use of a tubular gauze bandage.
17. Explain the principles underlying each step in the minor office surgery procedures.

Introduction

Various types of minor surgical operations may be performed in the medical office, such as insertion of sutures, sebaceous cyst removal, incision and drainage of infections, needle biopsies, cervical biopsies, and ingrown toenail removal. The physician explains the nature of the surgical procedure and any risks to the patient and offers to answer any questions. The medical assistant is responsible for helping to reassure the patient and may also be responsible for obtaining the patient's signature on a written consent form, which grants the physician permission to perform the surgery (Fig. 7–1).

Additional responsibilities of the medical assistant involve preparing the treatment room, preparing the patient, preparing the minor surgery tray, assisting the physician during the procedure, administering postoperative care to the patient, and cleaning the treatment room after the procedure.

The treatment room must be spotlessly clean, and the medical assistant should make sure the physician has adequate lighting for the procedure. The patient is positioned and draped according to the procedure to be performed. Sterile fenestrated drapes are often used. They have an opening that is placed directly over the operative area. The skin is prepared as specified by the physician. Hair around the operative site is considered a contaminant and may need to be removed by shaving. The skin is cleansed and an appropriate antiseptic is applied to the area to reduce the number of microorganisms present. The medical assistant prepares the minor surgery tray using sterile technique. The specific instruments and supplies included in each set-up will vary somewhat, depending on the physician's preference. Therefore, the medical assistant must become familiar with the instruments and supplies required for each surgical procedure performed in the medical office. During the operation, the medical assistant is present to assist the physician as needed and to lend support to the patient. The medical assistant should become completely familiar with each surgical procedure and learn to anticipate the needs of the physician, to help the operation proceed quickly and smoothly. After the operation, the medical assistant should remain with the patient as a safety precaution, to prevent accidental falls or other injuries and to make sure the patient understands the postoperative instructions. The medical assistant then removes and properly cares for all used instruments and supplies and cleans the treatment room in preparation for the next patient.

Surgical Asepsis

Surgical asepsis, also known as sterile technique, refers to those practices that keep objects and areas sterile, or free from all living microorganisms. Surgical asepsis protects the patient from pathogenic microorganisms that may enter the body and cause disease. It is always employed under the following circumstances: when caring for broken skin, such as open wounds and suture punctures; when a skin surface is being penetrated, such as by a surgical incision or the administration of an injection (the needle must remain sterile); or when a body cavity is entered that is normally sterile, such as during the insertion of a urinary catheter. Sterility of instruments and supplies is achieved through the use of disposable sterile items or by sterilizing reusable articles (see Chapter 6).

A sterile object that touches anything unsterile is automatically considered contaminated and must not be used. A medical assistant in doubt or who has a question concerning the sterility of an article, should consider it contaminated and replace it with a sterile article.

Sterility of the hands cannot be attained. Handwashing renders them medically aseptic and must be performed before and after each surgical procedure using proper technique (see Chapter 1). To prevent contamination of sterile articles, sterile transfer forceps or sterile gloves must be used to pick up or transfer articles during a sterile procedure.

The following guidelines must be observed during a sterile procedure to maintain surgical asepsis:

1. Take precautions to prevent sterile packages from becoming wet. Wet packages draw microorganisms into the package owing to the capillary action of the liquid, resulting in contamination of the sterile package. If a sterile package that has been prepared at the medical office becomes wet, it must be resterilized; if a disposable sterile package becomes wet, it must be discarded.
2. A 1-inch border around the sterile field is considered contaminated or unsterile, because this area may have become contaminated while the sterile field was being set up.
3. Always face the sterile field. If you must turn your back to it or leave the room, a sterile towel must be placed over the sterile field.

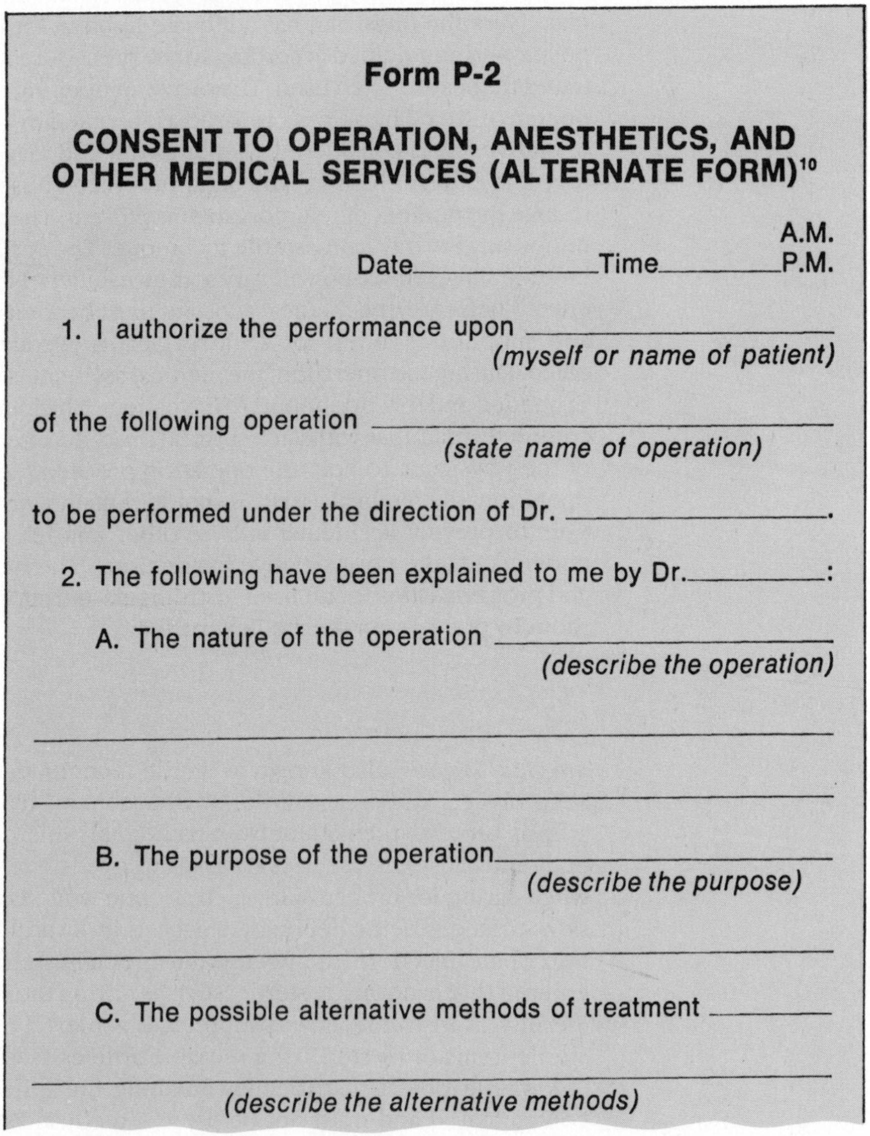

Form P-2

CONSENT TO OPERATION, ANESTHETICS, AND OTHER MEDICAL SERVICES (ALTERNATE FORM)[10]

Date__________ Time__________ A.M. / P.M.

1. I authorize the performance upon ________________
(myself or name of patient)

of the following operation ________________
(state name of operation)

to be performed under the direction of Dr. ____________.

2. The following have been explained to me by Dr.________:

A. The nature of the operation ________________
(describe the operation)

____

____

B. The purpose of the operation________________
(describe the purpose)

____

C. The possible alternative methods of treatment ________

____
(describe the alternative methods)

FIGURE 7–1

Illustration continued on opposite page

D. The possible consequences of the operation ________

____

(describe the possible consequences)

E. The risks involved ________________________

(describe the risks involved)

____

F. The possibility of complications ________________

____

(describe the possible complications)

3. I have been advised of the serious nature of the operation and have been advised that if I desire a further and more detailed explanation of any of the foregoing or further information about the possible risks or complications of the above listed operation it will be given to me.

4. I do not request a further and more detailed listing and explanation of any of the items listed in paragraph 2.

Signed ________________________

(Patient or person authorized to consent for patient)

Witness________________

FIGURE 7–1. Example of a written consent form. (From *Medicolegal Forms with Legal Analysis.* 3rd Edition, Office of the General Counsel, 1973, p. 59. Copyright © 1973, American Medical Association.)

4. Hold all sterile articles above waist level. Anything out of sight may become contaminated. The sterile articles should also be held in front of you and should not be allowed to touch your uniform.

5. To avoid contamination, all sterile items should be placed in the center of the sterile field and not around the edges.

6. Be careful not to spill water or solutions on the sterile field. The area beneath the field is contaminated, and microorganisms will be drawn up onto the field by the capillary action of the liquid, resulting in contamination of the field.

7. Do not talk, cough, or sneeze over a sterile field. Water vapor from the nose, mouth, and lungs will be carried out by the air and contaminate the sterile field.

8. Do not reach over a sterile field. Dust or lint from your clothing may fall onto it or your unsterile clothing may accidentally touch it.

9. Do not pass soiled dressings over the sterile field.

10. Always acknowledge if you have contaminated the sterile field, so that proper steps can be taken to regain sterility.

Instruments Used in Minor Office Surgery

A variety of surgical instruments are used for minor office surgery. Most instruments are made from stainless steel and have either a bright, highly polished finish or a dull finish. The medical assistant should become familiar with the name, use, and proper care of the instruments used in the medical office. Some of the more common instruments are described here and are illustrated in Figure 7–2.

A *scalpel* is a small, straight surgical knife consisting of a handle and a thin, sharp blade that has a convex edge. It is used to make surgical incisions and can divide

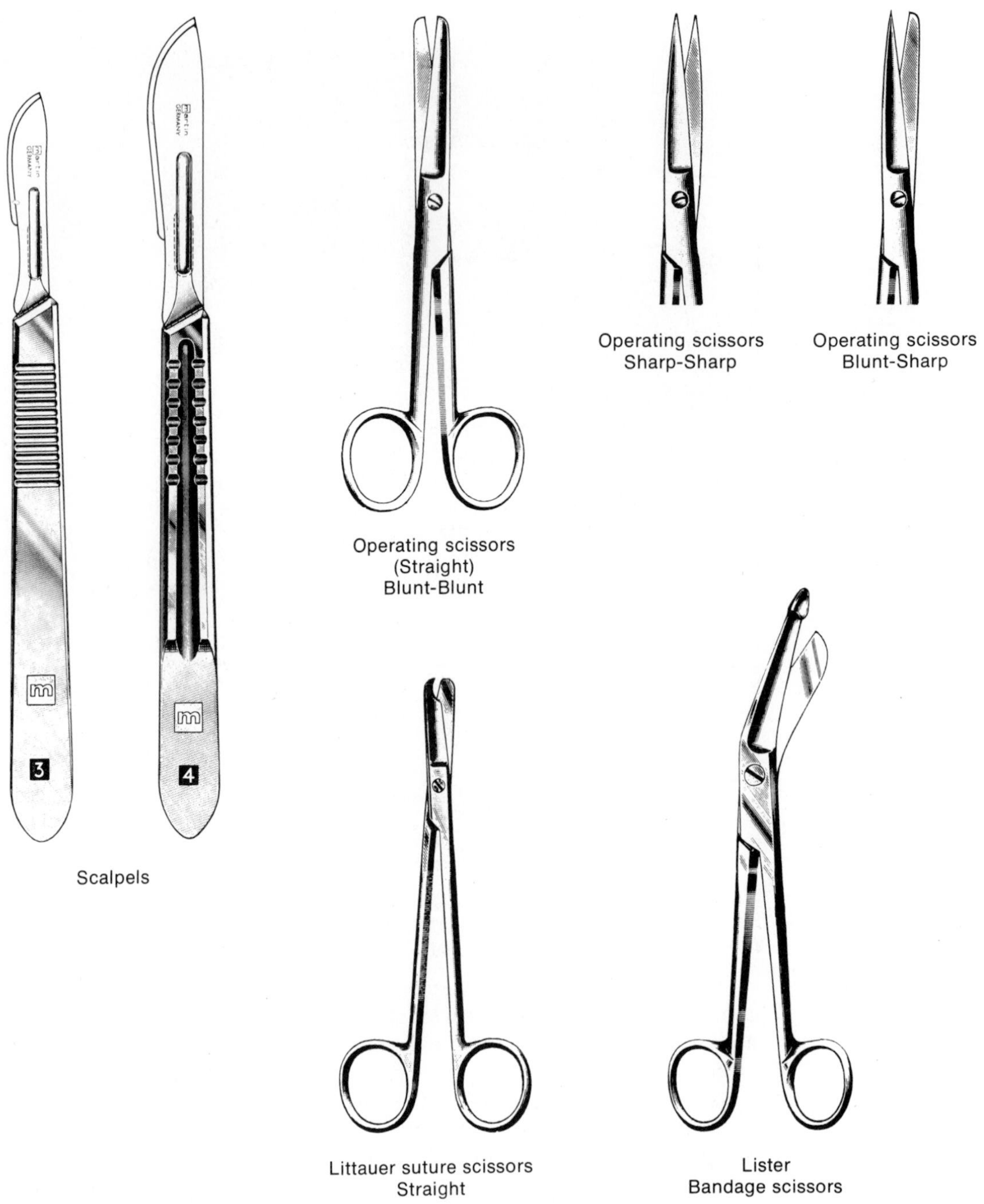

FIGURE 7 – 2. Instruments used in minor office surgery. (Courtesy of Elmed Incorporated, Addison, Illinois.)

tissue with the least possible trauma to the surrounding structures. Both reusable and disposable scalpels are available; scalpels having a reusable handle and a disposable blade are used most frequently.

Scissors are cutting instruments that have either straight (str) or curved (cvd) blades. Both blade tips may be sharp (s/s), both may be blunt (b/b), or one tip may be blunt and the other sharp (b/s). The two parts making up a pair of scissors come together at a hinge joint known as a box lock. The type of scissors employed depends on the intended use. *Operating scissors* have straight delicate blades that have a sharp cutting edge and are used for cutting through tissue. They are available with sharp/sharp, blunt/blunt, or blunt/sharp tips. *Suture scissors* are used to remove sutures. The hook on the tip aids in getting under a suture, and the blunt end prevents puncturing of the tissues. *Bandage scissors* are inserted beneath a

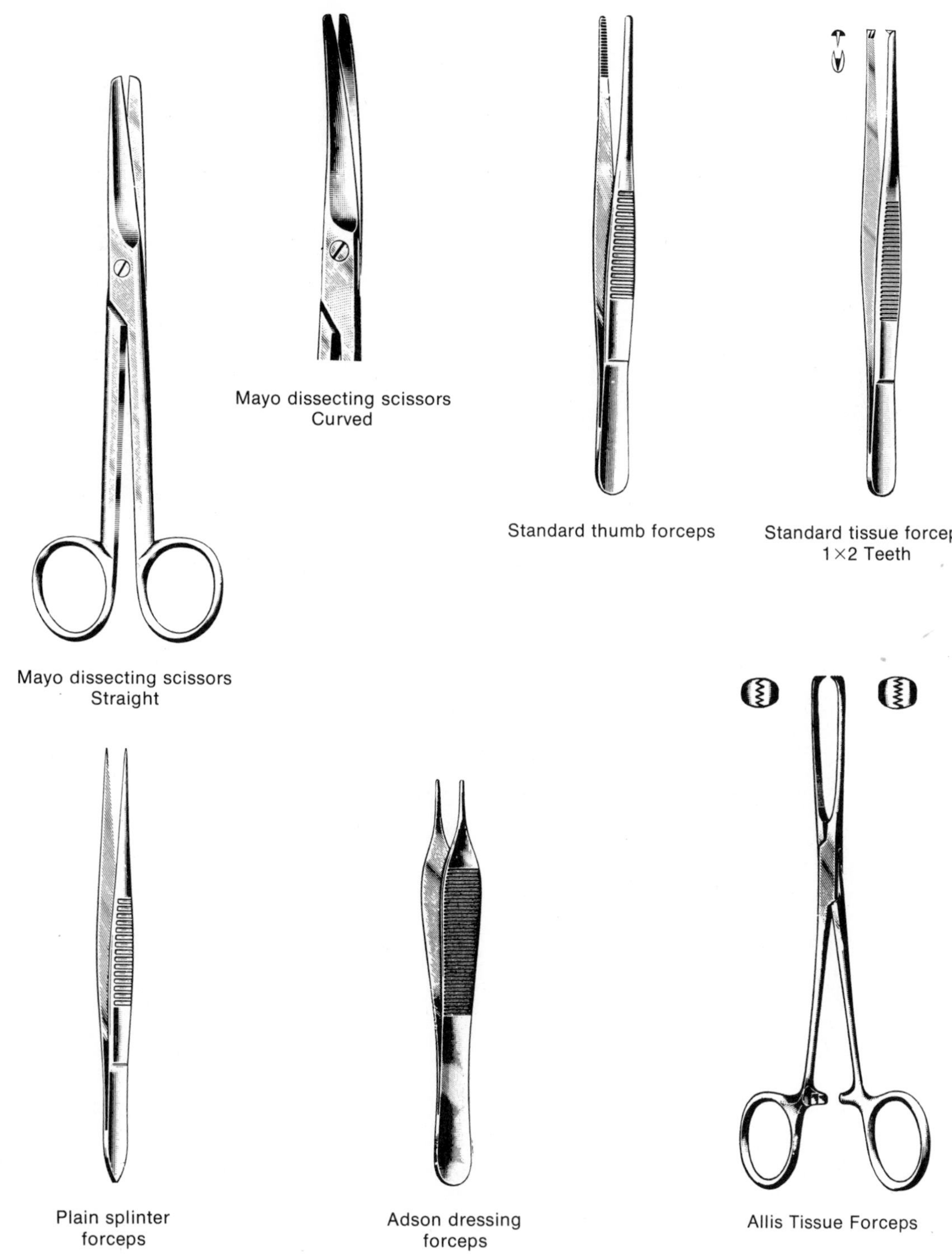

FIGURE 7–2 *Continued*

dressing or bandage to cut it for removal. The flat blunt prow can be inserted beneath a dressing without puncturing the skin. *Dissecting scissors* have a fine cutting edge used to divide tissue and are available with either straight or curved blades. Both blade tips of dissecting scissors are blunt.

Forceps are two-pronged instruments for grasping and squeezing. Some forceps have a spring handle (e.g., thumb, tissue, splinter, and dressing forceps) that provides the proper tension needed for grasping tissue. As you will note from Figure 7–2, some varieties have toothed clasps on the handle, known as ratchets, to hold the tips securely together (e.g., Allis tissue forceps, hemostatic forceps, and sponge forceps). The ratchets are designed to allow closure of the instrument

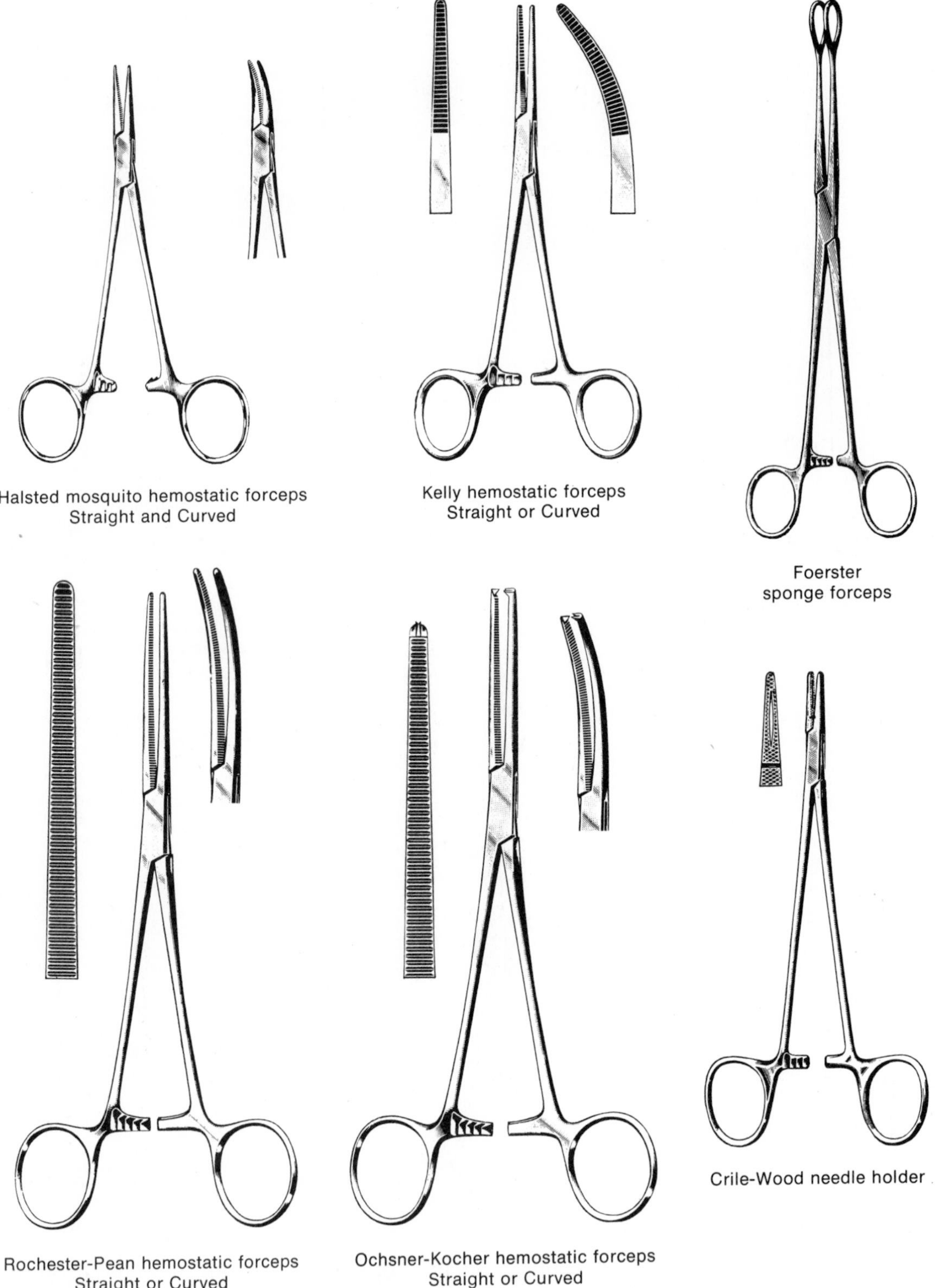

FIGURE 7-2 *Continued*

at three or more positions. *Thumb forceps* have serrated tips and are used to pick up tissue or to hold tissue between adjacent surfaces. Serrations are sawlike teeth that grasp tissue and prevent it from slipping out of the jaws of the instrument. *Tissue forceps* have teeth to prevent them from slipping and are used to grasp tissue. Tissue forceps are identified by the number of apposing teeth on each jaw (e.g., 1 × 2, 2 × 3, 3 × 4). The teeth should approximate tightly when the instru-

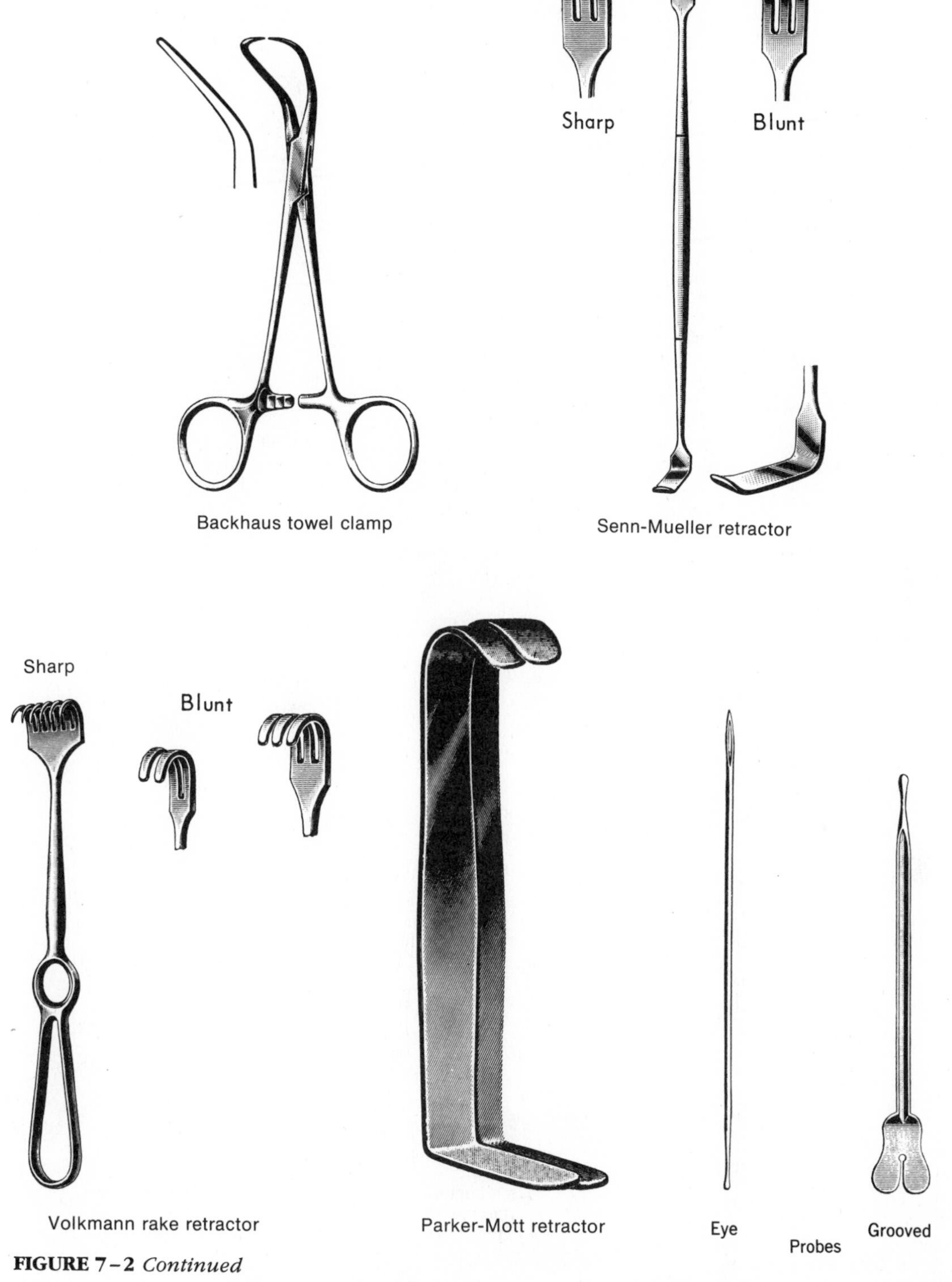

FIGURE 7-2 *Continued*

ment is closed. *Splinter forceps* have sharp points that are useful in removing foreign objects, such as splinters, from the tissues. *Dressing forceps* are used in the application and removal of dressings. They have a blunt end containing coarse cross striations used for grasping. *Hemostatic forceps* have serrated tips, ratchets, and box locks and are available with either straight or curved blades. Hemostats are used to clamp off blood vessels and to establish hemostasis until they can be closed with sutures. The ratchets keep the hemostat tightly shut when it is closed. They should mesh together smoothly when the instrument is closed; if they spring back open, the instrument is in need of repair. The serrations on a hemostat

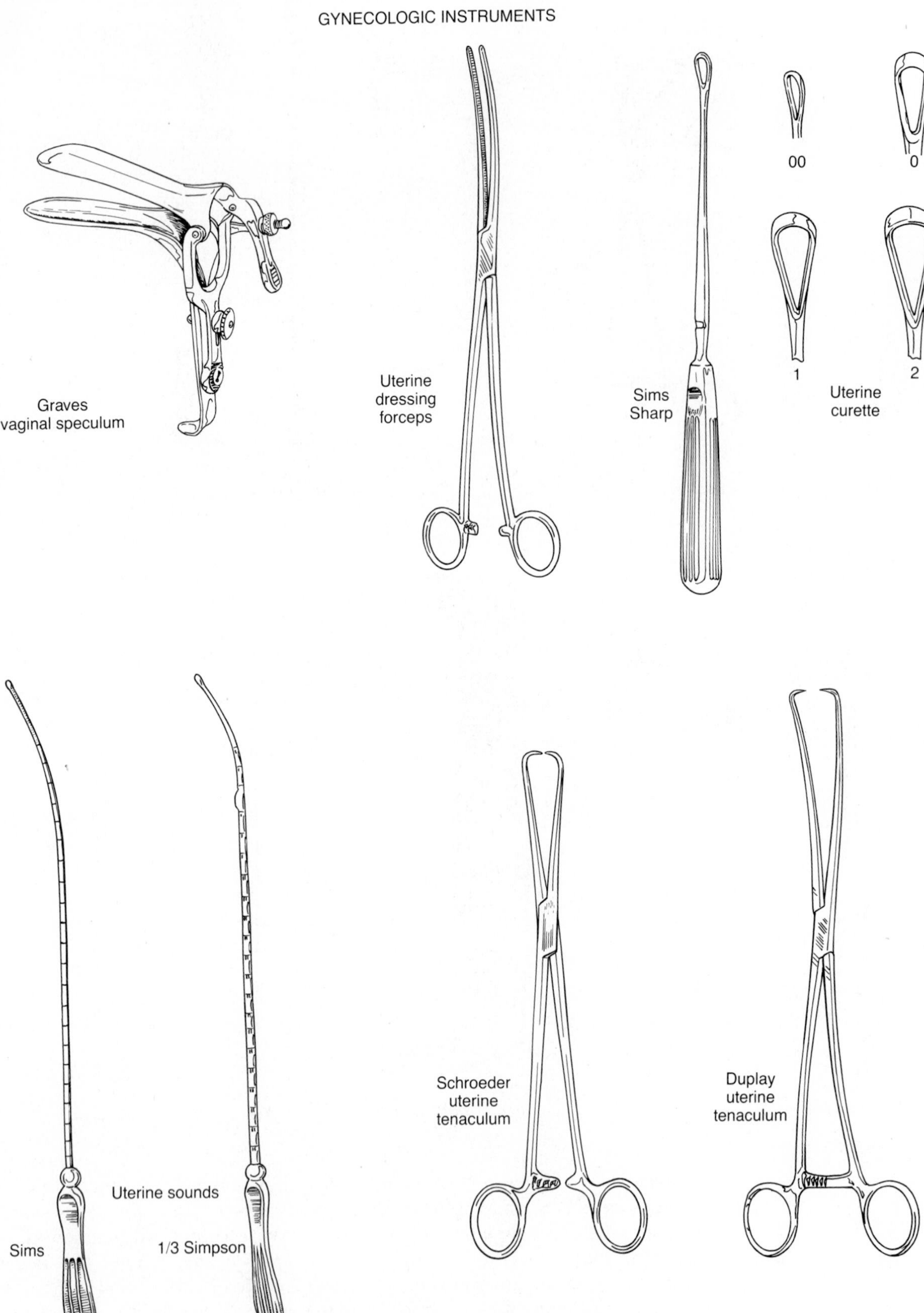
GYNECOLOGIC INSTRUMENTS
Graves
vaginal speculum
Uterine
dressing
forceps
Sims
Sharp
00
0
1
2
Uterine
curette
Uterine sounds
Sims
1/3 Simpson
Schroeder
uterine
tenaculum
Duplay
uterine
tenaculum

FIGURE 7–2 *Continued*

prevent the blood vessel from slipping out of the jaws of the instrument. *Sponge forceps,* as the name implies, have large serrated rings on the tips for holding sponges.

Needle holders have serrated tips, ratchets, and box locks and are used to grasp a curved needle firmly to insert it through the skin flaps of an incision. *Towel clamps* have two sharp points that are used to hold the edges of a sterile towel in place. *Retractors* are used to hold tissues aside to improve the exposure of the operative area. *Probes* are long slender instruments used to explore wounds or body cavities.

Gynecologic surgical procedures are often performed in the medical office; therefore, the medical assistant should be familiar with terms relating to gynecologic instruments described as follows. A *speculum* is an instrument used to open or distend a body orifice or cavity to permit visual inspection. A *tenaculum* is a hooklike instrument used to grasp and hold body parts. For example, a uterine tenaculum is used to grasp and hold the cervix. A *sound* is a long slender instrument that is introduced into a body passage or cavity for means of dilating strictures or to detect the presence of foreign bodies. A *curette* is a spoon-shaped instrument used to remove material from the wall of a cavity or other surface.

Surgical instruments are expensive, delicate yet durable, and able to last for many years if properly handled and maintained. The care an instrument receives depends to a large degree on the parts making up the instrument (e.g., box lock, ratchet, cutting edge, serrations). The medical assistant works with instruments while setting up a sterile tray, performing certain procedures such as suture removal or sterile dressing change, and cleaning up after minor office surgery and during the sanitization and sterilization process. During each of these procedures, the following guidelines must be followed to prolong the life span of each instrument and to ensure its proper functioning:

1. Always handle instruments carefully. Dropping an instrument on the floor or throwing an instrument into a basin may damage it.
2. Do not pile instruments in a heap, because they will become entangled and may be damaged when separated.
3. Keep sharp instruments separate from the rest of the instruments to prevent damaging and/or dulling the cutting edge. Also, keep delicate instruments, such as lensed instruments, separated, to protect them from damage.
4. Keep instruments with a ratchet in an open position when not in use, to prolong the proper functioning of the ratchet.
5. Rinse blood and body secretions off an instrument as soon as possible, to prevent them from drying and hardening on the instrument.
6. Check instruments for proper working order before sterilizing them, and alert the physician to instruments in need of repair. Specific areas that should be checked follow:
   a. The blades of an instrument should be straight and not bent.
   b. The tips of an instrument should approximate tightly and evenly when the instrument is closed.
   c. An instrument with a box lock should move freely but must not be too loose. The pin that holds the box lock together should be flush against the instrument.
   d. An instrument with a spring handle should have sufficient tension to grasp objects tightly.
   e. Scissors should cut cleanly and smoothly.
   f. The cutting edge of a sharp instrument should be smooth and devoid of nicks.
7. When performing procedures requiring surgical instruments, one should always use the instrument for the purpose for which it was designed. Substituting one type of instrument for another could damage it.
8. Sanitize and sterilize instruments using proper technique, as outlined in Chapter 6.

PROCEDURE 7-1

APPLYING STERILE GLOVES

The medical assistant must wear sterile gloves to perform a sterile procedure, such as a dressing change, or to assist the physician during minor office surgery. Disposable gloves are frequently utilized in the medical office. The medical assistant must learn to put on the gloves, using the principles of surgical asepsis so as not to contaminate them.

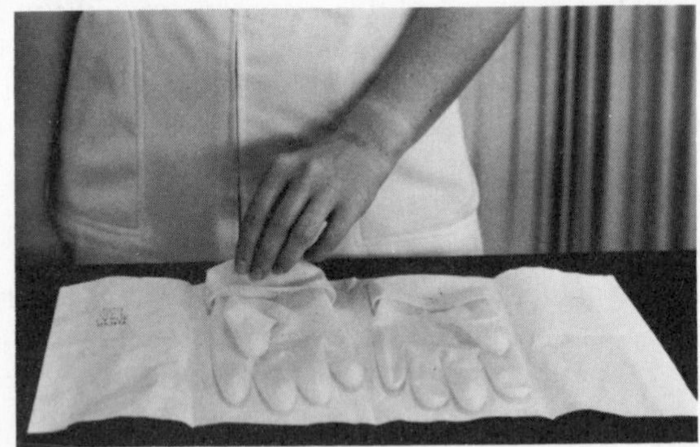

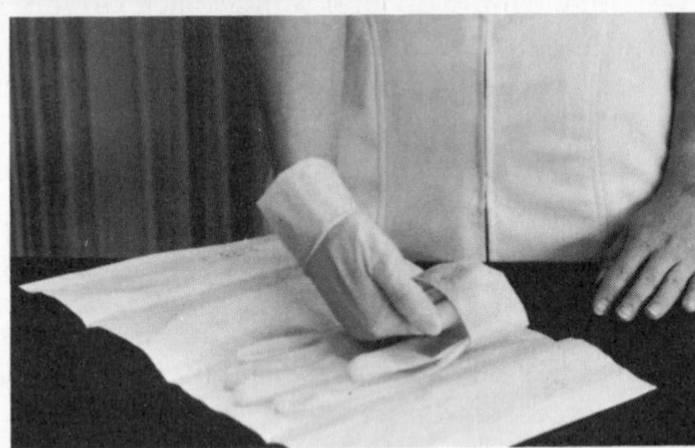

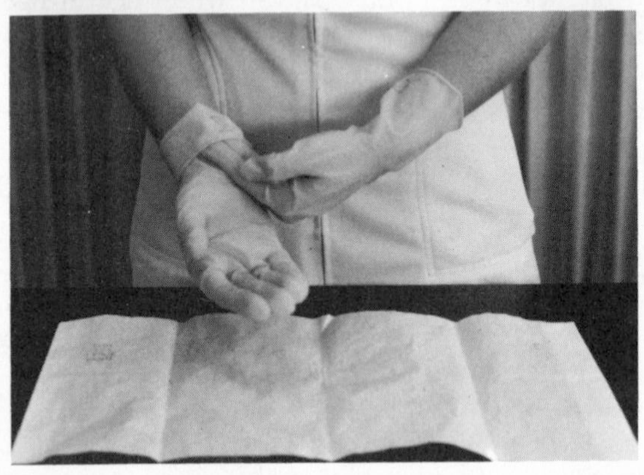

1. **PROCEDURAL STEP.** Remove all rings; wash the hands.

   PRINCIPLE. Rings may cause the gloves to tear.

2. **PROCEDURAL STEP.** Place the glove package on a flat surface. Open the glove package without touching the inside of the wrapper. The tops of the gloves are turned down to form a cuff that keeps them sterile during application.

   PRINCIPLE. The hands are unsterile and the inside of the wrapper is sterile.

3. **PROCEDURAL STEP.** Pick up the first glove on the inside of the cuff with the fingers of the opposite hand, making sure not to touch the outside of the glove with your ungloved hand.

   PRINCIPLE. The inside of the cuff will be lying next to your skin and does not remain sterile. Therefore, it is permissible to pick up the glove by the cuff. The outside of the glove is sterile and touching it will contaminate it. If a glove becomes contaminated, a new pair of gloves must be obtained and the procedure repeated, beginning with Procedural Step. 2.

4. **PROCEDURAL STEP.** Pull the glove on. Allow the cuff to remain turned back on itself.

5. **PROCEDURAL STEP.** Pick up the second glove by slipping your sterile gloved fingers under its cuff without touching the inside of the cuff.

   PRINCIPLE. The area under the folded cuff is sterile and may be touched by the sterile gloved hand.

6. **PROCEDURAL STEP.** Turn back the cuff of the first glove by reaching under the cuff with the other gloved hand. Do not allow the sterile glove to come in contact with the inside of the cuff. Adjust the gloves to a comfortable position. Inspect the gloves for tears.

   PRINCIPLE. The area under the folded cuff is sterile and may be touched by the sterile gloved hand. If a tear is present, a new pair of gloves must be applied.

PROCEDURE 7-2
REMOVING STERILE GLOVES

Gloves must be removed in a manner that protects the medical assistant from contaminating the clean hands with possible pathogens that may be present on the outside of the gloves. This is accomplished by not allowing the bare hands to come in contact with the outside of the gloves. The procedure follows.

1. Grasp the outside of the left glove 1 to 2 inches from the top with your gloved right hand.

2. Pull the glove off the hand. It will turn inside out as it is removed from your hand. Discard the glove in an appropriate container.

3. Place the tips of your fingers of the left hand on the *inside* of the right glove and grasp it near the top. Do not allow your clean hand to touch the outside of the glove.

4. Pull the second glove off the hand. It will turn inside out as it is removed from your hand. Discard the glove (touching only the inside) in an appropriate container.

PROCEDURE 7-3
OPENING A STERILE PACKAGE

A sterile package that has been wrapped following the procedure for wrapping presented in Chapter 6 (see Fig. 6–4) is opened, using the procedure outlined here. The sterile package may contain an instrument or supplies that need to be transferred to a sterile field, using sterile transfer forceps or sterile gloves or by "flipping" the article onto the field using sterile technique. The sterile package may also be in the form of either a commercially prepared disposable package or a pack that has been assembled and sterilized at the medical office; in both cases the inside of the sterile wrapper serves as the sterile field.

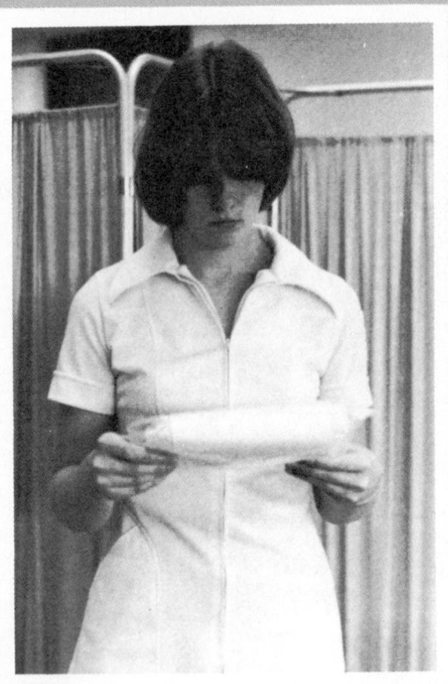

1. **PROCEDURAL STEP.** Wash the hands.

2. **PROCEDURAL STEP.** Assemble the equipment. The equipment needed includes the **sterile package containing the articles required** for the procedure. In addition, a **tray (such as a Mayo tray) or another clean flat surface** may be needed, on which to open the package.

3. **PROCEDURAL STEP.** Check the sterilization indicator and expiration date to make sure the wrapped package is sterile.
PRINCIPLE. Sterilization indicators are used to determine the effectiveness of the sterilization process. Articles wrapped in muslin or disposable paper are considered sterile for a period of 4 weeks. After this time, they should be resterilized.

4. **PROCEDURAL STEP.** Place the wrapped package in your hand or on the table so that the top flap of the wrapper will open away from you.
PRINCIPLE. Small packages containing an article to be transferred to a sterile field may be opened in your hand.

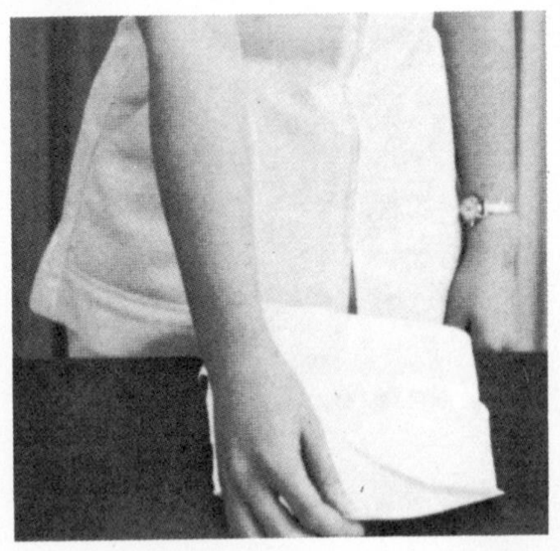

5. **PROCEDURAL STEP.** Loosen and remove the fastener on the wrapped package, and discard it in a waste container.

6. **PROCEDURAL STEP.** Open the first flap away from the body. Handle only the outside of the wrapper.
PRINCIPLE. The medical assistant should open the sterile package so as not to reach over the sterile contents. Otherwise, dust or lint from unsterile clothing may fall on the contents of the package and cause contamination.

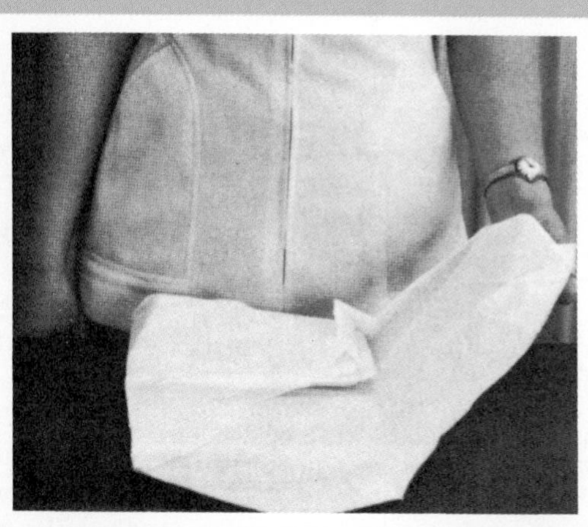

7. **PROCEDURAL STEP.** Open the left and right flaps without crossing over the sterile field.

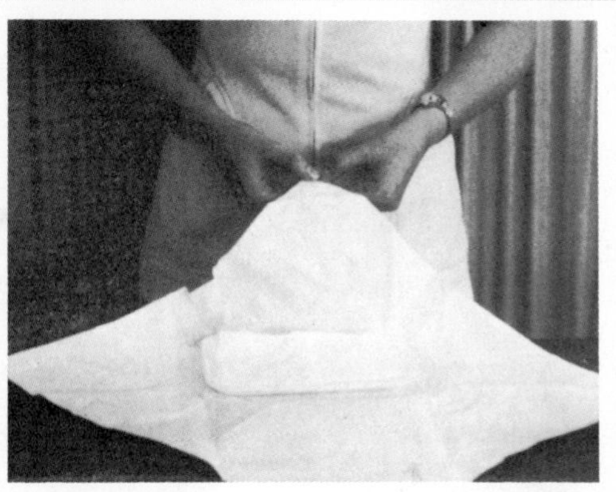

8. **PROCEDURAL STEP.** Open the flap closest to the body by lifting it toward you. Make sure to touch only the outside of the wrapper.

9. **PROCEDURAL STEP.** Transfer the contents of the package to the sterile field or utilize the package as a sterile set-up, according to your medical office procedure.

Commercially Prepared Sterile Packages

Commercially prepared disposable packages are frequently utilized and may contain one particular article (such as a sterile dressing) or a complete sterile set-up (such as one for the removal of sutures). The directions for opening the package are clearly stated on the outside of the package and should be carefully read to prevent contamination of the sterile contents.

One type of commercially prepared package is the peel-apart package (commonly referred to as a peel-pack). This type of sterile package has an edge with two flaps that can be pulled apart in the following manner: Grasp the two unsterile flaps between extended thumbs and, using a rolling-outward motion, pull the package apart (Fig. 7–3*A*). The inside of the wrapper and the contents are sterile and must not be touched with the bare hands, to prevent contamination. The contents of the package can be removed using sterile transfer forceps and placed onto a sterile field (Fig. 7–3*B*). The transfer forceps must not be permitted to touch the outside of the package or the edges of the package that have been

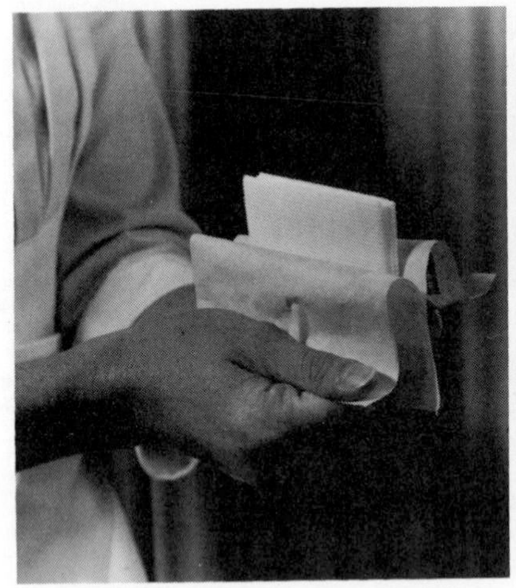

A, To open a peel-apart package, the two unsterile flaps are grasped between the thumbs and the package is pulled apart.

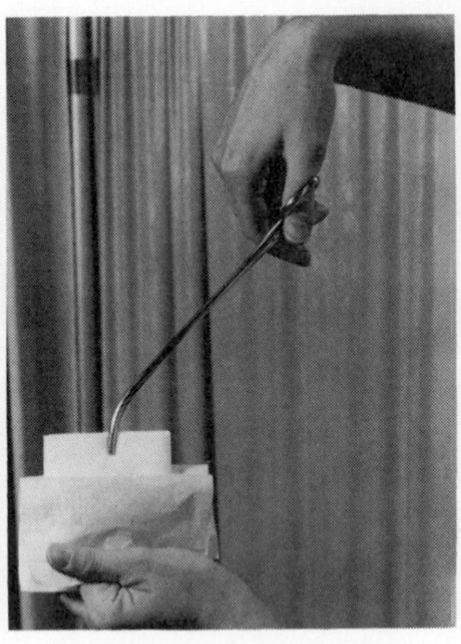

B, The sterile contents of a peel-apart package can be removed and placed on a sterile field by using sterile transfer forceps.

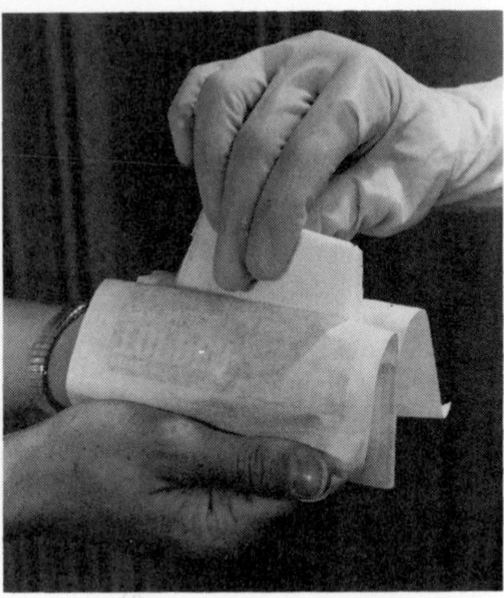

C, The sterile contents of a peel-apart package can be removed by using a sterile gloved hand.

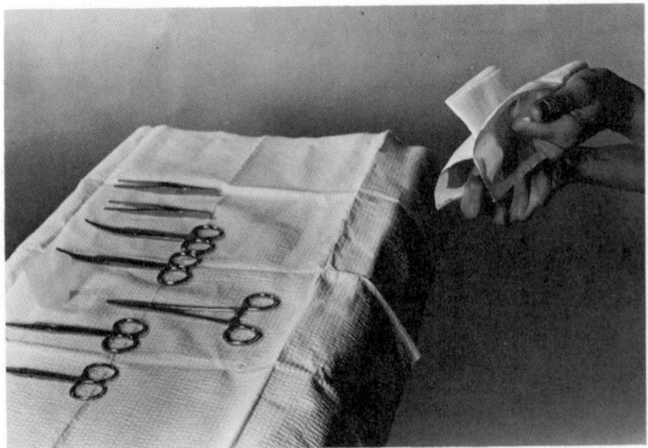

D, The contents of a peel-apart package can be placed directly on a sterile field by gently ejecting or "flipping" them onto the field.

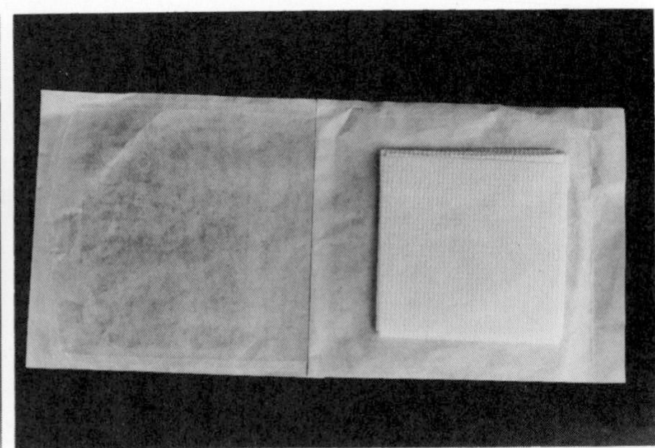

E, The inside of the package may be used as a sterile field by opening the package completely and laying it open flat on a clean dry surface.

FIGURE 7–3. Methods for removing the sterile contents of a peel-apart package in order to maintain sterility.

handled by the medical assistant, either of which would result in contamination of the forceps. The contents of the package may also be removed with a sterile gloved hand. This technique is useful during minor office surgery in which the physician needs additional supplies such as gauze pads, sutures, and so on. Using a gloved hand, the physician removes the sterile contents from the package, which is being held open by the medical assistant (Fig. 7–3*C*). The medical assistant may place the contents of the peel-pack directly on the sterile field by stepping back slightly from the field and then gently ejecting or "flipping" the contents onto it (Fig. 7–3*D*). Stepping back prevents the unsterile outer wrapper and the medical assistant's hands from crossing over the sterile field, which would result in contamination. The inside of the package may be used as a sterile field by opening the peel-apart package completely and laying it open flat on a clean dry surface (Fig. 7–3*E*).

Sterile Transfer Forceps

Sterile transfer forceps are used to transport sterile articles from one sterile area to another. The prongs of the forceps and the articles being transferred must remain sterile, whereas the handles are considered clean or medically aseptic. The transfer forceps are stored in a metal container in which there is a chemical disinfectant. The following guidelines for using sterile transfer forceps refer to forceps that are stored in a chemical disinfectant.

1. Lift the forceps out without letting the prongs touch any part of the container that is unsterile. The outside of the container and the part of the container above the disinfectant solution line are considered contaminated.
2. Place only one pair of transfer forceps in a container, to reduce the possibility of touching the unsterile handle of one pair of forceps with the sterile prongs of the other.
3. After removing the transfer forceps, allow the excess solution to drip back into the container by tapping the prongs together. Otherwise, it may drip onto the sterile field and contaminate it. *Note:* Do not tap the prongs on the edge of the container, because it is considered contaminated.
4. Hold the prongs downward at all times to prevent solution from running up the forceps and onto the unsterile handles and then running back down onto the sterile prongs and contaminating them. Always hold the transfer forceps above waist level to keep them in full view, to prevent accidental contamination.
5. Drop the sterile articles onto the sterile field without allowing the tips of the forceps to touch the field.
6. There should be enough disinfectant solution in the container to cover approximately two-thirds of the transfer forceps. The solution must be changed daily to ensure sterility of the forceps, because it may become contaminated by air currents or improper handling technique. Keep the container covered to prevent evaporation of the disinfectant; this could change its potency.

PROCEDURE 7-4

USING STERILE TRANSFER FORCEPS

This particular procedure shows how to transfer sterile cotton balls to a sterile field, using the principles of surgical asepsis. It can easily be adapted to meet the needs for transferring other sterile articles such as instruments, dressings, and so on.

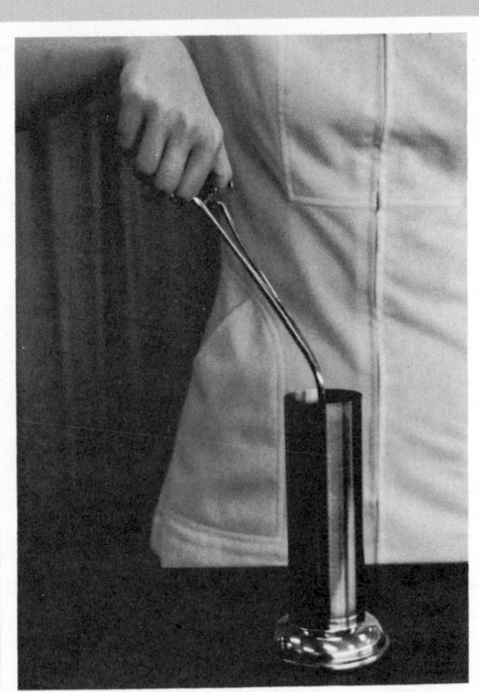

1. **PROCEDURAL STEP.** Wash the hands.

2. **PROCEDURAL STEP.** Grasp the transfer forceps by the handles and lift them vertically from the container, while keeping the prongs held downward. Do not allow the prongs to touch any part of the container that is unsterile. Allow the excess solution to drip back into the container by tapping the prongs together.

3. **PROCEDURAL STEP.** Open the lid of the cannister containing the sterile cotton balls, and hold it in your hand with the inside of the lid facing downward or place it on a solid surface with the inside facing upward.
PRINCIPLE. The inside of the lid must be held downward to prevent microorganisms in the air from settling on it, resulting in contamination. If the lid is placed on a solid surface, it must be positioned with the inside facing upward so it does not come in contact with an unsterile surface.

4. **PROCEDURAL STEP.** Keeping the prongs of the transfer forceps pointed downward, pick up the cotton balls without touching the outside of the cannister, because it is considered unsterile. Replace the lid of the cannister as soon as possible.
PRINCIPLE. Microorganisms in the air can settle on the sterile cotton balls, resulting in contamination.

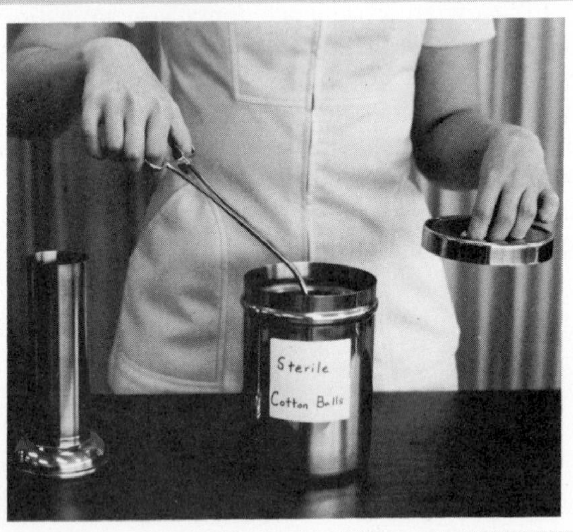

5. **PROCEDURAL STEP.** Drop the cotton balls onto the sterile field without letting the prongs of the transfer forceps touch the field. Do not return any unused cotton balls to the cannister.
PRINCIPLE. Unused cotton balls may have become contaminated after being exposed to the air.

6. **PROCEDURAL STEP.** Replace the transfer forceps in the metal container without allowing the prongs to touch any part of the container that is unsterile.

PROCEDURE 7-5
POURING A STERILE SOLUTION

The medical assistant may need to pour a sterile solution, such as an antiseptic, into a container located on a sterile field using the principles of surgical asepsis outlined in the following procedure:

1. **PROCEDURAL STEP.** Read the label to make sure you have the correct solution.

2. **PROCEDURAL STEP.** Check the expiration date on the solution. An outdated solution should not be used.

3. **PROCEDURAL STEP.** Palm the label of the bottle.
PRINCIPLE. Palming the label prevents the solution from dripping on the label and obscuring it.

4. **PROCEDURAL STEP.** Remove the cap by touching only the outside and place the cap on a flat surface with the open end facing up.
PRINCIPLE. Handling the cap by the outside prevents contamination of the inside. Placing the cap with the open end facing up prevents contamination of the inside of the cap by the unsterile surface.

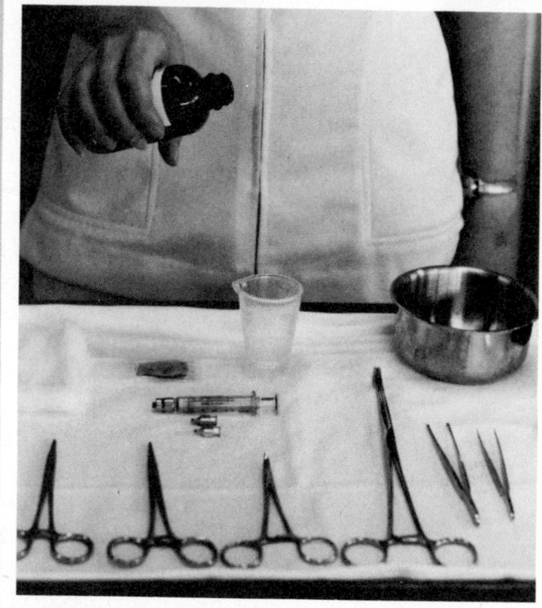

5. **PROCEDURAL STEP.** Rinse the lip of the bottle by pouring a small amount of solution into a separate container.
PRINCIPLE. Rinsing the lip washes away any microorganisms that may be on it.

6. **PROCEDURAL STEP.** Pour the proper amount of solution into the sterile container at a height of approximately 6 inches. Do not allow the neck of the bottle to come in contact with the sterile container, and be careful not to splash any solution onto the sterile field.
PRINCIPLE. Pouring from a height of approximately 6 inches helps to reduce splashing.

7. **PROCEDURAL STEP.** Replace the cap on the container without contaminating it.

Wounds

A *wound* is a break in the continuity of an external or internal surface caused by physical means. Wounds may be accidental or intentional (as when the physician makes an incision during a surgical operation). There are two basic types of wounds: closed and open. A *closed wound* involves an injury to the underlying tissues of the body without a break in the skin surface or mucous membrane; an example is a contusion or bruise. A *contusion* results when the tissues under the skin are injured and is often caused by a blunt object. Blood vessels rupture, allowing blood to seep into the tissues resulting in a bluish discoloration of the skin. After several days, the color of the contusion turns greenish or yellow, owing to oxidation of blood pigments. Bruising commonly occurs with injuries such as fractures, sprains, strains, and black eyes.

Open wounds involve a break in the skin surface or mucous membrane that exposes the underlying tissues; examples include incisions, lacerations, punctures, and abrasions. An *incision* is a clean, smooth cut caused by a sharp cutting instrument such as a knife, razor, or a piece of glass. Deep incisions are accompanied by profuse bleeding; in addition, damage to muscles, tendons, and nerves may occur. A *laceration* is a wound in which the tissues are torn apart, rather than cut, leaving ragged and irregular edges. Lacerations are caused by dull knives, large objects that have been driven into the skin, and heavy machinery. Deep lacerations result in profuse bleeding, and a scar often results from the jagged tearing of the tissues. A *puncture* is a wound made by a sharp-pointed object piercing the skin layers, for example, a splinter, needle, wire, knife, bullet, or animal bite. A puncture wound has a very small external skin opening, and for this reason bleeding is usually minor. A tetanus booster may be administered with this type of wound, because the tetanus bacteria grow best in a warm, anaerobic environment as would be found in a puncture. An *abrasion* or scrape is a wound in which the outer layers of the skin are scraped or rubbed off, resulting in an oozing of blood from ruptured capillaries. Abrasions are caused by falls such as floor burns and skinned knees and elbows. Figure 7–4 illustrates the specific wounds described above.

The Healing Process

The skin acts as a protective barrier for the body and is considered its first line of defense. Once the surface of the skin has been broken, it is easy for microorganisms to enter and cause infection. The body has a protective response to trauma such as cuts and abrasions and to the entrance of foreign matter such as microorganisms. This is known as *inflammation.* Inflammation is generally associated with an injury or infection that is localized or confined to one area. Inflammation destroys invading microorganisms and repairs injured tissue by healing or replacing it. The four local signs of inflammation include redness, swelling, pain, and warmth. The healing process of a wound serves to restore the structure and function of the damaged tissues and takes place in three phases. In the *lag phase* a fibrin network forms, resulting in a blood clot that "plugs" up the opening of the wound and stops the flow of blood. The blood clot eventually becomes the scab. During the *healing phase,* the fibrin threads making up the fibrin network pull the edges of the wound together. Next, there is growth of new capillaries to provide the damaged tissue with an abundant supply of blood. In addition, *fibroblasts* (immature cells from which connective tissue can develop) multiply and provide a basting to bind the edges of the wound together. They cause the wound to appear pinkish-red in color. If little tissue damage has occurred, the fibroblasts are no longer needed and are cleared away and disposed of by the body. If the wound is extensive or has uneven edges, a third phase occurs—the *maturation phase.* In this phase, fibrous connective tissue (arising from the fibroblasts) is deposited and acts as a bridge to fill the gap, because it is not feasible to pull the edges of an extensive or uneven wound together. The fibrous connective tissue eventually hardens into white scar tissue. Scar tissue is not true skin and does not contain nerves or have a blood supply. During a dressing change, the medical assistant should observe the wound for signs of inflammation. He or she should also note the amount of healing that has taken place and record this information in the patient's chart.

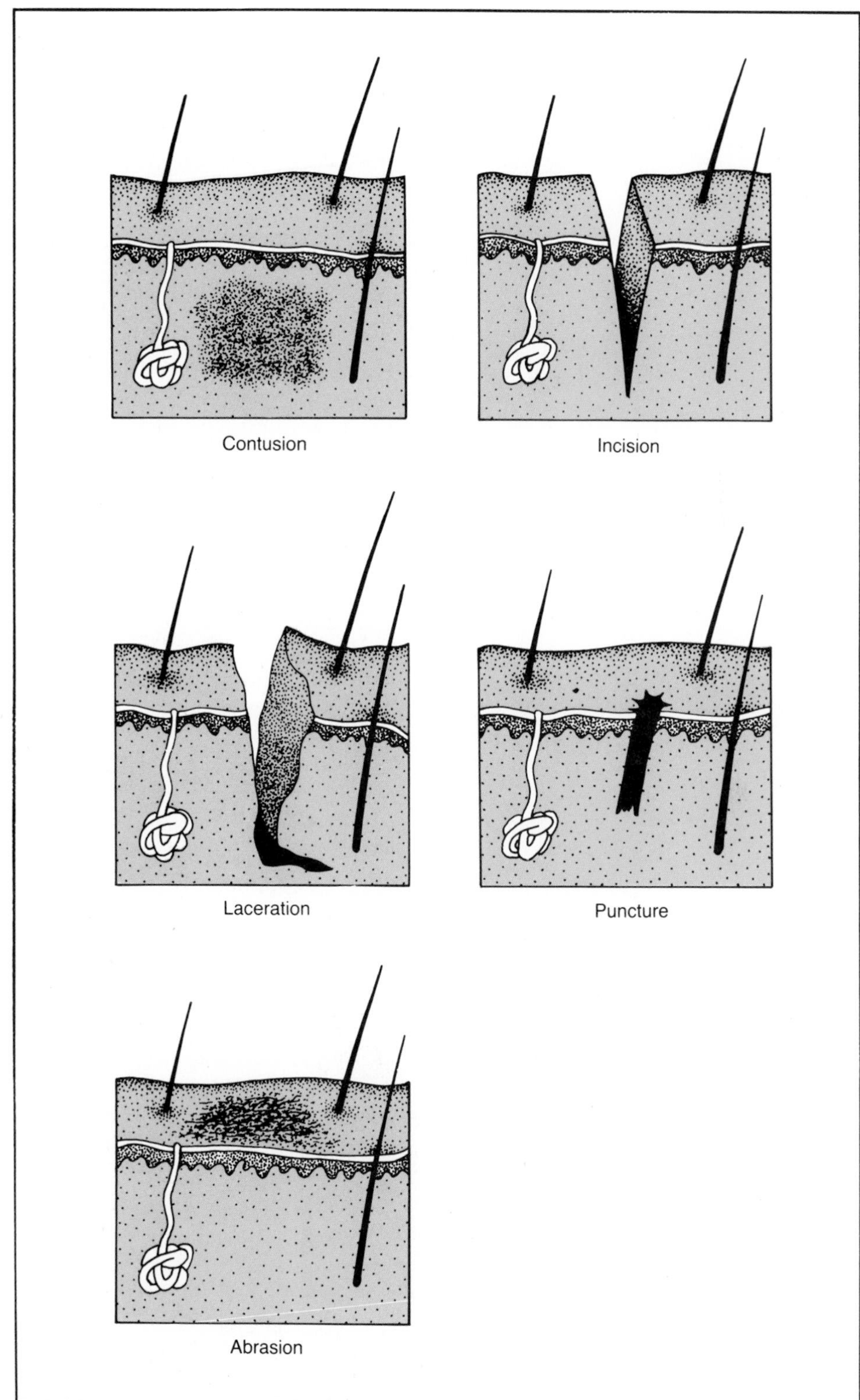

FIGURE 7–4. Types of wounds.

PROCEDURE 7-6
CHANGING A STERILE DRESSING

Surgical asepsis must be maintained when one is caring for and applying a sterile dressing to an open wound. The medical assistant must take care to prevent infection in clean wounds and to decrease infection in those wounds already infected. The function of a sterile dressing is to protect the wound from contamination and trauma, to absorb drainage, and to restrict motion, which may interfere with proper wound healing. The size, type, and amount of dressing material used depend on the size and location of the wound and the amount of drainage. Sterile folded gauze pads, often referred to as 4 × 4s (four by fours) are commonly used in the medical office for a sterile dressing change. This type of dressing functions well in absorbing drainage; however, the gauze has a tendency to stick to the wound when the drainage dries. Gauze pads come in a variety of sizes including 4 × 4, 3 × 3, and 2 × 2; the 4 × 4 size is used most frequently. Nonadherent pads are also used as a sterile dressing, having one surface that is impregnated with agents that prevent the dressing from sticking to the wound; a brand name for this type of dressing material is Telfa Pads. The nonadhering side, which is shiny in appearance, is placed next to the wound.

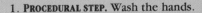

1. **PROCEDURAL STEP.** Wash the hands.

2. **PROCEDURAL STEP.** Assemble the equipment and prepare the sterile field using surgical asepsis. The equipment and supplies used vary with the type of wound and the medical office policy but generally include **gloves, forceps,** an **antiseptic solution and a container to hold** it, **cotton balls,** a **dressing,** a **waterproof waste bag,** and **adhesive tape.** These items are either contained in a prepackaged sterile set-up or placed onto a sterile field using sterile transfer forceps or sterile gloves. Position the waterproof waste bag in a convenient location for disposal of contaminated items.

3. **PROCEDURAL STEP.** Pour the antiseptic solution into the appropriate container on the sterile field without contaminating it (refer to Procedure 7-5: Pouring a Sterile Solution).

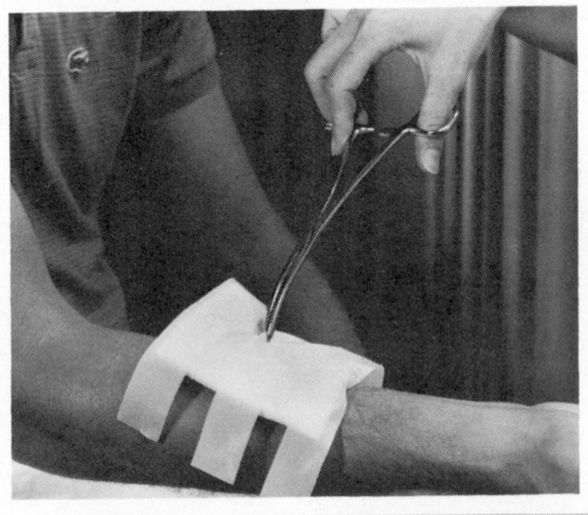

4. **PROCEDURAL STEP.** Identify the patient and explain the procedure. Instruct the patient not to move during the procedure and not to talk, laugh, sneeze, or cough over the sterile field.

   PRINCIPLE. By moving, the patient may accidentally contaminate the sterile field or touch the wound. Microorganisms are carried in water vapor from the mouth, nose, and lungs and can be transferred onto the sterile field.

5. **PROCEDURAL STEP.** Loosen the tape on the dressing, and pull it toward the wound. Carefully remove the soiled dressing with clean gloves or forceps. Do not pass the soiled dressing over the sterile field. Place the soiled dressing in the waste bag without allowing the dressing to touch the outside of the bag.

   PRINCIPLE. Passing the soiled dressing over the sterile field will contaminate it.

6. **PROCEDURAL STEP.** Inspect the wound and observe for the following: amount of healing, presence of inflammation, presence of drainage including the amount (scant, moderate, or profuse) and type of drainage.

PRINCIPLE. Drainage is classified as *serous* (containing serum); *sanguineous* (red and composed of blood); *serosanguineous* (containing serum and blood); or *purulent* (containing pus and appearing white, yellow, pink, or green, depending on the type of infecting microorganism). Purulent drainage is usually thick and has an unpleasant odor.

7. **PROCEDURAL STEP.** Discard the gloves or forceps without contaminating yourself. The gloves and disposable forceps should be placed in the waste bag. Reusable forceps should be placed in a basin.

PRINCIPLE. These items have touched the unsterile dressing and are considered contaminated.

8. **PROCEDURAL STEP.** Open a package of sterile gloves and apply them (refer to Procedure 7-1: Applying Sterile Gloves).

9. **PROCEDURAL STEP.** Cleanse the wound using an antiseptic pledget or cotton balls moistened with an antiseptic and held with sterile forceps. Cleanse the wound from the top to the bottom, working from the center to the outside of the wound. Use a new cotton ball for each cleansing motion. Discard the contaminated articles in the waste bag.

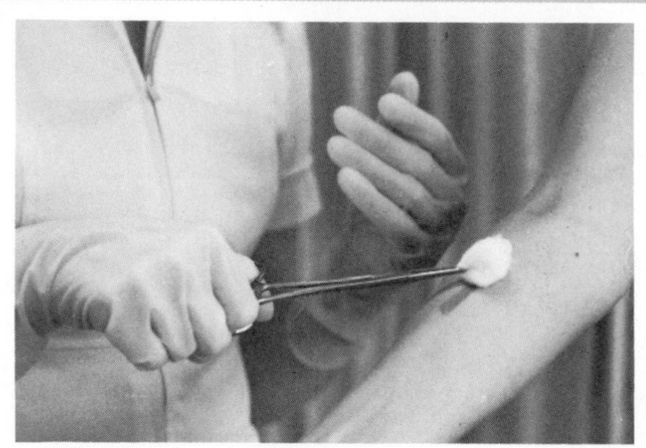

10. **PROCEDURAL STEP.** Place the sterile dressing over the wound by dropping it in place using sterile forceps or sterile gloves. Discard the gloves or forceps.

PRINCIPLE. Dropping the dressing over the wound prevents the possibility of transferring microorganisms from the skin to the center of the wound.

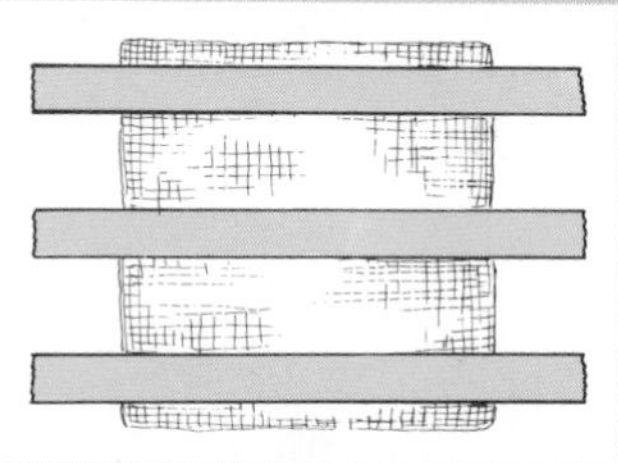

11. **PROCEDURAL STEP.** Apply adhesive tape to hold the dressing in place. The tape must be long enough to adhere to the skin but not so long that it will loosen during patient movement. The strips of tape should be evenly spaced, with strips at each end of the dressing.

12. **PROCEDURAL STEP.** Instruct the patient in the proper care of the dressing. The patient should be told to keep the dressing clean and dry and to contact the physician if signs of inflammation occur. Assist the patient off the examining table.

13. **PROCEDURAL STEP.** Return the equipment. Tightly secure the bag containing the soiled dressing and contaminated articles, and dispose of it in a covered trash container.

PRINCIPLE. The bag must be secured well to prevent the spread of infection.

14. **PROCEDURAL STEP.** Wash the hands.

Continued

15. **PROCEDURAL STEP.** Record the procedure. Include the patient's name, the date and time, location of the dressing, condition of the wound, type and amount of drainage, and any problems the patient may have experienced with the wound. Also, record the instructions given to the patient regarding the care of the drsssing. Place your initials next to the recording.

Record data below.

DATE	TIME	PATIENT'S NAME	RECORDING

Insertion of Sutures

The insertion and removal of sutures are commonly performed in the medical office. Sutures may be required to close a surgical incision or to repair an accidental wound. They approximate or bring together the edges of the wound with surgical stitches and hold them in place until proper healing can occur. A local anesthetic is necessary, to numb the area before the sutures are inserted.

Sutures are measured by their gauge, which refers to the diameter of the suturing material. The size ranges from numbers below 0 (pronounced "aught") to numbers above 0. The diameter of the suture material increases with each number above 0 and decreases with each number below 0. If the size of a particular suture material ranges from 6-0 to 4, the available sizes would include 6-0, 5-0, 4-0, 3-0, 2-0, 0, 1, 2, 3, and 4, with 6-0 being very fine sutures and the diameter of each size progressively increasing in sequence, with 4 being very heavy sutures. For example, size 2-0 (00) sutures have a smaller diameter than size 0 sutures.

Sutures are available in two different types: absorbable and nonabsorbable. *Absorbable* sutures consist of surgical gut, also known as catgut, made from the submucosa of sheep's intestine. This type of suturing material is gradually digested by tissue enzymes and absorbed by the body's tissues from 5 to 20 days after insertion, depending on the kind of surgical gut employed. Plain surgical gut has a rapid absorption time, whereas chromic surgical gut is treated to slow down its rate of absorption in the tissues. Absorbable sutures are frequently used to suture subcutaneous tissue, fascia, intestines, bladder, and peritoneum and to ligate vessels. Since the suturing of this type of tissue is generally done during surgery performed by the physician in a hospital setting with the patient under a general anesthetic, the medical office may not stock absorbable suture material.

Nonabsorbable suture material is not absorbed by the body and either remains permanently in the body tissues and becomes encapsulated by fibrous tissue or is removed (e.g., skin sutures). Nonabsorbable sutures are used to suture skin; therefore, this type of suture is frequently used in the medical office. Nonabsorbable sutures with a smaller gauge are used for suturing incisions in more delicate tissue such as the face or neck (5-0 to 6-0), whereas heavy sutures are used for firmer tissue such as the chest or abdomen. Finer sutures also leave less scar formation and are used when cosmetic results are desired.

Nonabsorbable sutures are made from materials that are not affected by tissue enzymes. These materials include silk, cotton, nylon, Dacron, stainless steel, and metal skin clips. The most commonly used nonabsorbable suture material is surgical silk, which is obtained from silkworms and is dyed black for easy visibility in the tissues. Nonabsorbable sutures used for skin closure must be removed. The length of time the sutures remain in place depends on their location and the amount of healing that must occur. Some areas of the body, such as the head and neck, have a good blood supply; there, the sutures do not need to remain in as long, because this area heals more rapidly. Sutures must always be left in place long enough for proper healing to take place. The physician decides on the length of time, but, in general, skin sutures inserted in the head and neck are removed in 3 to 5 days, and sutures inserted in other areas, such as the skin of the arms, legs, and hands, are removed in 7 to 10 days.

Sutures are commercially available in individual packages consisting of an outer peel-apart package and a sterile inner packet that are labeled according to the type of suture material (e.g., surgical silk), the size (e.g., 4-0), and the length of the suturing material (e.g., 18 inches). The type and size of material used are based on the nature and location of the tissue being sutured and the physician's preference. For example, to repair a laceration of the arm, the physician might use a 4-0 surgical silk suture. The physician informs the medical assistant as to the type and size of sutures needed.

Adhesive skin closures may be used for wound repair to approximate the edges of a laceration. Skin closures consist of sterile nonallergenic tape that is commercially available in a variety of widths and lengths and is strong enough to approxi-

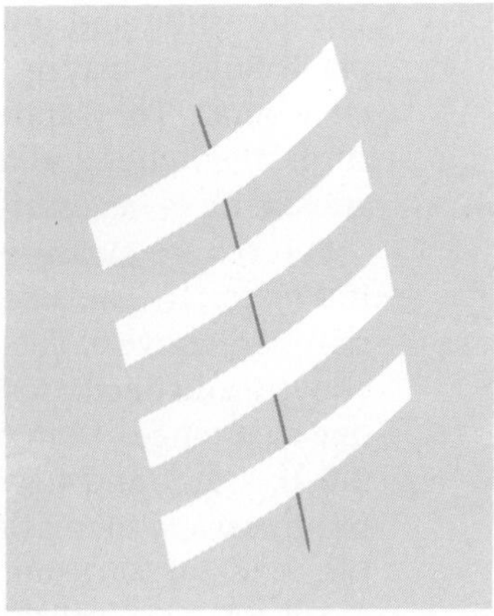

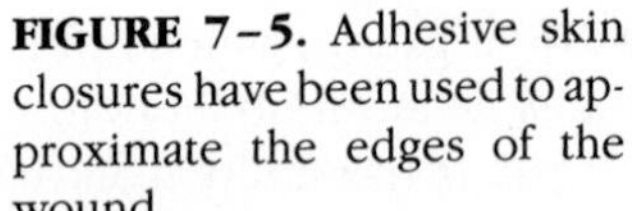

FIGURE 7–5. Adhesive skin closures have been used to approximate the edges of the wound.

mate a wound until healing takes place; Steri-Strips is one brand name of adhesive skin closures. Adhesive skin closures may be used when not much tension exists on the skin edges. The strips of tape are applied transversely across the line of incision (Fig. 7–5) to approximate the skin edges. The advantages of using adhesive skin closures are that they eliminate the need for skin sutures and a local anesthetic, they are easy to apply and remove, and they result in less scarring than skin sutures.

Needles used for suturing are categorized according to both their type of point and their shape. A needle with a sharp point is termed a *cutting* needle, and one with a round point is termed a *noncutting* needle. Cutting needles (Fig. 7–6*A*) are used for durable tissues such as skin; the sharp point helps to push the needle through the tissue. Noncutting needles are used to penetrate tissues that offer a

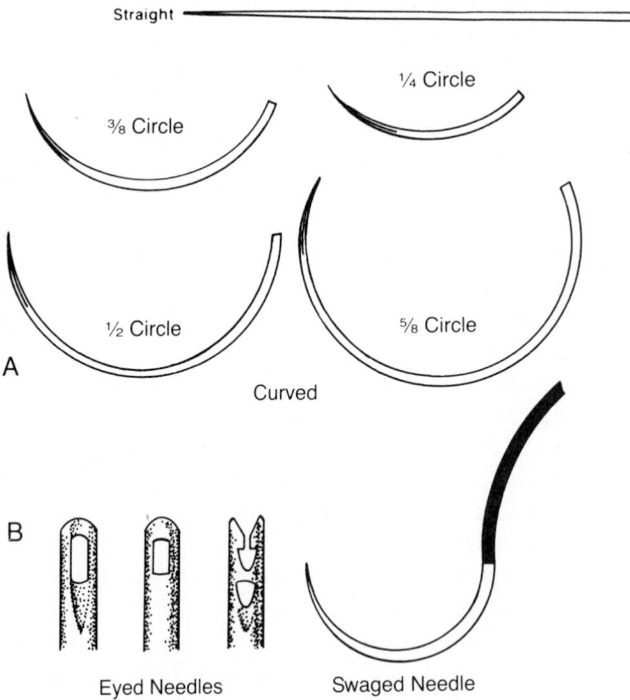

FIGURE 7–6. Common needle shapes. *A*, Examples of needles with a cutting point. *B*, Examples of eyed needles and a swaged needle. (*A*, from *Perspectives on Sutures,* courtesy of Davis & Geck. *B*, from Nealon, T. F., Jr. *Fundamental Skills in Surgery.* 3rd edition, Philadelphia, W. B. Saunders Company, 1980.)

small amount of resistance such as the viscera, subcutaneous tissue, muscle, and peritoneum.

The shape of the needle may be either curved or straight. (Fig. 7–6*A*). Curved needles permit the physician to dip in and out of the tissue. A needle holder must be used with a curved needle. A *straight* needle is used when the tissue can be displaced sufficiently to permit the needle to be pushed and pulled through the tissue. Straight needles do not require the use of a needle holder.

The needle may have an eye through which the suture material is inserted or it may be a *swaged* needle (Fig. 7–6*B*). Swaged means the suture and needle are one continuous unit; in other words, the needle is permanently attached to the end of the suture. Swaged needles are used frequently because they offer several advantages over eyed needles. One advantage is that the suture material does not slip off the needle, as might occur with suture material threaded through the eye of a needle. Another advantage is that tissue trauma is reduced because a swaged needle will have only a single strand of suture that must be pulled through the tissue compared with a double strand in an eyed needle. Therefore, the swaged needle can be pulled through the tissue with less trauma resulting. Swaged suture packets are labeled to specify the size, type, and length of suture material as well as the type of needle point (cutting or noncutting) and the needle shape (curved or straight) (Fig. 7–7).

The medical assistant may be responsible for preparing the suture tray and for assisting the physician during the insertion of the sutures. The physician designates the size and type of suture material and needle required. Since sutures, needles, and suture-needle combinations (swaged needles) are contained in peel-apart packages, they can be added to the sterile field using sterile transfer forceps or a gloved hand or by flipping them onto the sterile field (Fig. 7–8). The items required for suture insertion are listed on page 191.

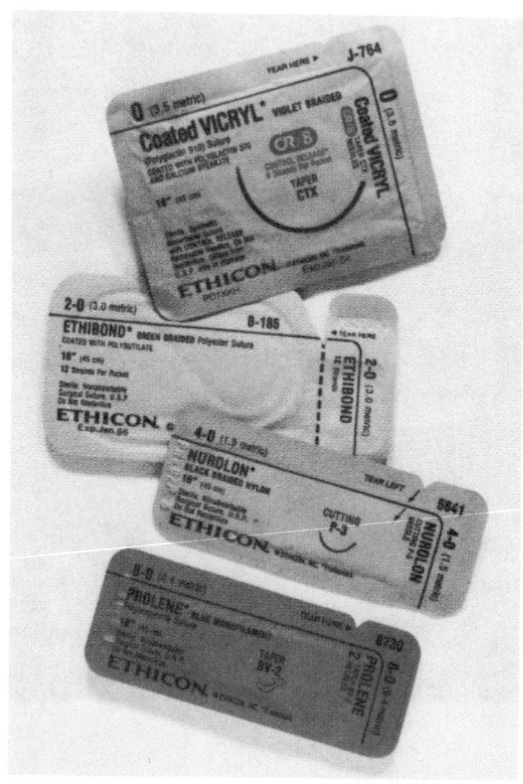

FIGURE 7–7. Swaged suture packets labeled according to the size, type, and length of suture material, the type of needle point, and the shape of the needle. Note: The second packet from the top consists of sutures only and does not contain a needle. (Courtesy of Ethicon, Incorporated.)

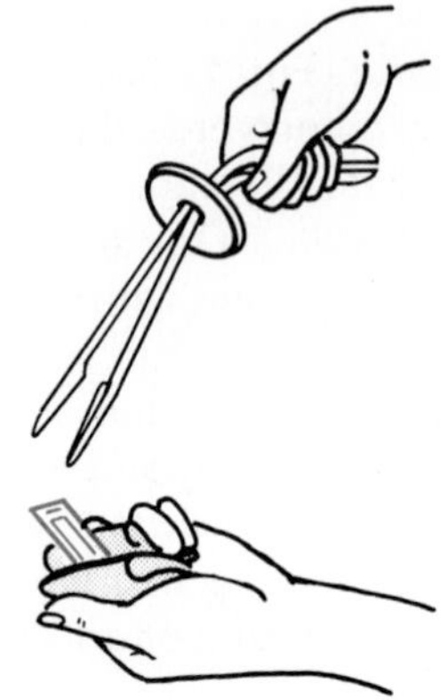

A, Removing sutures with sterile transfer forceps.

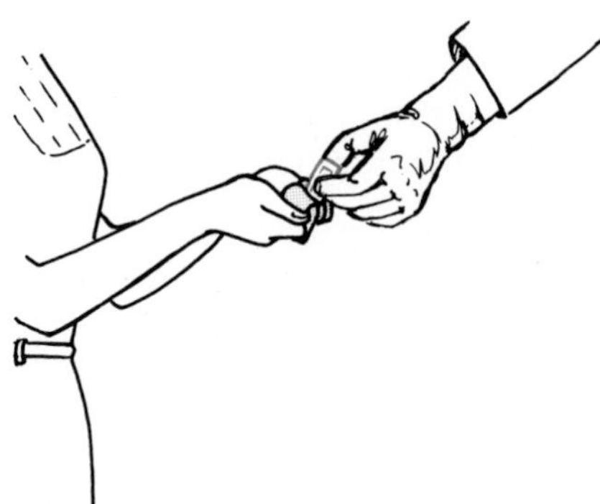

B, The physician removing the sutures with a sterile gloved hand.

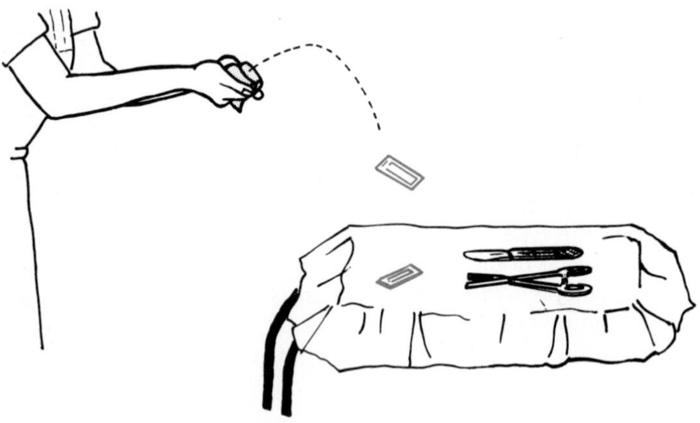

C, Flipping sutures onto the sterile field.

FIGURE 7–8. Adding sutures to a sterile field.

Items That Are Placed to the Side of the Sterile Field for Suture Insertion

- Brush and cleansing solution to clean the wound
- Sterile gloves
- Local anesthetic
- Alcohol pledget to cleanse the vial
- Tetanus toxoid with needle and syringe

Items That Are Included on the Sterile Field

- Antiseptic solution
- Sterile cotton tipped swabs or cotton balls
- Fenestrated drape
- Syringe and needle for drawing up the local anesthetic
- Hemostatic forceps
- Thumb forceps
- Tissue forceps
- Dissecting scissors
- Operating scissors
- Needle holder
- Sutures
- Sterile 4 × 4 gauze

Suture Removal

Some physicians delegate the responsibility for removing sutures to the medical assistant. The patient should be told that he or she will feel a pulling sensation as the suture is removed but that it will not be painful. In performing this procedure, the affected site should first be thoroughly cleansed with an appropriate antiseptic. The knot of the suture is picked up using thumb forceps, and the suture is cut below the knot on the side of the suture closest to the skin (Fig. 7–9*A*). Next, the suture is gently pulled out through the outer skin orifice using a smooth, continuous motion (Fig. 7–9*B*). To reduce the chance of an infection developing, the suture must be removed without allowing any portion that was previously outside to be pulled through the skin. After removing all of the sutures, the medical assistant should cleanse the site with an antiseptic and apply a dressing if indicated by the physician. The procedure should be recorded in the patient's chart, and should include the date and time, the number of sutures removed, the location of the suture site, and the condition of the wound. The medical assistant should be sure to place his or her initials next to the recording. The items that are required for suture removal are listed on the next page.

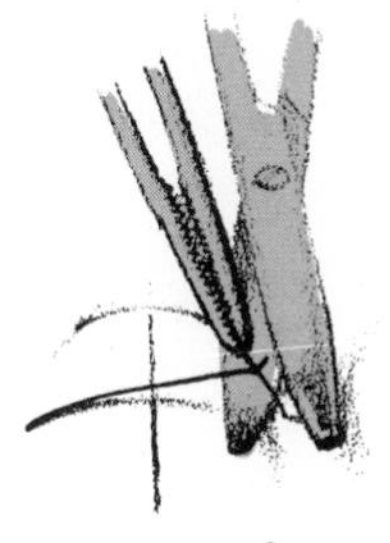

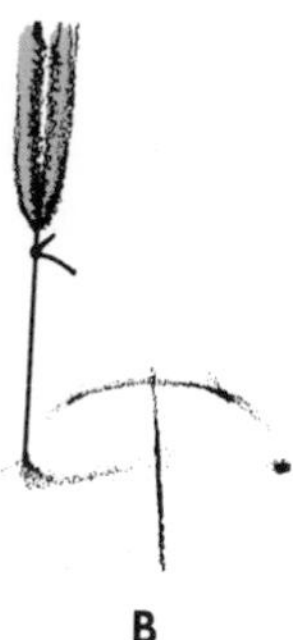

FIGURE 7–9. Technique for the removal of sutures. *A*, The suture is cut below the knot on the side of the suture closest to the skin. *B*, The suture is gently pulled out. (From Nealon, T. F., Jr.: *Fundamental Skills in Surgery.* 3rd edition, Philadelphia, W. B. Saunders Company, 1980.)

Items That Are Placed to the Side of the Sterile Field for Suture Removal

- Surgical tape

Items That Are Included on the Sterile Field

- Antiseptic solution
- Sterile cotton-tipped swabs or cotton balls
- Suture scissors
- Thumb forceps
- Sterile 4 × 4 gauze

Assisting with Minor Office Surgery

Tray Set-Up

Assisting with minor office surgery requires a thorough knowledge of the instruments and supplies for each tray set-up and the type of assistance required by the physician during the surgery. The medical assistant must be able to work quickly and efficiently and to anticipate the physician's needs.

The instruments and supplies for the surgery must be set up on a sterile field. Many offices maintain index cards indicating the appropriate instruments and supplies for each minor office surgery tray set-up. The card may also indicate information regarding the type of skin preparation, the position of the patient, the physician's glove size, the type of suture material, preoperative instructions, and postoperative instructions. The index cards are generally kept in a file box and are filed alphabetically by the type of surgery. The medical assistant should pull the card before setting up for the minor office surgery and use it as a guide to make sure all the required articles are placed on the sterile field. The medical assistant may set up the sterile tray either before or after preparing the patient's skin. The sterile tray set-up must not be permitted to become contaminated. If the medical assistant must turn away from the sterile tray or leave the room after setting up, a sterile towel must be placed over the tray to maintain sterility.

The current practice in setting up a sterile tray is to use prepackaged sterile set-ups wrapped in muslin (or other suitable wrapper) that are prepared by the medical office through autoclave sterilization. These set-ups are labeled according to their specific use (e.g., suture pack, cyst removal pack) and contain most of the instruments and supplies required for the minor office surgery indicated on the label. The medical assistant opens the wrapped package on a flat surface, such as a Mayo stand; the inside of the wrapper is sterile and serves as the sterile field. Several additional articles not contained in the prepackaged set-up (e.g., an antiseptic, sterile 4 × 4 gauze pads, disposable syringes and needles, and sutures) may need to be added to the sterile field, once the package is opened. The antiseptic is added to the sterile field, according to the procedure previously outlined in this chapter. Items in peel-apart packages are added by flipping them onto the sterile field or by using sterile transfer forceps. Another procedure, less commonly used, is to place all the necessary articles on a sterile field by using sterile transfer forceps or by flipping them onto the sterile field from peel-apart packages. In using this method, the sterile field is prepared by placing a sterile towel over a tray such as a Mayo stand or other flat surface. The sterile towel must be handled by the corners only so as not to contaminate it. It must not be fanned through the air but laid down gently and slowly to prevent airborne contamination.

Some articles required for minor office surgery are not placed on the sterile field but are set up off to the side on an adjacent table or stand. These articles, such as the label required for a specimen container, may be medically aseptic and therefore should not be placed on the sterile field, or they may be sterile but enclosed in a medically aseptic package or container. The local anesthetic, which is a sterile solution, is in a vial that is medically aseptic and therefore must not be placed on the sterile field. The physician needs to don gloves to perform the surgery. Although the gloves are sterile, the outside wrapper is not; therefore, the package of gloves must not be placed on the sterile field. In addition, it is easier for the physician to apply gloves from a side table or stand. The medical assistant opens the outside wrapper for the physician, to facilitate applying the gloves.

Skin Preparation

The patient's skin must be prepared prior to the minor office surgery, because the skin contains an abundance of microorganisms. If these microorganisms were to enter the body, a wound infection could develop. It is not possible to sterilize skin, because agents required to kill all living microorganisms are too strong to be placed on the skin surfaces. Therefore, the operative site and an area surrounding it must be cleaned and prepared in such a way as to remove as many microorganisms as possible to reduce the risk of surgical wound contamination.

Hair supports the growth of microorganisms and the physician may therefore want the medical assistant to shave the skin at and around the operative site. Disposable shave prep trays are commercially available and include several gauze sponges, a measured amount of antiseptic soap, a container for soapy water, and a disposable safety razor. The skin should be pulled taut as it is shaved, and the medical assistant must be careful to prevent nicks. Once all the hair has been removed, the shaved area should be rinsed and dried thoroughly and cleansed with an antiseptic soap such as pHisoHex. The medical assistant should clean the area using a firm circular motion, moving from the inside outward, and then rinse, if indicated, and finally blot the area dry with a sterile gauze pad. The effectiveness of some antiseptics is enhanced by a thin film of soap remaining on the patient's skin; therefore, the physician may not want the area rinsed but just blotted dry.

Once the patient's skin has been shaved (if required) and cleansed, an antiseptic is applied to the operative area followed by the application of a sterile drape. The physician generally performs this function after gloving. The antiseptic decreases the number of microorganisms on the patient's skin; an example of a commonly used antiseptic is povidone-iodine (Betadine). A disposable sterile fenestrated drape is most commonly used; it will cover a wide area of skin around the operative area, leaving only the operative site exposed. The drape provides a sterile area around the operative site and thereby decreases contamination of the patient's surgical wound.

Local Anesthetic

Minor office surgeries often require the use of a local anesthetic; examples of local anesthetics frequently used in the medical office include procaine hydrochloride (Novocain) and lidocaine hydrochloride (Xylocaine). The physician injects the local anesthetic into the tissue surrounding the operative site, a process termed *infiltration,* to produce a loss of sensation in that area and thereby prevent the patient from feeling pain during the surgery. Local anesthetics begin working in 5 to 15 minutes and have a duration of action from 1 to 3 hours, depending on the type of anesthetic used.

Some physicians may prefer to use a local anesthetic containing epinephrine, a vasoconstrictor that prolongs the local effect of the anesthetic and decreases the rate of systemic absorption of the local anesthetic by constricting blood vessels at the operative site. The physician will inform the medical assistant as to the type, strength, and amount of the local anesthetic needed for the minor office surgery. For example, Xylocaine is available in 0.5, 1.0, 1.5, and 2.0 per cent solutions. The physician may order 1 ml of Xylocaine 2.0 per cent with epinephrine to suture a laceration of the forearm.

The local anesthetic is drawn up into the syringe using the information presented in Chapter 8 (Procedure 8-3: Preparing the Injection). The vial must first be cleansed using an alcohol wipe. The correct amount of anesthetic solution is then withdrawn into the syringe. This may be performed by either the medical assistant or the physician. The medical assistant withdraws the anesthetic into the syringe and hands it to the physician, who has not yet donned gloves. The physician injects the anesthetic into the patient's tissues and then applies gloves to begin the surgery. The physician may prefer to draw the anesthetic solution into the syringe after he or she has applied gloves. The medical assistant should first show the label of the vial to the physician and then hold the vial securely with both hands while the physician withdraws the medication. The medical assistant must hold the vial, because the outside of the vial is medically aseptic and cannot be touched by the physician's sterile gloved hand. If the medical assistant prepares the anesthetic injection, the needle and syringe are not placed on the sterile field but assembled off to the side, using aseptic technique. If the physician withdraws the anesthetic, the needle and syringe are placed on the sterile field.

Assisting the Physician

The type of assistance required by the physician during minor office surgery is based on the type of surgery performed and physician's preference. Some physicians want the medical assistant to apply gloves and assist directly by handing instruments and supplies from the sterile field. An instrument should be handed to the physician in a firm, confident manner and should be placed in the physician's hand in its functional position, that is, the position in which it is to be used (Fig. 7-10). If handed correctly, the physician should not have to reposition the instrument to use it. The medical assistant is responsible for adding any instruments or supplies to the sterile field that are required by the physician after the surgery has begun, such as another hemostat, additional 4 × 4 gauze pads, or sutures. This is generally accomplished using peel-apart packages and either flipping the contents onto the sterile field or holding the package open and allowing the physician to remove the contents with a gloved hand. In assisting with minor office surgery, it is essential to know all steps in the procedure so that the physician's needs are anticipated and the surgery proceeds smoothly and efficiently.

The physician may obtain a tissue specimen that must be sent to the laboratory for histologic examination. The specimen must be placed in an appropriate-sized container with a preservative. The medical assistant is responsible for labeling the specimen container with the patient's name, the date, and the type of specimen.

Once the minor office surgery is completed, the physician may want the medical assistant to place a sterile dressing over the surgical wound to protect it from contamination or injury or to absorb drainage. The medical assistant is also responsible for assisting the patient and cleaning the examining room.

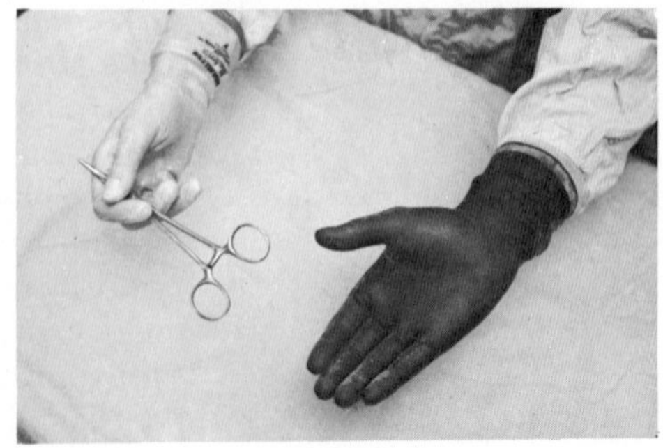

FIGURE 7-10. Handing a hemostat to the physician in its functional position. (From Nealon, T. F., Jr. *Fundamental Skills in Surgery.* 3rd edition, Philadelphia, W. B. Saunders Company, 1980.)

A general procedure for assisting with minor office surgery is outlined on the following pages. Specific instruments and supplies required for the minor office surgery depend on the type of surgery being performed and the physician's preference. Knowing the name and function of each of the surgical instruments presented in Figure 7–2 enables the medical assistant to set up for each type of minor surgery performed in the medical office. If the medical office utilizes prepackaged sterile set-ups, the medical assistant will have already assembled the instruments and supplies in the package during the sanitization and sterilization process; however, the instruments and supplies should be rechecked after the pack is opened to make sure all the sterile articles are included.

PROCEDURE 7-7
ASSISTING WITH MINOR OFFICE SURGERY

1. **Procedural step.** Determine the type of minor office surgery to be performed. The physician instructs the medical assistant as to the type of surgery as well as any additional information needed to set up for the surgery such as the appropriate anesthetic and suture material. If the medical office maintains a minor office surgery filing system, pull the file card indicating the **instruments and supplies that are required for the type of surgery to be performed.**

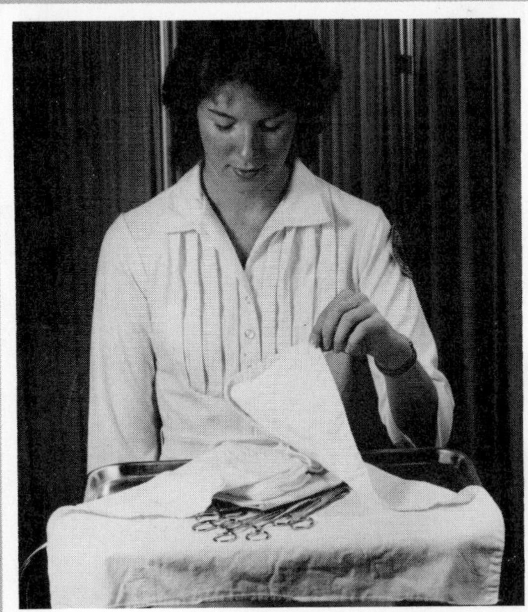

2. **Procedural step.** Prepare the examining room. Make sure the room is spotlessly clean and well lighted.

3. **Procedural step.** Wash the hands.

4. **Procedural step.** Set up any medically aseptic articles required on a side stand or table.
Principle. Articles that are medically aseptic cannot be placed on the sterile field because they would contaminate it.

5. **Procedural step.** Wash the hands and set up the minor office surgery tray on a clean, dry flat surface using the principles of surgical asepsis. The sterile tray can be set up as follows:

a. Use a prepackaged sterile set-up. Select the appropriate package from the supply shelf and place it on a Mayo stand or other flat surface. Open the set-up using the inside of the wrapper as the sterile field. Add any other articles to the sterile field that are needed for the surgery but not contained in the sterile package.

b. Place a sterile towel on a Mayo stand or other flat surface to provide a sterile field and transfer instruments and supplies to it using sterile transfer forceps or peel-apart packages. Pick up the folded sterile towel by two corner ends and allow it to unfold; make sure it does not touch an unsterile surface. Lay the sterile towel down gently and slowly over the Mayo stand, making sure it does not brush against an unsterile surface such as your uniform. Do not allow your arms to pass over the towel as you lay it down because this would result in contamination of the sterile field.

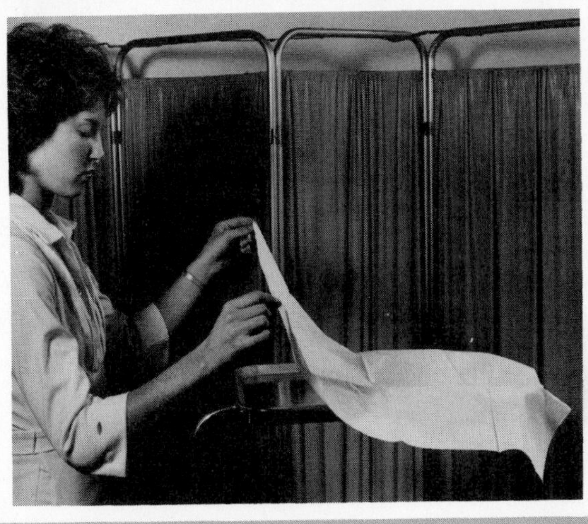

Continued

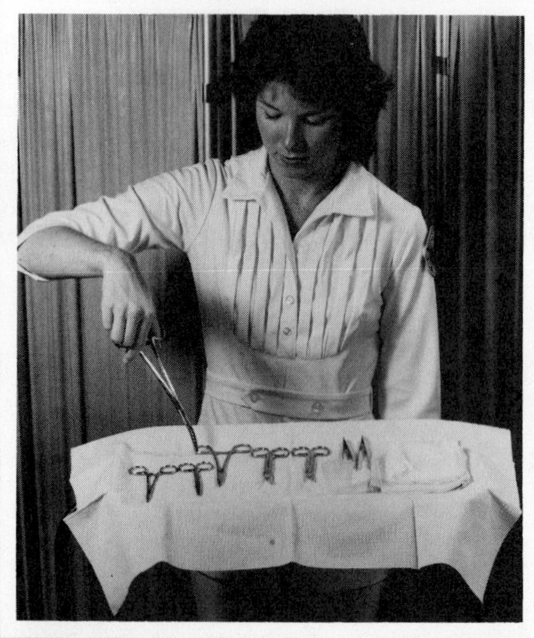

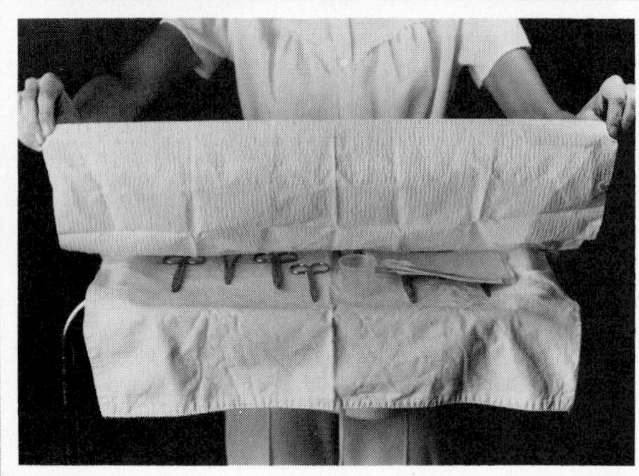

Sterile articles can be added to the sterile field using the following methods:

a. Use sterile transfer forceps to transport sterile articles to the sterile field from a sterile container or from a peel-apart package.
b. Flip the article onto the sterile field from a peel-apart package.

PRINCIPLE. The principles of surgical asepsis must be followed to prevent contamination of the sterile field.

6. **PROCEDURAL STEP.** Arrange the articles neatly on the sterile field using sterile transfer forceps or gloves. Do not allow one article to lie on top of another. Recheck to make sure all the instruments and supplies required for the surgery are available on the sterile field.

PRINCIPLE. Instruments and supplies can be located quickly and efficiently on a neat and orderly sterile field. Sterile transfer forceps or gloves must be used to prevent contamination of the sterile articles.

7. **PROCEDURAL STEP.** Cover the tray set-up with a sterile towel by picking up the towel by two corner ends and placing it gently and slowly over the set-up. Do not allow your arms to pass over the sterile field as you lay it down.

PRINCIPLE. The towel prevents the sterile tray from becoming contaminated. The towel must be picked up by the corner ends to prevent contaminating it and should be moved slowly and not fanned through the air to prevent airborne contamination. Passing the arms over the sterile field results in contamination of the field.

8. **PROCEDURAL STEP.** Identify the patient, explain the procedure, and prepare the patient for the minor office surgery. Help to allay patient fears. Ask the patient if he or she needs to void before the surgery. Provide instructions to the patient on any clothing that must be removed and on donning an examination gown, if required. Enough clothing must be removed to completely expose the operative area. Instruct the patient not to move during the procedure and not to talk, laugh, sneeze, or cough over the sterile field.

PRINCIPLE. Minor office surgery is often a frightening experience for the patient, and reassurance should be offered to help reduce apprehension. The amount of clothing that must be removed will depend on the type of minor office surgery being performed. By moving, the patient may accidentally contaminate the sterile field or touch the operative site. Microorganisms are carried in water vapor from the mouth, nose, and lungs and can be transferred onto the sterile field.

9. **PROCEDURAL STEP.** Position the patient. The type of position is determined by the type of minor office surgery to be performed. The patient is positioned in such a way as to provide the best possible exposure and accessibility to the operative site. *Note:* If a difficult position must be maintained, such as the knee-chest position, the patient should not be positioned until the physician is ready to begin the minor office surgery.

10. **PROCEDURAL STEP.** Adjust the light so that it is focused on the operative site.

11. **Procedural step.** Prepare the patient's skin as specified by the physician. The skin at and around the operative site may need to be shaved. The skin should be pulled taut as it is shaved. The area is then rinsed and dried thoroughly. Cleanse the patient's skin with an antiseptic soap, using a firm, circular motion and moving from the inside outward. Do not return to an area just cleansed. The area is then rinsed, if indicated, and blotted dry with a sterile gauze pad.

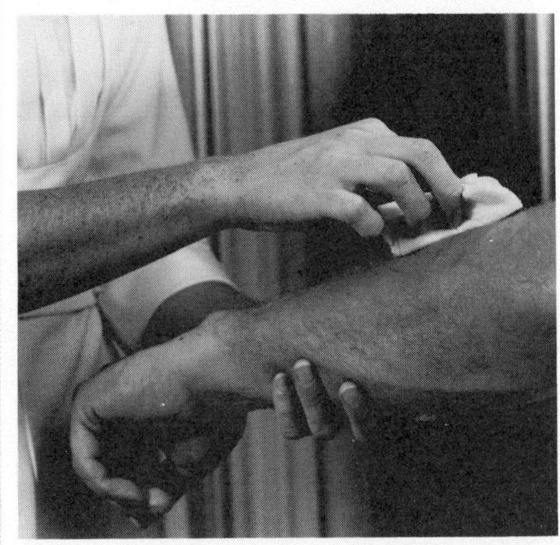

12. **Procedural step.** Check to make sure everything is prepared for the minor office surgery and inform the physician that the patient is ready.

13. **Procedural step.** Assist the physician as required during the minor office surgery following the principles of surgical asepsis. The physician will inject the local anesthetic, apply the antiseptic to the operative site, drape the patient, and perform the surgery.

The responsibilities of the medical assistant may include:

a. Uncovering the sterile tray set-up by picking up the sterile towel covering it. The towel should be picked up by two corner ends and removed slowly and gently, without allowing the arms to pass over the sterile field.
b. Withdrawing the local anesthetic into a syringe and handing it to the physician or holding the vial while the physician withdraws the local anesthetic.
c. Opening the outer glove wrapper for the physician to facilitate the application of sterile gloves.
d. Adjusting the light as needed by the physician for good visualization of the operative site.
e. Restraining patients such as children.
f. Relaxing and reassuring the patient during the minor office surgery.
g. Handing instruments and supplies to the physician. (The medical assistant must glove to perform this procedure.
h. Keeping the sterile field neat and orderly.
i. Holding a basin for the physician to deposit soiled instruments and supplies, such as hemostats and gauze sponges. Hold the basin by the outside to prevent a soiled article from touching your hand.
j. Retracting tissue from an area to allow the physician better access and visibility of the operative site. (The medical assistant must glove to perform this procedure.)
k. Sponging blood from the operative site. (The medical assistant must glove to perform this procedure.)
l. Adding additional instruments and supplies to the sterile field as required by the physician.
m. Holding the specimen container to accept a specimen received from the physician. Do not touch the inside of the container because it is sterile. Label the specimen container with the patient's name, the date, and the type of specimen.
n. Wash the hands and record information in the patient's chart as necessary and as indicated by the physician. Proper recording techniques provide for a complete patient record.

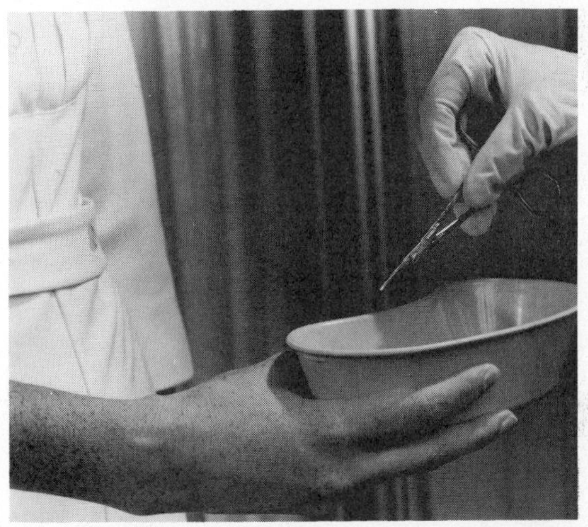

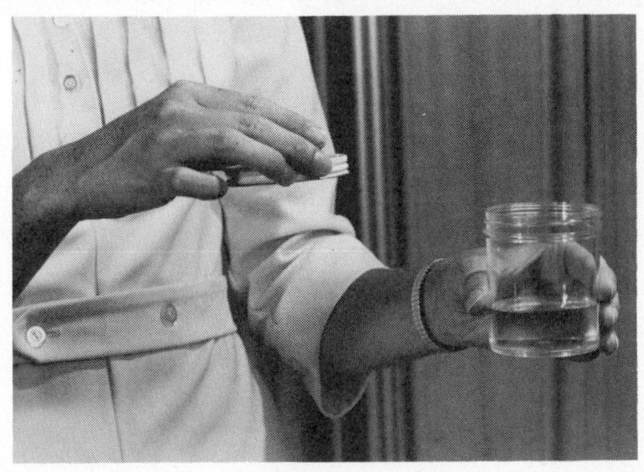

Continued

14. **PROCEDURAL STEP.** Apply a sterile dressing to the surgical wound, if ordered by the physician.

PRINCIPLE. The sterile dressing protects the wound from contamination and injury and helps to absorb drainage.

15. **PROCEDURAL STEP.** Stay with the patient as a safety precaution and to assist and instruct the patient. The patient may need to rest before getting off the examining table. Help the patient off the table to prevent falls. Instruct the patient to dress, offering assistance, if needed. Make sure postoperative instructions regarding any type of medical care to be administered at home are understood. Relay information regarding the return visit for postoperative care, such as the removal of sutures or a dressing change. If the patient has a wound or if sutures have been inserted, he or she should be told to keep the area clean and dry and to report any signs of inflammation such as redness, swelling, discharge, or increase in pain. Any instructions given must be charted in the patient's medical record.

PRINCIPLE. The patient (especially an elderly one) may become dizzy after the minor office surgery and should be allowed to rest before getting off the examining table. Patient instructions must be charted to protect the physician legally, in the event that the patient fails to follow instructions and causes harm or damage to the operative site.

16. **PROCEDURAL STEP.** If a specimen was collected, it must be transferred to the laboratory in a tightly closed, properly labeled specimen container. Complete a laboratory request form to accompany the specimen. Record information in the patient's chart, including the date the specimen was picked up or sent to the laboratory as well as the name of the laboratory.

PRINCIPLE. Recording information regarding the specimen transport documents that the specimen was sent to the laboratory.

17. **PROCEDURAL STEP.** Clean the examining room. Handle the instruments carefully so as not to damage them. Be especially careful with sharp instruments, to prevent cutting yourself. Blood and body secretions should be rinsed off the instruments immediately, to prevent them from drying and hardening. The instruments must then be sanitized and sterilized, when it is convenient to do so, following the procedures presented in Chapter 6. Discard disposable supplies, such as used gauze sponges, in an appropriate container.

PRINCIPLE. Surgical instruments are expensive and must be handled carefully to prolong their life span. Hardened blood and secretions on an instrument are difficult to remove. Disposable supplies must be discarded in an appropriate manner to prevent the spread of infection.

18. **PROCEDURAL STEP.** Wash the hands.

Record data below.

DATE	TIME	PATIENT'S NAME	RECORDING

Medical Office Surgical Procedures

The most common surgical procedures performed in the medical office are presented on the following pages. A discussion of the procedure and the items required for each tray set-up are included. The medical assistant should take into account, however, that the instruments and supplies may vary slightly from those listed below, based on the physician's preference.

Sebaceous Cyst Removal

A *sebaceous* cyst is a thin closed sac or capsule containing secretions from a sebaceous or oil gland. It forms when the outlet of the gland becomes obstructed. The built-up secretion of sebum from the gland causes swelling, and the lining of the cyst consists of the stretched sebaceous gland. Sebaceous cysts are soft to firm in consistency and are generally elevated and filled with an odorous cheesy material. This type of cyst may occur anywhere on the body except on the palms of the hands and the soles of the feet—these areas do not contain sebaceous glands. Sebaceous cysts tend to occur most frequently on the scalp, face, ears, neck, and back. A sebaceous cyst is usually painless and nontender, although it may become infected; to avoid this, the cyst should be excised by the physician. If it is already infected, the physician does not excise the cyst, but drains it and performs the removal at a later time. At the time of the minor surgery, a local anesthetic is used to numb the area. The physician makes an incision, removes the cyst, and sutures the surgical incision (Fig. 7–11). The cyst is placed in the specimen container with a preservative and sent to the laboratory for examination by a pathologist. A sterile dressing is then applied to the operative site. The items required for a sebaceous cyst removal are listed on the next page.

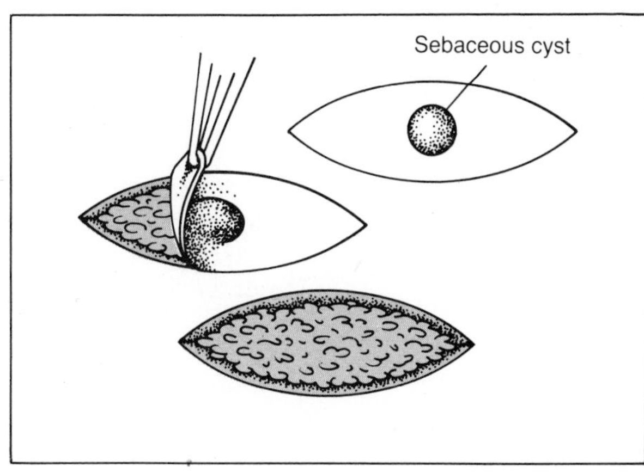

FIGURE 7–11. Sebaceous cyst removal. The physician makes an incision, removes the cyst, and sutures the surgical incision. (From Nealon, T. F., Jr.: *Fundamental Skills in Surgery.* 3rd edition, Philadelphia, W. B. Saunders Company, 1980.)

Items That Are Placed to the Side of the Sterile Field for Sebaceous Cyst Removal

- Sterile gloves
- Local anesthetic
- Alcohol pledget to cleanse the vial
- Specimen container with preservative and label
- Laboratory request form
- Surgical tape

Items That Are Included on the Sterile Field

- Antiseptic solution
- Sterile cotton-tipped swabs or cotton balls
- Fenestrated drape
- Needle and syringe for drawing up the local anesthetic
- Scalpel and blade
- Dissecting scissors
- Hemostatic forceps
- Tissue forceps
- Thumb forceps
- Operating scissors
- Needle holder
- Sutures
- Sterile 4 × 4 gauze

Surgical Incision and Drainage of Localized Infections

An *abscess* is a collection of pus in a cavity surrounded by inflamed tissue (Fig. 7–12). It is caused by a pathogen that invades the tissues, usually by way of a break in the skin. An abscess serves as a defense mechanism of the body to keep an infection localized by walling off the microorganisms, preventing them from spreading through the body. A *furuncle,* also known as a boil, is a localized staphylococcal infection that originates deep within a hair follicle. Furuncles produce pain and itching. The skin initially becomes red and then turns white and necrotic over the top of the furuncle. Erythema and induration usually surround it.

Localized infections, such as abscesses, furuncles, and infected sebaceous cysts that do not rupture and drain naturally may need to be incised and drained by the physician. A local anesthetic is generally used for the procedure. A scalpel is used to make the incision. Then either a rubber penrose drainage tube or a gauze wick is inserted into the wound to keep the edges of the tissues held apart, which facili-

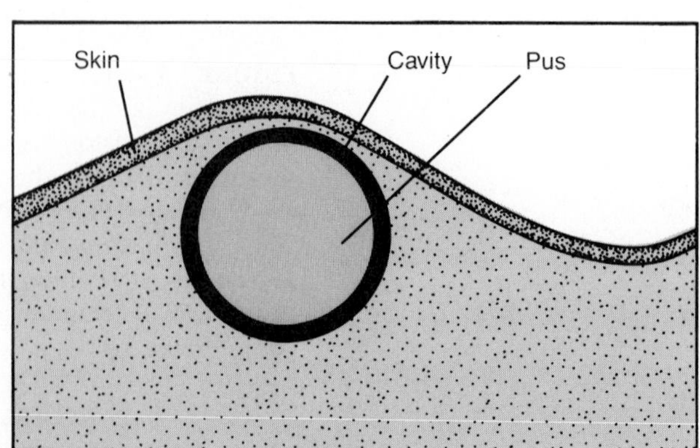

FIGURE 7–12. An abscess is a collection of pus in a cavity surrounded by inflamed tissue.

tates drainage of the exudate. The exudate contains pathogenic microorganisms; therefore, the medical assistant should be careful to avoid contact with the exudate while assisting with the minor surgery. A sterile dressing of several thicknesses is applied over the operative site to absorb the drainage. The patient may be instructed to apply warm moist compresses at home to promote healing. The items required for the incision and drainage of localized infections are listed below.

Items That Are Placed to the Side of the Sterile Field for Incision and Drainage

- Sterile gloves
- Local anesthetic
- Alcohol pledget to cleanse the vial
- Rubber penrose drain
- Idoform packing material
- Surgical tape

Items That Are Included on the Sterile Field

- Antiseptic solution
- Sterile cotton-tipped swabs or cotton balls
- Fenestrated drape
- Needle and syringe for drawing up the anesthetic
- Scalpel and blade
- Dissecting scissors
- Hemostatic forceps
- Tissue forceps
- Thumb forceps
- Operating scissors
- Sterile 4 × 4 gauze

Needle Biopsy

A *biopsy* is the removal and examination of tissue from the living body. The tissue is usually examined under a microscope. Biopsies are most often performed to determine whether a tumor is malignant or benign; however, a biopsy may also be used as a diagnostic aid for other conditions, such as infections. A *needle biopsy* is a type of biopsy in which tissue from deep within the body is obtained by the insertion of a biopsy needle through the skin. A biopsy needle consists of an outer needle for making the puncture and a forked inner needle for obtaining the tissue specimen (Fig. 7–13*A*). The inner needle detaches tissue from a part of the body and brings it to the surface through its lumen (Fig. 7–13*B*). The advantage of a needle biopsy is that a sample of tissue can be obtained that might otherwise require a major surgical operation. The procedure is performed under a local anesthetic, and, since an incision is not required, the patient does not have to undergo the discomfort and inconvenience of an operative recovery. The tissue specimen is placed in a container with a preservative and sent to the laboratory for examination by a pathologist. A small dressing, placed over the needle puncture site, is usually sufficient to protect the operative site and promote healing. After the procedure, the patient should be observed for any evidence of complications related to the procedure. The items required for a needle biopsy are listed below.

Items That Are Placed to the Side of the Sterile Field for Needle Biopsy

- Sterile gloves
- Local anesthetic
- Alcohol pledget to cleanse the vial

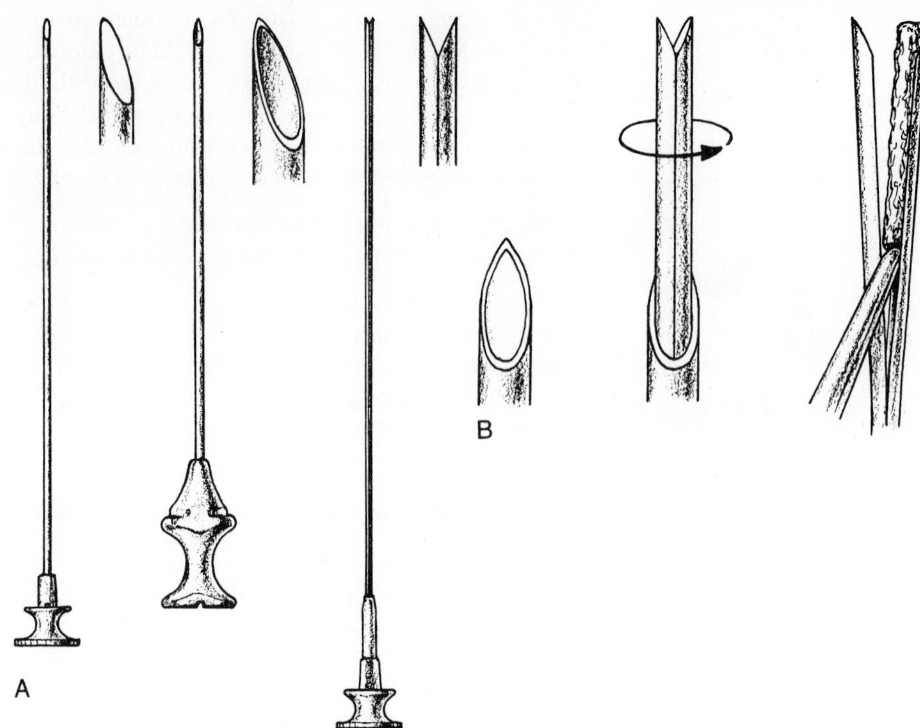

FIGURE 7–13. Biopsy needle. *A*, A biopsy needle consists of an outer needle for making the puncture and a forked inner needle for obtaining the specimen. *B*, The inner needle detaches tissue from a part of the body and brings it to the surface through its lumen. (From Nealon, T. F., Jr.: *Fundamental Skills in Surgery.* 3rd edition, Philadelphia, W. B. Saunders Company, 1980.)

- Specimen container with preservative and label
- Laboratory request form
- Surgical tape

Items That Are Included on the Sterile Field

- Antiseptic solution
- Sterile cotton-tipped swabs or cotton balls
- Fenestrated drape
- Needle and syringe for drawing up the local anesthetic
- Biopsy needle
- Sterile 4 × 4 gauze

Ingrown Toenail Removal

An ingrown toenail occurs when the edge of the toenail grows deeply into the nail groove and penetrates the surrounding skin, resulting in pain and discomfort to the patient (Fig. 7–14*A*). Ingrown toenails are caused by external pressure, such as from tight shoes or hose, or from trauma, improper nail trimming, or infection. The protruding nail acts as a foreign body, usually resulting in secondary infection and inflammation. The condition causes pain and discomfort to the patient. In mild cases, this condition is treated by inserting a small piece of cotton packing under the toenail to raise the nail edge away from the tissue of the nail groove (Fig. 7–14*B*). In severe and recurring cases, part of the nail must be surgically removed which relieves pain by decreasing the nail pressure on the soft tissues. To perform

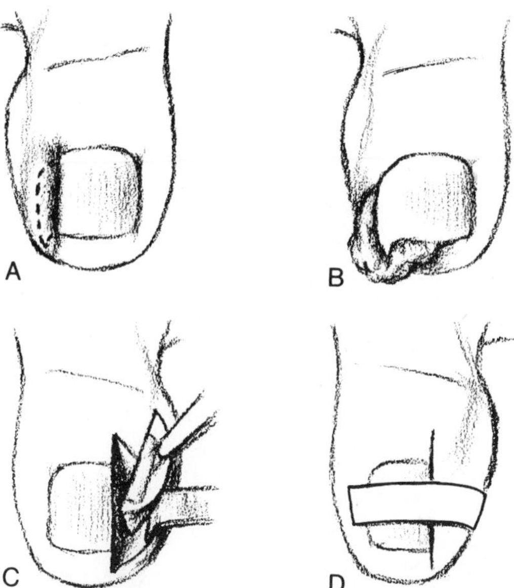

FIGURE 7–14. Ingrown toenail. *A*, The edge of the toenail grows deeply into the nail groove. *B*, In mild cases, treatment consists of inserting a small piece of cotton packing under the toenail. *C*, In severe and recurring cases, a wedge of the nail is surgically removed and *D*, a strip of surgical tape is applied over the area. (From Nealon, T. F., Jr.: *Fundamental Skills in Surgery.* 3rd edition, Philadelphia, W. B. Saunders Company, 1980.)

the surgical procedure, the affected foot must first be soaked in tepid water containing an antibacterial skin solution for 10 to 15 minutes to soften the nail plate and decrease the possibility of bacterial infection. The patient is then placed in a reclining position with the foot adequately supported, and the toe is shaved to remove hair, which would act as a contaminant. An antiseptic is applied to the affected toe, which is then numbed using a local anesthetic. The physician surgically removes a wedge of the nail using surgical toenail scissors (Fig. 7–14*C*). A sterile gauze dressing or a strip of surgical tape is then applied over the area to protect the operative site and to promote healing (Fig. 7–14*D*). The items required for the removal of an ingrown toenail are listed below.

Items That Are Placed to the Side of the Sterile Field for Ingrown Toenail Removal

- Sterile gloves
- Local anesthetic
- Alcohol pledget to cleanse the vial
- Surgical tape

Items That Are Included on the Sterile Field

- Antiseptic solution
- Sterile cotton-tipped swabs or cotton balls
- Fenestrated drape
- Needle and syringe for drawing up the local anesthetic
- Surgical toenail scissors
- Hemostatic forceps
- Operating scissors
- Sterile 4 × 4 gauze

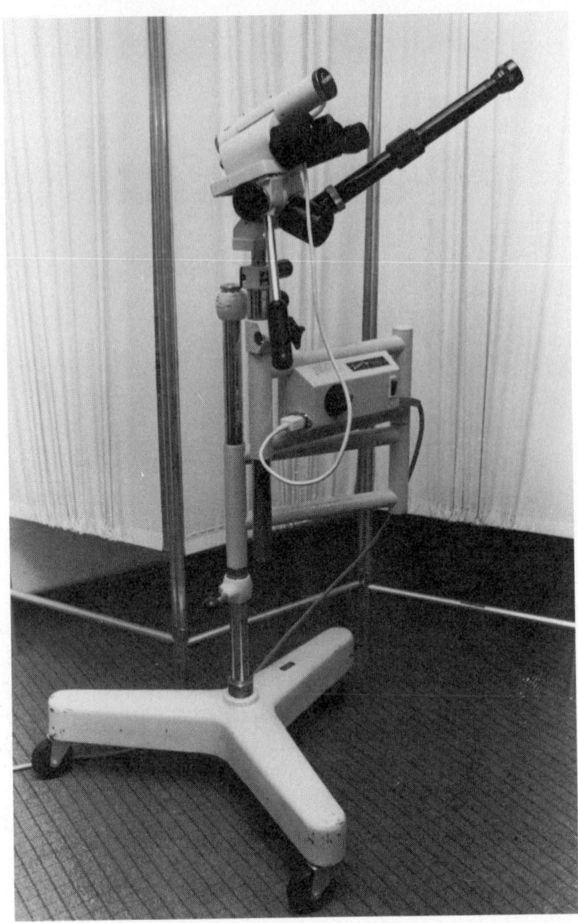

FIGURE 7–15. Colposcope.

Colposcopy

Colposcopy is the visual examination of the vagina and cervix by means of a lighted instrument with a binocular magnifying lens known as a *colposcope* (Fig. 7–15). The purpose of colposcopy is to examine the vagina and cervix to determine areas of abnormal tissue growth. Colposcopy is performed following an abnormal cytology report from a Pap smear, to evaluate a vaginal or cervical lesion observed during a pelvic examination, or after teatment for cancer of the cervix. The lens of the colposcope magnifies tissue, thereby facilitating the inspection of cervical cells and obtaining a biopsy. For a routine colposcopic examination, a magnification of 16× is generally used. The colposcope may be placed on an adjustable stand or attached to the side of the examining table and swung out prior to use.

For the examination, the patient is placed in a dorsal lithotomy position and prepared in a manner similar as for the pelvic examination. The physician inserts a warmed vaginal speculum that has not been lubricated into the vagina. A long cotton-tipped applicator moistened with saline is used to wipe the cervix to remove the mucus film that normally covers it. The saline also provides better visualization of the cervical epithelium, because dry cervical epithelium is not transparent and therefore does not allow satisfactory viewing of the vascular pattern of the cervix. The colposcope is focused on the cervix, and the physician inspects the saline-moistened cervix. Next, the cervix is swabbed with acetic acid, using a long cotton-tipped applicator. The acetic acid helps in dissolving cervical mucus and other secretions; furthermore, the acetic acid provides the best contrast between normal and abnormal tissue, allowing for easier visualization of dysplastic and neoplastic epithelium. The cervical epithelium may also be stained with a solution such as Lugol's solution or Gram's iodine, using a long-tipped applicator. The stain is another means to identify unhealthy epithelium. The healthy epithelium of the cervix contains glycogen, which is able to absorb these stains. Conversely, abnormal epithelium, such as would constitute a malignancy, does not contain glycogen and therefore is unable to absorb the stain. If an abnormal area is observed, the physician will obtain a cervical biopsy using punch biopsy forceps. The items required for colposcopy are listed below.

Items That Are Placed to the Side of the Sterile Field for Colposcopy

- Colposcope
- Sterile gloves
- Monsel's solution
- Specimen container with preservative and label
- Laboratory request form

Items That Are Included on the Sterile Field

- Vaginal speculum
- Normal saline
- Acetic acid (3 per cent)
- Staining solution (Lugol's solution or Gram's iodine)
- Long sterile cotton-tipped applicators
- Cervical punch biopsy forceps
- Uterine tenaculum
- Uterine dressing forceps

Cervical Punch Biopsy

A cervical biopsy is usually performed in combination with colposcopy to remove a cervical tissue specimen for examination by a pathologist. The purpose of the biopsy is to determine whether the specimen is benign or malignant. Cervical biopsies are often performed after an abnormal Pap smear cytology report. The procedure is usually performed a week after the end of the menstrual period, when the cervix is the least vascular. To perform the procedure, the patient is positioned and draped in a dorsal lithotomy position. An anesthetic is not needed; because the cervix has few pain receptors, the patient experiences little discomfort from the procedure. The physician inserts a vaginal speculum into the vagina for proper visualization of the cervix. To assist in obtaining the specimen, the physician may stain the cervix with Lugol's solution or Gram's iodine. If a colposcope is being used, it is focused on the cervix and utilized according to the information discussed on page 204. The physician obtains several tissue specimens (Fig. 7–16*A*) from the abnormal cervical epithelium, using cervical biopsy punch forceps (Fig. 7–16*B*). The specimen is placed in a container with a preservative and is sent to the laboratory for examination by a pathologist. If bleeding occurs, the physician controls it with gauze packing, a hemostatic solution (e.g., Monsel's solution), or electrocautery. A vaginal tampon is inserted after the procedure is finished to absorb drainage and should be left in place, usually for 8 to 24 hours. The patient should be instructed not to insert another tampon unless directed to do so by the physician, as it may irritate the cervix and could cause bleeding. The patient should be informed that a minimal amount of bleeding may follow the procedure; however, the patient should be instructed to contact the physician if bleeding is heavier than normal menstrual bleeding. A foul-smelling gray-green vaginal discharge may occur several days after the procedure and

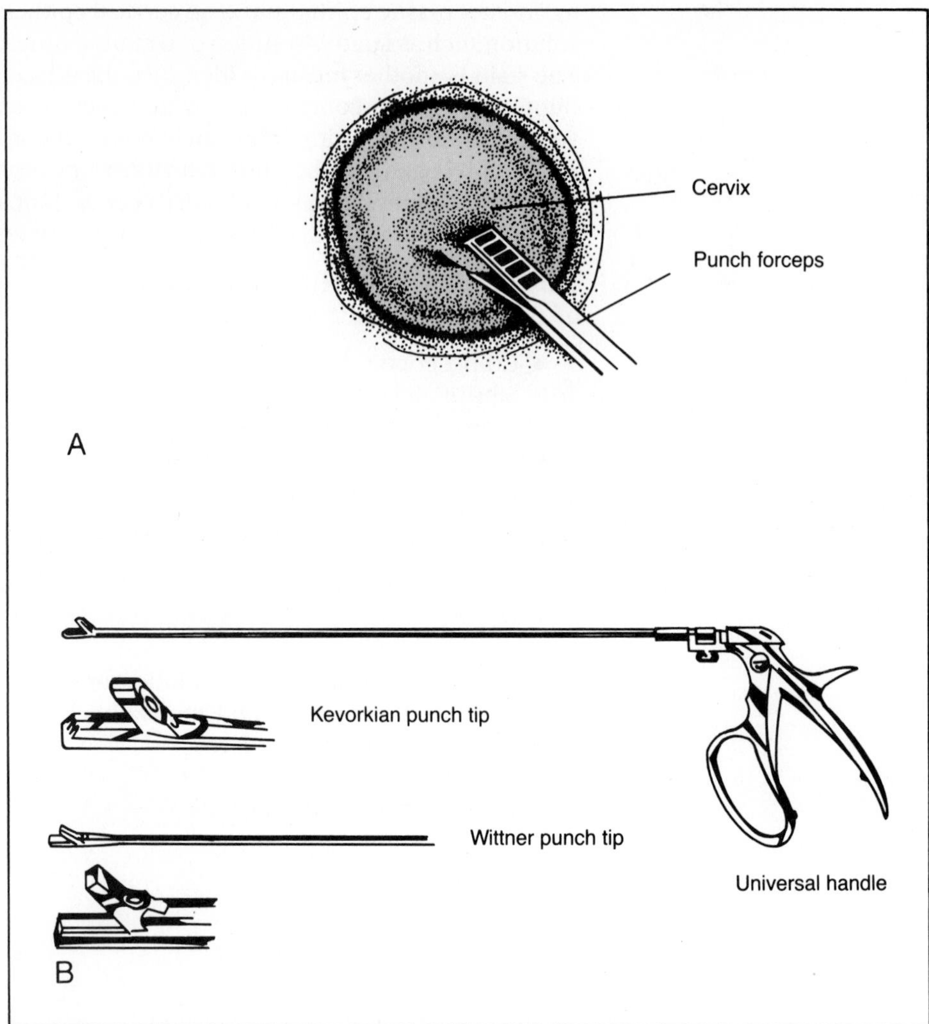

FIGURE 7–16. *A*, Obtaining a tissue specimen from the cervix, using cervical biopsy punch forceps. *B*, Cervical biopsy punch forceps. (Courtesy of Elmed Incorporated, Addison, Illinois.)

continue for a period of up to 3 weeks. The patient should be informed that this discharge results from normal healing of cervical tissue and will gradually diminish as the healing progresses. The items required for a cervical punch biopsy are listed below and at the top of page 207.

Items That Are Placed to the Side of the Sterile Field for Cervical Punch Biopsy

- Sterile gloves
- Monsel's solution
- Specimen container with preservative and label
- Laboratory request form
- Tampons
- Colposcope (if required)

Items That Are Included on the Sterile Field

- Vaginal speculum
- Staining solution (Lugol's solution or Gram's iodine)
- Long sterile cotton-tipped applicators
- Cervical punch biopsy forceps
- Uterine dressing forceps

- Uterine tenaculum
- Sterile 4 × 4 gauze

Cryosurgery

Cryosurgery, also known as *cryotherapy,* is generally used to treat chronic cervicitis and cervical erosion through the use of freezing temperatures. The procedure can be performed without an anesthetic, although occasionally a mild analgesia is necessary immediately afterward. The cryosurgery unit consists of a long metal probe attached to a cooling-agent tank (Fig. 7–17); examples of cooling agents include nitrous oxide, liquid nitrogen, and Freon. The probe is placed in contact with the infected area, and the cooling agent flows through the probe, freezing the cervical tissue to −40° to −80°C. This causes the cells to die and slough off so that the cervical covering can eventually be replaced with new healthy epithelial tissue. The regeneration of the new cervical tissue occurs within approximately 4 to 6 weeks after the procedure.

To perform cryosurgery, the patient is placed in the dorsal lithotomy position. The physician inserts a vaginal speculum for proper visualization of the cervix. The cervix is swabbed with an acid-saline solution to remove mucous and other contaminants. The metal probe is then placed in contact with the affected area, and the cryosurgery unit is turned on. The cooling agent is permitted to flow over the cervical area for approximately 3 minutes. During the procedure, the patient may experience some pain resembling menstrual cramping that usually lasts about 30 minutes. Once the procedure has been completed, the medical assistant should assist the patient as necessary and observe for any signs of discomfort or vertigo.

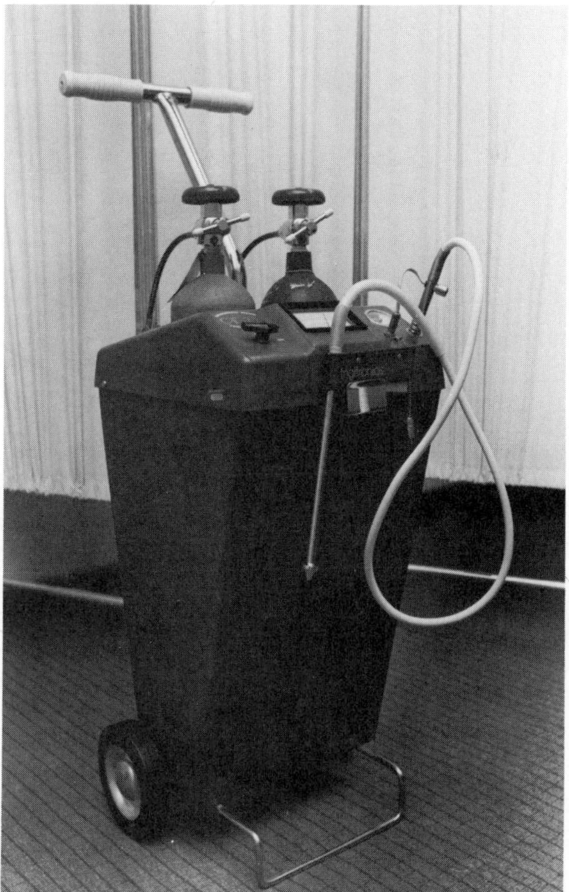

FIGURE 7–17. Cryosurgery unit.

The patient will be given a sanitary pad at the office following the procedure to absorb any discharge. On the first postoperative day following the procedure, the patient will develop a heavy, clear, watery vaginal discharge, which usually reaches its maximum by the sixth day. The patient should be told to use sanitary pads at home rather than tampons. In addition, a vaginal cream (e.g., Amino-Cerv) may be prescribed to promote wound healing and the formation of new epithelial tissue. The patient should be told that continuation of the discharge for approximately 4 weeks is normal, but that the development of a foul odor should be reported to the physician. In addition, the patient should be informed that the next menstrual period will be heavier than normal and may involve some cramping. The patient is usually instructed to abstain from intercourse for 4 weeks following the procedure and to douche with a solution of dilute vinegar and water. The patient will be required to schedule a return visit 6 weeks following the procedure to make sure proper wound healing has taken place.

Items That Are Placed to the Side of the Sterile Field for Cryosurgery

- Cryosurgery unit
- Sanitary pads

Items That Are Included on the Sterile Field

- Vaginal speculum
- Acid-saline solution
- Long cotton-tipped applicators

Bandaging

A bandage is a strip of woven material used to wrap or cover a part of the body. The function of the bandage may be as follows: to apply pressure to control bleeding; to protect a wound from contamination; to hold a dressing in place; or to protect, support, or immobilize an injured part of the body.

The bandage should be applied so that it feels comfortable to the patient, and it must be fastened securely with adhesive tape, metal clips, or safety pins. Guidelines for applying a bandage follow.

1. Observe the principles of medical asepsis during the application of a bandage.
2. Be sure that the area to which a bandage is applied is clean and dry.
3. Do not apply a bandage directly over an open wound. Rather, a sterile dressing should first be applied, and then the bandage. The dressing should be covered with the bandage by at least 2 inches (5 cm) beyond the edge of the dressing, to prevent contamination of the wound.
4. To prevent irritation, do not allow the skin surfaces of two body parts (for example, two fingers) to touch. In addition, the patient's perspiration provides a moist environment that encourages the growth of microorganisms. A piece of gauze should be inserted between the two body parts.
5. Be sure that joints and prominent parts of bones are padded to prevent the bandage from rubbing the skin and causing irritation.
6. Bandage the body part in its normal position with joints slightly flexed to avoid muscle strain.
7. Apply the bandage from the distal to the proximal part of the body to aid in the venous return of blood to the heart.
8. As you apply the bandage, ask the patient if it feels comfortable. The bandage should fit snugly enough so it does not fall off but not so tightly that it impedes circulation. If possible, the fingers and toes should be exposed when bandaging an extremity. This provides the opportunity to check them for signs of an impairment in circulation. Signs indicating that the bandage is too tight include coldness, pallor, numbness, cyanosis of the nailbeds, swelling, pain, or tingling sensations.

If any of these signs occur, the medical assistant should loosen the bandage immediately.

9. If a bandage roll is dropped during the procedure, obtain a new bandage and begin again.

Types of Bandages

Three basic types of bandages are utilized in the medical office. A *roller bandage* is a long strip of soft material wound on itself to form a roll. It ranges from ½ to 6 inches (1.3 to 15.2 cm) in width and from 2 to 5 yards (1.83 to 4.57 m) in length. The width used depends on the part being bandaged. Roller bandages are usually made of sterilized gauze. Gauze is porous and light in weight, molds easily to a body part, and is relatively inexpensive and easily disposed of. However, since it is made of a loosely woven cotton, it may slip and fray easily. *Kling* gauze is a special type of gauze that stretches; this allows it to cling, and, as a result, it molds and conforms better to the body part than does regular gauze.

Elastic bandages are made of woven cotton containing elastic fibers. One brand name for this bandage is the Ace bandage. Although elastic bandages are expensive, they can be washed and used again. The medical assistant must be extremely careful when applying an elastic bandage because it is easy to apply it too tightly and impede circulation, owing to its elastic nature. Elastic adhesive bandages may also be utilized; these have an adhesive backing to provide a secure fit.

Triangular bandages are usually made of muslin and measure approximately 55 inches across the base and 36 to 40 inches along the sides. A triangular bandage is often used as a sling to provide support and immobilization for an injured arm (Fig. 7–18). A *cravat* is formed by bringing the point of the triangular bandage to the center of its base and then folding the bandage lengthwise one or more times until the desired width is obtained (Fig. 7–19). During a medical emergency, a cravat can be used as a tie to hold a splint in place or as a tourniquet to control the flow of severe bleeding.

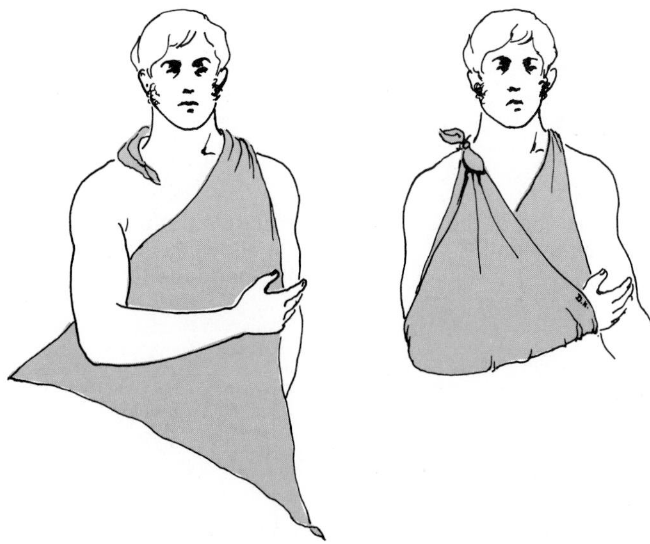

FIGURE 7–18. The procedure for applying a sling using a triangular bandage.

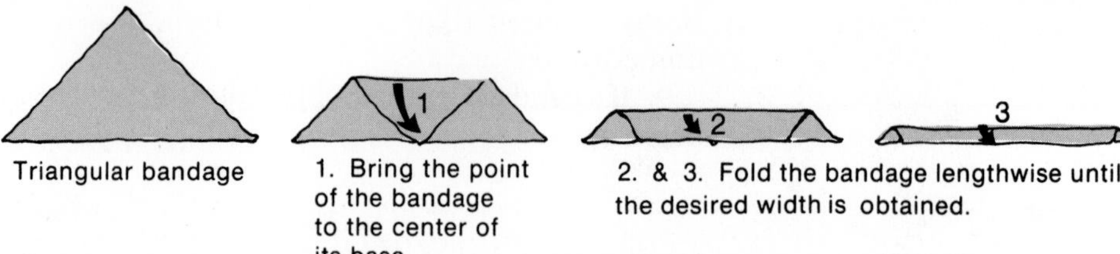

1
2
3
Triangular bandage
1. Bring the point of the bandage to the center of its base.
2. & 3. Fold the bandage lengthwise until the desired width is obtained.

FIGURE 7–19. The procedure for making a cravat from a triangular bandage.

Bandage Turns

Five basic bandage turns are used, alone or in combination with one another. The type of turn used depends on which body part to be bandaged and whether the bandage is used for support or immobilization or for holding a dressing in place.

The *circular turn* is applied to a part of uniform width, such as toes, fingers, or the head. Each turn completely overlaps the previous turn. Two circular turns are used to anchor a bandage at the beginning and end of a spiral, spiral-reverse, figure-eight, or recurrent turn (Fig. 7–20).

The *spiral turn* is applied to a part of uniform circumference, such as the fingers, upper arm, upper leg, chest, or abdomen. Each spiral turn is carried upward at a slight angle and should overlap the previous turn by one-half to two-thirds the width of the bandage (Fig. 7–21).

The *spiral-reverse turn* is useful for bandaging a part that varies in width, such as the forearm or lower leg. Reversing each spiral turn allows for a smoother fit and prevents gaping due to the variation in the contour of the limb. The thumb is used to make the reverse halfway through each spiral turn. The bandage is then directed downward and folded on itself while it is kept parallel to the lower edge of the previous turn. Each turn should overlap the previous one by two-thirds of the width of the bandage. The reverse turns are utilized as often as is necessary to provide a uniform fit (Fig. 7–22).

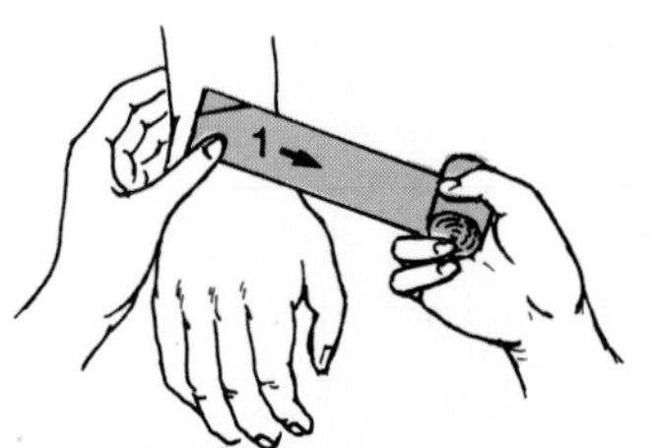

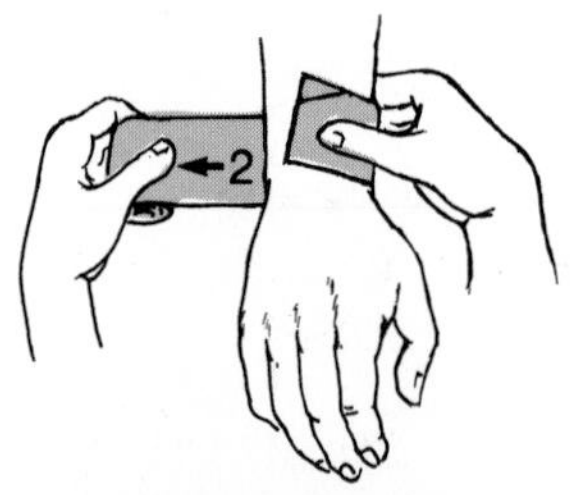

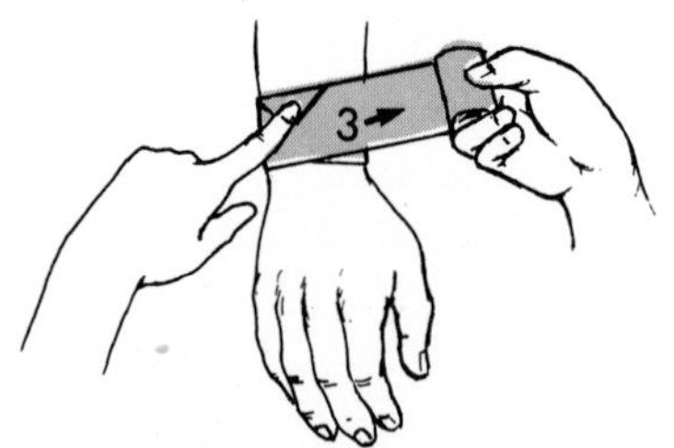

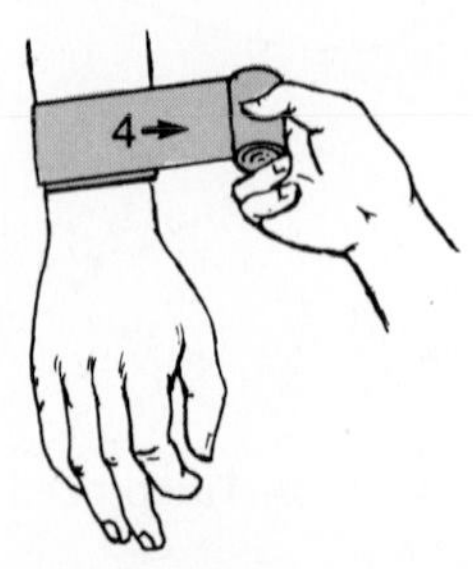

FIGURE 7–20. The procedure for anchoring a bandage.

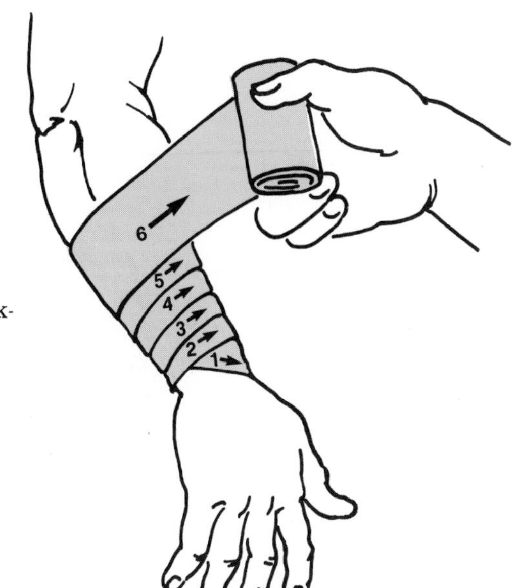

FIGURE 7–21. The procedure for making the spiral turn.

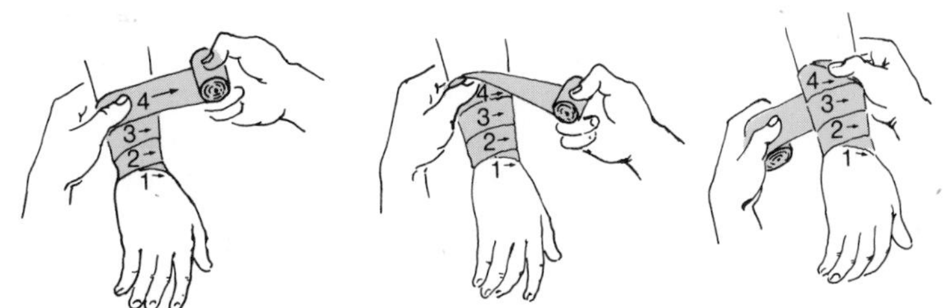

FIGURE 7–22. The procedure for making the spiral-reverse turn.

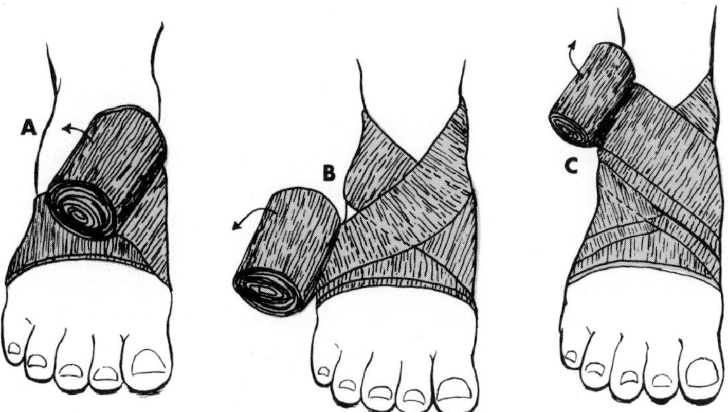

FIGURE 7–23. The procedure for applying an elastic bandage around the ankle using a figure-eight turn. (From Leake, M. J.: *A Manual of Simple Nursing Procedures.* Philadelphia, W. B. Saunders Company, 1971.)

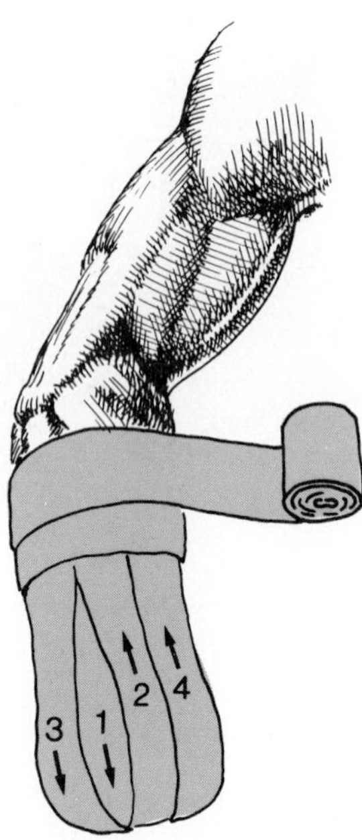

FIGURE 7–24. The procedure for using the recurrent turn to bandage the end of a stump.

The *figure-eight turn* is generally used to hold a dressing in place or to support and immobilize an injured joint, such as the ankle, knee, elbow, or wrist. The figure-eight consists of slanting turns that alternately ascend and descend around the part and cross over one another in the middle, resembling the figure 8. Each turn overlaps the previous one by two-thirds of the width of the bandage (Fig. 7–23).

The *recurrent turn* is a series of back-and-forth turns used to bandage the tips of fingers or toes, the stump of an amputated extremity, or the head. The bandage is anchored by using two circular turns and then is passed back and forth over the tip of the part to be bandaged, first on one side and then on the other side of the first center turn. Each turn should overlap the previous turn by two-thirds of the width of the bandage (Fig. 7–24).

Tubular Gauze Bandage

A tubular gauze bandage consists of seamless elasticized gauze fabric dispensed in a roll. It is used to cover round body parts such as fingers, toes, arms, and legs and resembles a sleeve in fit. This type of bandage is easier to apply than a roller bandage, and it also adheres more securely to the body part. Tubular gauze is not sterile and therefore should not be applied over open wounds; however, it can be applied over a sterile dressing to hold it in place. The gauze is available in varying widths; selection of the width is based upon the body part to be bandaged. Refer to Table 7–1 for a list of tubular gauze widths and the body parts each size can be used to bandage. The gauze is applied by means of a plastic or metal frame-like applicator, which comes in different sizes. The applicator selected must be somewhat larger than the part to be bandaged to allow the gauze to slide easily over the body part. To assist in selecting the proper gauze width, each applicator is marked with a size number that corresponds to the size number on the tubular gauze bandage box. The procedure for applying a tubular gauze bandage to a finger is outlined on the following pages.

TABLE 7-1. Tubular Gauze Bandage Widths and Recommended Application Sites

WIDTH	RECOMMENDED APPLICATION SITES
⅝ inch	Fingers and toes of infants Small fingers and toes of adults
1 inch	Hands and feet of infants Fingers and toes of adults Over bulky dressings
1½ inches	Arms and legs of infants Arms and feet of children Small hands, arms, and feet of adults
2⅝ inches	Legs, thighs and heads of children Arms and lower legs of adults Small thighs, small heads of adults
3⅝ inches	Legs, thighs, lower legs, shoulders, arms, heads of adults Trunks of infants
5 inches	Large heads, small trunks of adults
7 inches	Trunks of adults

PROCEDURE 7-8
APPLYING A TUBULAR GAUZE BANDAGE

1. **PROCEDURAL STEP.** Wash the hands. Identify the patient and explain the procedure.

2. **PROCEDURAL STEP.** Assemble the equipment. The equpment includes the **appropriate-size applicator** and **roll of tubular gauze** and **adhesive tape.** The applicator selected should be somewhat larger than the part to be bandaged.

PRINCIPLE. The applicator should be somewhat larger than the body part to allow the gauze to slide easily over the body part. The proper gauze width must be used to ensure a secure fit.

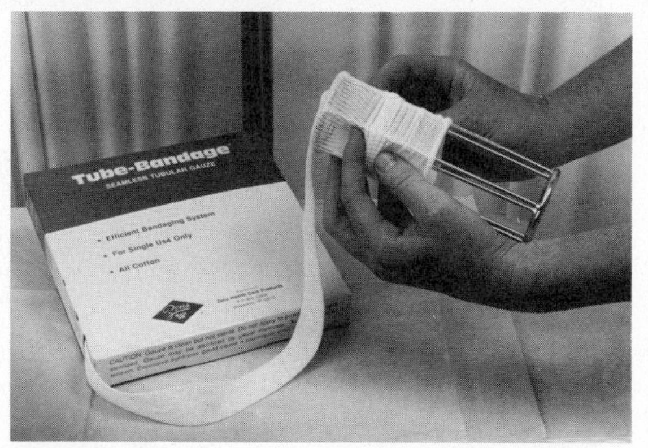

3. **PROCEDURAL STEP.** Place the gauze bandage on the applicator as follows:
   a. Place the applicator upright on a flat surface.
   b. Pull a sufficient length of gauze from the dispensing box roll.
   c. Spread apart the open end of the gauze, using your fingers.
   d. Slide the gauze over the upper end of the applicator. Continue loading the applicator by gathering enough gauze on the applicator to complete the bandage.
   e. Cut the roll of gauze near the opening of the box.

4. **PROCEDURAL STEP.** Place the applicator over the proximal end of the patient's finger.

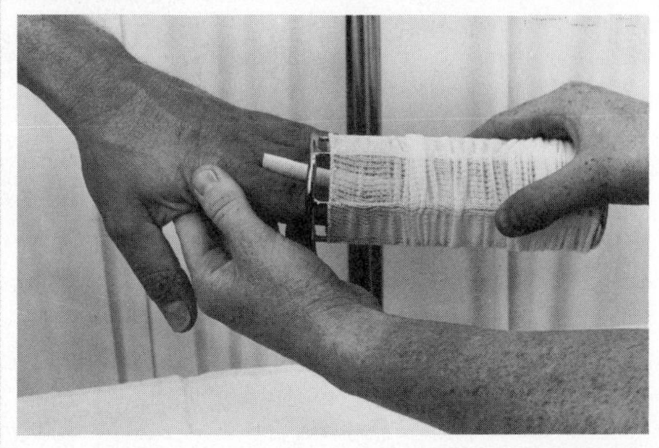

Continued

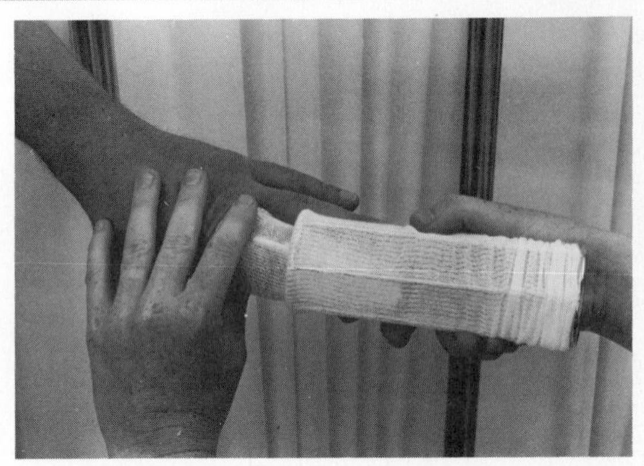

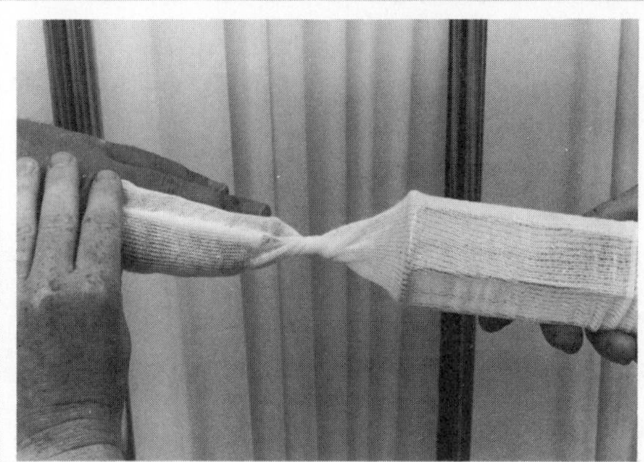

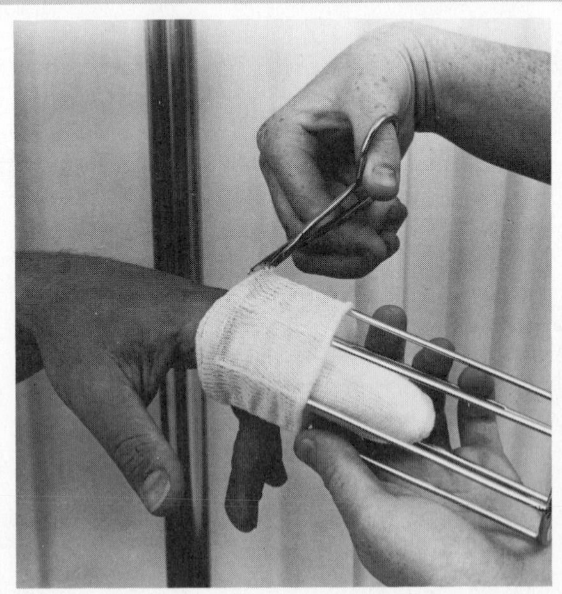

5. **PROCEDURAL STEP.** Move the applicator from the proximal end to the distal end of the patient's finger, while leaving the bandage on the length of the finger. The bandage should be held in place at the base of the patient's fingers with your fingers.

PRINCIPLE. The bandage should be held in place to prevent it from sliding, which would not ensure complete coverage of the affected part.

6. **PROCEDURAL STEP.** Pull the applicator 1 to 2 inches past the end of the patient's finger. Continue to hold the bandage in place with your fingers.

PRINCIPLE. The bandage must extend beyond the length of the patient's finger in order to secure it at the distal end.

7. **PROCEDURAL STEP.** Rotate the applicator one full turn to anchor the bandage.

PRINCIPLE. Anchoring the bandage holds it securely in place.

8. **PROCEDURAL STEP.** Move the applicator forward again toward the proximal end of the patient's finger.

PRINCIPLE. Moving the applicator forward applies a second layer of bandaging material to the patient's finger.

9. **PROCEDURAL STEP.** Move the applicator forward approximately 1 inch past the original starting point of the bandage, and anchor it using another rotating motion.

PRINCIPLE. Anchoring the bandage holds it securely in place.

10. **PROCEDURAL STEP.** Repeat this procedure for the number of layers desired. Finish the last layer at the proximal end. Cut any unused gauze from the applicator and remove the applicator.

11. **PROCEDURAL STEP.** Apply adhesive tape at the base of the finger to secure the bandage.

12. **PROCEDURAL STEP.** Wash the hands and record the procedure. Include the patient's name, date and time, and location of the bandage application. Place your initials next to the recording.

Record data below.

DATE	TIME	PATIENT'S NAME	RECORDING

Study Questions

1. What types of procedures require the use of surgical asepsis?
2. What guidelines should be observed during a sterile procedure to maintain surgical asepsis?
3. What is the difference between a closed wound and an open wound?
4. What are the three phases involved in the healing process?
5. What is the function of a dressing?
6. What guidelines should be followed when applying a bandage?

8

ADMINISTRATION OF MEDICATION

CHAPTER OUTLINE

Classification of Drugs Based on Preparation
Classification of Drugs Based on Action
Systems of Measurement Used to Administer Medication
Conversion Between Units of Measurement
The Prescription
Factors Affecting the Action of Drugs in the Body
Basic Guidelines for the Preparation and Administration of Medication
Oral Administration
Parenteral Administration
Tuberculin Skin Testing

COMPETENCIES

After completing this chapter, you should be able to demonstrate the proper procedures to perform the following:

1. Convert between the metric, apothecary, and household systems.
2. Prepare and administer oral medication and record the procedure.
3. Reconstitute a powdered drug for parenteral administration.
4. Withdraw medication from an ampule.
5. Withdraw medication from a vial.
6. Prepare and administer an intradermal injection and record the procedure.
7. Prepare and administer a subcutaneous injection and record the procedure.
8. Locate the following intramuscular injection sites: gluteus medius, deltoid, vastus lateralis, and ventrogluteal.
9. Prepare and administer an intramuscular injection and record the procedure.
10. Administer an injection using the Z-track method and record the procedure.
11. Administer a tine test and read, interpret, and record the test results.

LEARNING OBJECTIVES

After completing this chapter, you should be able to do the following:

1. Define the terms listed in the vocabulary.
2. List eight routes for administration of medication.
3. Explain the difference between administering, prescribing, and dispensing medication.
4. Classify drugs according to preparation.
5. Classify drugs according to the action they have on the body.
6. Explain why the metric system is used most often as a measurement system.
7. Identify the units of weight and volume in the metric and apothecary systems.
8. List the guidelines that should be followed in writing metric notations.
9. List the guidelines that should be followed in writing apothecary notations.
10. Describe the use of the household system in medication administration.
11. List and explain the different parts of a prescription.
12. Identify four factors that affect the action of drugs in the body.
13. List the six "rights" of preparing and administering medication.
14. State the advantages and disadvantages of using the parenteral route of administration.
15. Explain which tissue layers of the body are used for an intradermal, a subcutaneous, and an intramuscular injection.
16. Identify the parts of a needle and syringe and explain their function. Read correctly the calibrations on the syringe.
17. Explain the purpose for using the Z-track technique to administer medication.
18. Explain the purpose for performing tuberculin skin testing.
19. Explain the significance of a positive reaction to a tuberculin skin test and list the diagnostic procedures that will be performed as a result of a positive reaction.
20. Explain the principle underlying each step in the procedures for administering oral and parenteral medication and for performing a tine test.

• VOCABULARY •

ampule (am' pūl)—A small sealed glass container containing a single dose of medication.

aspirate (as' pi-rāt)—To remove by suction.

avoirdupois (av' er-dŭ-poiz")—A system of weight used in English-speaking countries for weighing heavy articles. This system is not used to weigh drugs and precious stones and metals.

conversion (kon-ver' zhun)—Changing from one unit of measurement to another.

cubic centimeter (kyōō' bik sĕn' tə-me' tər)—The amount of space occupied by 1 milliliter (1 ml = 1 cc).

dermis (der' mis)—The true skin; the main thickness of the skin, with an active blood supply.

dose (dōs)—The quantity of a drug to be administered at one time.

epidermis (ep" i-der' mis)—The outermost, nonvascular layer of the skin.

induration (in" du-ra' shun)—An area of hardened tissue.

inhalation administration (in" hah-la' shun ăd-mĭn" ĭs-tra' shun)—The administration of medication by way of air or other vapor being drawn into the lungs.

intradermal injection (in" trah-der' mal in-jek' shun)—Introducing medication into the dermal layer of the skin.

intramuscular injection (in" trah-mus' ku-lar in-jek' shun)—Introducing medication into the muscle layer of the body.

intravenous injection (in" trah-ve' nus in-jek' shun)—Introducing medication into the bloodstream directly through a vein.

length (length)—A unit of linear measurement used to measure length or distance.

oral administration (o' ral ăd-mĭn" ĭs-tra' -shun)—Administration of medication by mouth.

prescription (pre-skrip' shun)—Order for a drug or other therapy written by a physician.

subcutaneous injection (sub" ku-ta' ne-us in-jek' shun)—Introducing medication beneath the skin, into the subcutaneous or fatty layer of the body.

sublingual administration (sub-ling' gwal ăd-mĭn" ĭs-tra' shun)—Administration of medication by placing it under the tongue, where it dissolves and is absorbed through the mucous membrane.

topical administration (top' i-kal ăd-mĭn" ĭs-tra' shun)—Applying a drug to a particular spot, usually for a local action.

vesiculation (vē-sik" u-la' shun)—The formation of vesicles (fluid-containing lesions of the skin).

vial (vi' al)—A closed glass container with a rubber stopper.

volume (vol' ūm)—The amount of space occupied by a substance.

weight (wāt)—The measure of heaviness of a substance.

wheal (hwēl)—A small raised area of the skin.

Introduction

In the medical office, medication may be administered, prescribed, or dispensed. Medication that is *administered* is actually given to the patient at the office. Medication is *prescribed* when a physician provides the patient with a written prescription for a drug to be filled at a pharmacy. Prescriptions may also be telephoned to the pharmacy by the physician, depending on the preference of the patient. *Dispensed* medication is either given or sold to the patient at the office, to be taken at home.

An important responsibility of the medical assistant is the administration of medication. (However, one should first check the laws of the state to make sure it is legally permissible for the medical assistant to administer medication.) Common routes of administration are oral, sublingual, inhalation, rectal, urethral, vaginal, topical, intradermal, subcutaneous, intramuscular, and intravenous. The route of administration used depends on the type of drug being given, the intended action, and the rapidity of response desired. The routes by which medication is most commonly given in the medical office are the oral and the parenteral. *Parenteral* refers to sites outside the gastrointestinal tract; this term is most commonly used to indicate the administration of medication by injection.

The medical assistant is obligated to become familiar with the drugs that are most frequently used in his or her office. It is essential to have a knowledge of their indications, precautions, common side effects, adverse reactions, route of administration, dosage, and storage. With each drug, the manufacturer includes a package insert that contains valuable information regarding the drug. In addition, many drug references are available. The *Physician's Desk Reference* is frequently used in the medical office. A list of drugs commonly used in the medical office is included in Table 8–1.

The medical assistant should administer and dispense medication only under the instructions of the physician. It is unlawful to act without his or her consent.

Classification of Drugs Based on Preparation

The study of drugs is known as *pharmacology.* This discipline includes the preparation, use, and action of drugs. A *drug* is a chemical that is used for the treatment, prevention, or diagnosis of disease. Most drugs are produced synthetically, but they may also be obtained from other sources such as animals, plants, and minerals.

Drugs are available in two basic forms: liquid and solid. The following list includes the common categories of drugs available in these forms.

Liquid Preparations

Elixir — An elixir is a drug that is dissolved in a solution of alcohol and water. Elixirs are sweetened and flavored and are taken orally. Example: phenobarbital elixir.

Emulsion — An emulsion is a mixture of fats or oils in water. Example: cod liver oil emulsion.

Liniment — A liniment is a drug combined with oil, soap, alcohol, or water. Liniments are applied externally, using friction, to produce a feeling of heat or warmth. Example: camphor liniment.

TABLE 8-1. Drugs Commonly Utilized in the Medical Office*

ANALGESICS
Non-narcotic
Acetylsalicylic acid (ASA, Bayer Aspirin, Ascriptin, Bufferin)
Acetaminophen (Tylenol, Datril)
Propoxyphene (Darvon)
Ibuprofen (Advil, Medipren, Motrin)

Narcotic
Morphine sulfate
Codeine phosphate
Meperidine hydrochloride (Demerol)
Oxycodone hydrochloride; oxycodone terephthalate with ASA (Percodan)
Oxycodone with Tylenol (Percocet)

ANTACIDS
Magnesium and aluminum hydroxides (Maalox)
Magnesium and aluminum hydroxides with simethicone (Mylanta)
Aluminum hydroxide (Amphojel)

ANTIANEMICS (IRON PREPARATIONS)
Iron-dextran (Imferon)
Ferrous sulfate (Feosol)
Cyanocobalamin; Vitamin B_{12} (Sytobex)
Folic acid (Folvite)

ANTIANXIETY (MINOR TRANQUILIZERS)
Chlordiazepoxide (Librium)
Diazepam (Valium)
Alprazolam (Xanax)
Meprobamate (Equanil)

ANTIARRHYTHMICS
Verapamil (Calan, Isoptin)
Quinidine sulfate
Propranolol (Inderal)
Procainamide (Pronestyl)

ANTIARTHRITIC
Ibuprofen (Advil, Medipren, Motrin)
Acetylsalicylic acid (ASA, Bayer Aspirin, Ascriptin)
Indomethacin (Indocin)

ANTIBIOTICS
Penicillin V (Pen-Vee K, V-Cillin K)
Benzathine penicillin G (Bicillin)
Procaine penicillin G (Wycillin, Duracillin)
Ampicillin (Amcill, Omnipen)
Amoxicillin (Amoxil)
Tetracycline hydrochloride (Achromycin V; Sumycin)
Erythromycin (E-mycin, Erythrocin, Ilosone, Pediamycin)
Cephalexin (Keflex, Keflin)
Gentamicin sulfate (Garamycin)

ANTICOAGULANTS
Heparin sodium (Liquaemin)
Bishydroxycoumarin (Dicumarol)
Warfarin sodium (Coumadin)

ANTICONVULSANTS
Phenytoin (Dilantin)
Phenobarbital sodium (Luminal)
Carbamazepine (Tegretol)

ANTIDEPRESSANTS
Amitriptyline hydrochloride (Elavil)
Phenelzine sulfate (Nardil)
Trazodone (Desyrel)

ANTIDIARRHEALS
Diphenoxylate hydrochloride (Lomotil)
Kaolin/Pectin (Kaopectate)
Loperamide (Imodium)

ANTIEMETICS
Dimenhydrinate (Dramamine)
Meclizine (Antivert)
Hydroxyzine (Atarax, Vistaril)
Prochlorperazine (Compazine)

ANTIHISTAMINES
Diphenhydramine hydrochloride (Benadryl, Benylin)
Promethazine hydrochloride (Phenergan)
Brompheniramine (Dimetane)
Cyproheptadine (Periactin)
Terfenadine (Seldane)

ANTIHYPERTENSIVES
Captopril (Capoten)
Verapamil (Calan, Isoptin)
Nifedipine (Procardia)
Prazosin (Minipress)
Reserpine (Serpasil)
Methyldopa (Aldomet)
Atenolol (Tenormin)
Hydralazine (Apresoline)

ANTITUSSIVES
Codeine syrup (Cheracol)
Dextromethorphan (Pertussin, Romilar)
Diphenhydramine hydrochloride (Benadryl, Benylin Cough Syrup)

ANTIULCERS
Cimetidine (Tagamet)
Ranitidine (Zantac)

BRONCHODILATORS
Isoproterenol hydrochloride (Isuprel)
Aminophylline (Aminophyllin)
Metaproterenol (Alupent, Metaprel)
Epinephrine hydrochloride (Adrenalin Chloride)

CARDIOTONICS
Digoxin (Lanoxin)
Digitoxin (Crystodigin)

CATHARTICS AND LAXATIVES
Bisacodyl (Dulcolax)
Psyllium seed (Metamucil)
Magnesium hydroxide (Milk of Magnesia)
Docusate calcium (Colace, Surfak)
Mineral oil (Agoral, Neo-Cultol)

DIURETICS
Furosemide (Lasix)
Hydrochlorothiazide (Esidrix, Hydro-Diuril)
Chlorothiazide (Diuril)
Bumetanide (Bumex)

EMETICS
Ipecac syrup

EXPECTORANTS
Glyceryl guaiacolate (Robitussin)
Acetylcysteine (Mucomyst)

GLUCOCORTICOIDS
Cortisone (Cortone)
Hydrocortisone (Cortisol, Hydrocortone)
Prednisone (Deltasone)
Dexamethasone (Decadron)

INSULIN
Rapid Acting
Regular Iletin
Humulin R

Table continued on following page

TABLE 8–1. Drugs Commonly Utilized in the Medical Office* *(Continued)*

INSULIN *(Continued)*
Intermediate Acting
NPH Iletin
Humulin N
Lente Iletin

Long Acting
Protamine Zinc Iletin
Ultralente

Oral Hypoglycemics
Chlorpropamide (Diabinese)
Tolbutamide (Orinase)

MUSCLE RELAXANTS
Methocarbamol (Robaxin)
Cyclobenzaprine (Flexeril)
Diazepam (Valium)
Methocarbamol (Robaxin)

NASAL DECONGESTANTS
Phenylephrine hydrochloride (Neo-Synephrine)
Xylometazoline hydrochloride (Otrivin Spray)
Oxymetazoline hydrochloride (Afrin)

ORAL CONTRACEPTIVES
Norethindrone/ethinyl estradiol (Ortho-Novum)
Norgestrel/ethinyl estradiol (Ovral)
Norethindrone/mestranol (Norinyl)

SEDATIVE-HYPNOTICS
Phenobarbital sodium (Luminal)
Secobarbital sodium (Seconal)
Pentobarbital sodium (Nembutal)
Flurazepam (Dalmane)
Temazepam (Restoril)
Triazolam (Halcion)
Meprobamate (Equanil)
Alprazolam (Xanax)
Hydroxyzine (Atarax, Vistaril)

SULFONAMIDES
Sulfisoxazole acetyl (Gantrisin)
Sulfamethoxazole (Gantanol)
Trimethoprim/sulfamethoxazole (Bactrim, Septra)

VASODILATORS (CORONARY)
Nitroglycerin (Nitro-Bid, Nitroglyn, Nitrol, Nitrostat)
Erythrityl tetranitrate (Cardilate)
Dipyridamole (Persantine)

* The generic names are listed first and the trade names follow in parentheses.

Lotion — A lotion is an aqueous preparation that contains suspended ingredients. Lotions are used to treat external skin conditions. They work to soothe, protect, and moisten the skin and/or to destroy harmful bacteria. Example: calamine lotion.

Solution — A solution is a liquid preparation containing one or more completely dissolved substances. The dissolved substance is known as the solute, and the liquid in which it is dissolved is known as the solvent. Example: epinephrine solution.

Spirit — A spirit is a drug combined with an alcoholic solution that is volatile (a substance that is volatile evaporates readily). Example: aromatic spirit of ammonia.

Spray — A spray is a fine stream of medicated vapor and is usually used to treat nose and throat conditions. Example: ephedrine spray.

Syrup — A syrup is a drug dissolved in a solution of sugar, water, and a flavoring that may be added to disguise an unpleasant taste. Example: syrup of ipecac.

Tincture — A tincture is a drug dissolved in a solution of alcohol or alcohol and water. Example: tincture of iodine.

Solid Preparations

Capsule — A capsule is a drug contained in a gelatin capsule that is water soluble and functions to prevent the patient from tasting the drug. Example: diphenhydramine (Benadryl) capsules.

Lozenge — A lozenge is a drug contained in a candy-like base. Lozenges have a circular shape and are designed to dissolve on the tongue. Example: cough lozenges.

Ointment — An ointment is a drug combined with an oil or water-soluble base, resulting in a semisolid preparation. Ointments are applied externally to the skin. Example: sulfur ointment.

Suppository	A suppository is a drug mixed with a firm base, such as cocoa butter, that is designed to melt at body temperature. A suppository is shaped into a cylinder or a cone for easy insertion into a body cavity, such as the rectum or vagina. Example: glycerin suppository.
Tablet	Tablets are powdered drugs that have been pressed into discs. Some tablets are *scored,* meaning they are marked with an indentation so they can be broken into halves and/or quarters for proper dosage. Example: aspirin tablet.

Tablets and capsules may be *enteric-coated,* meaning that they are coated with a substance that prevents them from dissolving until they reach the intestines. The purpose of this is to protect the drug from being destroyed by gastric juices or to prevent it from irritating the stomach lining.

Classification of Drugs Based on Action

Drugs can also be classified according to the action they have on the body. The medical assistant should know in which category a particular drug belongs. The following is a classification of common categories of drugs based on action:

Analgesic	Drug that relieves pain.
Anesthetic	Drug that produces a loss of feeling and an inability to perceive pain. There are two types of anesthetics: general and local. A general anesthetic affects the whole body by producing a loss of consciousness. It is administered through inhalation of a gas or by an intravenous injection. A local anesthetic produces a loss of feeling in only a specific part of the body and is administered through an intradermal or intramuscular injection.
Anorectic	Drug that decreases the appetite.
Antacid	Drug that neutralizes acid, usually in the gastrointestinal tract.
Antianemic	Drug that prevents or cures anemia.
Antianxiety (minor tranquilizer)	Drug that reduces anxiety and tension but still allows the person to carry on normal activities.
Antiarrhythmic	Drug that helps prevent or alleviate cardiac arrhythmias.
Antiarthritic	Drug that relieves arthritis.
Antibiotic	Drug that inhibits the growth of or kills disease-producing bacteria.
Anticoagulant	Drug that inhibits blood clotting.
Anticonvulsant	Drug that suppresses convulsions or seizures.
Antidepressant	Drug that elevates the mood and relieves depression.
Antidiarrheal	Drug that counteracts diarrhea.
Antidote	Substance that neutralizes a poison or drug overdose.
Antiemetic	Drug that helps to prevent or stop vomiting.
Antihistamine	Drug that counteracts the production of histamine in the body to help relieve allergic symptoms.

Antihypertensive	Drug that reduces high blood pressure.
Antiseptic	Drug that inhibits the growth of or kills disease-producing microorganisms.
Antitussive	Drug that suppresses coughing.
Antiulcer	Drug that promotes the healing of ulcers.
Bronchodilator	Drug that dilates the bronchi.
Cardiotonic	Drug that has a tonic effect on the heart. (Tonic refers to producing and restoring normal tone.)
Cathartic and laxative	Drugs that promote defecation.
Decongestant	Drug that works to decrease congestion and swelling, usually of the nasal mucosa; it acts as a vasoconstrictor.
Diuretic	Drug that increases the output of urine.
Emetic	Drug that induces vomiting.
Expectorant	Drug that liquefies mucus and helps to expel it from the respiratory tract.
Hemostatic	Drug that stops blood flow.
Hypnotic	Drug that induces sleep.
Insulin (therapy)	Preparation used in the medical treatment of diabetes.
Muscle relaxant	Drug that works to relax muscles by decreasing muscle tone or spasms.
Oral contraceptive	Birth control drug that works by preventing ovulation.
Sedative	Drug that calms and quiets, without necessarily inducing sleep.
Tranquilizer	Drug that reduces anxiety and tension but still allows the person to carry on normal activities.
Vasoconstrictor	Drug that narrows the diameter of the blood vessels.
Vasodilator	Drug that widens the diameter of blood vessels.

Systems of Measurement Used to Administer Medication

Three systems of measurement are used in the United States for prescribing and administering medication: the metric system, the apothecary system, and the household system. The metric system is the most common, because it is more accurate and easier to use. However, some physicians originally trained in the apothecary system may still use it to order medication. Therefore, it is important for the medical assistant to be familiar with both of these systems. The third, the household system, is the least accurate and is generally used only when a patient takes liquid medication at home.

Systems of measurement have units of weight, volume, and length. *Weight* refers to the heaviness of an item, whereas *volume* refers to the amount of space occupied by a substance. *Length* is a unit of linear measurement used to measure the distance from one point to another. Although length is not used to administer medication, it is used in other aspects of the medical office. For example, the head circumference of infants is measured in centimeters (cm), a metric unit of linear measurement.

To properly prepare and administer medication and to avoid medication errors, the medical assistant must have a thorough knowledge of the specific units of measurement for each of these three systems and must be able to convert within each, as well as from one system to another. A basic discussion of the metric, apothecary, and household systems is presented below. A more thorough study of these systems, including conversion of units and dose calculation, is included in the *Student Manual* (Supplemental Education for Chapter 8: Drug Dosage Calculation).

The Metric System

The metric system was developed in France in the latter part of the eighteenth century in an effort to simplify measurement. Most European countries are required by law to use this system for the measurement of weight, volume, and length. Overall, the metric system is used for most scientific and medical measurements. All pharmaceutical companies now use the metric system for labeling medications. Those drugs originally manufactured using the apothecary system include both the apothecary and the metric equivalent on their labels; examples include aspirin, codeine, nitroglycerin, and phenobarbital.

The metric system employs a uniform decimal scale and is based upon units of 10, making it very flexible and logical. The basic metric units of measurement are the gram, liter, and meter. The gram is a unit of weight used to measure solids. The liter is a unit of volume used to measure liquids, and the meter is a linear unit used to measure length or distance. The metric units used most often in the administration of medication in the medical office are the milligram, gram, milliliter, and cubic centimeter. Because a *cubic centimeter* (cc) is the amount of space occupied by 1 milliliter (ml), these two units can be used interchangeably (i.e., 1 ml = 1 cc).

Prefixes added to the words gram, liter, and meter designate smaller or larger units of measurement in the metric system. The same prefixes are used with all three units. For example, *milli-* is used as follows: *milli*gram, *milli*liter, and *milli*meter. Each prefix changes the value of the basic unit of measurement by the same amount. The prefix milli- denotes a unit that is 1/1000 of the basic unit. Therefore, 1 gram is equal to 1000 milligrams, 1 liter is equal to 1000 milliliters and 1 meter is equal to 1000 millimeters. Table 8–2 lists the units of measurement in the metric system and equivalent values between the units.

TABLE 8–2. Metric System: Conversion of Equivalent Values

WEIGHT	
1000 micrograms	= 1 milligram
1000 milligrams	= 1 gram
1000 grams	= 1 kilogram
VOLUME	
1000 milliliters	= 1 liter
1000 liters	= 1 kiloliter
1 milliliter	= 1 cubic centimeter

Metric Notation Guidelines

Specific guidelines are used in the medical notation of metric units of measurement and dose quantity. In order to read prescriptions and medication orders, to record medication administration, and, most important, to avoid medication errors, the medical assistant must be familiar with and be able to use these guidelines as listed below.

1. The units of metric measurement are written using the following abbreviations:

Weight microgram: mcg
milligram: mg
gram: g
kilogram: kg

Volume milliliter: ml or mL
cubic centimeter: cc
liter: L

2. A period should not be used with the abbreviation of the units of measurement.

Example Correct: mg
ml
Incorrect: mg.
ml.

3. Arabic numerals (1, 2, 3, 4) are used to express the quantity of the dose.

Example Correct: 4 mg
Incorrect: $\overline{\text{iv}}$ mg

4. The numeral expressing the quantity of the dose is placed in front of the abbreviation. To make it easier to read, a (single) space should be left between the quantity and abbreviation.

Example Correct: 5 ml
Incorrect: ml 5 and 5ml

5. A fraction of a dose is written as a decimal.

Example Correct: 0.5 g
Incorrect: ½ g

6. If the dose is a fraction of a gram, a zero must be placed before the decimal as a means of focusing on the fractional dose. This reduces the possibility of misreading the dose as a whole number.

Example Correct: 0.5 g (This reduces the possibility of not seeing the decimal point and reading the dose as 5 grams.)
Incorrect: .5 g

7. A decimal point and a zero should not be placed after a whole number. The decimal point may be overlooked, resulting in a tenfold overdose error.

Example Correct: 1 ml (This reduces the possibility of not seeing the decimal point and reading the dose as 10 ml.)
Incorrect: 1.0 ml

TABLE 8-3. Apothecary System: Conversion of Equivalent Values

WEIGHT	
60 grains	= 1 dram
8 drams	= 1 ounce
12 ounces	= 1 pound
VOLUME	
60 minims	= 1 fluidram
8 fluidrams	= 1 fluidounce
16 fluidounces	= 1 pint
2 pints	= 1 quart
4 quarts	= 1 gallon

Apothecary System

The apothecary system is older and less accurate than the metric system. It was brought to the United States from England during the eighteenth century. Pharmacists used this system during the colonial period to compound and measure medications. This system is gradually being phased out in preference to the metric system. Until that process is completed, however, the medical assistant must be familiar with this system and be able to use it to administer medication.

The basic unit of weight in the apothecary system is the grain, derived from the weight of a large grain of wheat, which was used to balance the material being weighed. The next largest unit of measurement is the scruple; however, this unit is not used to administer medication. The remaining units, in order of increasing weight, are the dram, ounce, and pound. The pound is not generally used in the administration of medication. The medical assistant should note, however, that in the apothecary system the pound is equal to 12 ounces, in contrast to the more familiar *avoirdupois* pound used to measure body weight, which is equal to 16 ounces.

Measures of liquid volume in the apothecary system correlate closely with measures of dry weight in the same system. The smallest unit of measurement is the minim, meaning "the least." A minim is approximately equivalent to a volume of water weighing 1 grain. A minim glass or a syringe calibrated in minims must be used to measure with this unit. The remaining units of liquid volume in the apothecary system, in order of increasing volume, are the fluidram, fluidounce, pint, quart, and gallon. The basic unit of linear measurement is the inch, followed by the foot, yard, and mile. Most Americans are familiar with apothecary units of measurement because of their frequent use in everyday life. For example, milk is available in pints, quarts, and gallons, and height is measured in feet and inches. Table 8-3 lists the units of measurement in the apothecary system and equivalent values between units.

Apothecary Notation Guidelines

The following guidelines are used in the medical notation of apothecary units of measurement and dose quantity.

1. The units of apothecary measurement are usually written using abbreviations and symbols as follows:

Weight grain: gr
dram: ʒ
ounce: ℥

Volume minim: ♏
fluidram: fʒ
fluidounce: f℥
pint: pt
quart: qt
gallon: gal or C

2. When symbols and abbreviations are used to express apothecary units, lower-case roman numerals must be used to express the dose quantity.

Example Correct: ℥ vi (6 ounces)
Incorrect: 6 ℥; ℥ 6

3. The roman numeral expressing dose quantity must *follow* the symbol or abbreviation.

Example Correct: ʒ ii (2 drams); gr v (5 grains)
Incorrect: ii ʒ; v gr

4. A line may be placed over the roman numerals. Dots are placed above the line for emphasis as a safeguard against error.

Example Correct: fʒ iii (3 fluidrams)
Incorrect: fʒ 111

5. The symbol ss is used to designate ½ of a dose and must follow the apothecary symbol or abbreviation.

Example Correct: gr ss
Incorrect: gr ½

6. Fractions (other than ½) are written in arabic numerals and must follow the apothecary symbol or abbreviation.

Example Correct: gr ¼
Incorrect: gr 0.25; ¼ gr

(*Note:* If abbreviations and symbols are *not* used to express apothecary units of measurement, arabic numerals must be used to express dose quantity and are placed before the unit of measurement.)

Example Correct: 5 grains; ½ ounce
Incorrect: grains 5; ounce ½ or ounce ss

The Household System

The household system is more complicated and less accurate for administering liquid medication than either the metric or apothecary system. Nevertheless, most individuals are familiar with this system because of its frequent utilization in the United States. Thus, this system of measurement may be the only one the patient can fully relate to and therefore safely use to administer liquid medication at home. For example, most patients are more comfortable measuring medication in drops and teaspoons, rather than minims and milliliters. In addition, the patient is

TABLE 8-4. Household System: Conversion of Equivalent Values

ABBREVIATIONS

drop: gtt
teaspoon: t or tsp
tablespoon: T or tbs
ounce: oz
cup: c

VOLUME

60 drops	=	1 teaspoon
3 teaspoons	=	1 tablespoon
6 teaspoons	=	1 ounce
2 tablespoons	=	1 ounce
6 ounces	=	1 teacup
8 ounces	=	1 glass

more likely to have household measuring devices on hand than to have metric measuring devices. If a precise measurement is needed, however, the metric system must be used, and the medical assistant should instruct the patient in the use of the metric measuring device.

Volume is the only household unit of measurement used to administer medication. The basic unit of liquid volume in the household system is the drop (gtt), which is approximately equal to 0.6 ml in the metric system and 1 minim in the apothecary system. These units cannot be considered exact equivalents, because the size of the drop varies based upon temperature, the viscosity of the liquid, and the size of the dropper. The remaining units, in order of increasing volume, are the teaspoon, tablespoon, ounce (fluidounce), cup, and glass. Table 8-4 lists the units of liquid volume measurement in the household system and equivalent values between units.

Conversion Between Units of Measurement

Changing from one unit of measurement to another is known as *conversion*. Conversion is required when medication is ordered in one unit of measurement and the medication label expresses the drug strength in a different unit. The dose quantity must be mathematically translated or converted to the unit of measurement of the medication on hand. For example, if the physician orders 5 g of an oral solid medication and the medication label expresses the drug strength in milligrams, the medical assistant would need to convert the grams into milligrams to know how much medication to administer. Converting of units of measurement can be classified into the following categories: (1) conversion of units within a measurement system and (2) conversion of units from one measurement system to another.

Converting units within a measurement system allows a quantity to be expressed in a different, but equal, unit of measurement within the *same* system. An example of converting between units of weight within the metric system is as follows: 1 g is equal to 1000 mg. Converting from one measurement system to another allows a quantity to be expressed in a unit of measurement from *another* system. An example of a conversion between the apothecary and metric systems is as follows: 1 grain (apothecary system) is equivalent to 60 mg (metric system).

Conversion requires the use of a conversion table to indicate the equivalent values between various units of measurement. Conversion tables of equivalent values used to convert within each of the three measurement systems have previously been discussed and are included in the following tables:

- Metric Conversion—Table 8-2
- Apothecary Conversion—Table 8-3
- Household Conversion—Table 8-4

TABLE 8-5. Conversion Chart for Metric and Apothecary Systems (Commonly Used Approximate Equivalents)

METRIC SYSTEM TO APOTHECARY SYSTEM		APOTHECARY SYSTEM TO METRIC SYSTEM
Weight		**Weight**
	60 mg = 1 grain	15 grains = 1000 mg (1 g)
	1 g = 15 grains	10 grains = 600 mg
	4 g = 1 dram	7½ grains = 500 mg
	30 mg = 1 ounce	5 grains = 300 mg
	1 kg = 2.2 pounds	3 grains = 200 mg
Volume		1½ grains = 100 mg
	0.06 ml = 1 minim	1 grain = 60 mg
	1 ml (cc) = 15 minims	3/4 grain = 50 mg
	4 ml = 1 fluidram	1/2 grain = 30 mg
	30 ml = 1 fluidounce	1/4 grain = 15 mg
	500 ml = 1 pint	1/6 grain = 10 mg
	1000 ml (1 L) = 1 quart	1/8 grain = 8.0 mg
		1/12 grain = 5.0 mg
		1/15 grain = 4.0 mg
		1/20 grain = 3.0 mg
		1/30 grain = 2.0 mg
		1/40 grain = 1.5 mg
		1/50 grain = 1.2 mg
		1/60 grain = 1.0 mg
		1/100 grain = 0.6 mg
		1/120 grain = 0.5 mg
		1/150 grain = 0.4 mg
		1/200 grain = 0.3 mg
		1/300 grain = 0.2 mg
		1/600 grain = 0.1 mg

Tables used to convert between systems consist of approximate equivalents, rather than exact equivalents, and a 10 per cent error usually occurs in making these conversions. Conversion tables used to convert from one system to another are presented in Tables 8-5 and 8-6.

The medical assistant must be careful when using conversion tables to avoid errors in interpolation. The numbers on conversion tables are small and close together; therefore, it is possible to misread the chart from one column to the other. To reduce this possibility, a straight edge should be used when obtaining a value from a conversion table.

TABLE 8-6. Conversion Chart for Apothecary and Metric Equivalents of Household Measures (Volume)

HOUSEHOLD	APOTHECARY	METRIC
1 drop	= 1 minim	= 0.06 milliliter
15 drops	= 15 minims	= 1 milliliter (1 cc)
1 teaspoon	= 1 fluidram	= 5 (4) milliliter*
1 tablespoon	= 4 fluidrams	= 15 milliliter
2 tablespoons	= 1 fluidounce	= 30 milliliter
1 ounce	= 1 fluidounce	= 30 milliliter
1 teacup	= 6 fluidounces	= 180 milliliter
1 glass	= 8 fluidounces	= 240 milliliter

* The American standard teaspoon is accepted as 5 ml; however, 4 ml can be used as the equivalent to provide a more accurate conversion.

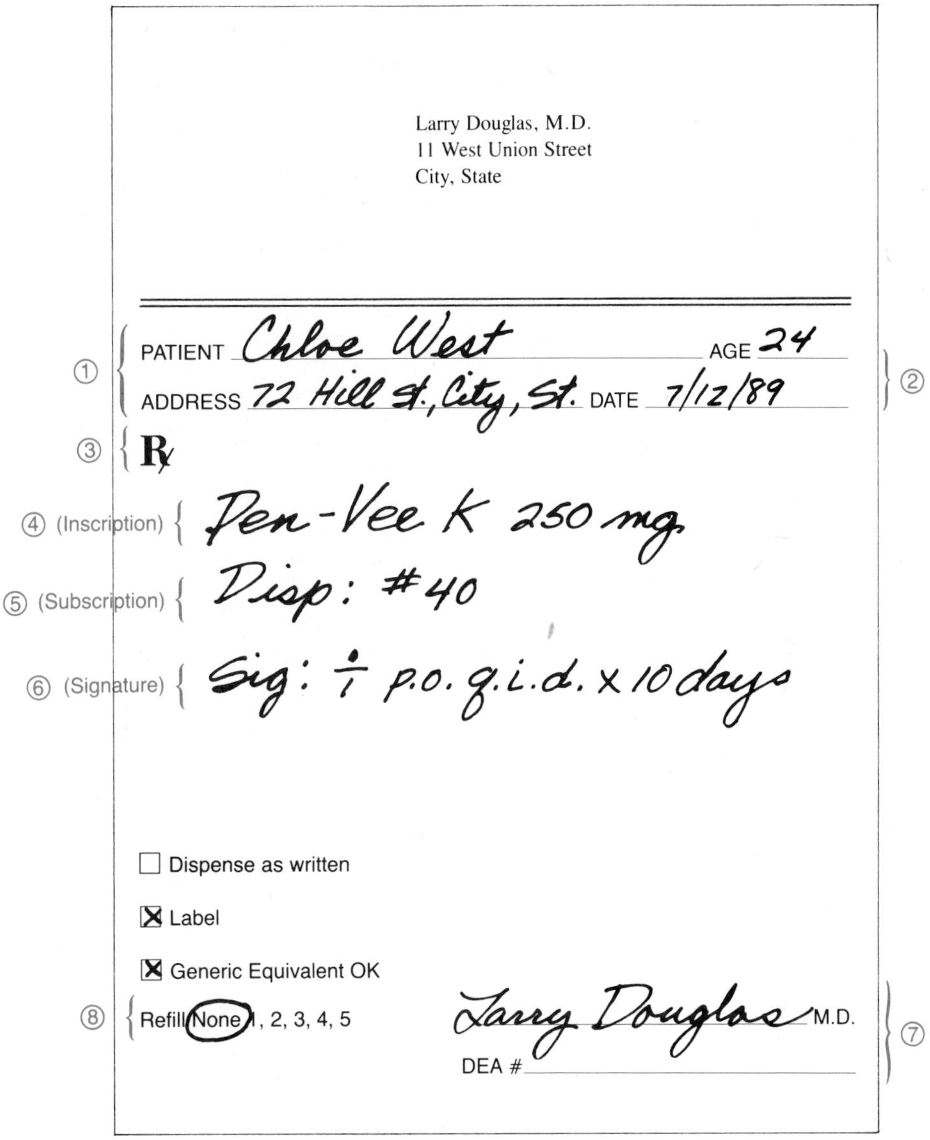

Larry Douglas, M.D.
11 West Union Street
City, State

① PATIENT Chloe West AGE 24
ADDRESS 72 Hill St., City, St. DATE 7/12/89 ②

③ ℞

④ (Inscription) Pen-Vee K 250 mg.

⑤ (Subscription) Disp: #40

⑥ (Signature) Sig: i p.o. q.i.d. x 10 days

☐ Dispense as written

☒ Label

☒ Generic Equivalent OK

⑧ Refill (None) 1, 2, 3, 4, 5 Larry Douglas M.D. ⑦

DEA #

FIGURE 8–1. An example of a prescription.

The Prescription

A *prescription* is an order written by a physician for the dispensing of drugs (or other forms of therapy). The prescription is written on a specially designed form. It includes directions to the pharmacist for filling the prescription and instructions to the patient for taking the medication (Fig. 8–1). The specific information that the prescription must include is as follows:

1. The patient's name and address.
2. The date.
3. The *superscription,* which consists of the symbol ℞. This symbol comes from the Latin word *recipe* and means "take."
4. The *inscription,* which states the name of the drug, the dosage form, and the amount per dose. Drug dosage is stated in either metric or apothecary units of measurement.
5. The *subscription,* which gives directions to the pharmacist. At present, it is generally used to designate the number of doses to be dispensed.
6. The *signature* (abbreviated S or Sig), which indicates the information to be included on the medication label. It consists of directions to the patient for taking the medication. Most physicians also prefer that the name of the drug be included on the label, since this helps the patient to identify the medication.

TABLE 8–7. Abbreviations and Symbols Commonly Used in the Medical Office

ABBREVIATION OR SYMBOL	MEANING	ABBREVIATION OR SYMBOL	MEANING
āā	of each	ml or mL	milliliter
ac	before meals	NPO	nothing by mouth
AD	right ear	non rep	do not repeat
ad lib	as desired	OD	right eye
AS	left ear	OS	left eye
aq	water	OU	in each eye
AU	in each ear	℥ or oz	ounce
bid	twice a day	pc	after meals
c̄	with	po	by mouth
cc	cubic centimeter	prn	as needed
caps	capsules	pt	patient
dil	dilute	qd	every day
ʒ	dram	qh	every hour
EENT	eye, ear, nose, and throat	q (2, 3, 4) h	Every (2, 3, 4) hours
elix	elixir	qid	four times a day
GI	gastrointestinal	qod	every other day
g	gram	qs	of sufficient quantity
GU	genitourinary	Rx	take
gr	grain	s̄	without
gtt (s)	drop (drops)	sol	solution
h	hour	SOS	if necessary
hs	at bedtime	ss	one half
IM	intramuscular	stat	at once
IV	intravenous	tab	tablet
kg	kilogram	tbs	tablespoon
L	liter	tsp	teaspoon
liq	liquid	tid	three times a day
♏	minim	tr	tincture
mg	milligram	ung	ointment

7. The physician's signature, address, and telephone number. The narcotic registry number (DEA number) must be included if a narcotic is being prescribed.
8. Instructions indicating the number of times the prescription may be refilled.

The medical assistant should make sure that all prescription pads are kept in a safe place and out of reach of individuals who may want to obtain drugs illegally. The stock supply of prescription pads should be locked in a drawer.

Abbreviations and symbols are used to write a prescription. They are also used when recording in the patient's chart. A list of the common abbreviations used in the medical office is included in Table 8–7. A more extensive list of medical abbreviations is included in Appendix B.

Controlled Drugs

By means of federal and state legislation, restrictions are placed upon drugs that have potential for abuse. These medications are known as *controlled drugs* and are classified into five categories, called schedules, which are based upon their abuse potential. Refer to Table 8–8 for a list and description of the schedules for controlled drugs. In order to prescribe or dispense controlled drugs, the physician must register each year with the *Drug Enforcement Agency (DEA)*. The physician is assigned a registration number known as the *DEA number*. Each time a prescription for a controlled drug is written, the DEA number must be indicated in the appropriate space on the prescription blank (Fig. 8–1).

Generic Prescribing

Recent changes in drug product selection laws have provided the pharmacist with more flexibility in filling prescriptions through generic prescribing. *Generic prescribing* means that the physician has written the prescription using the generic name, rather than the brand name, of the drug. Because a number of pharmaceutical manufacturers may produce the same generic drug (but by a different brand name), price competition often results. If the physician prescribes a drug using its generic name (rather than the brand name), the pharmacist is permitted to fill it with the drug offering the best savings to the patient. In addition, some states allow the pharmacist the option of filling the prescription with a generically equivalent drug, even if the prescription has been prescribed by brand name. In this case, if the physician desires the prescription to be filled with a specific brand of drug, instructions must be indicated on the prescription form, such as "dispense as written (DAW)" or words of a similar meaning (Fig. 8–1).

Factors Affecting the Action of Drugs in the Body

Certain factors affect the action of drugs in the body. Patients may respond differently to the same dosage of the same drug. The drug dosage may need to be adjusted to meet these individual variations.

The first factor to consider is *age*. Children and elderly people tend to respond more strongly to drugs than do young and middle-aged adults. The physician may calculate smaller doses for these very young and old patients.

TABLE 8–8. Classification of Controlled Substances

CLASSIFICATION	DESCRIPTION	EXAMPLES
Schedule I	Drugs having a high potential for abuse and no accepted medical use. (The drug container is marked C-I.)	Heroin LSD Marihuana Mescaline
Schedule II	Drugs having a high potential for abuse but with accepted medical use. Abuse may lead to severe psychologic or physical dependence. (The drug container is marked C-II.)	Amobarbital Amphetamine Cocaine Codeine Meperidine hydrochloride (Demerol) Morphine
Schedule III	Drugs having an accepted medical use with moderate or low potential for physical dependence and high potential for psychologic dependence. (The containers are marked C-III.)	Butabarbital Codeine-containing medications Nalorphine Paregoric
Schedule IV	Drugs having accepted medical use and that may cause mild physical or psychologic dependence. (The container is marked C-IV.)	Chloral hydrate (Noctec) Chlordiazepoxide (Librium) Diazepam (Valium) Flurazepam (Dolmane) Meprobamate (Equanil) Phenobarbital
Schedule V	Drugs having accepted medical use and that have limited potential for causing physical or psychologic dependence. (The container is marked C-V.)	Drug mixtures containing small quantities of narcotics such as cough syrups containing codeine (e.g., Robitussin A-C) Diphenoxylate and atropine preparations (e.g., Lomotil)

Medications administered by *different routes* will be absorbed at different rates. Drugs administered orally will be absorbed slowly, because they must first be digested. Parenterally administered drugs are usually absorbed more quickly than orally administered drugs, because they are injected directly into the body.

The *body size* of a patient has an effect on drug action. A thin person may require a smaller quantity of a drug, whereas an obese person may require more.

Time of administration has an effect on drug action. A drug administered through the oral route will be absorbed more rapidly when the stomach is empty than when food is present. A drug may not produce the desired effect or may be absorbed too slowly if it is taken when food is present. However, some drugs are irritating to the stomach lining and must therefore be taken with food. The medical assistant should check the drug insert or a drug reference to make sure that the drug is being administered at the proper time.

Another factor affecting drug action is *tolerance*. A patient taking a certain drug over a period of time may develop a tolerance to it. This means that the same dose of a drug no longer produces the desired effect after prolonged administration. The physician should be notified to determine whether a change of drug or alteration of dosage is needed.

When certain medications are used at the same time, *drug interactions* may occur, producing undesirable effects. The medical assistant should inquire about other medications the patient is taking and record this information in the patient's chart for review by the physician.

The patient may exhibit an *allergic reaction* to a drug after administration. The reaction may be mild and take the form of a rash, rhinitis, or pruritus. However, it may also be severe and may occur suddenly and immediately. It is then known as an *anaphylactic reaction*. Symptoms of an anaphylactic reaction begin with sneezing, edema, and itching. The symptoms quickly increase in severity and lead to dyspnea, cyanosis, and shock. Blood pressure decreases and the pulse becomes weak and thready. Convulsions, loss of consciousness, and death may occur, if treatment is not initiated promptly. To aid in preventing an allergic reaction from a drug or to reduce its danger, the medical assistant should stay with the patient after administration of the medication and should be especially alert for signs of a reaction after administering allergy skin tests or an allergy injection. If a drug reaction occurs, the physician should immediately be notified to begin treatment, which generally consists of one or more injections of epinephrine, depending on the severity of the reaction. The medical assistant must make sure that an ample supply of epinephrine is kept on hand at all times.

Basic Guidelines for the Preparation and Administration of Medication

The medical assistant should follow some basic rules when preparing and administering any drug.

1. Work in a quiet, well-lighted atmosphere that is free from distractions.
2. Know the drug to be given; be sure to give the correct drug at the proper dose. The term *dose* refers to the quantity of a drug to be administered at one time. Each medication will have a certain *dosage range,* or range of quantities of the drug, that can produce therapeutic effects. It is important to administer the exact dose of the drug. If the dose is too small, it will not produce a therapeutic effect, whereas a dose that is too large could be harmful or even fatal to the patient.
3. Read the label of the medication as it is taken from the shelf, before pouring the medication, and before replacing the medication on the shelf. Do not use a drug if the label is missing or difficult to read.
4. Do not use a drug if the color has changed, if a precipitate has formed, or if it has an unusual odor.
5. Check the expiration date before pouring the drug.
6. Check the patient's records or question the patient to make sure that he or she is not allergic to the medication before administering it.

7. Choose an appropriate site at which to administer an injection; the proper location is dictated by the type of injection being given. The site must be intact and free from abrasions, lesions, bruises, edema, and so on.
8. Make sure you give the drug to the correct patient.
9. Stay with the patient after giving the medication.
10. Record information properly in the patient's chart immediately after administering the drug. Make sure the recording is clear and written in legible handwriting to avoid confusion by individuals reading it. Include the date and time, the name of the medication, the dose given, the route of administration, the site of administration, and any unusual observations or patient reactions. Initial the entry. If you administer a medication that contains a fraction of a gram, place a 0 before the decimal point (e.g., 0.5 mg) so that the dosage is not misread as 5 mg. An example of a medication recording is as follows:

    9/15/8_, 10:30 AM, DPT, 0.5 ml, IM, left vastus lateralis JB

11. Follow the six "rights" of preparing and administering medication:
    Right drug
    Right dose
    Right route
    Right time
    Right patient
    Right technique

PROCEDURE 8-1

ADMINISTERING ORAL MEDICATION

The oral route is the most convenient and the most widely used method of administering medication. *Oral* means that the drug is given by mouth. Absorption of most oral medication takes place in the small intestines, although some may be absorbed in the mouth and stomach. Many patients find it easier to swallow a tablet or capsule with half a glass of water. However, water should not be offered after the patient has received a cough syrup, because the water would dilute its beneficial effects.

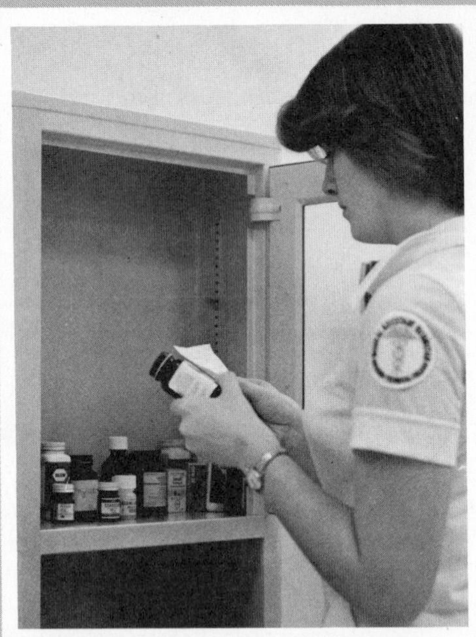

1. **PROCEDURAL STEP.** Wash the hands.

2. **PROCEDURAL STEP.** Assemble the equipment. The equipment needed includes a **medicine cup, a medication tray**, and the **physician's medication instructions.**

3. **PROCEDURAL STEP.** Work in a quiet, well-lighted atmosphere.
   PRINCIPLE. Good lighting aids the medical assistant in reading the medication label.

4. **PROCEDURAL STEP.** Select the correct medication from the shelf, and check the expiration date. Compare the medication with the physician's instructions. The drug label must be checked three times: before removing the medication from the shelf, while pouring the medication, and before returning it to its proper place.
   PRINCIPLE. If the medication is outdated, consult the physician, because it may produce undesirable effects for which the medical assistant could be held responsible. The medication should be carefully compared with the physician's instructions, to prevent a drug error.

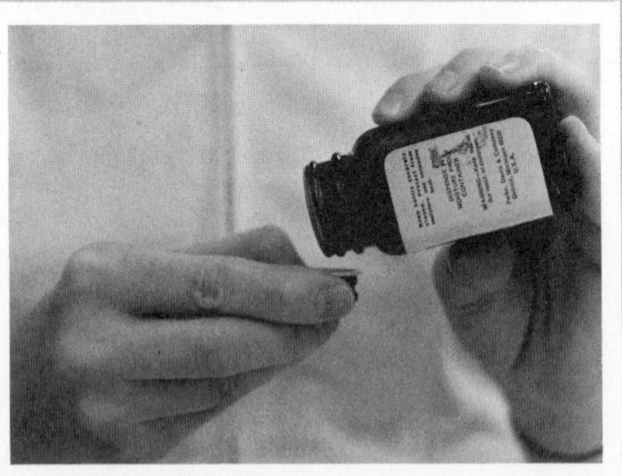

5. **PROCEDURAL STEP.** Calculate the correct dose to be given, if necessary.

6. **PROCEDURAL STEP.** Remove the bottle cap, touching the outside of the lid only.
   PRINCIPLE. Touching the inside of the lid will contaminate it.

7. **PROCEDURAL STEP.** Check the drug label and pour the medication.

Solid Medications. Pour the correct number of capsules or tablets into the bottle cap. Transfer the medication to a medicine cup, being careful not to touch the inside of the cup.

PRINCIPLE. Pouring the medication into the lid prevents contamination of the medication and lid.

Liquid Medications. Place the lid of the bottle upside down on a flat surface with the open end facing up. Palm the surface of the label. With the opposite hand, place the thumbnail at the proper calibration on the medicine cup, and hold the cup at eye level. Pour the medication and read the dose at the lowest level of the meniscus. (The meniscus is the curved surface of the liquid in a container. When a liquid is poured into a medicine cup, capillary action will cause the liquid in contact with the cup to be drawn upward, resulting in a curved surface in the middle.)

PRINCIPLE. Placing the bottle cap with the open end facing up prevents contamination of the inside of the cap. Palming the medication label prevents the medication from dripping on the label and obscuring it.

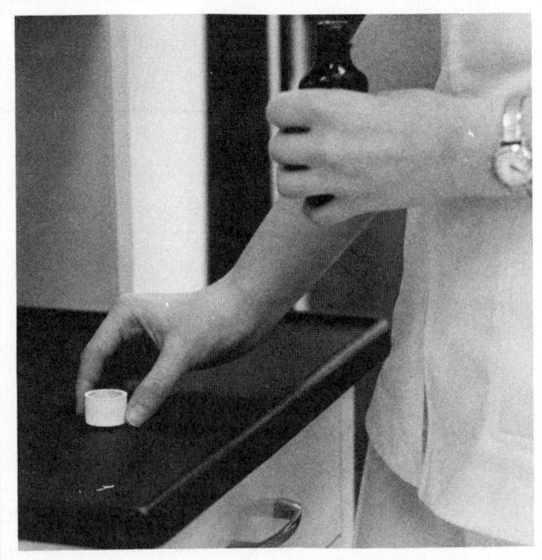

8. **PROCEDURAL STEP.** Check the drug label and return the medication to the shelf.

9. **PROCEDURAL STEP.** Identify the patient and explain the procedure. Explain the purpose of administering the medication.

PRINCIPLE. It is crucial that no error be made in patient identity.

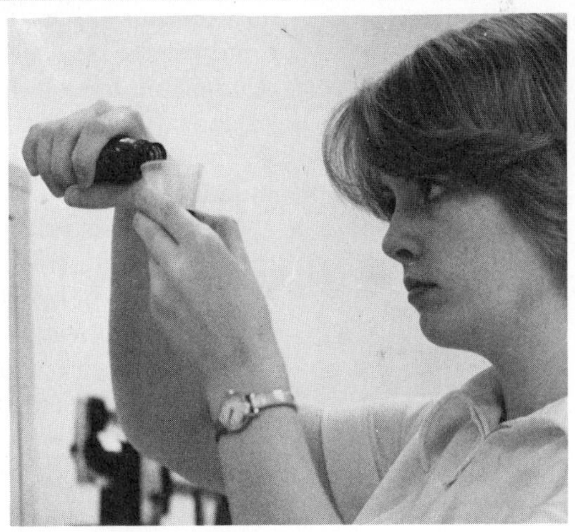

10. **PROCEDURAL STEP.** Hand the medicine cup containing the medication to the patient, along with a glass of water. (Water should not be offered if the medication is a cough syrup.)

PRINCIPLE. Water helps the patient to swallow the medication.

11. **PROCEDURAL STEP.** Remain with the patient until the medication is swallowed. If the patient experiences any unusual reaction, notify the physician.

12. **PROCEDURAL STEP.** Wash the hands.

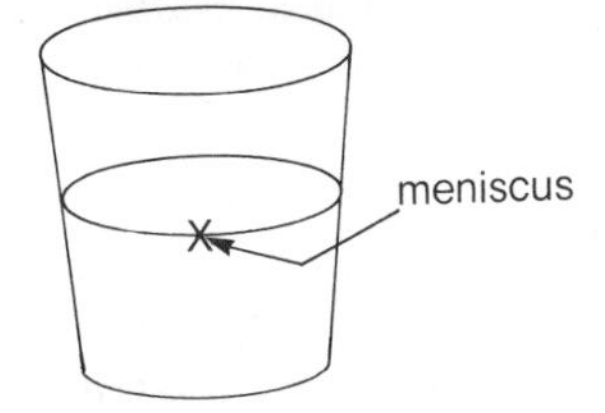

13. **PROCEDURAL STEP.** Record the procedure. Include the patient's name, the date and time, the name of the medication, the dosage given, the route of administration, and any significant observations or patient reactions. Initial the entry. The Latin abbreviation *po* (per os) can be used to indicate the route of administration. This abbreviation means *by mouth.*

Continued

Record data below.

DATE	TIME	PATIENT'S NAME	RECORDING

Parenteral Administration

There are several advantages to using the parenteral route of administration (intradermal, subcutaneous, intramuscular, intravenous). Medications are absorbed more rapidly and completely than through the oral route. In some cases, the parenteral route is the only way a drug can be given. For example, if the patient is unconscious or has a gastric disturbance such as nausea or vomiting, the parenteral route would be used. If the state laws permit, the medical assistant is usually responsible for administering intradermal, subcutaneous, and intramuscular injections. Intravenous injections are given when an immediate effect is needed; in the medical office, they are usually administered by the physician in an emergency situation.

There are also disadvantages with the parenteral route, such as pain and the chance that infection may result, owing to the break in the skin. The medical assistant can help to reduce pain by inserting and withdrawing the needle smoothly and by withdrawing the needle using the angle of insertion.

If injections are given repeatedly (e.g., allergy injections), the sites should be rotated to prevent the overuse of one particular site, which may result in irritation and tissue damage. Rotating sites also allows for better absorption of the drug. When recording the procedure in the patient's chart, the medical assistant must be sure to include the site of the injection (e.g., right or left gluteus medius, deltoid, vastus lateralis). This assists in proper site rotation for patients requiring more than one injection. In addition, the information provides a reference point, should a problem arise with the injection site.

Medical asepsis must be used when parenteral medications are administered. In addition, the needle, the inside of the syringe, and the outside of the lower end of the plunger should remain sterile. This reduces the danger of microorganisms entering the patient's body. The medical assistant must also be sure to follow the Center for Disease Control (CDC) recommended infection precautions as a means of protecting oneself from blood-borne pathogens. Refer to Chapter 1 to review medical asepsis and the CDC recommended precautions and to Chapter 7 to review sterile technique.

Parts of a Needle and Syringe

The needle consists of several parts (Fig. 8–2). The *hub* of the needle fits onto the top of the syringe. The *shaft,* also known as the cannula, is inserted into the body tissue. The opening in the shaft of the needle, known as the *lumen,* is continuous with the needle hub. Medication flows from the syringe and through the lumen of the needle. The *point* of the needle is located at the end of the needle shaft. The point is sharp so that it can penetrate the body tissues easily. The top of the needle is slanted and is called the *bevel.*

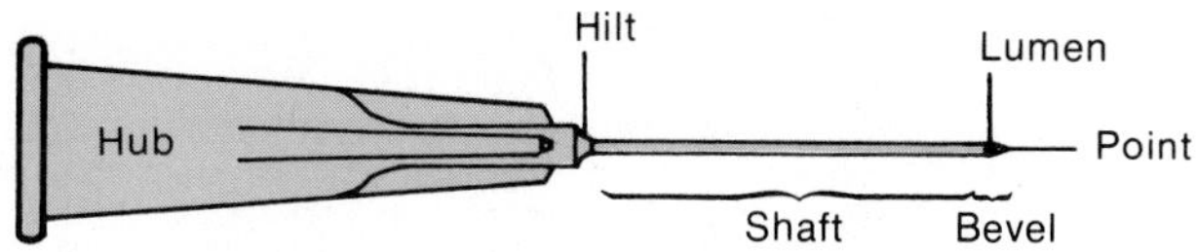

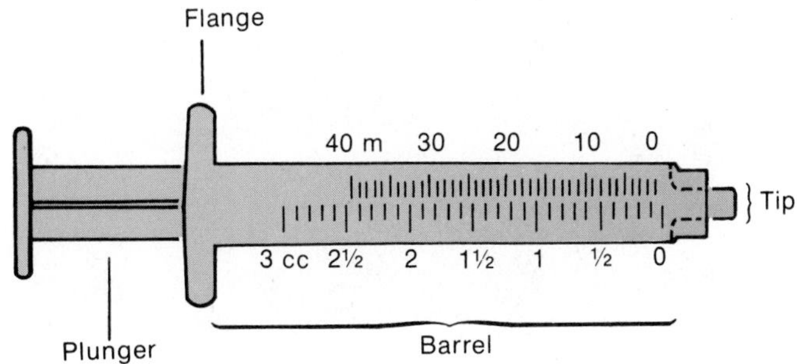

FIGURE 8–2. Diagrams of a needle and a 3-cc syringe, with parts identified.

Each needle has a certain *gauge;* needle gauges range between 14 and 27. The gauge of a needle is determined by the diameter of the lumen: as the size of the gauge increases, the diameter of the lumen decreases. Thus, a needle with a gauge of 21 has a smaller lumen diameter than a needle with a gauge of 16. Thick or oily preparations must be given with a large lumen, because they are too thick to pass through a smaller one. A needle with a larger lumen causes a larger needle track to be made in the tissues. To help reduce pain and tissue damage, a needle with the smallest gauge appropriate for the solution and route of administration is always chosen. The length of the needle ranges between ⅜ and 5 inches; the length used will be based on the type of injection being given. For instance, the needle used to give an intramuscular injection must be longer than one used for a subcutaneous injection so that it penetrates deeply enough to reach muscle tissue.

The syringe is used for inserting fluids into the body. Glass or plastic syringes are available. Glass syringes are sterilized after use and can be used again. Plastic syringes can be used only once and are disposed of after use. Plastic syringes are available individually packaged for sterility in a paper or cellophane wrapper or a rigid plastic container. The medical assistant needs to attach a needle to the syringe, which is available individually wrapped. Individually packaged syringes are also available with the needle already attached. Information regarding the syringe capacity and the length and gauge of the needle is found on the wrapper of the syringe and/or needle (Fig. 8–3). Most physicians prefer to use the disposable plastic syringes for administering medications in the medical office. Because glass syringes can be sterilized, they are commonly used in minor office surgery tray set-ups for administering a local anesthetic, draining fluid from a cyst, and so on.

Parts of a syringe include the barrel, flange, and plunger (see Fig. 8–2). The *barrel* of the syringe holds the medication and contains calibrated markings to measure the proper amount of medication. Most syringes are calibrated in both cubic centimeters (cc) and minims; cubic centimeters are used most often in administering medication. The medical assistant should become familiar with reading the graduated scales on syringes. At the end of the barrel is a rim known as the *flange,* which helps in injecting the medication. The flange also prevents the syringe from rolling when it is placed on a flat surface. The *plunger* is a movable cylinder that slides back and forth within the barrel. It is used to draw substances into and out of the barrel.

Various types of syringes are available to administer injections. The choice is based on the type of injection (e.g., allergy skin test, insulin, antibiotic) and the

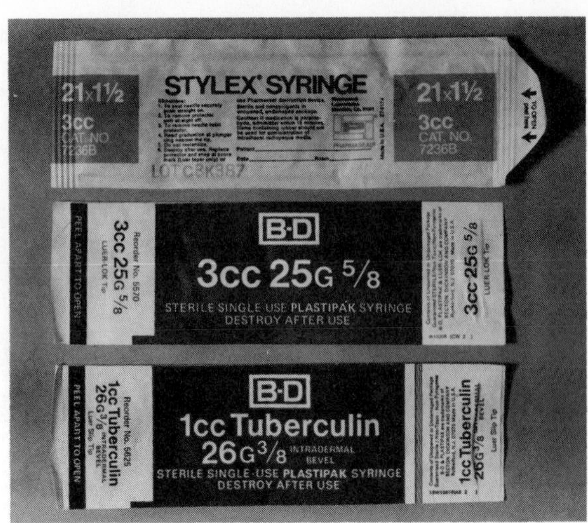

FIGURE 8–3. Examples of syringe/needle packages labeled according to contents.

amount of medication being administered. The types used most often in the medical office include hypodermic, insulin, and tuberculin (Fig. 8–4). *Hypodermic syringes* are available in 2-, 2.5-, 3-, and 5-cc sizes and have two sets of calibrations—cc and minims. They are commonly used to administer intramuscular injections. The *insulin syringe* is designed especially for the administration of an insulin injection, and the barrel is calibrated in units. The most commonly used type is the U-100 syringe, which is calibrated into 100 units and divided into increments of 2 units. Insulin syringes are also available in U-40 and U-80 syringes; however, today they are not used as commonly as the U-100, because U-100 insulin is rapidly becoming the only type of insulin used in many health-care facilities. The proper syringe must be selected when administering insulin; for example, a U-100 syringe is used to administer U-100 insulin, a U-40 syringe to administer U-40 insulin, and a U-80 syringe to administer U-80 insulin.

Tuberculin syringes are employed when a very small dose of medication is to be administered such as in the tuberculin skin test. The tuberculin syringe has a capacity of 1 cc, and the calibrations are divided into tenths (0.1) and hundredths (0.01) of a cubic centimeter.

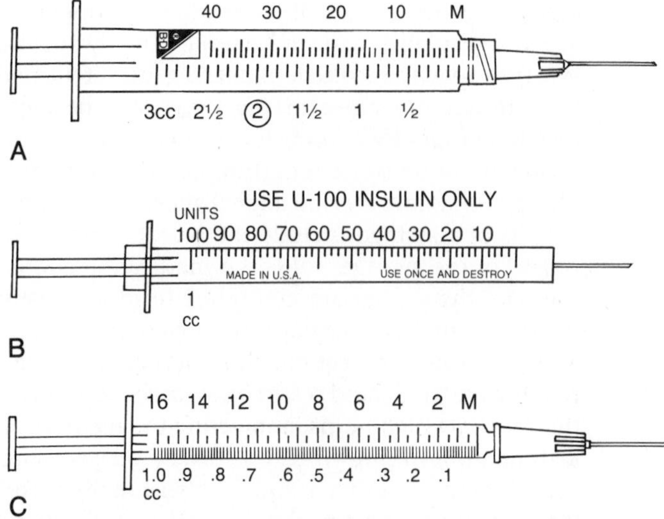

FIGURE 8–4. Various types of syringes used to administer injections. *A,* Hypodermic; *B,* Insulin (U-100); *C,* Tuberculin.

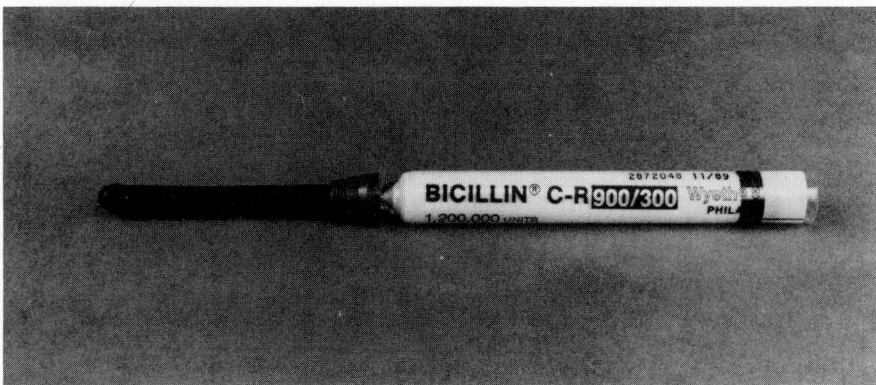

FIGURE 8–5. An example of a prefilled disposable cartridge containing medication. Disposable cartridges must be inserted into a specially designed metal syringe for administration of the injection.

Syringes are also available with capacities of 10, 20, and 50 cc; however, they are not generally used for administering medication, but rather for medical treatments such as irrigating wounds and draining fluid from cysts.

Preparation of Parenteral Medication

Medication used for injections is available in different types of dispensing units.

Some drugs come in *prefilled disposable syringes,* or *cartridges.* Using this type of dispensing unit does not require drawing up the medication. The name of the drug, the dose, and the expiration date are included on the syringe or cartridge (Fig. 8–5). An example is the Tubex closed injection system, consisting of a reusable metal hypodermic syringe that holds a disposable unit-dose cartridge-needle unit. The procedure for administering an injection using the Tubex system is presented in Figure 8–6.

An *ampule* is a small sealed glass container that holds a single dose of medication (Fig. 8–7). An ampule has a constriction in the stem, known as the neck, that helps in opening it. Before opening, make sure there is no medication in the stem by tapping it lightly. A sawtooth file is used to scratch the glass gently on the neck. If the ampule is prescored, filing is unnecessary. The ampule is opened by holding it firmly with gauze and breaking off the stem using moderate pressure. The needle opening is inserted into the base below the fluid level to withdraw medication. To prevent contamination, the needle should not touch the edge of the ampule. Air should never be injected into the ampule, because this may force out some of the medication.

Parenteral medication is also available in single-dose and multiple-dose vials (Fig. 8–7). A *vial* is a closed glass container with a rubber stopper; a soft metal cap protects the rubber stopper and must be removed the first time the medication is used.

Some vials may require mixing before the medication can be withdrawn (e.g., reconstituting a powdered drug or mixing a vial that separates upon standing). Vials requiring mixing should be rolled between the hands rather than shaken, because shaking will cause the medication to foam, thus creating air bubbles that may enter the syringe when the medication is withdrawn. To remove medication, an amount of air exactly equal to the amount of liquid to be removed is injected into the vial. The air should be inserted above the fluid level to avoid creating bubbles in the medication. If air is not injected first, a partial vacuum will be created and it will be difficult to remove the medication. During the withdrawal of medication, the needle opening should be inserted below the fluid level to pre-

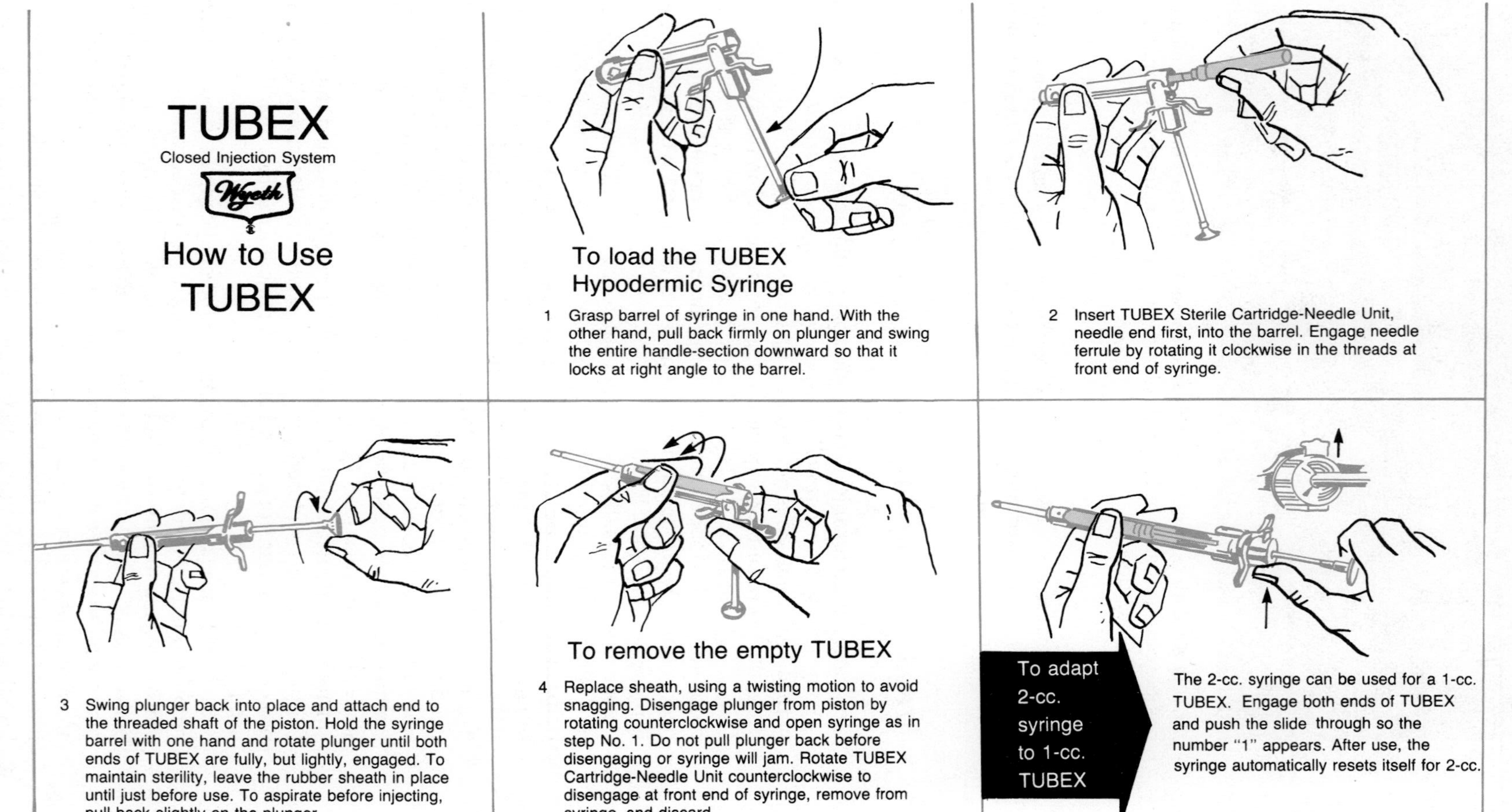

TUBEX
Closed Injection System
Wyeth
How to Use
TUBEX
To load the TUBEX
Hypodermic Syringe
1 Grasp barrel of syringe in one hand. With the other hand, pull back firmly on plunger and swing the entire handle-section downward so that it locks at right angle to the barrel.
2 Insert TUBEX Sterile Cartridge-Needle Unit, needle end first, into the barrel. Engage needle ferrule by rotating it clockwise in the threads at front end of syringe.
3 Swing plunger back into place and attach end to the threaded shaft of the piston. Hold the syringe barrel with one hand and rotate plunger until both ends of TUBEX are fully, but lightly, engaged. To maintain sterility, leave the rubber sheath in place until just before use. To aspirate before injecting, pull back slightly on the plunger.
To remove the empty TUBEX
4 Replace sheath, using a twisting motion to avoid snagging. Disengage plunger from piston by rotating counterclockwise and open syringe as in step No. 1. Do not pull plunger back before disengaging or syringe will jam. Rotate TUBEX Cartridge-Needle Unit counterclockwise to disengage at front end of syringe, remove from syringe, and discard.
To adapt 2-cc. syringe to 1-cc. TUBEX
The 2-cc. syringe can be used for a 1-cc. TUBEX. Engage both ends of TUBEX and push the slide through so the number "1" appears. After use, the syringe automatically resets itself for 2-cc.

FIGURE 8–6. Procedure for administering an injection using a Tubex closed injection system. The method of administration is the same as with a conventional syringe: Remove the rubber sheath, introduce the needle into the patient, aspirate, and inject.

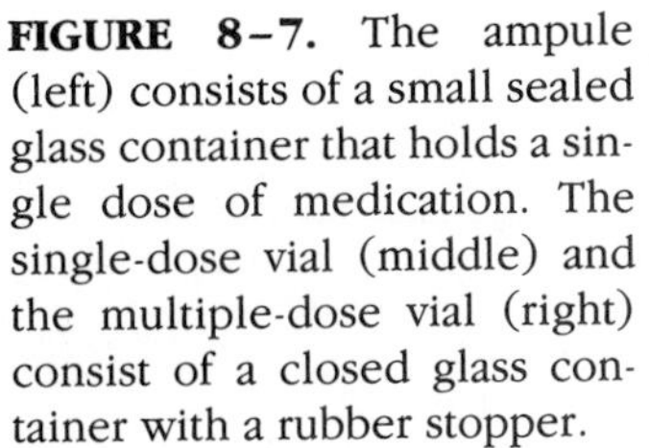

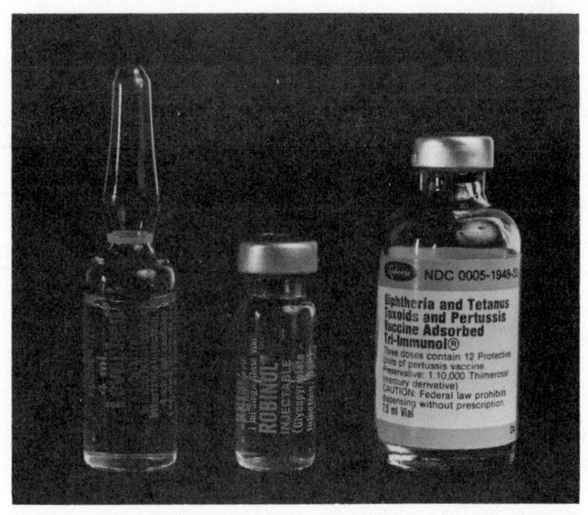

FIGURE 8-7. The ampule (left) consists of a small sealed glass container that holds a single dose of medication. The single-dose vial (middle) and the multiple-dose vial (right) consist of a closed glass container with a rubber stopper.

vent the entrance of air bubbles. Air bubbles can be removed by tapping the barrel of the syringe with the fingertips. If allowed to remain, they take up space that the medication should occupy.

The medical assistant should always read the manufacturer's instructions to determine the proper method for storing each parenteral medication, because improper storage may alter the effectiveness of the medication.

Reconstitution of Powdered Drugs

Some parenteral medications are stable for only a short period of time in liquid form; therefore, these medications are prepared and stored in a powdered form and require the addition of a liquid before administration. Examples include the measles, mumps, and rubella immunization (Fig. 8-8) and potassium penicillin G. The process of adding a liquid to a powdered drug is known as *reconstitution.* The liquid used is usually sterile water or sterile normal saline. The powdered drug is contained in a single-dose or multiple-dose vial and is accompanied by specific instructions for reconstitution. A general procedure for reconstituting powdered drugs is outlined on the next page.

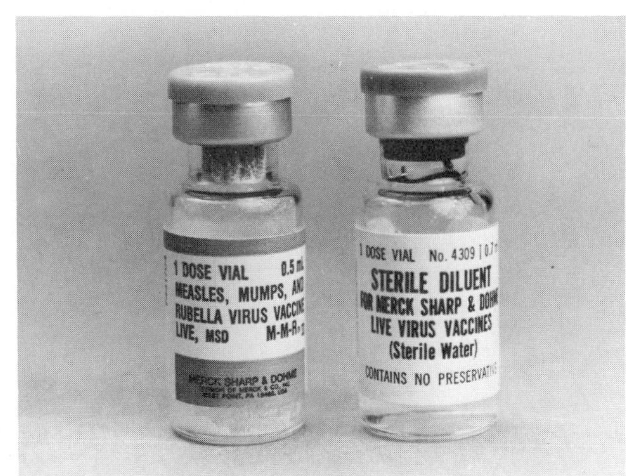

FIGURE 8-8. The M-M-R vaccine (measles, mumps, and rubella) is an example of a parenteral medication that requires reconstitution before administration. The vial on the left contains the medication in powdered form and the vial on the right contains the sterile diluent.

PROCEDURE 8-2

CONSTITUTING POWDERED DRUGS (GENERAL PROCEDURE)

1. From the vial containing the powdered drug, withdraw an amount of air equal to the amount of liquid to be injected into the vial.

2. Add the appropriate amount of reconstituting liquid to the powdered drug.

3. Roll the vial between the hands to mix the powdered drug and liquid.

4. Label multiple-dose vials with the name of the medication, the date of preparation, and your initials.

5. Store multiple-dose vials as indicated by the manufacturer's instructions. Because reconstituted drugs are stable for a short period of time, be sure to carefully check the date of preparation on the multiple-dose vial before administering it.

PROCEDURE 8-3
PREPARING THE INJECTION

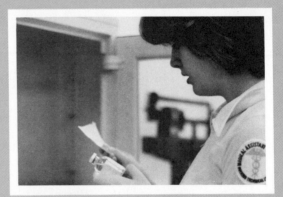

1. **PROCEDURAL STEP.** Wash the hands.

2. **PROCEDURAL STEP.** Assemble the equipment. The equipment needed includes an **antiseptic wipe,** a **medication tray,** the **appropriate needle and syringe** required for the injection, and the **physician's medication instructions.**

3. **PROCEDURAL STEP.** Work in a quiet, well-lighted atmosphere.
PRINCIPLE. Good lighting aids the medical assistant in reading the medication label.

4. **PROCEDURAL STEP.** Select the proper medication and check the expiration date. Compare the medication with the physician's instructions. The drug label must be checked three times: while removing the medication from the shelf, before withdrawing the medication into the syringe, and before returning it to its proper place.
PRINCIPLE. If the medication is outdated, consult the physician; it may produce undesirable effects and the medical assistant could be held responsible. The medication should be carefully compared with the physician's instructions, to prevent a drug error.

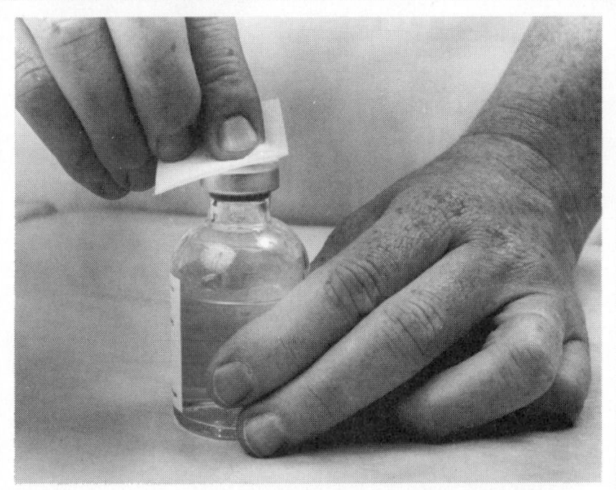

5. **PROCEDURAL STEP.** Calculate the correct dose to be given, if necessary.

6. **PROCEDURAL STEP.** Open the antiseptic; wipe and cleanse the ampule or vial.
PRINCIPLE. Cleansing the ampule or vial removes dust and bacteria.

7. **PROCEDURAL STEP.** Open the syringe and needle package. Assemble the needle and syringe if necessary.
PRINCIPLE. Disposable needles and syringes may come together in a package, already assembled, or in separate packages, requiring assembly of the needle and syringe.

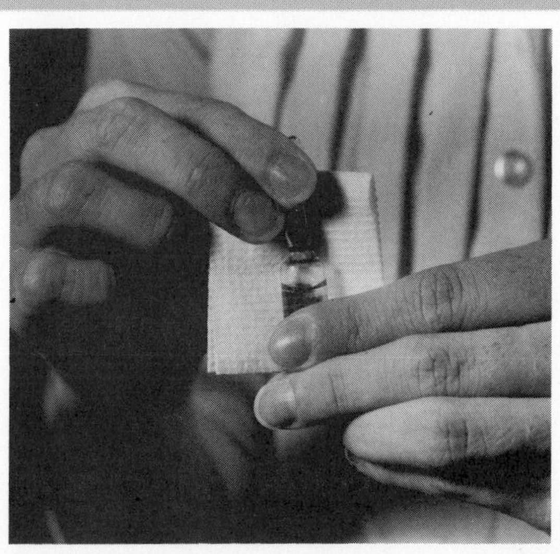

8. **PROCEDURAL STEP.** Remove the needle guard and check to make sure that the needle is attached firmly to the syringe by grasping the needle at the hub and turning it clockwise.

9. **PROCEDURAL STEP.** Check the drug label, and withdraw the proper amount of medication from the ampule or vial as follows:

A. Ampule
   a. Tap the stem of the ampule lightly to remove any medication in the neck of the ampule.
   b. Place a piece of gauze around the neck of the ampule.

Continued

c. Using both hands, hold the ampule firmly between the fingers.
d. Break off the stem by snapping it quickly and firmly away from the body.
e. Insert the needle opening below the fluid level.
f. Withdraw the proper amount of medication by pulling back on the plunger. Be sure to keep the needle opening below the fluid level to prevent the entrance of air bubbles into the syringe. Air bubbles take up space the medication should occupy, resulting in an inaccurate measurement of medication.
g. Remove the needle from the ampule without allowing the needle to touch the edge of the ampule.
h. If air bubbles are in the syringe, hold the syringe in a vertical position and tap the barrel with the fingertips until they disappear. Draw back slightly on the plunger and slowly push the plunger forward to eject the air. Do not eject the fluid.

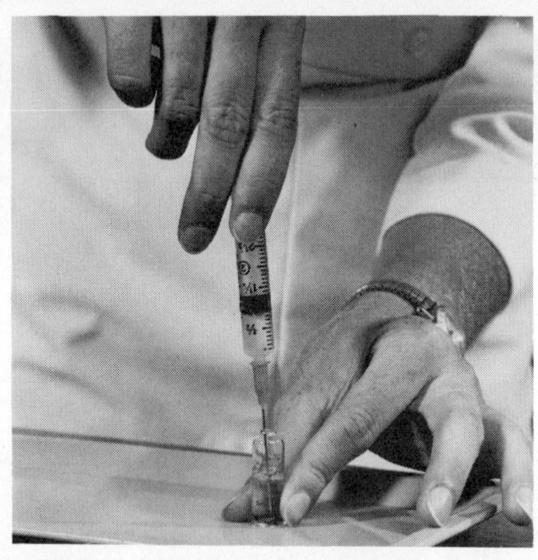

B. Vial
a. Pull back on the plunger to draw an amount of air into the syringe equal to the amount of medication to be withdrawn from the vial. Air must first be injected into the vial to prevent the formation of a partial vacuum in the vial, making it difficult to remove medication.
b. Using moderate pressure, insert the needle through the center of the rubber stopper, until it reaches the empty space between the stopper and fluid level.
c. Push down on the plunger to inject the air into the vial, making sure to keep the needle opening above the fluid level. The air must be inserted above the fluid level to avoid creating air bubbles in the medication.
d. Invert the vial while holding onto the syringe and plunger.
e. Hold the syringe at eye level, and withdraw the proper amount of medication. Keep the needle opening below the fluid level to prevent the entrance of air bubbles into the syringe.
f. Remove any air bubbles in the syringe by holding the syringe in a vertical position and tapping the barrel with the fingertips until they disappear. Air bubbles take up space the medication should occupy.
g. Remove any air remaining at the top of the syringe by slowly depressing the plunger and allowing the air to flow back into the vial.
h. Carefully remove the needle from the rubber stopper.

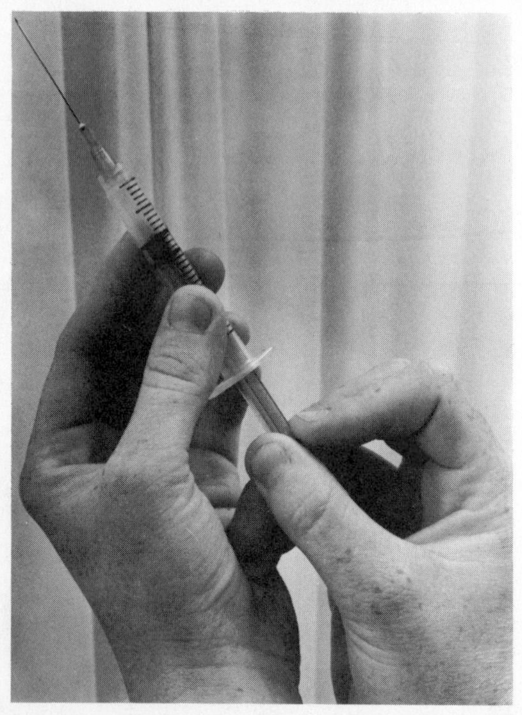

10. **PROCEDURAL STEP.** Replace the needle guard, and place the syringe on a medication tray with an antiseptic wipe.

PRINCIPLE. The needle must remain sterile. The needle guard prevents the needle from becoming contaminated.

11. **PROCEDURAL STEP.** Check the drug label and return the medication to its proper storage compartment.

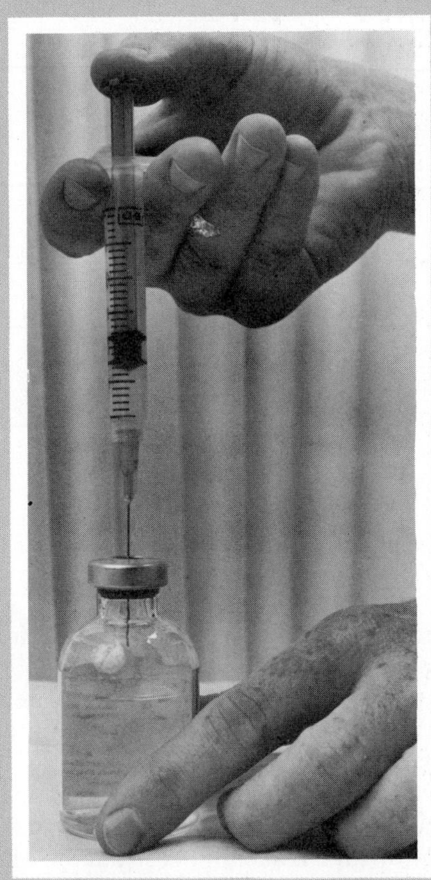

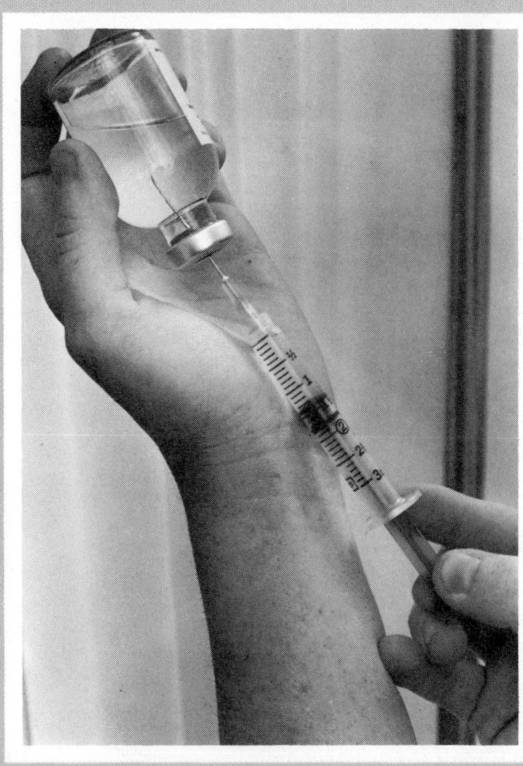

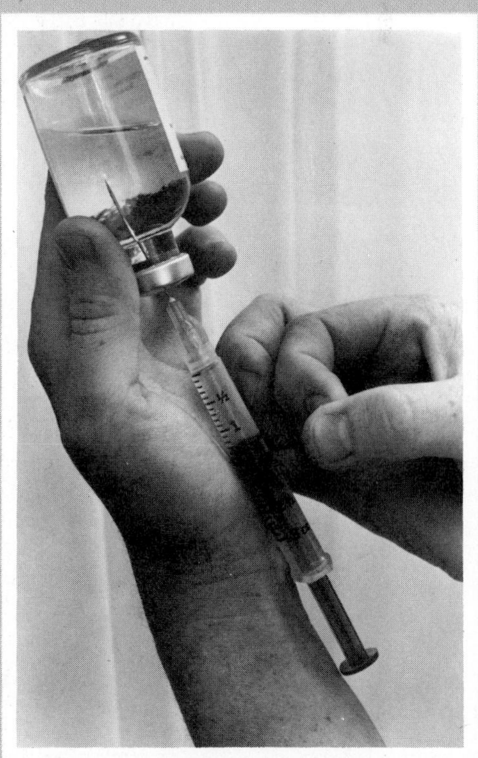

Continued

Record data below.

DATE	TIME	PATIENT'S NAME	RECORDING

Intradermal Injections

An intradermal injection is given into the dermal layer of the skin, at an angle almost parallel to the skin (Fig. 8–9). Absorption is slow; therefore, only a small amount of medication may be injected (0.1 to 0.3 cc). The sites most often used for an intradermal injection are areas where the skin is thin, such as the anterior forearm and the middle of the back.

The needle used is short, usually ⅜ to ⅝ inch long, and the lumen has a small diameter, usually 25 to 27 gauge. A tuberculin syringe is often used for administering the injection. The capacity of the syringe is small (1 cc), and the calibrations are divided into tenths and hundredths of a cubic centimeter. The fine calibrations allow for a very small amount of medication to be administered, which is required with an intradermal injection.

The most frequent use of intradermal injections is to administer a skin test such as an allergy skin test or a tuberculin skin test. The medication for the appropriate test is placed into the skin layers, and a small raised area known as a wheal is

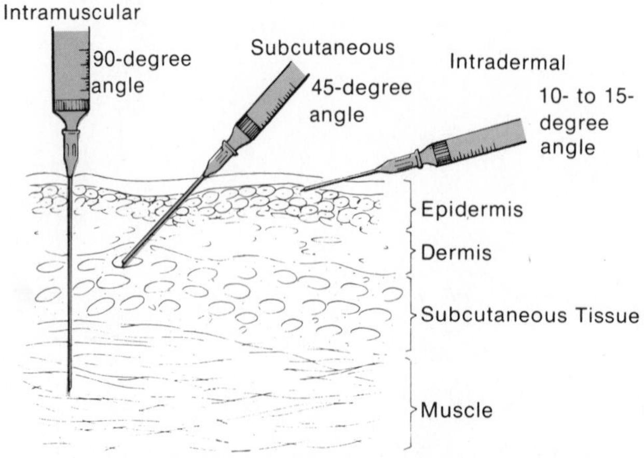

FIGURE 8–9. Angle of insertion for intradermal, subcutaneous, and intramuscular injections.

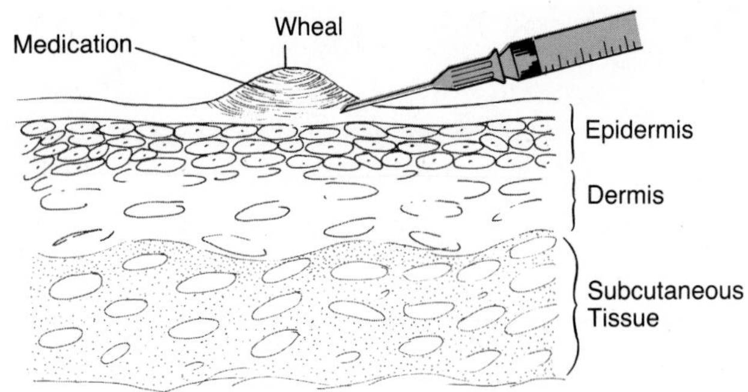

FIGURE 8–10. Intradermal injections are used to administer skin tests. Enough medication must be deposited in the skin layers to form a wheal.

produced at the injection site, owing to distention of the skin (Fig. 8–10). At a time dictated by the type of test being administered, the results are read and interpreted. For example, the majority of allergy skin tests may be read and interpreted at the medical office within a short period of time (usually 15 to 20 minutes) after administration of the test, whereas tuberculin skin testing requires 48 hours before the test results may be read. The skin testing medication interacts with the body tissues; if no reaction occurs, the wheal disappears within a short period of time, and the only visible sign left is the puncture site. If a reaction to the skin test occurs, induration results, indicating a positive reaction. Erythema may also be present at the test site; however, for most skin tests, the extent of induration is the only criterion used to assess a positive reaction. Examples of allergy skin test reactions are illustrated on the inside front cover.

PROCEDURE 8-4
ADMINISTERING AN INTRADERMAL INJECTION

1. **PROCEDURAL STEP.** Identify the patient and explain the procedure.

PRINCIPLE. It is crucial that no error be made in patient identity. Explain the purpose of the injection to help reassure an apprehensive patient.

2. **PROCEDURAL STEP.** Select an appropriate injection site. The anterior forearm and the middle of the back are recommended sites for an intradermal injection.

PRINCIPLE. The entire area should be exposed, to ensure a safe and comfortable injection.

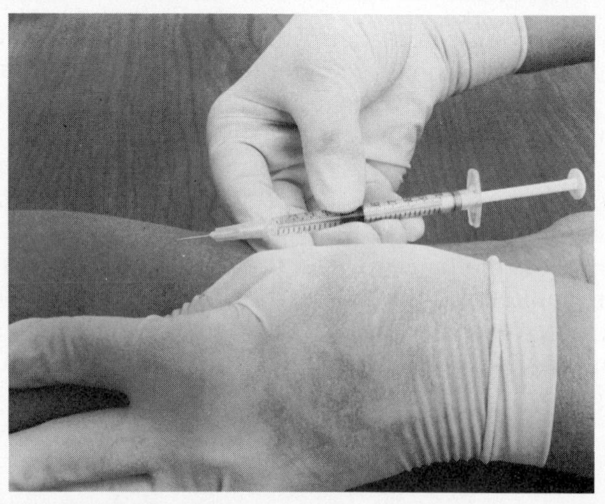

3. **PROCEDURAL STEP.** Prepare the injection site. Cleanse the area with an antiseptic wipe. Using a circular motion, start with the injection site and move outward. Touching the site after cleansing will contaminate it, and the cleansing process will need to be repeated. If the site is grossly soiled, wash the area with soap and water first.

PRINCIPLE. Using a circular motion will carry material away from the injection site.

4. **PROCEDURAL STEP.** Apply gloves and remove the needle guard. With the nondominant hand, stretch the skin taut at the proposed site of administration. Insert the needle at a 10- to 15-degree angle, with the bevel upward. The lumen should just penetrate the skin. No aspiration is needed.

PRINCIPLE. Gloves provide a barrier precaution against contaminated blood. Stretching the patient's skin taut will permit easier insertion of the needle. The needle should be inserted at an angle almost parallel to the skin, to ensure penetration within the dermal layer of the skin. The needle must be inserted with the bevel facing upward to allow for proper wheal formation. If the needle is inserted with the bevel facing downward, the medication will be absorbed and a wheal will not form.

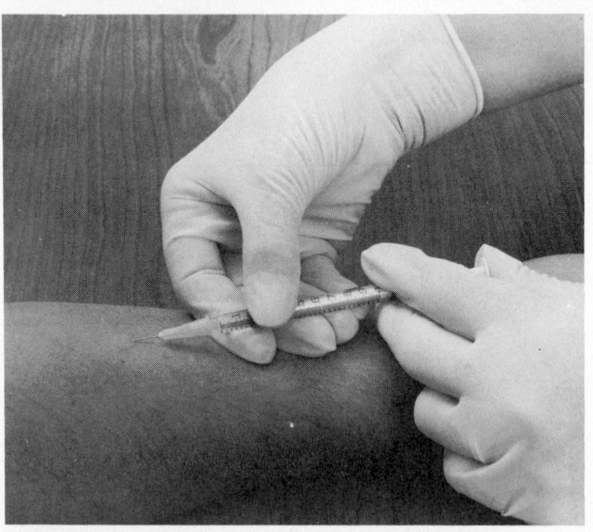

5. **PROCEDURAL STEP.** Hold the syringe steady, and inject the medication slowly and steadily by depressing the plunger until a wheal forms (approximately 6 mm in diameter). Expect to feel a certain amount of resistance as you inject the medication; this helps in indicating that the needle is properly located in the superficial skin layers rather than in the deeper subcutaneous tissue.

PRINCIPLE. Moving the syringe once the needle has entered the skin causes patient discomfort.

6. **PROCEDURAL STEP.** Place the antiseptic wipe gently over the injection site; remove the needle quickly and at the same angle as for insertion. Properly dispose of the needle and syringe.

PRINCIPLE. Withdrawing the needle quickly and at the angle of insertion reduces patient discomfort. The antiseptic wipe placed over the injection site helps to prevent tissue movement as the needle is withdrawn, also reducing patient discomfort. Proper disposal of the needle and syringe protects the medical assistant from being pricked by a contaminated needle.

7. **PROCEDURAL STEP.** Do not massage the injection site. Place an adhesive bandage over the site if needed.

PRINCIPLE. Massaging is not needed because the medication is not intended to be distributed into the tissues. In addition, massaging may cause leakage of the testing solution through the needle puncture site, which could interfere with the test results.

8. **PROCEDURAL STEP.** Remove the gloves and wash the hands.

9. **PROCEDURAL STEP.** Stay with the patient to make sure that he or she is not experiencing any unusual reactions. Perform *one* of the following, based on the type of skin test being administered, the length of time required for the body tissues to react to the test, and the medical office policy.

a. Read the test results, using inspection and palpation at the site of the injection to assess the presence of and/or to determine the amount of induration.

or

b. Inform the patient of a date and time to return to the medical office to have the results read.

or

c. Instruct the patient in the proper procedure for reading and interpreting the results at home and reporting them to the medical office.

In all cases, the results must be read and interpreted according to the manufacturer's instructions that accompany the test. Assist the patient off the examining table. (*Note:* The medical assistant should be especially careful and alert for any sign of a patient reaction when administering allergy skin tests.) If the patient experiences an unusual reaction, notify the physician.

10. **PROCEDURAL STEP.** Record the procedure. Include the patient's name, the date and time, the name of the medication, the dosage given, the route of administration, the injection site used, the skin test results, and any significant observations or patient reactions. Initial the entry. (*Note:* If the skin test results are to be recorded at a later date, the test results will not be recorded at this time.)

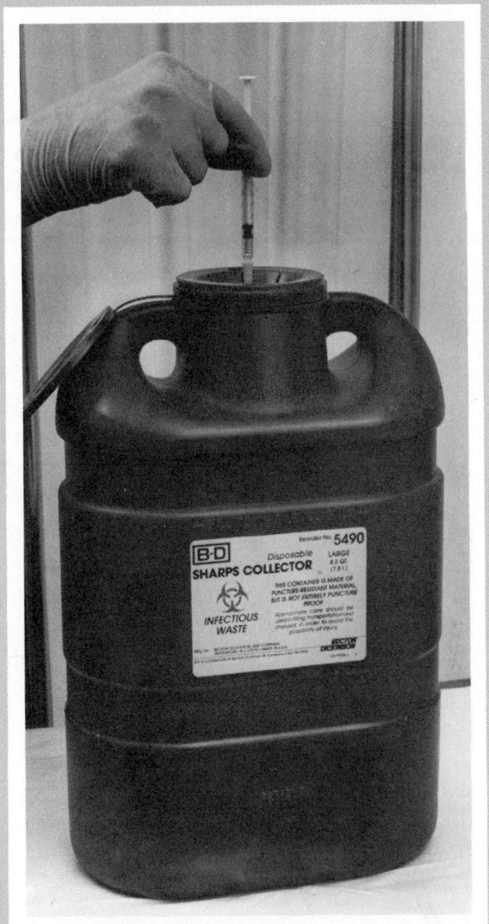

Record data below.

DATE	TIME	PATIENT'S NAME	RECORDING

Subcutaneous Injections

A subcutaneous injection is made into the subcutaneous tissue, which is located just under the skin (see Fig. 8–9). This consists of adipose (fat) tissue. Subcutaneous tissue is located all over the body; however, certain sites are more commonly used, in which bones and blood vessels are not near the surface of the skin. These include the upper lateral part of the arms, the anterior thigh, the upper back, and the abdomen (Fig. 8–11). Tissue that is grossly adipose, hardened, inflamed, or edematous should not be used as an injection site.

The needle length varies from ½ to ⅝ inch, and the gauge ranges from 23 to 25. Elderly and dehydrated patients tend to have less subcutaneous tissue, whereas obese patients will have more. The length of the needle should be adjusted accordingly, to make sure the injection is given into the subcutaneous tissue and not into muscle tissue.

Subcutaneous tissue is sensitive to irritating solutions and large volumes of medications; therefore, drugs given subcutaneously must be isotonic, nonirritating, nonviscous, and water soluble. The amount of medication injected through the subcutaneous route should not exceed 2 cc. More than this amount results in pressure on sensory nerve endings, causing discomfort and pain.

Medications commonly administered through the subcutaneous route include epinephrine, insulin, and allergy injections. Patients receiving an allergy injection must wait in the medical office for 15 to 20 minutes following the injection to be observed for the occurrence of any unusual reactions.

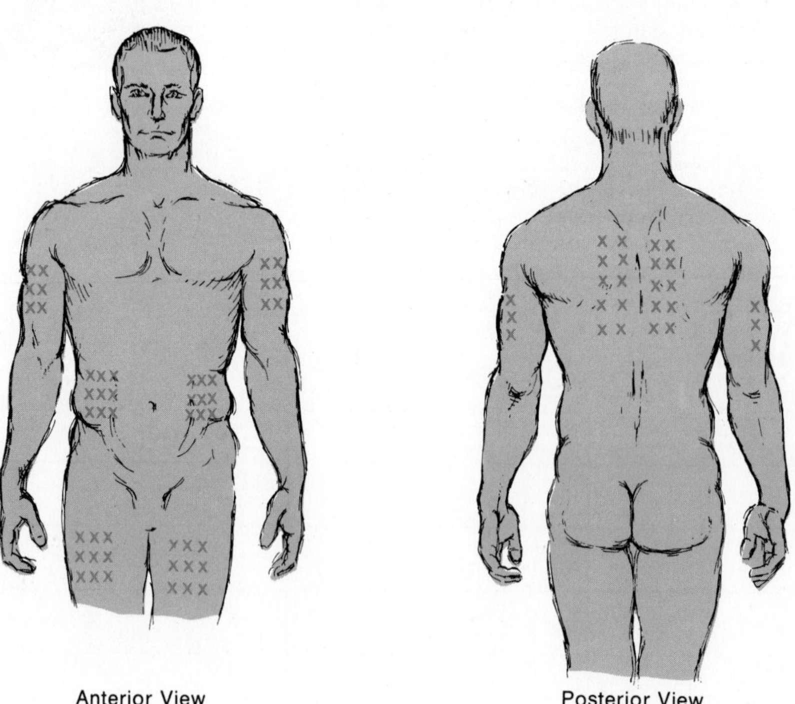

FIGURE 8–11. Sites on the body where a subcutaneous injection can be given.

PROCEDURE 8-5

ADMINISTERING A SUBCUTANEOUS INJECTION

1. **PROCEDURAL STEP.** Identify the patient and explain the procedure and purpose of the injection.

PRINCIPLE. It is crucial that no error be made in patient identity. An apprehensive patient may need reassurance.

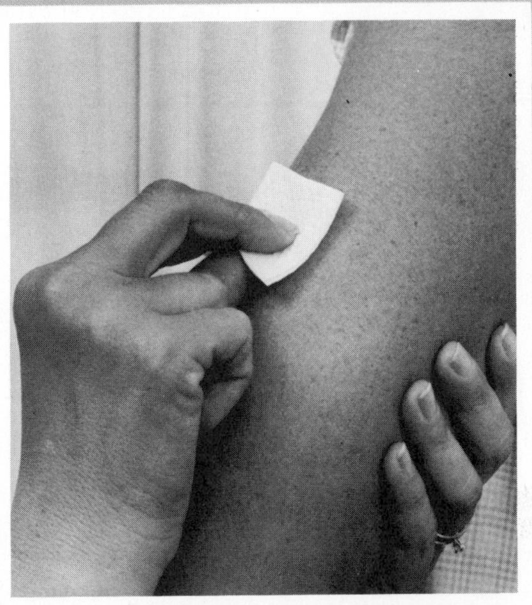

2. **PROCEDURAL STEP.** Select an appropriate injection site. The upper arm, thigh, back, and abdomen are recommended sites for a subcutaneous injection. Refer to Figure 8-11.

PRINCIPLE. The entire area should be exposed, to ensure a safe and comfortable injection.

3. **PROCEDURAL STEP.** Prepare the injection site. Cleanse the area with an antiseptic wipe. Using a circular motion, start with the injection site and move outward. Touching the site after cleansing will contaminate it, and the cleansing process will need to be repeated. If the site is grossly soiled, wash the area with soap and water first.

PRINCIPLE. Using a circular motion carries contaminants away from the injection site.

4. **PROCEDURAL STEP.** Apply gloves and remove the needle guard. Position your nondominant hand on the area surrounding the injection site. The skin may be held taut or the area surrounding the injection site may be grasped and held in a cushion fashion.

PRINCIPLE. Gloves provide a barrier precaution against contaminated blood. In normal adults, the needle will enter the subcutaneous tissue when the skin is held taut. Grasping the area around the injection site is recommended for a thin or dehydrated patient. It will assure that the subcutaneous tissue, and not muscle tissue, is entered.

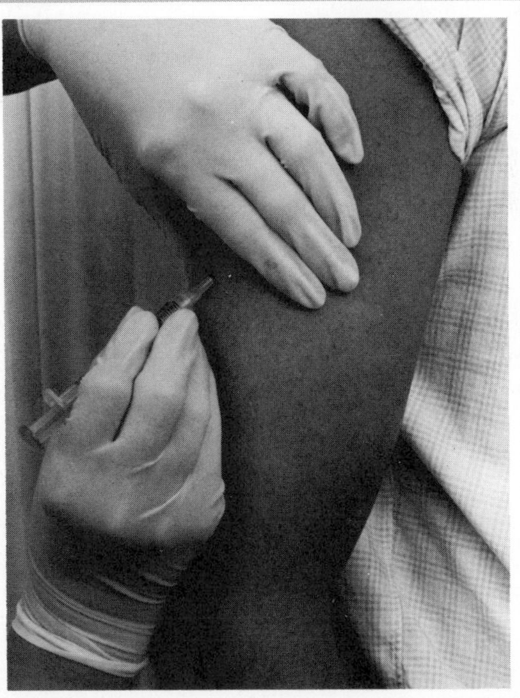

5. **PROCEDURAL STEP.** Insert the needle at a 45-degree angle with a firm motion. The barrel of the syringe should be held between the thumb and index finger. Insert the needle to the hub.

6. **PROCEDURAL STEP.** Remove your hand from the skin.

PRINCIPLE. Medication injected into compressed tissue causes pressure against nerve fibers and is uncomfortable for the patient.

7. **PROCEDURAL STEP.** Hold the syringe steady and pull back gently on the plunger to determine whether the needle is in a blood vessel, in which case blood will appear in the syringe. If blood appears, withdraw the needle, prepare a new injection, and begin again.

PRINCIPLE. Moving the syringe once the needle has entered the tissue causes patient discomfort. Drugs intended for subcutaneous administration but injected into a blood vessel are absorbed too quickly, and undesirable results may occur.

Continued

8. **PROCEDURAL STEP.** Inject the medication slowly and steadily by depressing the plunger.

PRINCIPLE. Rapid injection creates pressure and destroys tissue, which are uncomfortable for the patient.

9. **PROCEDURAL STEP.** Place the antiseptic wipe gently over the injection site and remove the needle, keeping it at the same angle as for insertion. Properly dispose of the needle and syringe.

PRINCIPLE. Withdrawing the needle quickly and at the same angle as for insertion reduces patient discomfort. The antiseptic wipe placed over the injection site helps to prevent tissue movement as the needle is withdrawn, reducing patient discomfort. Proper disposal of the needle and syringe protects the medical assistant from being pricked by a contaminated needle.

10. **PROCEDURAL STEP.** Massage the injection site with an antiseptic wipe. Apply pressure and place an adhesive bandage over the site if needed.

PRINCIPLE. Massaging helps to distribute the medication so that it is more completely absorbed.

11. **PROCEDURAL STEP.** Remove the gloves and wash the hands.

12. **PROCEDURAL STEP.** Stay with the patient to make sure he or she is not experiencing any unusual reactions. Assist the patient off the examining table. (*Note:* If an allergy injection has been given, the patient should remain at the medical office for at least 15 minutes to make sure that a reaction does not occur.) If the patient experiences an unusual reaction, notify the physician.

13. **PROCEDURAL STEP.** Record the procedure. Include the patient's name, the date and time, the name of the medication, the dosage given, the route of administration, the injection site used, and any significant observations or patient reactions. Initial the recording.

Record data below.

DATE	TIME	PATIENT'S NAME	RECORDING

Intramuscular Injections

Intramuscular injections are made into the muscular layer of the body, which lies below the skin and subcutaneous layers (see Fig. 8–9). The amount of medication injected into muscle tissue may be larger (up to 5 cc) than the amount injected into subcutaneous tissue. Absorption is more rapid by this route than by the subcutaneous route, because there are more blood vessels in muscle tissue. Medication that is irritating to subcutaneous tissue is often given intramuscularly, because there are fewer nerve endings in deep muscle tissue.

The length of the needle varies from 1 to 3 inches, and the gauge ranges from 18 to 23.

The sites chosen for intramuscular injections are away from large nerves and blood vessels. The medical assistant should practice locating these sites to become familiar with them. The area should always be fully exposed to permit clear visualization of the injection site. Intramuscular injection sites are described in the following sections.

Gluteus Medius

The gluteus medius is the site most commonly used for intramuscular injections. It is considered a good site because the gluteus medius is a large muscle and can absorb a large amount of medication. The patient should lie on the abdomen with the toes pointed inward, which aids in relaxation of the gluteus muscles. The injection is made into the upper outer quadrant of the gluteal area, in the area located above and outside a diagonal line drawn from the greater trochanter to the posterior superior iliac spine. These landmarks should be identified through palpation. The medical assistant must be extremely careful to maintain the proper boundary lines to avoid injection into the sciatic nerve or superior gluteal artery (Fig. 8–12).

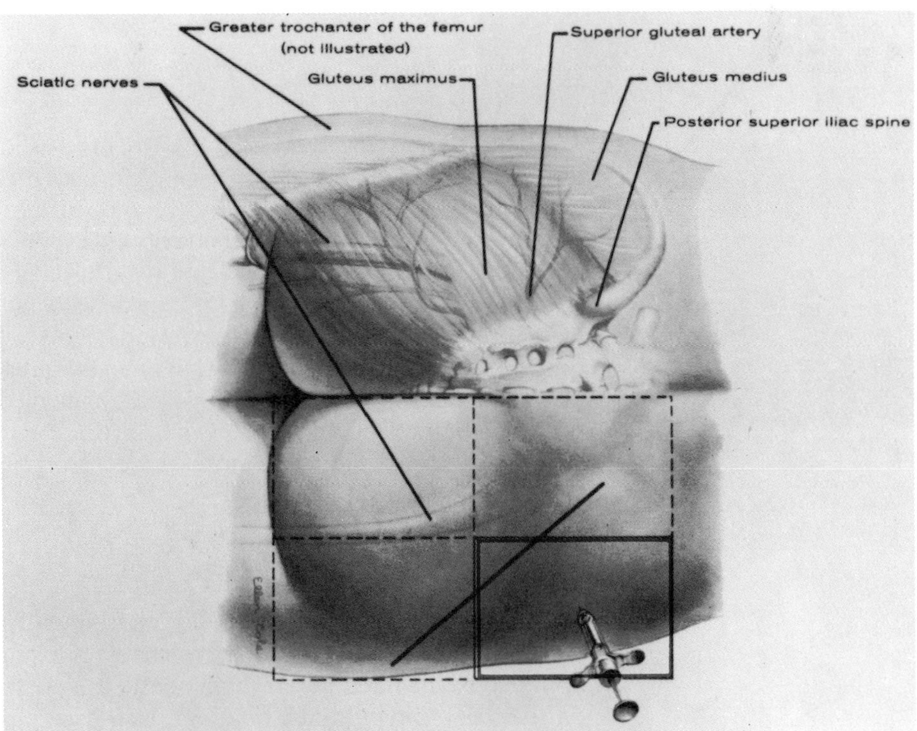

FIGURE 8–12. The proper insertion of the needle into the gluteus medius intramuscular injection site. (Courtesy Wyeth Laboratories, Philadelphia, Pennsylvania.)

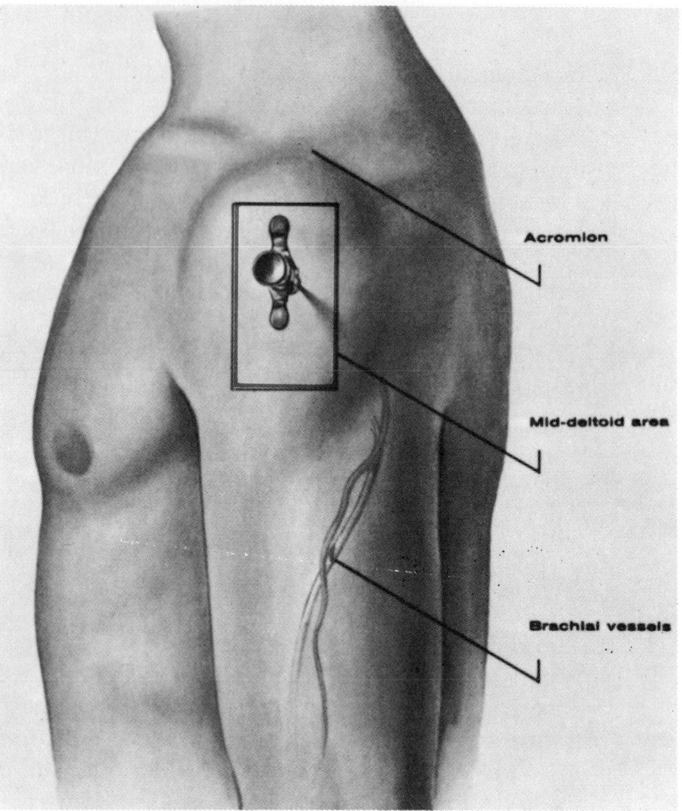

FIGURE 8–13. The proper insertion of the needle into the deltoid intramuscular injection site. (Courtesy Wyeth Laboratories. Philadelphia, Pennsylvania.)

Deltoid

The deltoid area is easily accessible and can be used when the patient is in a sitting or lying position (Fig. 8–13). This area forms a rectangle, bounded on top by the lower edge of the acromion process and on the bottom by the lateral side of the arm, opposite the axilla. The side boundaries of the rectangle are parallel to the arm. They are located one-third and two-thirds of the way around the site of the arm. The medication is injected into the deltoid muscle. This site is small, because major nerves and blood vessels surround it, and large amounts of medication and repeated injections should not be given in this area. The medical assistant should make sure that the entire arm is exposed by having the patient's sleeve completely pulled up or by removing the sleeve from the arm if it cannot be pulled up. A tight sleeve constricts the arm and causes unnecessary bleeding from the puncture site.

Vastus Lateralis

The vastus lateralis is now utilized more frequently, because it is away from major nerves and blood vessels and is a relatively thick muscle (Fig. 8–14). The area is bounded by the midanterior thigh on the front of the leg and the midlateral thigh on the side. The proximal boundary is a hand's breadth below the greater trochanter, and the distal boundary is a hand's breadth above the knee. It is easier to give an injection in the vastus lateralis if the patient is lying down, but a sitting position may also be used.

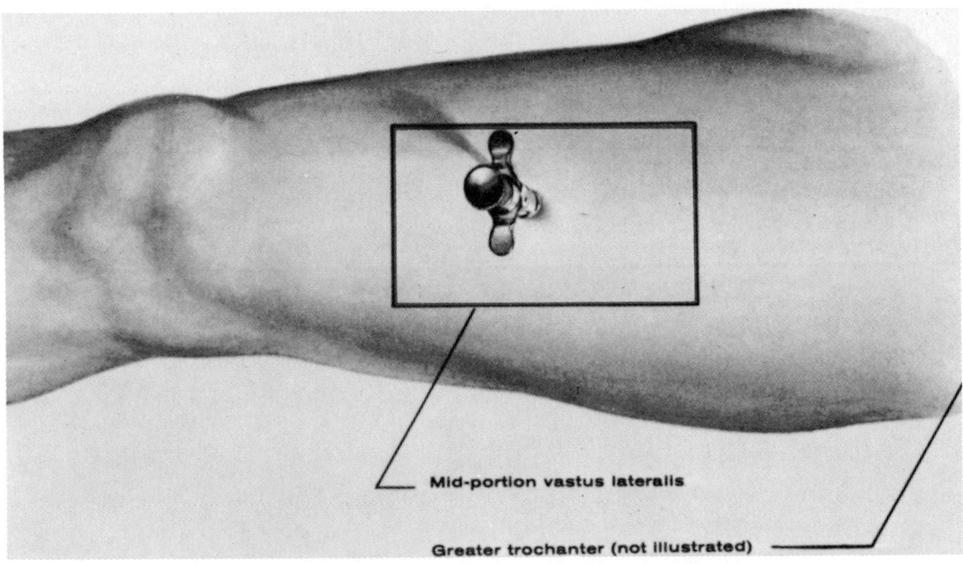

FIGURE 8–14. The proper insertion of the needle into the vastus lateralis intramuscular injection site. (Courtesy Wyeth Laboratories, Philadelphia, Pennsylvania.)

Ventrogluteal

Also growing in acceptability is the ventrogluteal site. The subcutaneous layer is relatively small and the muscle layer is thick. The site is located away from major nerves and blood vessels. Through palpation, the greater trochanter of the femur, the anterior superior iliac spine, and the iliac crest can be located. If the injection is being made into the left side of the patient, the palm of the right hand is placed on the greater trochanter, and the index finger is placed on the anterior superior iliac spine. The middle finger is spread posteriorly as far as possible away from the index finger, to touch the iliac crest. The hand position is reversed if the injection is being made into the right side of the patient. The triangle formed by the fingers is the area into which the injection is given. An injection into the ventrogluteal site can be administered when the patient is lying prone or on one side (Fig. 8–15).

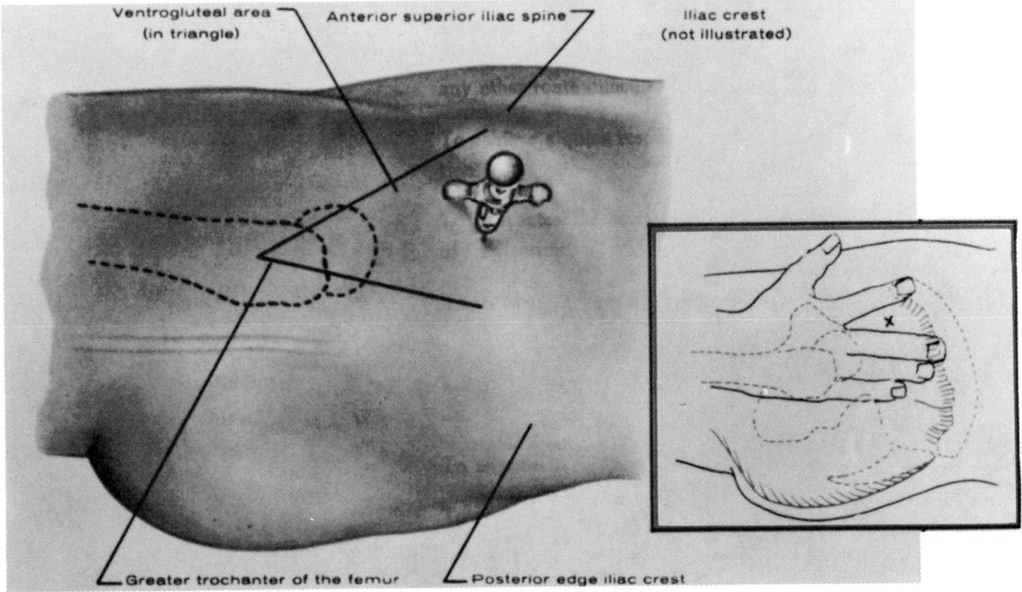

FIGURE 8–15. The proper insertion of the needle into the ventrogluteal intramuscular injection site. (Courtesy Wyeth Laboratories, Philadelphia, Pennsylvania.)

PROCEDURE 8-6
ADMINISTERING AN INTRAMUSCULAR INJECTION

1. **PROCEDURAL STEP.** Identify the patient and explain the procedure.
PRINCIPLE. Make sure you are giving the medication to the right patient. Explain the purpose of the injection. Assistance may be needed for restraining infants and children.

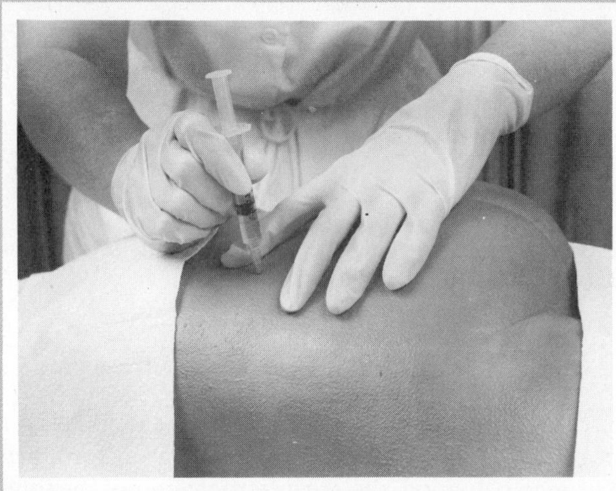

2. **PROCEDURAL STEP.** Select an appropriate injection site. Refer to pages 253 to 255 for the recommended intramuscular injection sites. Remove the patient's clothing as necessary to make sure the entire area is exposed.
PRINCIPLE. Major nerves and blood vessels may lie in close proximity to the intramuscular injection sites. The medical assistant should develop skill and accuracy in locating the proper sites.

3. **PROCEDURAL STEP.** Prepare the injection site. Cleanse the area with an antiseptic wipe. Using a circular motion, start with the injection site and move outward. Touching the site after cleansing will contaminate it, and the cleansing process will need to be repeated. If the site is grossly soiled, wash the area with soap and water first.

4. **PROCEDURAL STEP.** Apply gloves and remove the needle guard. Stretch the skin taut over the injection site, using the thumb and first two fingers of the nondominant hand.
PRINCIPLE. Gloves provide a barrier precaution against contaminated blood. Stretching the skin taut permits easier insertion of the needle and helps to ensure that the needle enters muscle tissue.

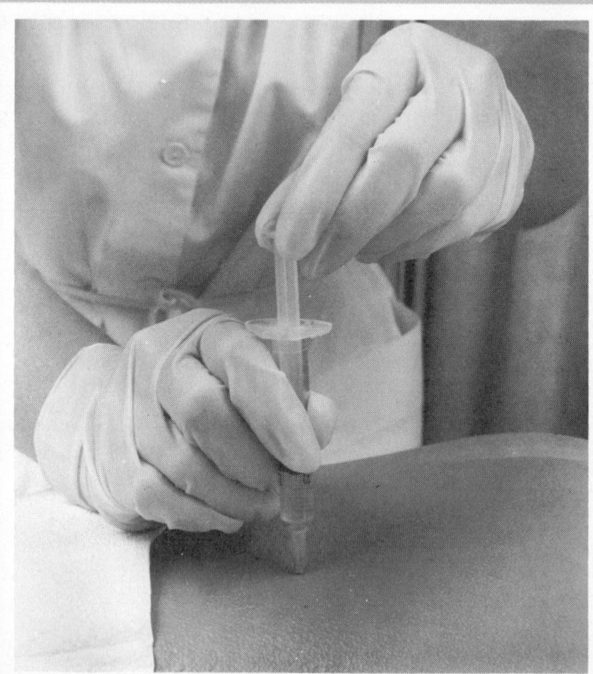

5. **PROCEDURAL STEP.** Hold the barrel of the syringe like a dart and insert the needle at a 90-degree angle with a firm motion. Insert the needle to the hub.
PRINCIPLE. The needle is inserted at a 90-degree angle to ensure that it reaches muscle tissue.

6. **PROCEDURAL STEP.** Hold the syringe steady and pull back gently on the plunger to determine whether the needle is in a blood vessel. If blood appears, withdraw the needle, prepare a new injection, and begin again.
PRINCIPLE. Moving the syringe once the needle has penetrated the tissue causes patient discomfort. If drugs that are intended for intramuscular administration are injected into a blood vessel, the result is faster absorption of the medication. This may produce undesirable results.

7. **PROCEDURAL STEP.** Inject the medication slowly and steadily by depressing the plunger.
PRINCIPLE. Rapid injection creates pressure and destroys tissue, thus causing discomfort for the patient.

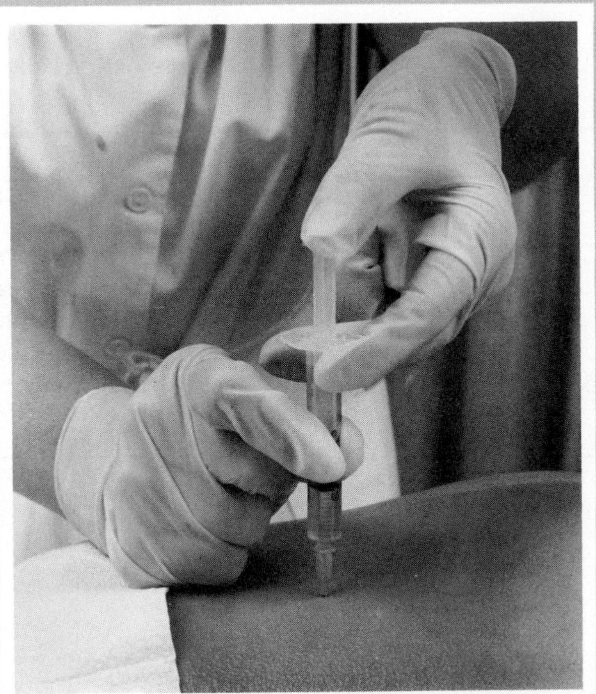

8. **PROCEDURAL STEP.** Place the antiseptic wipe gently over the injection site, and remove the needle quickly, keeping it at the same angle as for insertion. Properly dispose of the needle and syringe.
PRINCIPLE. Withdrawing the needle quickly and at the same angle as for insertion reduces patient discomfort. Placing the antiseptic wipe over the injection site helps to prevent tissue movement as the needle is withdrawn, also reducing patient discomfort. Proper disposal of the needle and syringe protects the medical assistant from being pricked by a contaminated needle.

9. **PROCEDURAL STEP.** Massage the injection site with an antiseptic wipe. Apply pressure and place an adhesive bandage over the site if needed.
PRINCIPLE. Massaging helps to distribute the medication so that it is absorbed by the muscle tissue.

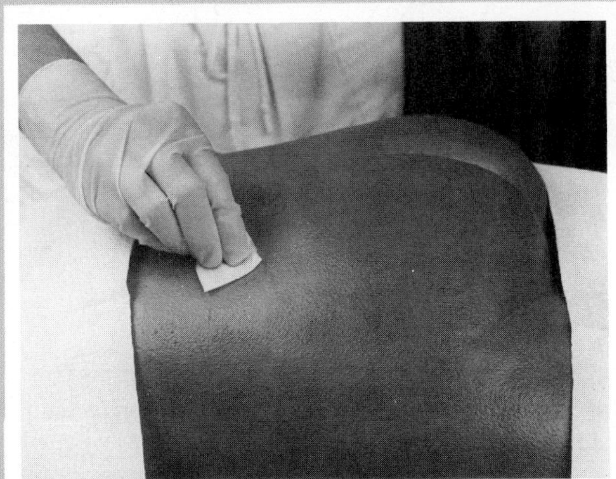

10. **PROCEDURAL STEP.** Remove the gloves and wash the hands.

11. **PROCEDURAL STEP.** Stay with the patient to make sure he or she is not experiencing any unusual reactions. Assist the patient off the examining table.
PRINCIPLE. If the patient experiences an unusual reaction, notify the physician.

12. **PROCEDURAL STEP.** Record the procedure. Include the patient's name, the date and time, the name of the medication, the dosage given, the route of administration, the injection site used, and any significant observations or patient reactions. Initial the recording.

Record data below.

DATE	TIME	PATIENT'S NAME	RECORDING

Z-Track Method

Medications that are irritating to subcutaneous and skin tissue and/or that discolor the skin must be given intramuscularly using the Z-track method; an example of a medication that is administered by this method is iron-dextran (Imferon). The Z-track method is very similar to the intramuscular injection procedure, except that the skin and subcutaneous tissue at the injection site are pulled to the side before the needle is inserted. This causes a zigzag path through the tissues once the skin is released, preventing the medication from reaching the subcutaneous layer or skin surface by sealing off the needle track (Fig. 8–16). The procedure for administering medication using the Z-track method is presented below, utilizing concepts previously presented in the intramuscular injection procedure.

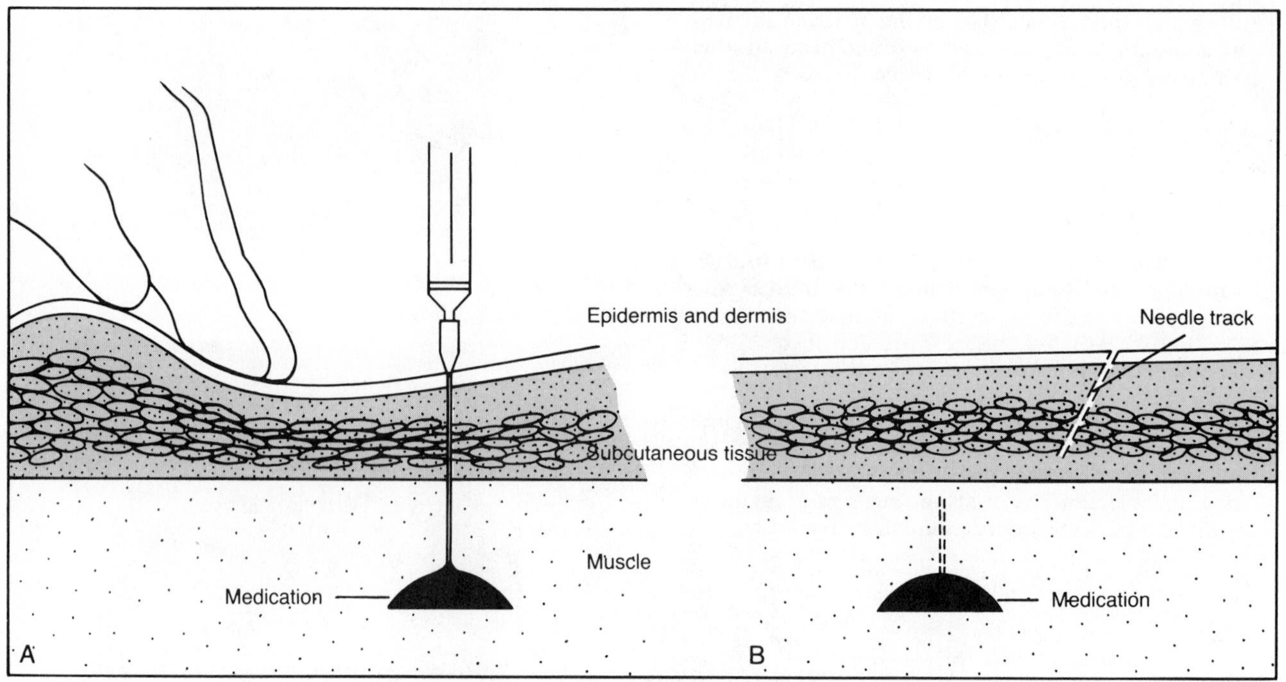

FIGURE 8–16. The Z-track intramuscular injection technique. *A*, The skin and subcutaneous tissue are pulled to the side before the needle is inserted. *B*, This causes a zigzag path through the tissue once the skin is released, which seals off the needle track.

PROCEDURE 8-7
Z-TRACK INTRAMUSCULAR INJECTION TECHNIQUE

1. Follow Steps 1 to 3 of the intramuscular injection procedure.

2. Apply gloves and remove the needle guard. With the nondominant hand, pull the skin away laterally from the injection site approximately 1 to 1½ inches.

3. Insert the needle at a 90-degree angle.

4. Aspirate to determine whether the needle is in a blood vessel (refer to Step 6 of the intramuscular injection procedure.)

5. Inject the medication slowly and steadily.

6. After injecting the medication, wait 10 seconds before withdrawing the needle to allow initial absorption of the medication.

7. Withdraw the needle at the same angle of insertion.

8. Release the traction on the skin in order to seal off the needle track; doing so prevents the medication from reaching the subcutaneous tissue and skin surface. Properly dispose of the needle and syringe.

9. Do not massage the site; massaging may cause the medication to seep out.

10. Complete the procedure by following Steps 10 to 12 of the intramuscular injection procedure (Procedure 8-6).

Tuberculin Skin Testing

Tuberculosis is an infectious disease that usually attacks the lungs, although it may occur in almost any other part of the body. The causative agent of tuberculosis is the tubercle bacillus *(Mycobacterium tuberculosis),* which is a rod-shaped bacterium.

The purpose of tuberculin skin testing is to detect the presence of a tuberculin infection. The test is often performed as a screening measure to assist in the early detection of unsuspected cases of tuberculosis before the patient becomes symptomatic. In this way, appropriate therapeutic measures can be instituted, leading to early treatment, which also helps to prevent the spread of the disease. Tuberculin skin testing is usually included as part of a regular health screen or it may be required as a prerequisite for employment, college entrance, entrance into the military service, and so on. The medical assistant is responsible for administering the tuberculin skin test and for interpreting the test results. Although tuberculin skin testing is relatively easy to perform, the procedure must be followed exactly to ensure accurate results. A patient with a tuberculous infection may fail to react to the test, if it is performed inaccurately.

The substance used in the skin test is tuberculin, which consists of a protein or protein derivative extracted from a culture of tubercle bacilli (the causative agent of tuberculosis) to test for sensitivity to the microorganism. Tuberculin, when introduced into the skin of an individual with an active or dormant case of tuberculosis, will cause a localized thickening of the skin, resulting in an abnormally hard spot termed *induration.* Induration is caused by an accumulation of small sensitized lymphocytes and occurs in the area in which the tuberculin was injected into the skin. Tuberculin skin test reactions are based on the amount of induration present and are interpreted according to the manufacturer's instructions, which accompany the test.

A positive reaction to a tuberculin skin test indicates the presence of a tuberculous infection; however, it does not differentiate between the active and dormant states of the infection. This means the individual had or now has a tuberculous infection but does not necessarily mean that the patient has the active tuberculosis disease. Therefore, a positive reaction will warrant further diagnostic procedures before the physician can make a final diagnosis. Additional procedures used to detect the presence of an active tuberculous infection include microbiologic examination of the patient's sputum for the presence of tubercle bacilli and an x-ray study of the patient's chest.

Several methods are used for tuberculin skin testing; the most commonly used methods are the Mantoux test and the tine test. The Mantoux test is administered using an intradermal needle and syringe, whereas the tine test utilizes a sterile plastic unit containing four stainless steel tines for puncturing the skin. The Mantoux test and the tine test have similar guidelines for administering and reading the tests, which are presented here. Procedures specific to each test are presented following these general guidelines.

Administering the Tuberculin Skin Test

1. The anterior forearm, approximately 4 inches below the bend in the elbow, should be used as the site of administration of the test; hairy areas of the skin, scar tissue, and areas without adequate subcutaneous tissue should be avoided.
2. The skin must be cleansed thoroughly and allowed to dry completely before the test is administered. Commonly used cleansing agents include alcohol, acetone, and ether.

3. The tuberculin must be deposited in the superficial layers of the skin. If blood appears at the puncture site once the test has been administered, it is not significant and will not interfere with the test.

4. Once the test has been administered, it must be read within 48 to 72 hours. The patient may be instructed to return to the medical office to have it read, or the medical assistant may need to instruct the patient in the proper procedure for reading the test at home.

Reading the Tuberculin Test Results

1. The test results must be read in good lighting (within 48 to 72 hours).
2. The medical assistant must instruct the patient to flex the arm at the elbow.
3. The test results are read using both inspection and palpation. If induration is present, the medical assistant should rub her finger lightly from the area of normal skin (without induration) to the indurated area to assess its size. The area of induration is then measured in millimeters. The extent of induration present is the only criterion used in determining a positive reaction. If erythema is present without induration, the results are interpreted as negative.

Mantoux Test

The Mantoux test is administered through an intradermal injection using a tuberculin syringe with a capacity of 1.0 ml and a short (⅜ to ½ inch) needle with a gauge of 26 to 27. The amount of solution that is injected is 0.1 ml, which is drawn into the syringe from a multiple-dose vial containing the Mantoux tuberculin solution. It is important that the medical assistant draw up the proper amount of tuberculin solution. Injecting too much of the solution might elicit a reaction not caused by a tuberculous infection, whereas injecting too little of the solution results in not enough solution being injected into the skin to elicit a reaction. This will invalidate the test, because if no reaction occurs, it cannot be accepted as a negative reaction. Procedure 8-3, Preparing the Injection, and Procedure 8-4, Administering an Intradermal Injection, should be followed to prepare and administer the Mantoux test. The medical assistant must make sure to inject the solution into the superficial skin layers to form a wheal. If the injection is made into the subcutaneous layer, a wheal will not form and the test will yield a false-negative result, whereas a too-shallow injection may cause leakage of the tuberculin solution onto the skin. In either case, the medical assistant must repeat the test again at another site at least 2 inches away. The medical assistant should not massage the site after injecting the solution, because the solution is not intended to be absorbed into the tissues. In addition, massaging may cause leakage of the tuberculin solution out through the needle puncture site.

The test results must be read in good lighting within 48 to 72 hours. The diameter of induration should be measured transversely to the long axis of the forearm, and the results should be recorded in millimeters. Mantoux tuberculin skin test results are interpreted as follows:

Positive — Induration of 10 mm or more constitutes a positive reaction and warrants further diagnostic procedures to determine whether active tuberculosis is present.

Doubtful — Induration measuring 5 to 9 mm means that retesting is recommended, using a different site of injection.

Negative — Induration of less than 5 mm constitutes a negative reaction.

Tine Test

The tine test, a multiple puncture test, is convenient and easy to administer; therefore, it is especially useful for tuberculin screening. A sterile disposable intradermal test device is used that consists of a stainless steel disc attached to a plastic handle. Four triangle-shaped prongs or tines, approximately 2 mm long, project from the disc; these tines have been impregnated with tuberculin. The patient is inoculated intradermally to a depth of 1 to 2 mm by simple pressure on the skin, and the tuberculin on the tines is deposited into the skin layers. The medical assistant frequently administers the tine test in the medical office and is also responsible for reading the test results in the office and/or instructing the patient in reading the results at home and reporting them to the office. If the tine test reaction is positive, most physicians confirm the positive reaction by performing the Mantoux test. The procedure for administering and reading a tine test is outlined on the following pages.

PROCEDURE 8-8
ADMINISTERING A TINE TEST

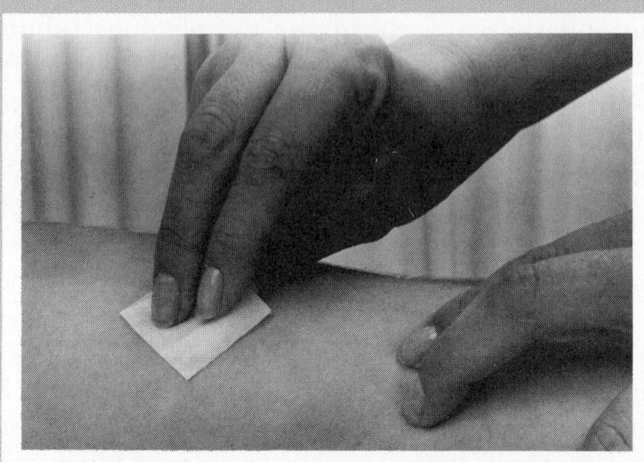

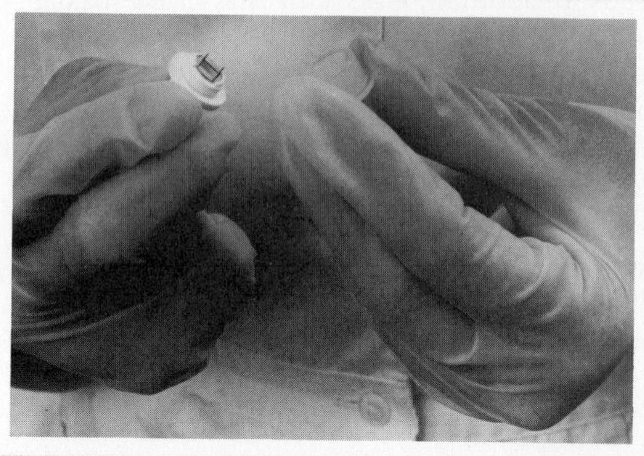

1. **PROCEDURAL STEP.** Wash the hands.

2. **PROCEDURAL STEP.** Identify the patient and explain the procedure.

3. **PROCEDURAL STEP.** Select an appropriate site to administer the tine test. The anterior surface of the forearm, approximately 4 inches below the bend of the elbow, is recommended. Hairy areas of the skin, areas with blemishes, scar tissue, and areas without adequate subcutaneous tissue should be avoided.
   PRINCIPLE. Hairy areas of the skin and areas with blemishes make it difficult to read the test results.

4. **PROCEDURAL STEP.** Prepare the site. Cleanse the area with an appropriate agent such as alcohol, acetone, or ether. Allow the area to dry completely. Do not touch the site once it has been cleansed.
   PRINCIPLE. Touching the site after cleansing contaminates it, and the cleansing process will need to be repeated.

5. **PROCEDURAL STEP.** Apply gloves. Expose the four tuberculin-coated tines using the following technique: Hold the protective plastic cap with one hand and, with the other hand, use a twisting pulling motion on the cap covering the tines, thereby removing the cap and exposing the tines.
   PRINCIPLE. Gloves provide a barrier precaution against contaminated blood.

6. **PROCEDURAL STEP.** Grasp the forearm with the nondominant hand immediately behind the proposed site of administration of the test and stretch the skin of the forearm tightly to prevent the patient's arm from jerking during administration.

PRINCIPLE. If the patient jerked the arm during the administration of the test, it could result in a scratch on the arm. Stretching the skin will permit easier insertion of the tines.

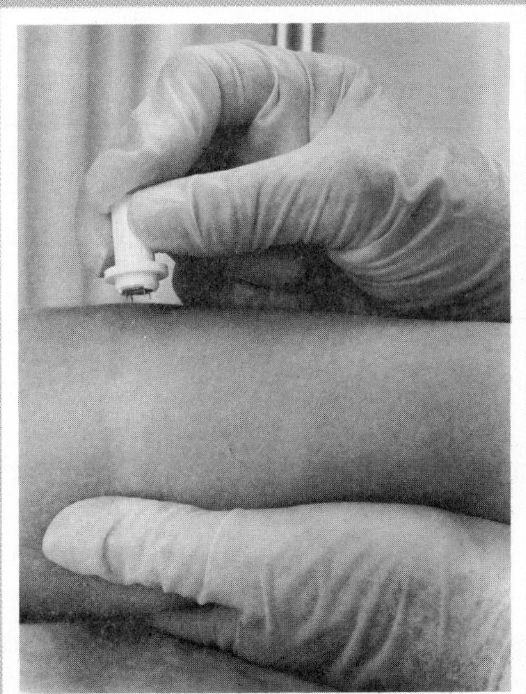

7. **PROCEDURAL STEP.** Hold the tine test device in the dominant hand, place the plastic disc (with the four tines) on the patient's skin, and hold for at least 1 second (between 1 and 2 seconds is recommended) to allow the tines to pierce the skin. Sufficient pressure should be exerted so that the four puncture sites and the circular depression from the plastic base are visible on the patient's skin.

PRINCIPLE. The tines penetrate the skin, thereby introducing the tuberculin on the tines into the patient's skin.

8. **PROCEDURAL STEP.** Release the tension from the grasp on the patient's forearm and withdraw the tine test unit. Do *not* massage or rub the test site after application of the tines.

PRINCIPLE. The incidence of bleeding at the test site is reduced if the tension on the forearm is released before the tines are withdrawn. The test site should not be massaged because the tuberculin is intended to be deposited into the skin layers and not absorbed into the tissues.

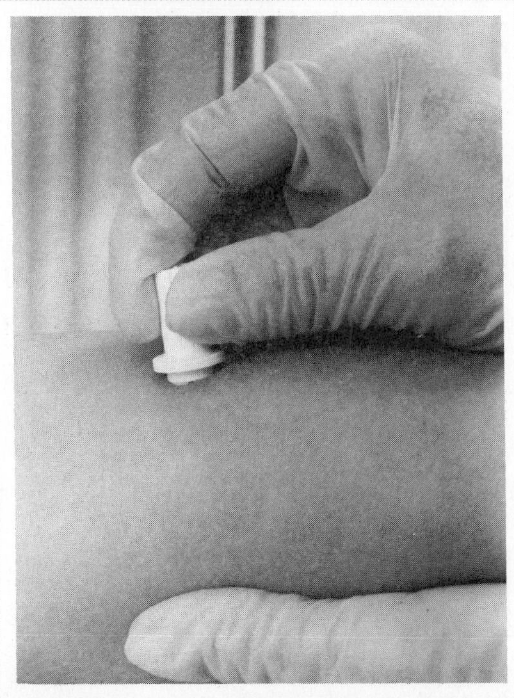

9. **PROCEDURAL STEP.** Discard the plastic disc. Local care of the skin is not necessary. Some minor bleeding may occur but this does not interfere with the test results.

PRINCIPLE. Once used, the tine test unit is contaminated and should never be reused.

10. **PROCEDURAL STEP.** Remove gloves and wash the hands.

11. **PROCEDURAL STEP.** Instruct the patient to return for reading of the test in 48 to 72 hours or instruct the patient in reading the test at home and reporting results.

PRINCIPLE. The response to the tuberculin deposited in the patient's skin occurs within 24 to 72 hours; therefore, the skin test results must be read within 48 to 72 hours.

12. **PROCEDURAL STEP.** Record in the patient's chart. Include the patient's name, the date and time, the name of the test administered (tine test), the site of administration, and any unusual patient reactions. Place your initials next to the recording.

PRINCIPLE. Recording the site of administration facilitates locating the test site if the patient will be returning to the medical office to have the test read.

Continued

Record data below.

DATE	TIME	PATIENT'S NAME	RECORDING

PROCEDURE 8-9
READING THE TINE TEST RESULTS

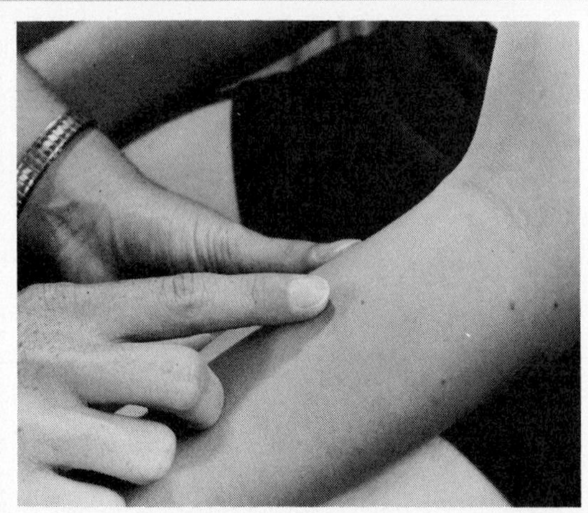

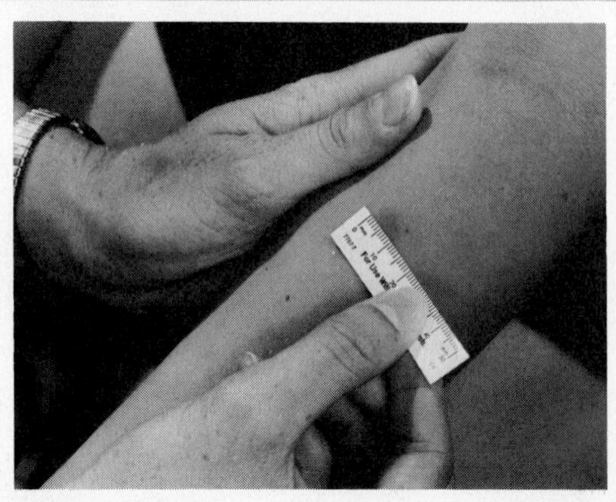

1. **PROCEDURAL STEP.** Wash the hands.

2. **PROCEDURAL STEP.** Work in a quiet, well-lighted atmosphere.

3. **PROCEDURAL STEP.** Ask the patient to flex the arm at the elbow.

4. **PROCEDURAL STEP.** Locate the application site by inspecting the patient's arm for the presence of the four-point pattern.

5. **PROCEDURAL STEP.** Read the test results. Gently rub your finger over the test site to palpate for the presence of induration. If induration is present, the area should be lightly rubbed from the area of normal skin (without induration) to the indurated area to assess the size of the area of induration present. Measure the diameter of the largest single reaction around one of the puncture sites with a millimeter ruler (supplied by the manufacturer). The results of the tine test are interpreted as follows:

A. Positive Reactions
   a. Vesiculation: *Vesiculation* is the formation of vesicles, which are fluid-containing lesions of the skin. If vesiculation is present, the test is interpreted as positive and will warrant further diagnostic procedures to determine if active tuberculosis is present.
   b. Induration 2 mm or greater is interpreted as a positive reaction. Most physicians confirm the positive reaction by performing the Mantoux test (before performing further diagnostic procedures).

B. Negative Reaction: Induration less than 2 mm constitutes a negative reaction.

PRINCIPLE. Vesiculation or induration 2 mm or greater is the only criterion used to determine a positive reaction. Erythema without the presence of vesicles or induration constitutes a negative reaction.

6. **PROCEDURAL STEP.** Wash the hands.

7. **PROCEDURAL STEP.** Record results in the patient's chart. Include the patient's name, the date and time, the name of the test (tine test), and the test results (recorded in millimeters). Initial the recording.

Record data below.

DATE	TIME	PATIENT'S NAME	RECORDING

Study Questions

1. What is the difference between administering, prescribing, and dispensing medication?
2. What factors affect the action of drugs in the body?
3. What are the advantages and disadvantages of using the parenteral route of administration?
4. What tissue layers of the body are used for an intradermal, a subcutaneous, and an intramuscular injection?
5. What is the purpose of using the Z-track technique to administer medication?
6. What is the purpose for performing tuberculin skin testing?

9

INTRODUCTION TO THE CLINICAL LABORATORY

CHAPTER OUTLINE

Laboratory Tests
Purpose of Laboratory Testing
Relationship Between the Medical Office and the Clinical Laboratory
Laboratory Requests
Laboratory Reports
Patient Preparation and Instructions
Collecting, Handling, and Transporting Specimens
Testing the Specimen
Quality Control
Laboratory Safety

COMPETENCIES

After completing this chapter, you should be able to demonstrate the proper procedure to perform the following:

1. Complete a laboratory request form.
2. Use a laboratory directory.
3. Read a laboratory report.
4. Instruct a patient in the preparation necessary for a laboratory test requiring fasting.
5. Collect a biologic specimen.
6. Handle and store a biologic specimen.
7. Transport a biologic specimen to an outside laboratory.
8. Employ quality control methods.
9. Practice laboratory safety.

LEARNING OBJECTIVES

After completing this chapter, you should be able to do the following:

1. Define the terms listed in the vocabulary.
2. Explain the general purpose of a laboratory test.
3. List and explain five specific uses of laboratory test results.
4. Describe the relationship between the medical office and an outside laboratory.
5. List the information included in a laboratory directory.
6. Identify the purpose of a laboratory request form. List and explain the function of each type of information included on the form.
7. Identify the general use of the following profiles and list the tests included in each: SMA-12, liver function profile, thyroid profile, prenatal profile, electrolyte profile, rheumatoid profile, coronary assessment profile, lipid profile.
8. Identify the purpose of the laboratory report and list the information included on it.
9. Explain the purpose of advance patient preparation for the collection of a laboratory specimen.
10. List 10 examples of biologic specimens.
11. Identify and explain five guidelines that should be followed during specimen collection.
12. Explain why specimens must be handled and stored properly. Identify the proper handling and storage techniques for the following specimens: blood, urine, microbiologic specimen, stool specimen.
13. Identify the general guidelines that must be followed when a specimen is sent through the mail.
14. Identify and define the eight categories of laboratory tests based on function. List examples of three tests included under each category.
15. List the six basic steps involved in testing a biologic specimen.
16. Describe the three methods (manual, automated, semiautomated) that can be used to test a biologic specimen. Identify the advantages and disadvantages of each method.
17. Explain the purpose of quality control in the laboratory and list quality-control methods that should be employed for each of the following: advance patient preparation; specimen collection, handling, and transportation; laboratory testing.
18. List 10 laboratory safety guidelines that should be followed in the medical office to prevent accidents.

• VOCABULARY •

automated method (aw-to-ma' ted mĕth' ud) (for testing laboratory specimens)—A method of laboratory testing in which the series of steps in the test method is performed by an automated analyzer.

fasting (fast' ing)—Abstaining from food or fluids (except water) for a specified amount of time prior to the collection of a specimen.

homeostasis (ho" me-o-sta' sis)—The state in which body systems are functioning normally and the internal environment of the body is in equilibrium; the body is in a healthy state.

in vivo (in ve' vo)—Occurring in the living body or organism.

laboratory test (lab' o-rah-tor" e test)—The clinical analysis and study of materials, fluids, or tissues obtained from patients to assist in diagnosing and treating disease.

manual method (man' u-al mĕth' ud)—A method of laboratory testing in which the series of steps in the test method is performed by hand.

normal range (nor' mal rānj) (for laboratory tests)—A certain established and acceptable parameter or reference range within which the laboratory test results of a healthy individual are expected to fall.

plasma (plaz' mah)—The liquid part of the blood consisting of a clear yellowish fluid that makes up approximately 55 per cent of the total blood volume.

profile (pro' fīl)—A combination of laboratory tests providing related or complementary information used to determine the health status of a patient.

quality control (kwol' ĭ-te kon-trōl')—The application of methods to ensure that test results are reliable and valid and that errors are detected and eliminated.

routine test (ro͞o-tēn' test)—Laboratory tests performed on a routine basis on apparently healthy patients to assist in the early detection of disease.

serum (se' rum)—Plasma from which the clotting factor fibrinogen has been removed.

specimen (spes' ĭ-men)—A small sample of something taken to show the nature of the whole.

Introduction

Clinical laboratory test results are often used along with a thorough health history and physical examination (refer to Chapter 3) to provide essential data needed by the physician to accurately diagnose and manage a patient's condition. Clinical laboratory tests provide objective and quantitative information regarding the status of body conditions and functions. When the body is in a healthy state, its systems will be functioning normally and a state of equilibrium of the internal environment is said to exist; this is termed *homeostasis.* When the body is in a state of homeostasis, the physical and chemical characteristics of the body substances (e.g., fluids, secretions, excretions) will be within a certain acceptable range known as the normal or reference range. On the other hand, when a pathologic condition exists, biologic changes take place within the body, altering the normal physiology or functioning of the body and resulting in an imbalance. These changes cause the patient to experience the symptoms of that particular pathologic condition; for example, iron-deficiency anemia will usually cause the patient to experience weakness, fatigue, pallor, irritability, and, in some cases, shortness of breath on exertion. In addition, these changes in the body's biologic processes may cause an alteration in the physical and chemical characteristics of body substances such as an alteration of the chemical content of the blood or urine; an alteration in the antibody level; an alteration in cell counts or cellular morphology, and so on.

The physical and chemical alterations of body substances are evidenced through abnormal values or results occurring in laboratory tests — in other words, values lying outside the accepted normal range or limit for that particular test. Just as certain pathologic conditions cause specific symptoms to occur, certain pathologic conditions cause abnormal values to occur for specific laboratory tests; for example, iron-deficiency anemia causes an alteration in normal red blood cell morphology and a decreased hemoglobin level. It is important to realize, however, that an abnormal value for a particular test may be seen with more than one pathologic condition. For example, a decrease in the hemoglobin level also is found with hyperthyroidism and cirrhosis of the liver. In this regard, the physician cannot rely solely on laboratory test results to make a final diagnosis, but rather upon the combination of the data obtained from the health history, the physical examination, and diagnostic and laboratory test results.

Laboratory Tests

The number of laboratory tests ordered on a patient will vary depending on the physician's clinical impressions. A clinical diagnosis of a urinary tract infection, for example, usually requires only a urine culture to confirm the clinical diagnosis. Many diseases, however, exhibit more than one alteration in the physical and chemical characteristics of body substances; therefore, it is often necessary to order a series of laboratory tests to establish the pattern of abnormalities characteristic of a particular disease. For example, with a clinical diagnosis of infectious hepatitis, the physician will order a liver function profile. (See Table 9–2 for a list of the tests included in a liver function profile.) A patient with infectious hepatitis has an alteration in normal values on a number of test results. There is an abnormal increase in the SGOT (AST), SGPT (ALT), and bilirubin, and there may be a slight elevation in alkaline phosphatase. When the clinical signs and symptoms of the patient are vague, a number of laboratory tests may be necessary to provide a wide range of data on the overall status of the patient's body functions. As a result of testing, any abnormal values become apparent and assist in pinponting the patient's condition.

The medical assistant should realize that not all pathologic conditions require the use of laboratory test results to arrive at a final diagnosis; the information obtained from the patient's clinical signs and symptoms is sufficient to make a final diagnosis of some conditions. In these instances, the physician is so certain of the clinical diagnosis that therapy can be instituted without laboratory confirmation. For example, most physicians diagnose acute purulent otitis media using the information obtained from patient symptoms (earache, fever, feeling of fullness in the ear) and from an otoscopic examination of the tympanic membrane (the tympanic membrane is red and bulging). The information obtained through the clinical signs and symptoms is sufficiently specific to otitis media to allow the physician to make a final diagnosis and to prescribe treatment.

The medical assistant must acquire both knowledge and skill in basic clinical laboratory methods and techniques. It is important that the medical assistant have a knowledge of those laboratory tests that are performed most often, including the purpose of these tests, how to perform them, the normal value or range for each test, any advance patient preparation or special instructions, and any substances that might interfere with accurate test results, such as food or medication. The medical assistant frequently works with this information when collecting, handling, and storing biologic specimens; performing laboratory tests; typing health histories; and receiving and filing laboratory reports. It is essential that the medical assistant appreciate the value of laboratory tests and alert the physician to any abnormal results as soon as the test is performed or the laboratory report is received. This chapter is intended to serve as an introduction to the clinical laboratory by providing an overview of methods and general guidelines to follow and by focusing on the relationship between the medical office and an outside laboratory. Specific information for collection, handling, storing, and testing of biologic specimens is presented in the following chapters: Urinalysis, Venipuncture, Hematology and Blood Chemistry, Microbiology and Disease, and Specialty Examinations and Procedures.

Purpose of Laboratory Testing

The most frequent use of laboratory test results is to assist in the diagnosis of a patient's condition; however, they also have a number of other significant medical uses. A summary of the purpose and function of laboratory testing follows:

1. Laboratory tests are most frequently ordered by the physician to *assist in the diagnosis of pathologic conditions.* Along with the health history and the physical examination, laboratory test results provide the physician with essential data needed to arrive at the final diagnosis and to prescribe treatment. Following the health history and physical examination, the physician may order laboratory tests for these reasons:

a. *To confirm a clinical diagnosis.* The patient's signs and symptoms may provide a strong clinical diagnosis of a particular condition, and the physician may order laboratory tests simply to confirm that diagnosis. For example, the patient may exhibit the typical signs and symptoms of diabetes mellitus, providing the physician with a fairly certain clinical diagnosis. In this instance, a glucose tolerance test is ordered to confirm the diagnosis and to institute therapy.

b. *To assist in the differential diagnosis of a patient's condition.* Two or more diseases may have similar signs and symptoms; therefore, the physician will order laboratory tests to assist in the differential diagnosis of the patient's condition. For example, a final diagnosis of streptococcal sore throat must be made by a laboratory test to differentiate it from other pathologic conditions having similar signs and symptoms.

c. *To obtain information regarding a patient's condition when there is not enough concrete evidence to support a clinical diagnosis.* At times, the patient may exhibit vague signs and symptoms, and laboratory tests are ordered to provide information on what may be causing the patient's problem. For example, the patient may complain of nonspecific abdominal pain, and the physical examination may not yield enough information to support a clinical diagnosis.

In this case, the physician may order a series of tests that may include a number of laboratory tests, usually in the form of a profile(s), x-ray studies, and special diagnostic procedures to assist in pinpointing the cause of the patient's problems.

2. Once the final diagnosis has been made, laboratory testing may be performed to *evaluate the patient's progress and to regulate treatment.* Based on the laboratory results, the therapy may need to be adjusted or further treatment prescribed. For example, a patient on iron therapy for iron-deficiency anemia should have a complete blood count (CBC) performed every month to assess response to the treatment and to make sure the condition is improving. Another example would be a patient with thrombophlebitis who is taking warfarin sodium (Coumadin), an anticoagulant used to inhibit blood clotting. The patient must have a prothrombin time test at regular intervals to assess the clotting ability of the blood. Based on the test results, the medication may need to be adjusted to make sure the dosage is at a safe level. The diabetic patient who measures his or her blood glucose level each day to regulate insulin dosage is another example of the utilization of laboratory tests to regulate treatment.

3. Based on such factors as age, sex, race, and geographic location, individuals will have different normal levels within the established normal range for a particular test. In this respect, laboratory tests can also serve *to establish each patient's baseline or normal level* against which future results can be compared. For example, a patient who is going to be placed on warfarin sodium therapy should have a blood specimen drawn for a prothrombin time test prior to administration of this anticoagulant. The results serve as a baseline recording for that particular patient against which future prothrombin time test results can be compared.

4. Laboratory tests can also help *prevent or reduce the severity of disease* by early detection of abnormal findings. Certain conditions, such as anemia and diabetes, are relatively common disorders and at times may exist undetected in a patient, especially early in the development of the disease. Laboratory tests known as *routine tests* are performed on a routine basis on apparently healthy patients (usually as part of a general physical examination) to assist in the early detection of disease. These tests are relatively easy to perform and present a minimal hazard to the patient. The most commonly used routine tests include urinalysis, CBC, and routine blood chemistries.

5. Another reason for performing a laboratory test is its *requirement by state law.* The statutes of most states require a gonorrhea culture and serology for syphilis to be performed on pregnant women. The purpose of these tests is to protect the mother and fetus from harm by screening for the presence of these venereal diseases. Many states also require a premarital serology to screen individuals for the presence of syphilis.

Relationship Between the Medical Office and the Clinical Laboratory

The medical office may use an outside laboratory for testing, and/or the office may contain its own laboratory in which the medical assistant performs various tests; most medical offices utilize a combination of the two to fulfill the physician's needs for test results. Generally speaking, laboratory tests that are convenient to execute, and commonly required, such as the hematocrit and urinalysis, are performed in the medical office. Most physicians consider it too time-consuming and expensive in terms of equipment, supplies, medical laboratory personnel, and quality control to perform in the medical office highly sophisticated and complex tests such as serologic studies and microbiologic studies. Therefore, these tests are usually performed at an outside laboratory. These laboratories utilize automated equipment to perform the tests, providing the medical offices with fast and reliable test results at a relatively low cost. Because the medical assistant usually works closely with an outside laboratory, it is important that she or he have a basic knowledge of the relationship between the medical office and the laboratory, as described in the following paragraphs.

Outside laboratories include hospital and privately owned commercial laboratories, which employ individuals specifically trained in clinical laboratory techniques and methods. The laboratory usually supplies the medical office with the equipment and forms necessary to collect and transport biologic specimens. The medical assistant is responsible for checking these supplies periodically and for reordering them from the laboratory as needed. The outside laboratory performs most of the tests ordered by the physician; however, some tests not performed very often and requiring sophisticated equipment and specialized knowledge may be referred to a larger laboratory for analysis. These *reference laboratories* serve a number of smaller laboratories.

The outside laboratory provides the medical office with a directory that serves as a valuable reference source for the proper collection and handling of specimens. Directories vary in organization, depending on the laboratory; however, the following information is generally included: names of the tests performed by the laboratory, the normal range for each test, instructions on completion of forms, patient preparation required for each test, supplies required for the collection of each specimen, amount and type of specimen required by the laboratory, techniques to employ for the collection of the specimen, proper handling and storage of the specimen, and instructions for transporting specimens. Table 9–1 is a sample of some representative tests taken from a laboratory directory. If the medical assistant has a question regarding any aspect of the collection and handling of the specimen, she or he should call the laboratory before proceeding.

The collection and testing of a biologic specimen with respect to a medical office setting can be categorized according to the following modes: (1) the specimen is collected and tested at the medical office; (2) the specimen is collected at the medical office and transferred (through hand pick-up or mail) to an outside medical laboratory for testing; (3) the patient is given a laboratory request to have the specimen collected and tested at an outside laboratory. The responsibilities of the medical assistant with respect to the clinical laboratory depend largely on the modes utilized in the medical office to collect and test the specimen. For example, a specimen collected at the medical office and transferred to an outside laboratory for testing will involve a series of individual steps different from those followed when it is both collected and tested at the medical office. The following clinical laboratory methods are presented in the remainder of this chapter to provide the student with the information needed to function competently in all three modes just described.

1. Completing laboratory request forms and reviewing laboratory reports.
2. Informing the patient of any necessary advance preparation or special instructions.
3. Collecting, handling, and transporting biologic specimens.
4. Testing the specimen in the medical office.
5. Practicing quality control and laboratory safety.

Laboratory Requests

Laboratory requests are printed forms containing a list of the most frequently ordered laboratory tests (refer to Figure 9–1). A laboratory request is required when the specimen is collected at the medical office and transferred to an outside laboratory for testing or when the specimen will be collected and tested at an outside laboratory, in which case the request is given to the patient at the medical office to take to the laboratory. The request provides the outside laboratory with essential information required for accurate testing, reporting of results, and billing. The organizational formats for the request forms vary, depending on the

TABLE 9-1. Representative Tests from a Laboratory Directory

TEST	SPECIMEN REQUIREMENTS	NORMAL VALUES
A/G ratio (includes total protein, albumin, and globulin)	2 ml serum in a white top transfer tube.	1.1-2.5
Albumin, serum	2 ml serum in a white top transfer tube.	3.0-5.5 gm/dl
Bilirubin, total	2 ml serum in a white top transfer tube. Protect from light.	0.2-1.2 mg/dl
Blood group (ABO)	1-5 ml red stoppered tube.	
Blood group and Rh type	1-5 ml red stoppered tube.	
BUN, serum	2 ml serum in a white top transfer tube or 1-5 ml red stoppered tube.	10-26 mg/dl
Calcium, serum	2 ml serum in a white top transfer tube. DO NOT USE CORKS!	8.5-10.5 mg/dl
Carbon dioxide (CO_2)	2 ml serum in a white top transfer tube.	25-32 mEq/L
CBC (complete blood count) (includes differential)	1-5 ml lavender stoppered tube. Tube should be inverted 6-8 times immediately after drawing. 2 blood smears.	Values given with report
Chloride, serum	2 ml serum in a white top transfer tube.	96-106 mEq/L
CPK (CK) (creatine phosphokinase)	1 ml serum in a white top transfer tube. If mailed, specimens must be frozen. If local, send immediately.	Normal: 0-12 sigma units/ml Borderline: 12-20 sigma units/ml
CRP (C-reactive protein)	1 ml serum in a white top transfer tube. Avoid hemolysis.	Negative
Creatinine, serum	2 ml serum in a white top transfer tube.	0.7-1.5 mg/dl
Glucose, blood	1-5 ml gray stoppered tube. Tube should be inverted 6-8 times immediately after drawing.	60-110 mg/dl
LDH (LD) (lactic dehydrogenase)	2 ml serum in a white top transfer tube. Hemolysis invalidates results.	Adult: 75-225 U/L Child, 3-17 year: approx. 2 × adult values
Potassium, serum	2 ml serum in a white top transfer tube. Hemolysis invalidates results.	3.5-5.0 mEq/L
Sedimentation rate (ESR)	1-5 ml lavender stoppered tube. Tube should be inverted 6-8 times immediately after drawing.	Male: 0-10 mm/hour Female: 0-20 mm/hour
Serology (VDRL)	1 ml serum in a white top transfer tube or 1-5 ml red stoppered tube.	Nonreactive
SGOT (AST)	2 ml serum in a white top transfer tube. Separate serum from clot within 1 hour after venipuncture.	0-41 U/L
SGPT (ALT)	2 ml serum in a white top transfer tube. Separate serum from clot within 1 hour after venipuncture.	0-45 U/L
Sodium, serum	2 ml serum in a white top transfer tube.	136-145 mEq/L
T_3 updake	1 ml serum in a white top transfer tube.	26-35%
T_4 (thyroxine) by RIA	2 ml serum in a white top transfer tube.	4.5-13.0 μg/dl
Total protein, serum	2 ml serum in a white top transfer tube.	6.0-8.5 g/dl
Triglycerides	2 ml serum in a white top transfer tube. Patient should be fasting 12-18 hours.	Values given with report.
Uric acid, serum	1 ml serum in a white top transfer tube.	Male: 3.9-9.0 mg/dl Female: 2.2-7.7 mg/dl
Urinalysis	Random sample. First morning specimen preferred. Yellow top urine container(s) with preservative.	

Biomedical Laboratories, Inc.

SIGNIFICANT CLINICAL INFORMATION

ACCOUNT NAME AND ADDRESS	ACCOUNT NO.

SPECIMEN DATE MO DAY YR | SPECIMEN TIME HR MIN | PATIENT NAME (LAST) | (FIRST) | SEX | AGE YRS MOS

TYPE BILLING | PATIENT I.D. | PHYSICIAN I.D. | PATIENT TELEPHONE NO. ( )

RESPONSIBLE PARTY (LAST) | (FIRST)

MAILING ADDRESS

CITY | STATE | ZIP CODE

MEDICAID NUMBER | MEDICARE TYPE: REGULAR, RAILROAD, UMW | MEDICARE NUMBER

PHYSICIAN NAME (LAST) | FI | PROVIDER/LICENSE NUMBER | DATE OF BIRTH MO. DAY YR | DIAGNOSIS (CODE)

PHYSICIAN SIGNATURE (MEDICAID ONLY)

For Medicare and other insured patients: I authorize any holder of medical or other information about me to release to the Social Security Administration or its intermediaries or carriers or any other government agency or insurance carrier responsible for payment any information needed for this or related Medicare or other claim. I permit a copy of this authorization to be used in place of the original, and request payment of medical insurance benefits either to myself or to the party who accepts assignment above.

PATIENT'S SIGNATURE

* CHECK SCHEDULE	INDICATE TOTAL VOLUME ______ ml. †	(R) RED	(L) LAVENDER	(G) GREY	(GN) GREEN	(RB) ROYAL BLUE	(B) LIGHT BLUE	(★) EDTA PLASMA	(S) SERUM	(U) URINE	(AF) AMNIOTIC FLUID	(GF) GASTRIC FLUID	(F) FROZEN SPECIMEN

PROFILES

- 27623 DIAGNOSTIC MULTI-CHEM / 37267 (SEE BACK FOR OPTIONS) (S)
- 00570 EXECUTIVE PROFILE A (L)(S)
- 95091 EXECUTIVE PROFILE B (L)(S)
- 57224 EXECUTIVE PROFILE C (U)(L)(2-S)
- 00018 Health Survey (SMA 12/60) (S)
- 00109 SMA 12/60 PLUS CBC (NO DIFF) (L)(S)
- 22020 SMA 12/60 PLUS CBC & DIFF (L)(S)
- 00067 SMA 12/60 PLUS ELECTROLYTES (S)
- 00026 SMA 12/60 PLUS T_4 (S)
- 00125 SMA 12/60 PLUS T_4 & CBC (NO DIFF) (L)(S)
- 00042 SMA 12/60 PLUS T_4 & TRIGLYCERIDES (S)
- 25239 DIABETES MANAGEMENT PROFILE (L)(S)
- 00604 ELECTROLYTE PROFILE (S)
- 90415 GLUCOSE/INSULIN RESPONSE (F)(S)
- 58560 HEPATITIS PROFILE I (Diagnostic) (S)
- 46938 HEPATITIS PROFILE II (S)
- 58537 HEPATITIS PROFILE IV (S)
- 58545 HEPATITIS PROFILE VI (S)
- 00315 HYPERTENSION SCREEN (U)(S)
- 00406 LIPID PROFILE A (S)
- 23358 LIPID PROFILE B (S)
- 33886 LIPID PROFILE C (S)
- 00505 LIVER PROFILE A (S)
- 00513 LIVER PROFILE B (S)
- 00893 MYOCARDIAL INFARCTION PROFILE (2-S)
- 00778 PRENATAL PROFILE A (2-L)(S)
- 00745 PRENATAL PROFILE B (2-L)(S)
- 43083 RHEUMATOID PROFILE A (S)
- 97279 RHEUMATOID PROFILE B (S)
- 00455 THYROID PROFILE A (S)
- 00620 THYROID PROFILE B (S)
- 09993 THYROID PROFILE C (S)

CHEMISTRY

- 4747 ACID PHOS., PROSTATIC (F)(S)
- 1107 ALKALINE PHOSPHATASE (S)
- 1396 AMYLASE (S)
- 1099 BILIRUBIN, TOTAL (S)
- 1214 BILIRUBIN, DIRECT & TOTAL (S)
- 1040 BUN (BLOOD UREA NITROGEN) (S)
- 1016 CALCIUM (S)
- 2139 CEA (★)
- 1206 CHLORIDE (S)
- 1065 CHOLESTEROL (S)
- 1362 CPK (S)
- 2154 CPK ISOENZYMES (F)(S)
- 1370 CREATININE (S)
- 2014 FOLIC ACID (FOLATE) (F)(S)
- 100800 FRUCTOSAMINE (S)
- 1958 GAMMA G T (S)
- 1818 GLUCOSE (G)
- 1255 GLUCOSE SCREEN (2-G)
- 1289 GLUCOSE TOLERANCE (3-G)
- 1453 GLYCO-HEMOGLOBIN (A1c) (L)
- 1925 HDL CHOLESTEROL (S)
- 1768 IMMUNOGLOBULINS QUANT. (S)
- 1321 IRON AND IBC (S)
- 1115 LDH (S)
- 1842 LDH ISOENZYMES (S)
- 1404 LIPASE (S)
- 1024 PHOSPHORUS (S)
- 1180 POTASSIUM (S)
- 1487 PROTEIN ELECTROPHORESIS (S)
- 1073 PROTEIN, TOTAL (S)
- 1123 SGOT (S)
- 1545 SGPT (S)
- 1198 SODIUM (S)
- 1172 TRIGLYCERIDES (S)
- 1057 URIC ACID (S)
- 1503 VITAMIN B_{12} (S)
- 0810 VITAMIN B_{12} & FOLATE (F)(S)

HEMATOLOGY

- 5017 CBC (L)
- 5009 CBC WITH DIFFERENTIAL (Include Slide) (L)
- 5058 HEMATOCRIT (L)
- 5041 HEMOGLOBIN (L)
- 5249 PLATELET COUNT (Include Slides) (L)
- 5199 PROTHROMBIN TIME (B)
- 5215 SEDIMENTATION RATE (L)
- 5223 SICKLE CELL TEST (L)

ENDOCRINOLOGY

- ALDOSTERONE ☐ 4374 (S) ☐ 4291 †(U)
- 4184 CATECHOLAMINES, TOTAL †(U)
- 4051 CORTISOL, SERUM OR PLASMA (★)(S)
- FSH ☐ 4309 (S) ☐ 4085 †(U)
- 4390 GASTRIN (RIA) (F)(S)
- HCG (BETA) ☐ 4416 (S) ☐ 4093 †(U)
- LH (RIA) ☐ 4283 (S) ☐ 4408 †(U)
- 4010 17-KETOGENIC STEROIDS †(U)
- 4002 17-KETOGENIC AND KETOSTEROIDS †(U)
- 4028 17-KETOSTEROIDS †(U)
- 4234 METANEPHRINES †(U)
- 4242 17-OHCS (PORTER-SILBER) †(U)
- 4150 PARATHYROID HORMONE (R)(F)(S)
- 4077 PLACENTAL ESTRIOL (IN PREGNANCY) †(U)
- 4556 PREGNANCY SERUM (RIA) (HCG-BETA) (S)
- 4036 PREGNANCY TEST (U)
- 4069 SEROTONIN (5-HIAA) †(U)
- 1149 T_4 (RIA) (S)
- 1156 T_3 UPTAKE (S)
- 2188 T_3 (RIA) (S)
- 4226 TESTOSTERONE (RIA) (S)
- 4259 TSH (RIA) (S)
- 4143 VMA, QUANTITATIVE †(U)

SEROLOGY

- 6015 ANTIBODY SCREEN (R)
- 6221 ANTIBODY TITER (ANTIBODY PREVIOUSLY IDENTIFIED AS ______) (R)
- 6254 ANTI-NUCLEAR ANTIBODY (FANA) (S)
- 6031 ASO TITER (S)
- 6049 BLOOD GROUP AND Rh FACTOR (L)
- 6353 COLD AGGLUTINATION (S)
- 6452 COMPLEMENT C'3 *(F)(S)
- 1834 COMPLEMENT C'4 (F)(S)
- 6270 COOMBS, DIRECT (R)
- 6098 FEBRILE GROUP (S)
- 6510 HEPATITIS B SURFACE ANTIGEN (S)
- 6395 HEPATITIS B SURFACE ANTIBODY (S)
- 6569 HETEROPHILE ABSORPTION (S)
- 6171 LATEX RA (NO TITER) (S)
- 6502 LATEX RA (TITER IF POSITIVE) (S)
- 6189 MONO TEST (S)
- 6072 RPR (FOR SYPHILIS) (S)
- 6197 RUBELLA (S)
- 96297 UROGENITAL GC ASSAY

TOXICOLOGY

- 7740 ACETAMINOPHEN (S)
- 7062 ALCOHOL, BLOOD (GN)
- 7385 DIGOXIN (RIA) (LANOXIN[R]) (S)
- 7401 DILANTIN[R] (S)
- 72033 DRUG SCREEN COMPREHENSIVE (U)
- 41780 DRUG SCREEN COMPREHENSIVE (S)
- 7492 HEAVY METALS SCREEN †(U)
- 7625 LEAD, BLOOD (L)
- 7708 LITHIUM (S)
- 7906 PHENOBARBITAL AND DILANTIN[R] (S)
- 7849 SALICYCLATES (ASA) (S)

URINE CHEMISTRY

- 3277 ALBUMIN (TOTAL PROTEIN) †(U)
- 3004 CREATININE CLEARANCE (S)†(U)
- 3012 CREATININE, URINE †(U)
- 3038 URINALYSIS (U)

OTHER PROFILES AND TESTS (PLEASE PRINT)

FIGURE 9–1. Laboratory request form.

laboratory. In general, most outside laboratories find it more convenient and economic to provide the medical office with one form for designating all tests, with the possible exception of the Pap test, in which case a separate form, known as a cytology request, is provided.

Specific information that is required on the laboratory request form follows. This information should always be recorded in legible handwriting to avoid confusion or incomprehension by laboratory personnel.

1. *Physician's name and address.* The physician's name and address should be clearly indicated on the laboratory request form to facilitate the reporting of test results to the physician. Some laboratories provide request forms with the physician's name and address preprinted on the form. In addition, the forms may be prenumbered with the physician's account number, which assists in identification, reporting, and billing of laboratory tests.

2. *Patient's name.* The patient's name should be printed as requested by the laboratory; for example, the laboratory may want the patient's name written with the last name first, middle initial, first name. If the laboratory will be billing the patient directly or billing a third party, the patient's address is also required, including the city, state, and zip code.

3. *Patient's age and sex.* The normal ranges for some tests vary, depending on the patient's age and sex. For example, the normal range for total cholesterol and triglycerides varies according to age. The normal range for hemoglobin concentration varies according to sex; it is 12 to 16 gm/100 ml for a female, whereas for a male it is 14 to 18 gm/100 ml.

4. *Date and time of collection of the specimen.* The date of the specimen collection indicates to the laboratory the number of days that have passed since the collection, thus providing the laboratory with information regarding the freshness of the specimen. Too long a time lapse between collection and testing of a specimen may affect the accuracy of some test results. The time of collection is significant with respect to selected laboratory tests. For example, the normal range for serum cortisol varies depending on whether the specimen is an AM specimen (collected in the morning) or a PM specimen (collected in the afternoon).

5. *Laboratory tests desired.* The tests desired by the physician are usually indicated by checking a box adjacent to those tests (see Fig. 9–1). The boxes should be clearly marked to avoid any confusion. A space designated as *additional tests* or *other tests* on the laboratory request form provides for writing in a test that is desired but that is not listed on the request form. As previously indicated, most laboratory request forms include only those tests most frequently ordered. The laboratory directory contains a complete listing of all the tests performed.

Laboratory tests termed *profiles* contain a number of different tests; the profiles performed by the laboratory and the tests included in each are listed in the directory. A profile may be specific in nature; that is, all the tests included relate to a specific organ of the body or a particular disease state. A specific profile is usually ordered when the physician does not have a definite clinical diagnosis but has a good idea of what organ or organs are involved in the patient's condition. Most of these profiles are termed function tests, and the physician will order a function test of the organ in question. An example of this type of profile is the liver function profile, which is used to assess liver function and to assist in the diagnosis of a pathologic condition affecting the liver.

A profile may also be general in nature. A general profile contains a number of routine laboratory tests and is primarily used in a routine health screen of a patient. General profiles are used to detect any changes in the body's biologic processes that may be present, even though the patient may not have experienced any symptoms to indicate that these changes have occurred. General profiles are also used when the patient's symptoms are so vague that the physician does not have enough concrete evidence to support a clinical diagnosis of a specific organ or disease state. An example of a profile used for screening purposes is the SMA-12 profile, which contains 12 blood chemistry tests. SMA is an abbreviation for *sequential multiple autoanalyzer* and is named for the automated analyzer (SMA-12/60) used to perform the tests; the number 12 refers to the number of tests performed by the autoanalyzer on the (serum) blood specimen. (It should be noted that the SMA-12 is also utilized as a specific profile; some diseases exhibit a definite pattern of abnormal values that become apparent through the SMA-12 test results.) The advantage of using the SMA-12/60 analyzer and other types of automated equipment is that numerous tests can be performed on one sample of blood in a relatively short period of time, with accurate test results. In this regard, the patient can be screened for numerous diseases at a very low cost.

The medical assistant should have a knowledge of the names of common profiles and the tests generally contained in each, which are listed in Table 9–2. The specific tests contained in each profile may vary slightly from one laboratory to another, based on physicians' needs and the type of equipment utilized by the laboratory to perform the tests.

6. *Source of the specimen.* Certain tests such as cultures require that the source of the specimen (e.g., throat, wound, ear, eye, urine, vagina) be recorded on the laboratory request form. The purpose of this is to identify the origin of the specimen for the laboratory because it is not possible to obtain this information by looking at the specimen. In many instances, the source dictates the test method used by the laboratory to evaluate the specimen for the presence of a possible pathogen. For example, the test method used to detect the presence of *Streptococcus* in a specimen obtained from the throat will be different from that used to detect *Candida albicans* in a vaginal specimen.

7. *Physician's clinical diagnosis.* The clinical diagnosis assists the laboratory in correlating the clinical laboratory data with the needs of the physician. In some instances, further testing is performed by the laboratory if one test method proves inconclusive with respect to providing the physician with the information necessary to confirm or reject the clinical diagnosis. Another function of the clinical diagnosis is to assure laboratory personnel that the test results are within the framework of the diagnosis. When the results of a test disagree with the physician's clinical diagnosis of the patient, the laboratory repeats the test on the same or another specimen. The clinical diagnosis also alerts laboratory personnel to the possibility of the presence of a potentially dangerous pathogen, such as the hepatitis virus. In addition, it is required for third-party billing by the laboratory. If the laboratory is billing an insurance company for the tests, the clinical diagnosis will be required on the insurance form. This facilitates the processing of insurance forms by having the information at hand and not having to contact the medical office to obtain it.

8. *Medications.* Certain medications the patient is taking may interfere with the accuracy and validity of the test results. Therefore, the laboratory should be notified of any medications being taken by the patient by listing them on the request form.

9. *STAT.* At times the physician will want the laboratory test results reported as soon as possible. In this case, STAT should be clearly written in bold letters (or the appropriate STAT box checked) on the laboratory request form. Requests that are marked STAT are performed as soon as possible after being received by the laboratory, and the results are telephoned to the physician as soon as they are available.

Once the specimen has been collected, the completed request form must be placed with the specimen for transport to the outside laboratory. The medical assistant should realize the significance of this simple but important step.There are numerous possible tests that can be performed on one particular specimen, and without the request form, the laboratory does not have the information it needs to carry out the physician's orders, which causes delays in completing the tests and reporting results.

TABLE 9–2. Laboratory Profiles

PROFILE	TESTS INCLUDED	USE
SMA-12 profile (Health screen profile) Diabetes assessment Assessment of kidney function Assessment of infection and nutrition Assessment of liver function Assessment of tissue disease and cardiac function	Glucose Blood urea nitrogen (BUN) Uric acid Calcium Phosphorus Total protein Albumin Alkaline phosphatase Serum glutamic-oxalo-acetic transaminase [SGOT (AST)] Lactic dehydrogenase (LDH; LD) Bilirubin Cholesterol	General health screen Assessment of diseases of specific organs or disease states
Liver function profile	Total bilirubin Direct bilirubin Total protein Albumin Globulin A/G ratio Alkaline phosphatase SGOT (AST) SGPT (ALT)	Detection of pathologic conditions affecting the liver
Thyroid function profile	Triiodothyronine (T_3) Tetraiodothyronine (T_4)	Detection of pathologic conditions affecting the thyroid gland
Prenatal profile	Complete blood count ABO blood type Rh factor Serology (VDRL or RPR) Rubella titer Rh antibody titer Antibody screen if Rh– Urinalysis GC culture (if required by state law)	Establishment of baseline recordings and screening of prenatal patients for disease of potential problems
Electrolyte profile	Sodium Potassium Chloride	
Rheumatoid profile	Antistreptolysin O (ASO) titer Rheumatoid factor (RA) test C-reactive protein (CRP) Uric acid	Detection of rheumatoid arthritis
Coronary assessment profile	Cholesterol Triglycerides High-density lipoprotein (HDL) Low-density lipoprotein (LDL) Total cholesterol/HDL Cholesterol ratio	Detection of coronary heart disease
Lipid profile	Cholesterol Triglycerides	

PATIENT NAME					PATIENT I.D.
Judith Johnson					08575
ACCESSION NO.	AGE	SEX	T.V./SOURCE		DATE RECEIVED
1235-G8	26	F			4/10/84
REFERRING PHYSICIAN			CLIENT NO.		DATE REPORTED
J. Camerson, M.D.			HC-343		4/12/84
ORDER STATUS	COLLECTION DATE/TIME				CLIENT DATA
Routine	4/9/84 10:30 a.m.				

DAMON CLINICAL LABORATORIES
NEEDHAM HEIGHTS, MASS. 02194

SMAC
CBC w/o differential
Completed Report

TEST NAME	RESULT	UNITS	GEN. REF.
Hemogram			
WBC	11.8	thou.	(4.3 - 10.0)
RBC	4.27	millions	(3.60 - 5.40)
Hgb	13.4	gm/dl	(12.0 - 18.0)
Hct	39.1	%	(37.0 - 54.0)
MCV	91.	u-3	(81 - 99)
MCH	31.3	uug	(27.0 - 31.0)
MCHC	34.5	%	(32.0 - 36.0)
Differential			
Neutrophils		%	(50 - 65)
Bands		%	(0 - 1)
Lymphs		%	(25 - 40)
Monos		%	(4 - 10)
Eos		%	(1 - 3)
Basos		%	(0 - 1)
Blasts		%	
Promyelocytes		%	
Myelocytes		%	
Metamyelocytes		%	
Nuc. RBC's/100 WBC's			
Other			
Platelet Est:		RBC MORPH:	
Platelet Ct.		thou.	150 - 400
Protime Patient		seconds	
Control		seconds	
Activity		%	
LAB SCAN			
Calcium	9.0	mg/dl	(8.5 - 10.5)
Phosphorus	3.3	mg/dl	(2.5 - 4.5)
Glucose	91.	mg/dl	(65 - 120)
BUN	9.	mg/dl	(8 - 25)
Creatinine	1.00	mg/dl	(0.4 - 1.5)
B/C Ratio	9.0		
Uric Acid	3.6	mg/dl	(2.2-9.0)
Cholesterol	159.	mg/dl	(140 - 320)
Tot. Protein	6.8	gm/dl	(6.0 - 8.0)
Albumin	4.1	gm/dl	(3.0 - 5.0)
Globulin		gm/dl	(1.0 - 3.5)
A/G Ratio	1.5		(1.0 - 3.0)
T. Bilirubin	0.3	mg/dl	(0.1 - 1.2)
D. Bilirubin		mg/dl	(0.0 - 0.4)
I. Bilirubin		mg/dl	(0.0 - 0.8)
Alk. Phos.	82.	mU/ml	(30 - 115)
LDH	158.	mU/ml	(100 - 225)
SGOT	9.	mU/ml	(0 - 41)
SGPT	14.	mU/ml	(0 - 45)
Sodium	140	meq/l	(135 - 145)
Potassium	3.4	meq/l	(3.5 - 5.5)
Chloride	105.	meq/l	(96 - 110)
Carbon Diox.		meq/l	(20.0 - 30.0)
Triglyceride	69.	mg/dl	(40 - 170)

TEST NAME	RESULT
Urinalysis, Routine	
Color	
Appearance	
Spec. Gravity	
pH	
Protein	
Glucose	
Ketones	
Bile	
Occult Blood	
Epith Cells	
Bacteria	
Mucus	
Cells/HPF	
Crystals	
Casts/LPF	
Other	
Pregnancy	
STS (RPR)	
Hetero (monospot)	

Other Tests

FIGURE 9–2. Laboratory report form. (Courtesy Damon Clinical Laboratories, Needham Heights, Massachusetts.)

Laboratory Reports

The purpose of laboratory report forms is to relay the results of the laboratory tests to the physician (Figure 9–2). The report may be in the form of a computer printout or it may be a preprinted form with the test results written in by the laboratory technologist performing the tests. It will include certain types of information listed as follows:

1. Name, address, and telephone number of the laboratory
2. Physician's name and address
3. Patient's name, age, and sex
4. Patient accession number
5. Date the specimen was received by the laboratory
6. Date the results were reported by the laboratory
7. Names of the tests performed
8. Results of the tests
9. Normal range for each test performed
10. Initials or code number of the technologist performing the tests

A patient accession number or laboratory number is assigned to each specimen received by the laboratory. Its purpose is to provide positive identification of each specimen within the laboratory and to allow easy access to the patient's laboratory records should a test result need to be located again. If the physician desires to have the laboratory test repeated, the accession number listed on the original report form must be included on the laboratory request form.

A normal range, rather than a single value, is necessary for laboratory test results because of individual differences among a general population due to factors such as age, sex, race, and geographic location. In addition, no test can be so accurate that a single value is possible. The normal range for each test varies slightly from one laboratory to another, depending on the test method, equipment, and reagents used to perform the test. In this regard, it is essential that the medical assistant compare the test results with the normal values supplied by the laboratory performing the test, rather than with a reference source such as a medical laboratory test.

Laboratory reports are either hand-delivered or mailed to the medical office by the laboratory. Abnormal results posing a threat to the patient's health and laboratory reports marked STAT are telephoned to the medical office as soon as the tests are completed, and a written report follows immediately thereafter. The laboratory usually supplies the medical office with telephone reporting pads to transcribe the results from the telephone report to reduce errors.

The medical assistant may be responsible for reviewing the laboratory reports as they are received. He or she should compare the patient's test results with the normal ranges supplied by the laboratory and notify the physician of any abnormal test results. Many computer systems automatically identify abnormal results on the laboratory report; if not, the physician may want the medical assistant to identify them by circling them with a red pen. The reports are then reviewed by the physician and the data obtained are correlated with the information obtained from the health history and physical examination of the patient. The physician indicates, usually by placing his or her initials on the report, when he or she is finished with it. The medical assistant is then responsible for filing the laboratory report in the patient's chart, according to the medical office policy.

Patient Preparation and Instructions

Factors such as food consumption, medication, activity, and time of day affect the laboratory results of certain tests. Therefore, for some laboratory tests advance patient preparation is necessary to obtain a quality specimen suitable for testing, which leads to accurate results and, in turn, assists the physician in accurate diagnosis and treatment. It is important to realize that the quality of the laboratory test results can only be as good as the quality of the specimen obtained from the patient. A specimen obtained from a patient who has not prepared properly may invalidate the test results and necessitate calling the patient back to collect the specimen again.

The medical assistant is usually responsible for instructing the patient in any advance preparation that might be required. A complete and thorough explanation of the instructions should clearly be relayed to the patient. The medical assistant should explain the reason for the advance preparation; in this way, the patient will be more likely to comply with the preparation required. It should be emphasized to the patient that the preparation is essential to obtain accurate test results and to avoid having to collect the specimen again. Once the instructions have been explained, it is important to check to make sure the patient completely understands them and offer to answer any questions. It is also advisable to provide the patient with written instructions to serve as a reference, should he or she forget some of the information after leaving the medical office. Some specimen collections may require that the patient remain at the collection site for a specified period of time; an example of this is the glucose tolerance test, which requires several hours for the collection of multiple, timed specimens. The patient should be told in advance of the time requirement so that he or she can make any necessary arrangements with an employer, babysitter, and so on.

At times, the patient will be collecting the specimen himself or herself, either at home or at the medical office. The medical assistant is responsible for explaining detailed instructions to the patient on the proper techniques to use to collect the specimen. For example, if a first-voided morning urine specimen is required for the laboratory test, the medical assistant will need to provide the patient with the appropriate specimen container and to instruct the patient in the proper collection, handling, and storage of the specimen until it reaches the medical office. A clean-catch midstream urine collection also requires detailed patient instructions to obtain a quality specimen from the patient. As with advance patient preparation, the medical assistant should take the time to completely explain the instructions to facilitate accurate test results.

The specific type of preparation required for a particular test depends on the test ordered and the method used to run it. If the medical office utilizes an outside laboratory, the patient preparation required for each test will be found in the laboratory directory. If the test is to be performed in the medical office, the medical assistant should consult the manufacturer's instructions that accompany the testing materials to obtain specific information regarding patient preparation. Advance patient preparation is usually in the form of a diet modification (e.g., low-fat diet), fasting, or medication restrictions.

Fasting

Many venous blood specimens require the patient to fast before collection. The composition of blood is altered by consumption of food because the digested food is absorbed into the circulatory system, thus changing the results of certain laboratory tests. For example, food intake causes the blood glucose and triglyceride laboratory tests to yield falsely high results, whereas it causes phosphorus values to be falsely low. Therefore, any individual test or profile including these tests, such as fasting blood sugar (FBS), a glucose tolerance test (GTT), or an SMA-12 profile, requires the patient to fast before the specimen is collected.

Fasting involves abstaining from food and fluids (except water) for a specified amount of time prior to the collection of the specimen (usually 12 to 14 hours). Fasting specimens are usually collected in the morning, to allow the food from the previous evening meal to be completely digested and absorbed. In addition, collecting the specimen in the morning causes the least amount of inconvenience to the patient in terms of abstaining from food and fluid. The medical assistant must be sure to give detailed instructions to the patient, making certain the patient understands that fasting includes abstaining from both food and fluid; however, the patient should be told that it is permissible—in fact advisable—to drink water, because dehydration caused by water abstinence can also alter certain test results. The medical assistant should indicate a specific time to the patient for initiating the fast; if the specimen will be collected in the morning, the patient should be instructed to begin fasting at 6:00 PM on the previous evening. The patient must also be told the time to report for collection of the specimen.

Medication Restrictions

Many medications affect the physical and chemical characteristics of body substances; therefore, medications the patient is taking may lead to inaccurate test results. For example, antibiotic therapy administered prior to collection of a throat specimen for culture may cause a falsely negative report. The physician generally asks the patient to avoid taking medication for a period of time before the collection of the specimen, if discontinuing the medication will not cause any health threat or serious discomfort to the patient. Because medication is more likely to interfere with test results on urine than on blood, it is recommended that the patient discontinue medication 48 to 72 hours prior to the collection of a urine specimen and 4 to 24 hours prior to the collection of a blood specimen. If the patient cannot be taken off medication, the information should be recorded on the laboratory request form for those specimens being transported to an outside laboratory for testing. This alerts the laboratory personnel to the presence of the medication. If the medication being taken by the patient interferes with the method normally used to perform the test, the laboratory may be able to utilize an alternate method to obtain valid results. If the test is being performed in the medical office, the medical assistant should consult the manufacturer's instructions that accompany the testing materials for the names of the medications that interfere with test results.

The physician determines the need for abstinence from the medication prior to specimen collection. The medical assistant is responsible for making sure the patient understands any instructions regarding restrictions on medication and for recording medications the patient is taking on the laboratory request form.

Collecting, Handling, and Transporting Specimens

Clinical laboratory tests are performed on biologic specimens obtained from the body. A *specimen* is a small sample or part taken from the body to represent the nature of the whole. The majority of laboratory tests are performed on specimens that are easily obtained from the body such as blood, urine, feces, sputum, a cervical and vaginal scraping of cells, or a sample of a secretion or discharge from various parts of the body (e.g., nose, throat, wound, ear, eye, vagina, urethra) for microbiologic analysis. Other examples of biologic specimens analyzed in the laboratory but more difficult to obtain from the body include gastric juices, cerebrospinal fluid, pleural fluid, peritoneal fluid, synovial fluid, and tissue biopsies. The source of the specimen may not necessarily be indicative of the pathologic condition in question; for example, triiodothyronine (T_3) and tetraiodothyronine (T_4) tests are performed on blood serum but are used to detect a condition affecting the thyroid gland.

The medical assistant is responsible for the collection of the majority of the biologic specimens obtained from patients in the medical office; of these, blood and urine will constitute the largest percentage of specimens collected. Certain specimens, such as a sample of vaginal or urethral discharge, cerebrospinal fluid, or a tissue biopsy, must be collected by the physician; in this case, the medical assistant assists with the collection.

The most important aspect of specimen collection and handling is to provide the laboratory with a sample that is as biologically representative as possible of the body substance collected. If it is collected or handled improperly, the in vivo characteristics of the specimen may be adversely affected, which in turn may cause inaccurate and unreliable test results; this may interfere with accurate diagnosis and treatment of the patient's condition.

Guidelines

Specific guidelines that should be used regarding specimen collection and handling follow:

1. *Review and follow the CDC recommended precautions* for specimen collection (see Chapter 1, Precautions for Laboratories, page 10).

2. *Review the requirements for collection and handling of the specimen,* which include the collection materials required, the type of specimen to be collected (e.g., serum, plasma, whole blood, clotted blood, urine), the amount required for laboratory analysis, the procedure to follow in collecting the specimen, and its proper handling and storage.

3. *Assemble the equipment and supplies.* Use only the appropriate specimen containers as specified by the medical office or laboratory. Substituting containers may not yield the proper type of specimen required or may affect the test results, as shown by the following examples: If serum is required and a tube containing an anticoagulant is used (instead of a plain tube not containing an anticoagulant), the blood separates into plasma and cells, rather than serum and cells, and the wrong type of blood specimen is obtained, which results in having to draw another specimen from the patient. Collecting a microbiologic specimen that may contain anaerobic pathogens with supplies meant for aerobic pathogens results in death of the anaerobic pathogen.

The specimen container should be sterile, to prevent contamination of the specimen. Many specimens, especially microbiologic ones, are adversely affected by contaminants, such as extraneous microorganisms, which may affect the accuracy of the test results.

The medical assistant should check each container before using it to make sure it is not broken, chipped, cracked, or otherwise damaged. Damaged containers are unsuitable for specimen collection and should be discarded. The medical assistant should be sure to label each tube and/or specimen container with the patient's name, the date, his or her own initials, and any other information required by the laboratory, such as the source of the specimen, which is required with microbiologic specimens. The information should be legibly printed and the medical assistant should be certain that the information is accurate, to avoid a mix-up of specimens.

4. *Identify the patient and explain the procedure.* It is important for the medical assistant to identify the patient to avoid collecting a specimen from the wrong patient by mistake. If not discovered, this could lead to invalid test results and possibly affect the patient's diagnosis and treatment. Explaining the procedure helps to relax and reassure the patient and gains confidence and cooperation, especially if it is the first time the patient has had a specimen collected.

If the patient was required to prepare before having the specimen collected, determine whether this has been done properly. Improper preparation may lead to inaccurate test results. For example, if a test requiring fasting, such as an FBS, is performed on a nonfasting specimen, the results are altered; in this case, they are falsely high. If the patient has not prepared properly, inform the physician; the physician may want the patient to prepare properly and return, or the physician may tell the medical assistant to go ahead with the collection but to alert the laboratory to the situation by marking the information on the laboratory request. In the example just given, *nonfasting specimen* would be written on the request form.

5. *Collection of the specimen* involves a set of specific techniques for each type of specimen obtained. The information in this section is presented in general terms; the specific procedures for the collection of biologic specimens are included in this text in the following chapters: Urinalysis, Venipuncture, Hematology and Blood Chemistry, Microbiology and Disease, and Specialty Examinations and Procedures.

Specimen collection involves a combination of medical and surgical aseptic techniques. Certain parts of collection materials, such as needles, swabs, and the inside of the specimen containers, must remain sterile. If a culture medium (e.g., blood agar) is being used to collect a microbiologic specimen, the medical assistant must make sure that the lid of the container is removed only when the specimen is being spread on the culture medium. Unnecessary removal of the lid results in contamination of the culture medium with extraneous microorganisms, which interferes with accurate test results. During the collection and handling of the specimen, the medical assistant must also be careful to utilize medical and surgical asepsis to prevent contamination of the specimen, the patient, or the self.

The medical assistant must collect the specimen using proper technique. The procedure should be followed exactly to ensure a high-quality and reliable specimen. The proper type of specimen must be collected as designated either by the outside laboratory or by the instructions that accompany the testing materials. For example, the collection of a random urine specimen when a clean-catch midstream specimen is required will affect the accuracy of the test results.

The medical assistant must make sure to collect the amount required for the test, which varies, depending on the type of specimen being collected and the number of laboratory tests ordered. The medical assistant must refer to the appropriate reference material to determine the amount required for each test ordered by the physician. If the specimen is being transported to an outside laboratory, the amount required is listed next to each test in the laboratory directory (see Table 9–1). The amount required for those specimens being tested in the medical office is found in the manufacturer's instructions that accompany the testing materials. It is important that the medical assistant strictly observe the stipulated amount requirements, especially for specimens being transported to an outside laboratory. If the medical assistant fails to collect the specified amount, the laboratory will be unable to perform the test and the laboratory request will be returned marked QNS (quantity not sufficient). This situation warrants calling the patient back in for collection of another specimen.

Some specimens may require further processing, once collected. For example, if serum is required for the laboratory test, it must be separated from the whole blood and placed in a separate tube called a transfer tube. The medical assistant must be sure to place lids and caps tightly on containers to prevent contamination or leakage of the specimen.

Once the specimen has been collected, the medical assistant records the following information in the patient's chart: the date and time of the collection, any unusual patient reaction, the laboratory tests ordered by the physician, the type of specimen, and (for microbiologic specimens) the source of the specimen. If the specimen is being transported to an outside laboratory, this information should be indicated in the patient's chart, including the date the specimen was transported to the laboratory, if it is different from the date of collection.

6. *Properly handle and store the specimen* with care to preserve its in vivo qualities. Some specimens, such as microbiologic specimens, are more sensitive to environmental influences and must be handled with special care. Whenever possible, it is best to perform laboratory tests on fresh specimens (for most specimens, within 1 hour after collection), because they yield the most reliable test results. When this is not practical, as is usually the case, the specimen must be stored; it may require storage until pick-up by an outside laboratory, mailing, or until testing at the medical office. Storing a specimen involves properly preserving it so as to maintain its in vivo physical and chemical characteristics until it is analyzed. General guidelines for handling and storing biologic specimens most frequently collected in the medical office are presented in Table 9–3.

7. *Transport the specimen.* Specimens that are tested at an outside laboratory require transport, either by a laboratory pick-up service or by mail. The method

TABLE 9-3. Handling and Storage of Biologic Specimens

SPECIMEN	HANDLING	STORAGE
Blood	*All Blood Specimens:* Prevent hemolysis Collect the specimen in a tube that is at room temperature *Serum:* Separate serum from blood within 30 to 45 minutes after collection *Plasma:* Mix anticoagulant gently but thoroughly with the blood specimen immediately after collection	For most blood specimens, refrigerate at 4°C (39°F) to retard alterations in the physical and chemical composition of the specimen Plasma and serum may be frozen; however, whole blood should not be frozen because it will cause hemolysis
Urine	Avoid contamination of the inside of the specimen container Do not leave the specimen standing out for more than 1 hour after collection	If the urine specimen cannot be tested within 1 hour after collection, refrigerate it or add an appropriate preservative
Microbiologic specimens	Avoid contamination of the swab used to collect the specimen Avoid contamination of the inside of the microbiologic specimen container Protect yourself from contamination from the microbiologic specimen Protect anaerobic specimens from exposure to air	Transport the specimen as soon as possible. If not possible, place the specimen in a transport medium or inoculate it on the appropriate culture medium and (for most specimens) place it in the refrigerator at 4°C (39°F) to prevent drying and death of the specimen or overgrowth of the specimen with extraneous microorganisms
Stool	Collect the specimen in a clean container For the detection of ova and parasites, keep the stool warm	For the most accurate test results, deliver the specimen to the laboratory immediately. If there will be a delay in transporting the specimen, mix the stool with an appropriate preservative or place it in a transport medium

For all specimens: Do not expose to extreme temperature changes.

used depends on the proximity of the laboratory to the medical office; the pick-up service covers a designated area within the locale of the laboratory. If the medical office is outside this area, the specimen needs to be mailed.

The outside laboratory provides the mailing containers, which consist of protective material such as corrugated cardboard and styrofoam to protect the specimen from breakage during mailing. The specimen container must be wrapped carefully and placed in the appropriate mailing container; to avoid breakage, it should never be forced into a mailing container. The outside of the container must bear a label indicating the presence of a biologic specimen. The specimen should be placed into a mailbox as close as possible to postal pick-up time. It is important not to allow the specimen to lie in the mailbox for a prolonged period of time, especially in extreme weather conditions. The laboratory will pick up specimens from the post office several times daily to ensure that they are fresh and reliable.

PROCEDURE 9-1

COLLECTING SPECIMEN FOR TRANSPORT TO AN OUTSIDE LABORATORY

There is a growing trend toward medical offices utilizing the services of an outside laboratory for performing tests. A summary of the series of individual steps required for collecting a specimen in the medical office and transporting it to an outside laboratory is presented in this procedure.

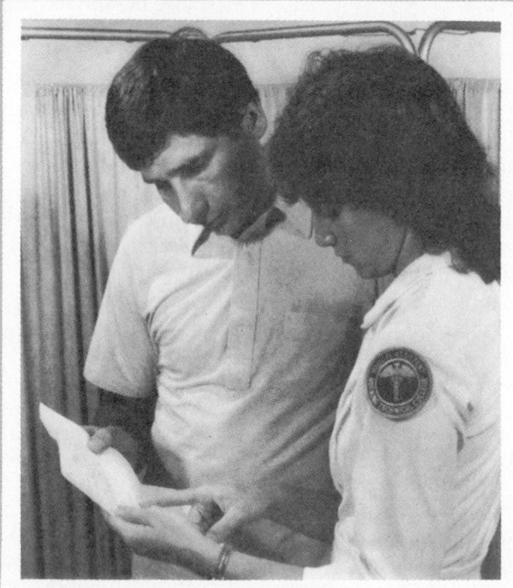

1. **PROCEDURAL STEP.** Inform the patient of any advance preparation or special instructions, which may include
a. Diet modification
b. Fasting
c. Medication restriction
d. Collection of a specimen at home
Explain the instructions thoroughly and provide the patient with written instructions to take home as a reference. Notify the patient of the time to report to the medical office for the specimen collection.
PRINCIPLE. The patient must prepare properly in order to obtain a quality biologic specimen that will lead to accurate test results and avoid having to return to have another specimen collected.

2. **PROCEDURAL STEP.** Review the requirements in the laboratory directory for the collection and handling of the specimens ordered by the physician, which include
a. Collection materials required
b. Type of specimen to be collected
c. Amount of the specimen required for laboratory analysis
d. Procedure to follow to collect the specimen
e. Proper handling and storage of the specimen
Telephone the laboratory with any questions you have regarding any aspect of the collection or handling of the specimen.
PRINCIPLE. Reviewing the requirements beforehand prevents errors in collection and handling of the specimen.

3. **PROCEDURAL STEP.** Complete the laboratory request form, which must include the following information printed in legible handwriting:
a. Physician's name and address
b. Patient's name (and address if required)
c. Patient's age and sex
d. Date and time of the collection
e. Laboratory tests ordered by the physician
f. Type of specimen
g. Source of specimen (for microbiologic specimens)
h. Physician's clinical diagnosis
i. Any medications the patient is taking
j. When applicable, third-party billing information (e.g., Blue Cross, Blue Shield, Medicare, and so on)
If the test results are needed by the physician as soon as possible, mark STAT on the request in bold letters.
PRINCIPLE. The completed form provides the laboratory with the information necessary to accurately perform the tests.

4. **PROCEDURAL STEP.** Wash the hands.
PRINCIPLE. Practicing medical asepsis helps protect the specimen from becoming contaminated.

5. **PROCEDURAL STEP.** Assemble the equipment and supplies. Be sure to use the appropriate specimen container required by the outside laboratory. Make sure the container is sterile and check to make sure it is not broken, chipped, or cracked.
PRINCIPLE. The appropriate specimen container must be used to assure the collection of the proper type of specimen required by the laboratory. Damaged specimen containers are unsuitable for collection and should be discarded.

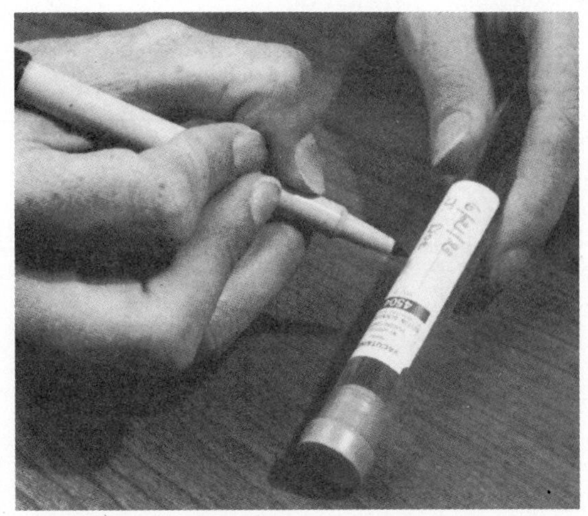

6. **PROCEDURAL STEP.** Clearly label the tubes and containers with the patient's name, the date, your initials, and any other information required by the laboratory, such as the source of the specimen (for microbiologic specimens).
PRINCIPLE. Properly labeled tubes and containers prevent mix-up of specimens.

7. **PROCEDURAL STEP.** Identify the patient and explain the procedure. Make sure you have the correct patient. If the patient was required to prepare for the test, determine if he or she has prepared properly.
PRINCIPLE. Identifying the patient prevents collecting a specimen from the wrong person by mistake. Specimen collection is often an anxiety-producing experience for the patient, and reassurance should be offered to help reduce apprehension.

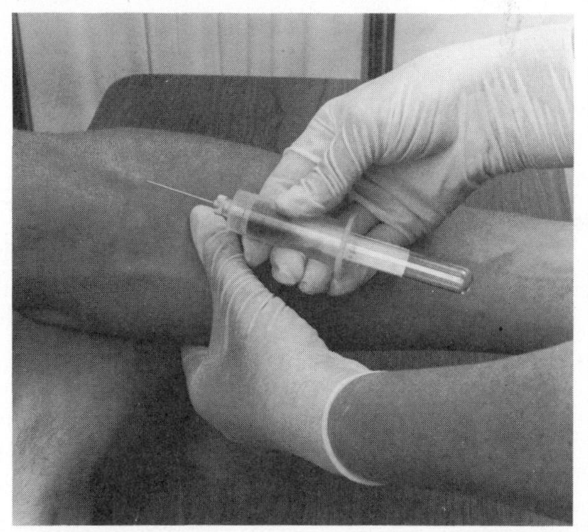

8. **PROCEDURAL STEP.** Collect the specimen, using the following guidelines:
a. Use medical and surgical asepsis.
b. Collect the specimen using proper technique.
c. Collect the proper type and amount of the specimen required for the test.
d. Process the specimen further, if required by the outside laboratory.
e. Place the lid tightly on the specimen container.
f. Record information in the patient's chart, including the patient's name, the date and time of the collection, any unusual patient reaction, the laboratory tests ordered by the physician, the type and source of the specimen, and information indicating its transport to the outside laboratory.

PRINCIPLE. Proper collection of a specimen maintains its in vivo qualities and provides the laboratory with a biologically representative sample of the body substance collected.

9. **PROCEDURAL STEP.** Properly handle and store (if necessary) the specimen, according to the laboratory specifications.
PRINCIPLE. The specimen must be handled and stored properly to maintain the in vivo characteristics of the specimen.

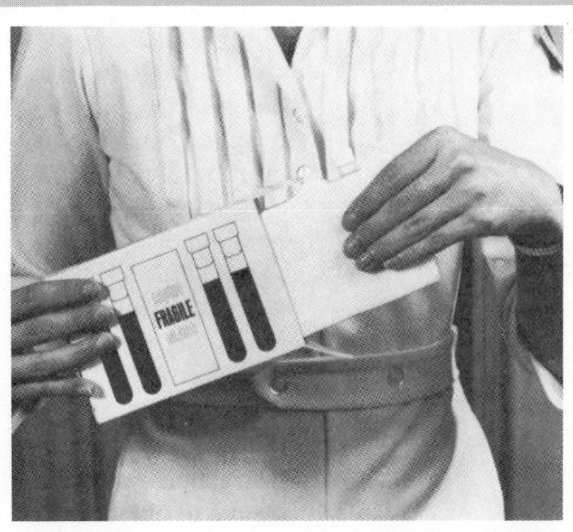

10. **PROCEDURAL STEP.** Prepare the specimen for transport to the outside laboratory. If the specimen is to be mailed, wrap the specimen container in protective materials and carefully place it in its appropriate mailing container. Be sure to include the completed laboratory request with the specimen.
PRINCIPLE. The specimen container must be handled carefully to prevent breakage during mailing. The outside laboratory must have the completed request form to know which laboratory tests have been ordered by the physician.

Continued

11. **Procedural step.** Review the laboratory report when it is returned to the medical office. Compare each test result with the normal range provided by the laboratory, and notify the physician of any abnormal results. File the laboratory report in the patient's chart once it has been reviewed by the physician.

Record data below.

DATE	TIME	PATIENT'S NAME	RECORDING

Testing the Specimen

Testing a biologic specimen involves following a series of steps to measure or identify the presence of a specific substance in the specimen, such as the measurement of a chemical or the identification of a microorganism. The medical assistant may be responsible for performing the laboratory tests and recording results, or the physician may employ a medical laboratory technician or a medical technologist to perform the tests. The decision is based on the number of tests performed in the medical office and the complexity of these tests. The medical assistant is trained to perform basic laboratory tests; the more sophisticated tests require the knowledge and skill of the medical laboratory technician.

Laboratory tests can be classified by function into one of the following categories: hematology, clinical chemistry, serology and blood banking, urinalysis, microbiology, parasitology, cytology, and histology. Table 9–4 lists the definition of each of these categories and provides examples of commonly performed tests in each. Using these classifications makes it easier to refer to laboratory tests.

Specimens can be analyzed by manual, automated, or semiautomated methods. The method (or methods) the physician utilizes to test biologic specimens in the medical office is based on the number and type of laboratory tests performed in the office and the cost involved in purchasing the laboratory equipment and supplies. For example, a physician who orders a large number of blood chemistry tests may be able to justify the purchase of an automated blood chemistry analyzer for the medical office. Regardless of the method used, a series of basic steps must be followed in testing each specimen; these are as follows:

1. The specific amount of the specimen required for the test method is measured out of the specimen sample.
2. The necessary chemical reagents required for the test are combined with the specimen.
3. The specimen/reagents may require further processing, such as centrifugation, incubation, heating in a water bath, air drying or heat fixing.
4. The substance undergoing assessment is manually or automatically measured or identified.
5. The results of the laboratory testing are obtained from a direct readout or by a mathematic calculation.

TABLE 9-4. Categories of Laboratory Tests

Categories of laboratory tests are listed, including the definition of each and commonly performed tests or pathologic condition in each category. Those tests that are commonly known by their abbreviations are listed as such.

HEMATOLOGY

Hematology is the science dealing with the study of blood and the blood-forming tissues. Laboratory analysis in hematology deals with the examination of blood for the detection of pathologic conditions and includes areas such as blood cell counts, cellular morphology, the clotting ability of the blood, and identification of cell types.

- White blood cell count (WBC)
- Red blood cell count (RBC)
- Differential white blood cell count (Diff)
- Hemoglobin (Hgb)
- Hematocrit (HCT)
- Prothrombin time (PT)
- Erythrocyte sedimentation rate (ESR)
- Platelet count

CLINICAL CHEMISTRY

Laboratory analysis in clinical chemistry involves detecting the presence of chemical substances or determining the amount of substances present in body fluids, excreta, and tissues (e.g., blood, urine, cerebrospinal fluid). The largest area in clinical chemistry is blood chemistry.

- Glucose
- Blood urea nitrogen (BUN)
- Creatinine
- Total protein
- Albumin
- Globulin
- Calcium
- Inorganic phosphorus
- Chloride
- Sodium
- Potassium
- Bilirubin
- Cholesterol
- Triglycerides
- Uric Acid
- Lactic dehydrogenase LDH (LD)
- Serum glutamic-oxaloacetic transaminase SGOT (AST)
- Serum glutamic-pyruvic transaminase SGPT (ALT)
- Alkaline phosphatase
- Phospholipids

SEROLOGY AND BLOOD BANKING

Laboratory analysis in serology and blood banking deals with studying antigen-antibody reactions to assess the presence of a substance and/or to determine the presence of disease.

- Syphilis detection tests (VDRL, RPR)
- C-reactive protein test (CRP)
- ABO blood typing
- Rh typing
- Rh antibody titer test
- Crossmatch
- Direct Coombs test
- Cold agglutinins
- Rheumatoid factor (RA factor)
- Monospot
- Heterophil antibody titer test
- Hepatitis B Surface Antigen (HBsAg)
- Anti-streptolysin O Titer (ASO)
- Pregnancy tests

URINALYSIS

Urinalysis involves the physical, chemical, and microscopic analysis of urine.

A. Tests included in the physical analysis of urine:
   - Color
   - Transparency
   - Specific gravity

B. Tests included in the chemical analysis of urine:
   - pH
   - Glucose
   - Protein
   - Ketone bodies
   - Blood
   - Bilirubin
   - Urobilinogen
   - Nitrite
   - Leukocytes

C. Tests included in the microscopic analysis of urine:
   - Red blood cells
   - White blood cells
   - Epithelial cells
   - Casts
   - Crystals

MICROBIOLOGY

Microbiology is the scientific study of microorganisms and their activities. Laboratory analysis in microbiology deals with the identification of pathogens present in specimens taken from the body (i.e., urine, blood, throat, sputum, wound, urethra and vagina, cerebrospinal fluid). Examples of infectious diseases diagnosed through identification of the pathogen present in the specimen include

- Candidiasis
- Chlamydia
- Diphtheria
- Gonorrhea
- Meningitis
- Pertussis
- Pharyngitis
- Pneumonia
- Streptococcal sore throat
- Tetanus
- Tonsillitis
- Tuberculosis
- Urinary tract infection

PARASITOLOGY

Laboratory analysis in parasitology deals with the detection of the presence of disease-producing human parasites or eggs present in specimens taken from the body (e.g., stool, vagina, blood). Examples of human diseases caused by parasites include

- Amebiasis
- Ascariasis
- Hookworm disease
- Malaria
- Pinworm disease (enterobiasis)
- Scabies
- Tapeworm disease (cestodiasis)
- Toxoplasmosis
- Trichinosis
- Trichomoniasis

CYTOLOGY

Laboratory analysis in cytology deals with the detection of the presence of abnormal cells.

- Chromosome studies
- Pap test

HISTOLOGY

Histology is the microscopic study of the form and structure of the various tissues making up living organisms.Laboratory analysis in histology deals with the detection of diseased tissues.

- Tissue analysis
- Biopsy studies

6. The results are recorded on a laboratory report form or in the patient's chart; the entry includes the patient's name, the date, the time, the name of each laboratory test, the results of the tests, and the name of the individual performing the tests.

These steps are stated in general terms, but they provide a basis for understanding the process of laboratory testing. Textbooks such as this one and/or the manufacturer's instructions included with testing equipment should be consulted as a reference source to obtain the procedure for performing specific tests. The medical assistant must be sure to follow the procedure exactly to ensure accurate and reliable test results.

Manual Method

The *manual method* of laboratory testing involves performing the series of steps included in the test method by hand, rather than using a self-operating system that performs them automatically. Testing kits, especially in the area of urinalysis, are available to speed the process, making it less time-consuming and more convenient to perform the procedure using the manual method. (Table 10–1 lists examples of commercially available testing kits.) The manual method may require a mathematic calculation to arrive at the test results; for example, performing a manual white blood cell count involves counting the cells and then multiplying this number by a conversion factor to determine the test results. Because each step in the procedure requires a physical manipulation and the application of clinical laboratory theory, the manual method requires a more thorough knowledge and skill in testing procedures and mathematic calculations than does the automated method. The medical assistant must be especially careful to avoid errors in technique, which may lead to inaccurate test results. The majority of the clinical laboratory testing procedures included in this text utilize the manual method. This will provide the medical assistant with the knowledge and skill in performing the individual series of steps included in the procedures commonly performed in the medical office. In addition, the medical assistant will understand what is occurring when an automated analyzer is operating.

Automated Analyzers

In the past decade, there has been tremendous growth in the development of automated and semiautomated analyzer systems for performing laboratory tests, especially in the area of blood chemistry; automated systems are also available for certain tests in the areas of hematology, blood banking, serology, urinalysis, and microbiology. The highly sophisticated automated analyzers such as the SMA-12/60, SMAC, and Coulter Counter are almost always confined to an outside laboratory setting, because the smaller laboratory workload of the medical office does not justify the expense of such systems. However, automated systems have been developed that are more practical and economical for the medical office.

Automated systems designed for use in the medical office permit the processing of a large number of specimens in a short period of time with accurate test results. Automated equipment takes less time and provides greater precision than the manual method, because the series of steps in the testing procedure are automatically performed by the analyzer. Such procedures include the measurement of the amount of the specimen required, the addition of the chemical reagents, further processing of the specimen, and so on. In addition, many automated systems can perform two or more tests on the same specimen simultaneously. The test results are obtained by a direct (usually digital display) readout, which does not require mathematic calculations, thus eliminating a potential source of human error. Automated systems designed for the medical office usually do not require an individual with high technical skill to operate the system. The ease in operating these systems, however, should not lead to a false sense of security, because these systems have limitations that must be recognized, the most critical one being the mechanical failure of the equipment. Therefore, one of the most important aspects of utilizing an automated system is to be able to recognize signs that indicate the system is malfunctioning, because this may lead to inaccurate test resuts. Some examples of automated analyzer systems include the QBC II (a hematology analyzer by Becton Dickinson), the Reflotron (blood chemistry analyzer by Boehringer Mannheim), and Clinitek (urine analyzer by Ames Corporation).

Semiautomated equipment utilizes a combination of automated and manual procedures to test the specimen; some of the steps in the procedure are performed automatically and others are performed by hand. For example, a semiautomated analyzer may require the manual addition of chemical reagents to the specimen but will automatically measure and directly read out the amount of the substance being analyzed in the specimen.

There are numerous automated systems available; they are continually growing in number and are being modified as new technology becomes available. Therefore, it is not possible or practical within the scope of this text to include specific procedures for operating automated systems. The manufacturer of each automated system provides a detailed operating manual with the equipment that includes the essential information needed to collect, handle, and test the specimen. In addition, the manufacturer has a laboratory specialist available for on-site training and service. It is important that the medical assistant become completely familiar with all aspects of any automated system used to perform laboratory tests in his or her medical office.

Each of the three methods for testing the laboratory specimens (manual, automated, and semiautomated) requires the use of specific laboratory supplies and chemical reagents. The medical assistant must keep a running inventory of these materials, and reorder them as needed.

Quality Control

The ultimate goal in the clinical laboratory is to make sure the laboratory test is accurately measuring what it is supposed to measure; this involves practicing and maintaining a quality control program. *Quality control* may be defined as the application of methods and means to ensure that test results are reliable and valid and that errors that may interfere with obtaining accurate test results are detected and eliminated. Quality control is an ongoing process that encompasses every aspect of patient preparation and specimen collection, handling, transport, and testing. The quality control methods that should be employed to obtain precision and accuracy in these areas have already been presented in this chapter under their respective headings, with the exception of testing, which is discussed here.

Quality control methods employed in testing the biologic specimen include

1. Using standards and controls to check the precision and accuracy of laboratory equipment and to detect any errors in technique of the individual performing the test.
2. Discarding outdated reagents.
3. Following the procedure exactly to test the specimen.
4. Performing tests in duplicate.
5. Periodically checking the accuracy of the test results with a reference laboratory.
6. Maintaining equipment by having it checked periodically for proper working order.

Practicing quality control methods ensures that the test results represent the true status of the patient's condition and body functions and provides the physician with reliable information with which to make a diagnosis and prescribe treatment.

Laboratory Safety

Laboratory safety is an important aspect of clinical laboratory testing in the medical office. Many of the laboratory tests performed in the medical office involve the use of strong chemical reagents, the handling of specimens that may contain pathogens, and the use of laboratory equipment. Practicing good techniques in testing laboratory specimens and recognizing potential hazards help to reduce accidents in the laboratory. Some areas specifically related to laboratory safety in the medical office are described here.

Carefully handle and store glassware to prevent breakage as follows:

1. Carefully arrange glassware in storage cabinets, to prevent breakage.
2. Carefully remove glassware from storage cabinets.
3. If glassware does break, dispose of it in a special container, to protect trash handlers from being cut.

The medical assistant should handle all chemical reagents carefully by adhering to the following:

1. Make sure all reagent bottles are clearly and properly labeled.
2. If a label bcomes loose, reattach it immediately.
3. Recap reagent bottles immediately after using, to prevent spills.
4. Do not pipet reagents by mouth, to avoid ingesting hazardous chemicals.

Laboratory specimens should be handled carefully as follows:

1. Follow the CDC recommended precautions when collecting and handling laboratory specimens (see Chapter 1, Precautions for Laboratories, page 10).
2. Wash hands frequently before and after handling specimens. The hands should be washed immediately if the medical assistant accidentally touches some of the material contained in the specimen.
3. Avoid hand-to-mouth contact while working with biologic specimens.
4. Do not pipet any specimen by mouth (e.g., serum, plasma, blood).
5. Immediately clean up any specimen spilled on the work table and cleanse the table with a disinfectant.
6. Properly dispose of all contaminated needles, syringes, specimen containers, and infectious waste.
7. Cover any break in the skin, such as a cut or scratch, with a bandage.
8. Make sure all specimen containers are tightly capped, to prevent leakage.

Handle all laboratory equipment and supplies properly and with care, as indicated by the manufacturer. For example, when using a centrifuge, wait until it comes to a complete stop before opening it.

Study Questions

1. What is the purpose of a laboratory test?
2. What is the purpose of a laboratory request and a laboratory report?
3. What is the purpose of advance patient preparation for the collection of a laboratory specimen?
4. What guidelines should be followed during specimen collection?
5. What is the purpose of maintaining quality control in the laboratory?

10

URINALYSIS

CHAPTER OUTLINE

Structure and Function of the Urinary System
Composition of Urine
Terms Relating to the Urinary System
Methods of Urine Collection
Analysis of Urine
Urine Pregnancy Testing

COMPETENCIES

After completing this chapter, you should be able to demonstrate the proper procedure to perform the following:

1. Instruct an individual in the procedure for obtaining a clean-catch midstream urine specimen.
2. Assess the color and turbidity of a urine specimen, and record the results.
3. Measure the specific gravity of urine, and record the results using a urinometer.
4. Measure the specific gravity of urine, and record the results using a refractometer.
5. Perform a chemical assessment of a urine specimen using a reagent strip and record the results.
6. Determine the amount of glucose present in a urine specimen, and record the results using the Clinitest testing kit.
7. Prepare the specimen, and identify the structures present in a microscopic examination of urine sediment and record the results.
8. Perform a urine pregnancy test and record the results.

LEARNING OBJECTIVES

After completing this chapter, you should be able to do the following:

1. Define the terms listed in the vocabulary.
2. Describe the structures forming the urinary system and state the function of each.
3. List three conditions that may cause polyuria and three conditions that may cause oliguria.
4. Define the terms used to describe symptoms of the urinary system.
5. Explain the purpose of collecting a clean-catch midstream specimen.
6. Explain why a first-voided morning specimen is often preferred for urinalysis, and list three changes that may occur if urine is allowed to remain standing for more than 1 hour.
7. List three factors that may cause urine to have an unusual color or to become cloudy.
8. Identify the various tests that are included in the physical and chemical examination of urine.
9. Explain the basis for urine pregnancy tests.
10. List the guidelines that must be followed in performing a urine pregnancy test to ensure accurate test results.
11. Explain the principle underlying each step in the urinalysis procedures.

• VOCABULARY •

agglutination (ah-gloo" ti-na' shun)—The aggregation or uniting of separate particles into clumps or masses.

bilirubinuria (bil" i-roo" bi-nu' re-ah)—The presence of bilirubin in the urine.

glycosuria (gli" ko-su' re-ah)—The presence of sugar in the urine.

ketonuria (ke" to-nu' re-ah)—The presence of ketone bodies in the urine.

ketosis (ke" to' sis)—An accumulation of large amounts of ketone bodies in the tissues and body fluids.

meniscus (mĕ-nis' kus)—The curved upper surface of a liquid in a container. The surface is convex if the liquid does not wet the container and concave if it does.

micturition (mik" tu-rish' un)—The act of voiding urine.

nephron (nef' ron)—The functional unit of the kidney.

oliguria (ol" i-gu' re-ah)—Decreased or scanty output of urine.

pH—The unit that describes the acidity or alkalinity of a solution.

polyuria (pol" e-u' re-ah)—Increased output of urine.

proteinuria (pro" te-i-nu' re-ah)—The presence of protein in the urine.

refractive index (re-frak' tiv in' deks)—The ratio of the velocity of light in air to the velocity of light in a solution.

refractometer (clinical) (re" frak-tom' ĕ-ter)—An instrument used to measure the refractive index of urine, which is an indirect measurement of the specific gravity of urine.

renal threshold (re' nal thresh' old)—The concentration at which a substance in the blood that is not normally excreted by the kidneys begins to appear in the urine.

specific gravity (spĕ-sif' ik grav' i-te)—The weight of a substance as compared with the weight of an equal volume of a substance known as the standard. In urinalysis, the specific gravity refers to the measurement of the amount of dissolved substances present in the urine, as compared with the same amount of distilled water.

supernatant (soo" per-na' tant)—The clear liquid that remains at the top after a precipitate settles.

urinalysis (u" ri-nal' i-sis)—The physical, chemical, and microscopic analysis of urine.

urinometer (u" ri-nom' ĕ-ter)—A device for measuring the specific gravity of urine.

void (void)—To empty the bladder.

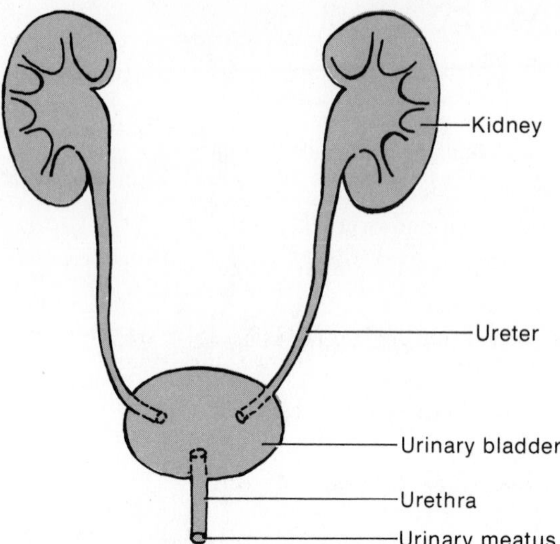

FIGURE 10–1. Structure of the urinary system.

Structure and Function of the Urinary System

The function of the urinary system is to regulate the fluid and electrolyte balance of the body and to remove waste products. The structures making up the urinary system are the kidneys, the ureters, the urinary bladder, and the urethra (Fig. 10–1). The *kidneys* are bean-shaped organs approximately 4.5 inches (11.5 cm) long and 2 to 3 inches (5 to 8 cm) wide; they are located in the lumbar region of the body. Urine drains from the kidneys into the urinary bladder through two tubes known as *ureters.* Each ureter is approximately 10 to 12 inches in length and ½ inch in diameter. The urine produced by the kidneys is propelled into the urinary bladder by the force of gravity and the peristaltic waves of the ureters. The *urinary bladder* is a hollow, muscular sac that can hold approximately 500 milliliters (ml) of urine. Its function is to store and expel urine. The *urethra* is a tube that extends from the urinary bladder to the outside of the body. The *urinary meatus* is the external opening of the urethra. In males, the urethra functions in transporting urine and reproductive secretions. In females, the urethra functions in urination only.

Each kidney is composed of approximately one million smaller units known as nephrons. The *nephron* is considered the functional unit of the kidney. It filters waste substances from the blood and dilutes them with water to produce urine. Another function of the nephron is reabsorption. Some substances filtered by the nephron, such as water, glucose, and electrolytes, are needed by the body and are reabsorbed or returned to the body for future use.

Composition of Urine

A physiologic change in the body, such as that caused by disease, can cause a disturbance in one or more of the functions of the kidney. Detection of such a disturbance can be made through the examination of urine as well as other body fluids such as blood.

Urine is composed of 95 per cent water and 5 per cent organic and inorganic waste products. Organic waste products consist of urea, uric acid, ammonia, and creatinine. Urea is present in the greatest amounts and is derived from the breakdown of proteins. Inorganic waste products include chloride, sodium, potassium, calcium, magnesium, phosphate, and sulfate.

The normal adult excretes approximately 1000 to 1500 ml of urine per day. This amount varies according to the amount of fluid consumed and the amount of fluid lost through other means, such as perspiration and feces and water vapor from the lungs. An excessive increase in urine output is known as *polyuria,* with the urine volume exceeding 2000 ml in 24 hours. Polyuria may be caused by the excessive intake of fluids or the intake of fluids that contain a mild diuretic, such as coffee and tea. Certain drugs, such as diuretics, and the pathologic conditions of diabetes mellitus, diabetes insipidus, and renal disease in which the kidney is unable to concentrate the urine may also result in polyuria. A decreased or scanty urine output is known as *oliguria.* In the case of oliguria, the urine volume will be less than 400 ml in 24 hours. Oliguria may occur with dehydration, profuse perspiration, vomiting, diarrhea, or kidney disease. The normal act of voiding urine is known as *micturition.*

Terms Relating to the Urinary System

The medical assistant should have a thorough knowledge of the following terms used to describe symptoms associated with the urinary system:

Anuria refers to the failure of the kidneys to produce urine.

Diuresis refers to the secretion and passage of large amounts of urine.

Dysuria refers to difficult or painful urination.

Enuresis refers to involuntary urination or the inability of the patient to control urination, especially at night during sleep (nocturnal enuresis or bedwetting).

Frequency is the condition of having to urinate often.

Hematuria refers to blood present in the urine.

Nocturia refers to excessive (voluntary) urination during the night.

Pyuria refers to pus present in the urine.

Retention refers to the inability to empty the bladder. The urine is being produced normally but is not being voided.

Urgency is the immediate need to urinate.

Urinary incontinence is the inability to retain urine.

Methods of Urine Collection

In order to obtain accurate test results, the medical assistant must adhere to proper urine collection procedures as well as obtain the proper specimen as ordered by the physician. The medical assistant must make sure to obtain an adequate volume of urine as required for the type of test being run and to properly label each specimen with the patient's name, the date and time of collection, and the type of specimen (i.e., urine) to avoid any mix-ups in specimens. Any medication the patient is taking should be recorded on the laboratory requisition and in the patient's chart because some medications may interfere with the accuracy of the test results. If possible, the collection of a urine specimen should be avoided in women during menstruation and for several days thereafter, because the specimen may become contaminated with blood. The medical assistant should take into consideration that it is difficult for some patients to void under stress and anxiety. In these instances, understanding and patience should be relayed to the patient. It may be difficult to obtain a urine specimen from a child, even with the assistance of the parents. In this case, the physician should be informed, because another collection method may be used, such as a urine collection bag or catheterization of the patient.

Urine testing in the medical office is often done on freshly voided, random specimens. The medical assistant instructs the patient to void into a clean, dry, wide-mouth, properly labeled container, and the urine is tested immediately at the medical office. At times, the patient may be responsible for collecting a urine specimen at home and bringing it to the medical office. It is helpful to provide the patient with a specimen container to prevent him or her from using a container that might harbor contaminants. The medical assistant should explain fully any special instructions that are necessary to ensure a reliable specimen. The medical office policy may require that the patient collect a *first-voided morning specimen,* which means the patient must collect the first specimen voided in the morning after rising. This type of specimen contains the greatest concentration of dissolved substances and is not affected by dietary consumption and physical activity. The medical assistant also needs to give the patient instructions on preserving a first-voided morning specimen until it is brought to the office.

Clean-Catch Midstream Specimen

The urinary bladder and most of the urethra are normally free of microorganisms, whereas the distal urethra and urinary meatus normally harbor microorganisms. If the urine is being cultured and examined for bacteria, a *clean-catch midstream specimen* is required to prevent contamination of the specimen with these normally present microorganisms. Only those microorganisms that may be causing the patient's condition are desired in the urine specimen. A clean-catch midstream collection may be ordered for both the detection of a urinary tract infection (UTI) and the evaluation of the effectiveness of drug therapy in a patient being treated for such an infection.

The purpose of the clean-catch midstream collection is to remove microorganisms from the urinary meatus by thoroughly cleansing the area surrounding it and to flush out microorganisms in the distal urethra. The urine specimen is collected in a sterile container under medically aseptic conditions. A properly collected specimen reduces the possibility of having to perform a bladder catheterization or a suprapubic aspiration of the bladder. Bladder catheterization involves passing a sterile tube (the catheter) through the urethra and into the bladder to remove urine. Suprapubic aspiration involves passing a needle through the abdominal wall into the bladder to remove urine. Both of these procedures must be performed using sterile technique.

A clean-catch midstream specimen is collected by the patient at the medical office. The medical assistant must provide complete instructions for the collection of this specimen. Failure to adequately instruct the patient may necessitate his or her having to return to the medical office for the collection of another specimen, owing to bacterial contamination. For reliable test results, the specimen should immediately be tested and not be allowed to stand. If this is not possible, the specimen should be refrigerated or a preservative should be added.

To assist the patient in obtaining a clean-catch midstream specimen, the medical assistant must first assemble the supplies needed by the patient for the specimen collection. The supplies include a sterile specimen container, a soap solution, and cotton balls. Midstream urine specimen kits are commercially available and include a sterile specimen container and label, antiseptic wipes (e.g., povidone-iodine wipes), and absorbent tissues (Fig. 10–2). The medical assistant should prepare the supplies for the patient by setting them out on a work surface

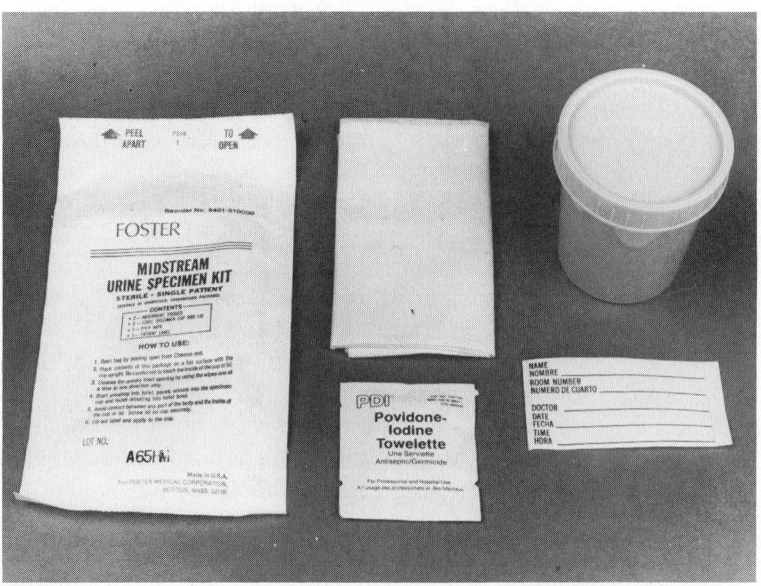

FIGURE 10–2. Clean-catch midstream urine specimen kit.

near the toilet. The lid should be removed from the specimen container and placed with the open end facing up just prior to the collection of the specimen. Early removal of the lid could result in contamination of the sterile container with extraneous microorganisms present in the air, which interferes with accurate test results.

Once the specimen has been collected, the medical assistant should immediately cap and label the container with the patient's name, the date, the time of the collection, and the type of specimen (clean-catch midstream specimen). If the specimen will be tested at an outside laboratory, it is necessary to complete a requisition to accompany it. Refer to Figure 10–3 for an example of a urinalysis laboratory request form. The procedure is then completed by washing the hands and recording the procedure in the patient's chart. The information to be recorded includes the patient's name, date and time, type of specimen, and the laboratory tests ordered. Patient instructions for obtaining a clean-catch midstream specimen are presented in Procedure 10-1.

PROCEDURE 10-1
CLEAN-CATCH MIDSTREAM SPECIMEN COLLECTION INSTRUCTIONS

Instruct the female patient as follows:

1. Wash the hands and remove undergarments.

2. Expose the urinary meatus by spreading apart the labia with one hand.

3. Cleanse each side of the urinary meatus with a front-to-back motion (from pubis to anus), using a fresh cotton ball on each side of the meatus. With the midstream specimen kit, an antiseptic wipe is used to cleanse each side of the meatus. A front-to-back motion must be used for cleansing to avoid drawing microorganisms from the anal region into the area that is being cleansed.

4. Cleanse directly across the meatus (front to back), using a third cotton ball (or antiseptic wipe).

5. Rinse with water to remove all traces of the soap. The soap solution must be completely removed to prevent its entrance into the urine specimen, which could affect the accuracy of the test results.

6. Dry the area with a cotton ball, using a single front-to-back motion. (*Note:* With the midstream specimen kit, Steps 5 and 6 are not required.)

7. Continue to hold the labia apart, and void a small amount of urine into the toilet.

8. Collect the next amount of urine by voiding into the sterile container. Be careful not to touch the inside of the container to prevent contaminating it.

9. Void the last amount of urine into the toilet. This means that the first and last portion of the urine flow is not included in the specimen.

10. Wipe the area dry with a tissue.

Continued

11. Provide the patient with instructions about what to do with the specimen, once it has been collected (e.g., placing it on a designated shelf or directly handing it to the medical assistant).

Instruct the male patient as follows:

1. Wash the hands and remove undergarments.

2. Retract the foreskin of the penis (if uncircumcised).

3. Cleanse the area around the meatus (glans penis) and the urethral opening (meatal orifice) by washing each side of the meatus with a separate cotton ball. With the midstream specimen kit, an antiseptic wipe is used to cleanse each side of the meatus.

4. Cleanse directly across the meatus, using a third cotton ball (or antiseptic wipe).

5. Rinse with water to remove all traces of the soap.

6. Dry the area with a cotton ball using a single front-to-back motion. (*Note:* If the midstream specimen kit is used, Steps 5 and 6 are not required.)

7. Void a small amount of urine into the toilet.

8. Collect the next amount of urine by voiding into the sterile container without touching the inside of the container with the hands or penis.

9. Void the last amount of urine into the toilet.

10. Wipe the area dry with a tissue.

11. Provide the patient with instructions about what to do with the specimen, once it has been collected.

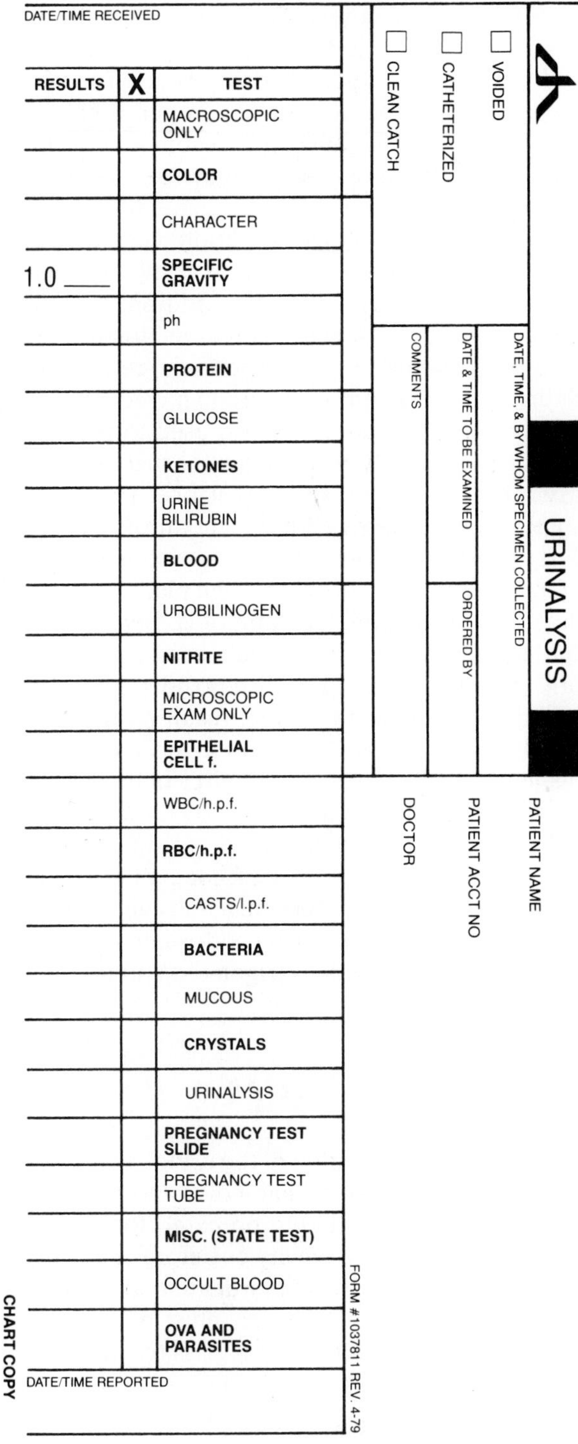

URINALYSIS

VOIDED
CATHETERIZED
CLEAN CATCH

DATE, TIME, & BY WHOM SPECIMEN COLLECTED
DATE & TIME TO BE EXAMINED
ORDERED BY
COMMENTS

PATIENT NAME
PATIENT ACCT NO
DOCTOR

DATE/TIME RECEIVED

RESULTS	X	TEST
		MACROSCOPIC ONLY
		COLOR
		CHARACTER
1.0 ____		SPECIFIC GRAVITY
		ph
		PROTEIN
		GLUCOSE
		KETONES
		URINE BILIRUBIN
		BLOOD
		UROBILINOGEN
		NITRITE
		MICROSCOPIC EXAM ONLY
		EPITHELIAL CELL f.
		WBC/h.p.f.
		RBC/h.p.f.
		CASTS/l.p.f.
		BACTERIA
		MUCOUS
		CRYSTALS
		URINALYSIS
		PREGNANCY TEST SLIDE
		PREGNANCY TEST TUBE
		MISC. (STATE TEST)
		OCCULT BLOOD
		OVA AND PARASITES

DATE/TIME REPORTED

CHART COPY

FORM #1037811 REV 4-79

URINALYSIS

FIGURE 10–3. Urinalysis laboratory request (and report) form.

Analysis of Urine

Urinalysis is the analysis of urine and is usually the laboratory test most commonly performed in the medical office, because a urine specimen is readily obtainable and can easily be tested. Urinalysis consists of a *physical, chemical,* and *microscopic* examination. A deviation from normal in any of the three areas assists the physician in the diagnosis and treatment of pathologic conditions, not only of the urinary system but of other body systems as well. Urinalysis may be performed as a screening measure as part of a general physical examination or to assist in the diagnosis of a pathologic condition when the patient presents with symptoms. It may also assist in the evaluation of effectiveness of therapy once treatment has been initiated for a pathologic condition. The urinalysis should be performed on a fresh or preserved specimen. If a specimen cannot be examined within 1 hour of voiding, it should be preserved in the refrigerator in a closed container and later returned to room temperature and mixed before testing. Chemical additives, such as toluene and thymol, are also used to preserve urine specimens, but they are generally used only with specimens that require prolonged storage, such as those that must be shipped a long distance. This is because the chemical preservative sometimes interferes with the chemicals used to perform the urine test.

If the urine is allowed to stand at room temperature for more than 1 hour, some of the following changes may take place: (1) Bacteria work on the urea present in the urine, converting it to ammonia. Because ammonia is alkaline, this causes an acid urine to become alkaline, raising the pH measurement. In addition, an alkaline pH may result in a false-positive result on the protein test. (2) Bacteria multiply rapidly in the urine, resulting in a cloudy specimen and a rise in the nitrite. (3) If glucose is present in the specimen, it will be reduced as microorganisms utilize the glucose as a source of food. (4) If any red or white blood cells are present, they may break down. (5) Casts decompose after several hours.

In many cases, a first-voided morning specimen may be desired for testing because it contains the greatest concentration of dissolved substances. Therefore, a small amount of an abnormal substance that is present would be more easily detected. If testing cannot be performed within 1 hour after voiding, the specimen should immediately be refrigerated and then returned to room temperature before testing.

Physical Examination of the Urine

The physical examination of the urine involves determination of the color, turbidity, and specific gravity. The color and turbidity of the urine specimen may be evaluated while it is being prepared for another testing procedure such as the evaluation of specific gravity or before centrifuging the specimen in preparation for microscopic analysis. In order to make an accurate evaluation of the color and turbidity, the urine specimen must be in a transparent container such as the urinometer glass cylinder or a glass test tube.

Color

The normal color of urine ranges from pale to dark yellow. Dilute urine tends to be a lighter yellow in color, whereas concentrated urine is a darker yellow. The first-voided morning specimen is usually the most concentrated because consumption of fluids is decreased during the night. The urine becomes more dilute as the day progresses and more fluids are consumed. The color of the urine is due to the presence of a yellow pigment known as *urochrome,* produced by the breakdown of hemoglobin. It is not uncommon for the color of urine to vary among different shades of yellow within the course of a day. Classifications that can be used to describe the normal color of urine include: light straw, straw, dark straw, light amber, amber, and dark amber.

Abnormal colors may be due to the presence of hemoglobin or blood (resulting in a red or reddish color), bile pigments (resulting in a yellow-brown or greenish color), and fat droplets or pus (resulting in a milky color). Some drugs and foods may also cause the urine to change to an abnormal color. The color of the specimen assists in determining additional tests that may be required.

Turbidity

The evaluation of the turbidity of urine is usually performed at the same time as the color evaluation. Fresh urine is usually clear, or transparent, but becomes cloudy on standing. Cloudiness in a freshly voided specimen may be due to the presence of bacteria, pus, blood, fat, yeast, sperm, mucous threads, or fecal contaminants. A microscopic examination of the urine sediment should be performed on all cloudy specimens to determine what is causing the cloudiness. Cloudiness due to bacteria may be caused by a urinary tract infection. Terms that may be used to describe the turbidity of urine include: clear, slightly cloudy, cloudy, and very cloudy. The medical assistant should develop skill in recognizing the varying degrees of urine turbidity.

Specific Gravity

The specific gravity of urine measures the weight of the urine as compared with the weight of an equal volume of distilled water. Specific gravity indicates the amount of dissolved substances present in the urine, thus providing information on the ability of the kidneys to dilute or concentrate the urine. Specific gravity is decreased in conditions in which the kidneys cannot concentrate the urine such as with diabetes insipidus, renal disease, glomerulonephritis, and pyelonephritis. The specific gravity is increased in patients with hepatic disease, diabetes mellitus with glycosuria, and conditions causing dehydration such as fever, vomiting, and diarrhea.

Normal specific gravity may range from 1.001 to 1.030 but is usually between 1.010 and 1.025 (the specific gravity of distilled water is 1.000). Dilute urine contains less dissolved substances and thus has a lower specific gravity. Concentrated urine, on the other hand, will have a higher specific gravity, owing to the increased amount of dissolved substances.

Specific gravity can be measured using several different methods. One method involves a color comparison determination using a reagent strip that contains a reagent area for specific gravity. The reagent strip is dipped into the urine specimen, and the results are compared with a color chart (refer to Procedure 10-3, Chemical Testing of Urine Using the Multistix 10 SG Reagent Strip).

The amount of dissolved substances in urine can also be measured using a clinical refractometer, which is a hand-held optical instrument consisting of a lens and prism system (Fig. 10–4). The refractometer measures the refractive index of

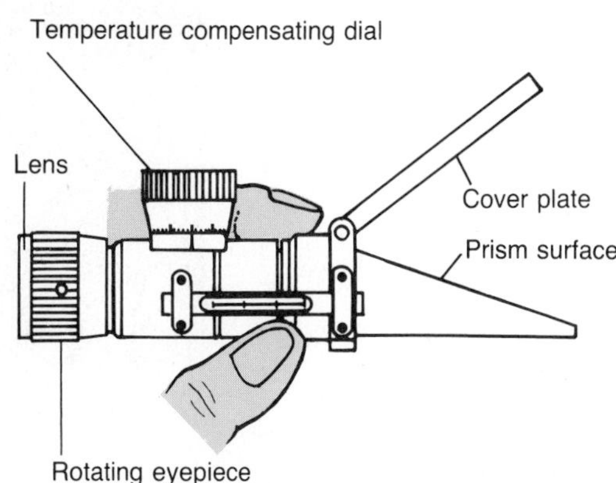

FIGURE 10–4. A clinical refractometer.

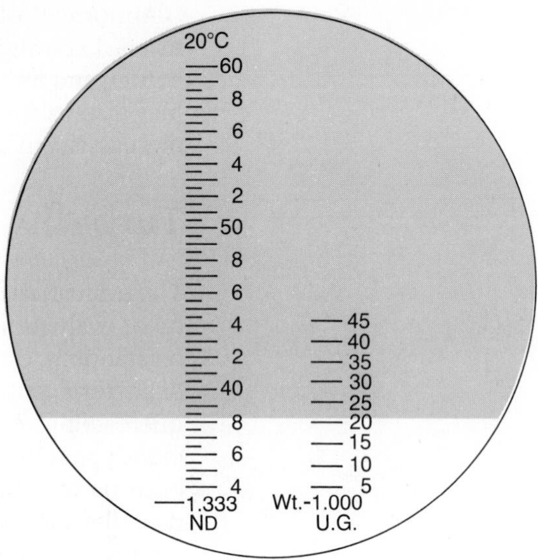

FIGURE 10–5. Calibrated scale of a clinical refractometer. The ND scale is the refractive index of urine and the UG scale is the specific gravity of urine. Specific gravity is read on the UG scale at the boundary line between the light and dark areas. The specific gravity of this urine specimen is 1.020.

urine, which is directly correlated with the specific gravity of urine; the results are read directly from a calibrated scale (Fig. 10–5). The advantage of using a refractometer is that only 1 to 2 drops of urine are required to perform the test and if the instrument has a temperature compensating dial, a temperature correction is not required. The procedure is easy to perform and is outlined as follows:

1. Using a Wintrobe pipet or an eye dropper, place a drop of urine on the surface of the prism. Depending on the brand of refractometer, this is accomplished in one of two ways:
   a. One alternative is to open the cover plate and place a drop of urine directly on the prism. Tightly close the cover plate.
   b Another alternative is to close the cover plate and place a drop of urine at its notched part. The urine will be drawn across the prism surface (between the cover plate and prism) by capillary action.
2. Point the instrument toward a light source and rotate the eyepiece to bring the calibrated scale clearly into view. A light area (bottom) and a dark area (top) will be observed through the eyepiece. Read the value on the scale at the boundary line that shows the distinct division of the light and dark areas.
3. Record the results. Include the patient's name, the date and time, and the specific gravity reading.
4. Clean the prism surface with a soft tissue, being careful not to scratch the prism.

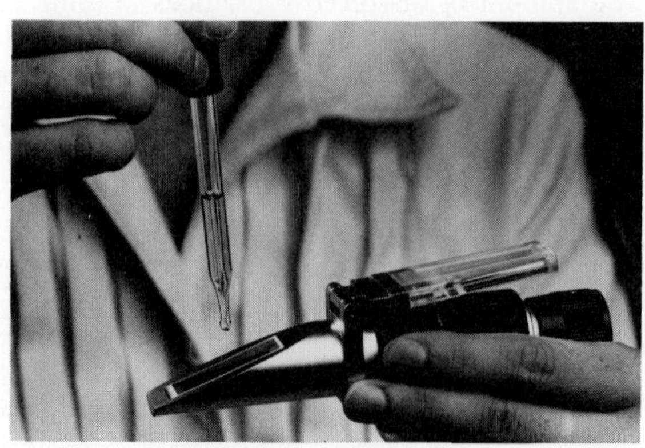

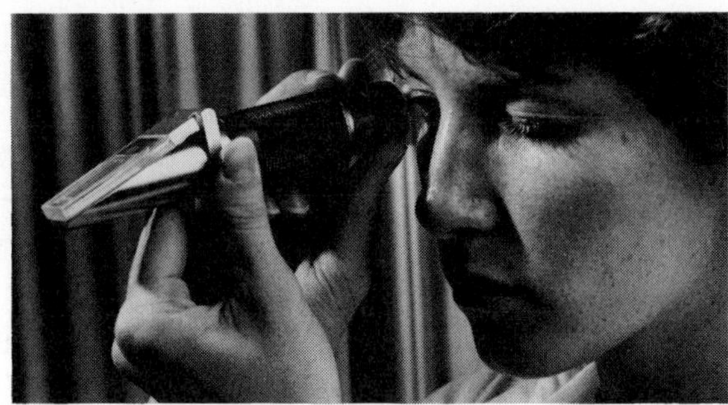

If the refractometer does not have a temperature compensating dial, it should be calibrated each day to compensate for temperature variations to ensure accurate test results. The refractometer is calibrated by checking the zero point using a drop of distilled water and following Steps 1 and 2 as just listed (except that distilled water is used instead of urine). If the calibration of the refractometer is correct, the boundary line should fall exactly on the weight (wt) line. If not, the boundary line must be corrected to coincide with the weight line by turning an adjusting screw with a small screwdriver, which is supplied by the manufacturer. Once the calibration of the refractometer has been checked, wipe off the distilled water with a soft tissue.

Specific gravity can also be measured with a type of hydrometer known as a *urinometer.* The urinometer consists of a weighted float with a stem containing a scale with gradations corresponding to the range of specific gravities for urine (1.000 to 1.045). The urinometer will sink in the urine to a depth proportional to the specific gravity of the urine. The procedure for measuring specific gravity using a urinometer is outlined on the following pages.

PROCEDURE 10-2

MEASURING THE SPECIFIC GRAVITY OF URINE — URINOMETER METHOD

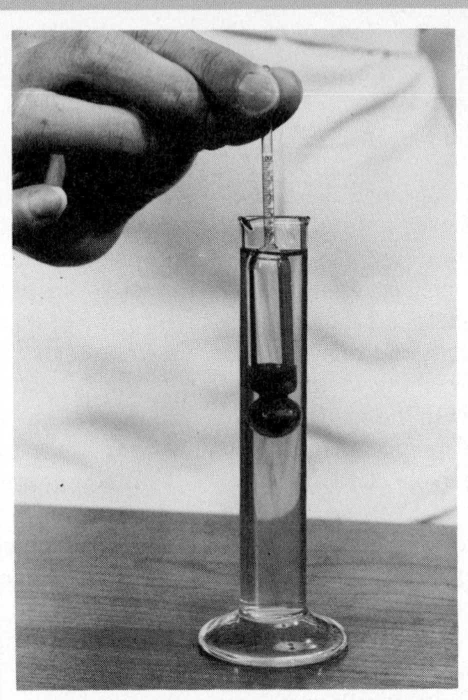

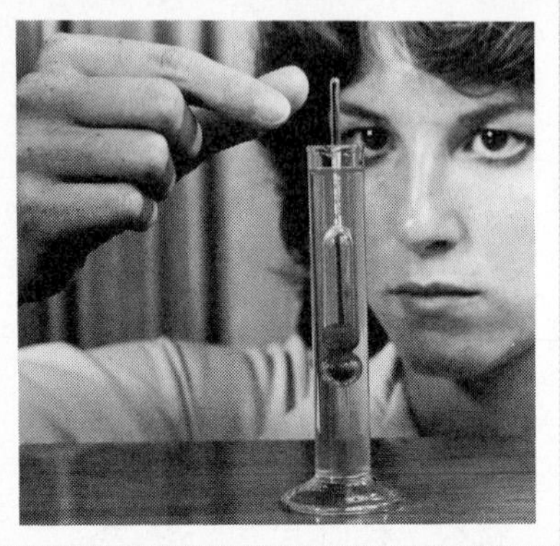

1. **PROCEDURAL STEP.** Wash the hands.

2. **PROCEDURAL STEP.** Assemble the equipment. The equipment needed includes a ***urinometer*** (stem and cylinder) and the ***urine specimen*** (at room temperature). Make sure the urinometer is clean.

PRINCIPLE. It is difficult to read the meniscus of a dirty urinometer. (The meniscus is the curved surface of a liquid in a container. When the urine is poured into the urinometer cylinder, capillary action causes the urine in contact with the cylinder to be drawn upward, resulting in a curved surface in the middle.)

3. **PROCEDURAL STEP.** Place the urinometer cylinder on a flat surface and fill the cylinder about three-fourths full with well-mixed urine (to within 1 inch from the top of the cylinder). If there is not enough urine in the specimen, record ***qns*** (quantity not sufficient) in the patient's chart.

PRINCIPLE. The urine should be well mixed to ensure a representative sample of dissolved substances in the specimen that is being tested. If there is not enough urine to fill the cylinder properly, the specific gravity measurement cannot be made, because there will not be enough urine to float the urinometer stem.

4. **PROCEDURAL STEP.** Grasp the urinometer stem at the top, and slowly insert it into the urine with a slight spinning motion. The stem should not be allowed to become wet above the liquid line.

PRINCIPLE. Allowing the stem to become wet above the liquid line causes it to sink below its true test reading.

5. **PROCEDURAL STEP.** Read the scale of the urinometer at eye level and at the lowest level of the meniscus. Do not allow the float to touch the sides of the cylinder.

PRINCIPLE. Allowing the float to touch the sides of the urinometer cylinder results in an inaccurate reading.

6. **PROCEDURAL STEP.** Wash the hands.

7. **PROCEDURAL STEP.** Record the results. The medical assistant may have to make a temperature correction, because the urinometer is calibrated at a specific temperature. Refer to the instructions that come with the urinometer to obtain this temperature. There is a change in the specific gravity of .0001 for each 3°C above and below this temperature.

8. **PROCEDURAL STEP.** Rinse the urinometer cylinder and stem and dry the stem before testing the next specimen.

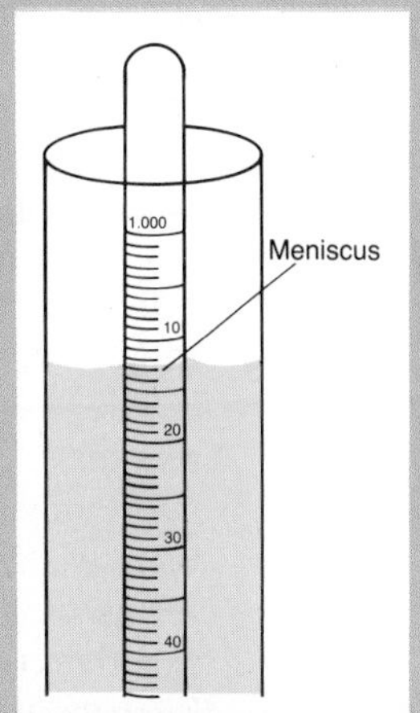

The scale of the urinometer is read at the lowest level of the meniscus. The reading on this scale is 1.013.

Record data below.

DATE	TIME	PATIENT'S NAME	RESULTS

Chemical Examination of the Urine

Substances present in excess (abnormal) amounts in the blood are usually removed by the urine. Therefore, the chemical testing of urine is an indirect means of detecting abnormal amounts of chemicals in the body, indicating a pathologic condition. The chemical examination of urine can also be used to detect the presence of substances that, in the absence of disease, do not normally appear in the urine, such as blood and nitrite.

The chemical analysis of urine involves the use of both qualitative and quantitative tests. *Qualitative tests* provide an approximate indication of whether or not a substance is present in abnormal quantities. The interpretation of qualitative tests usually involves the utilization of a color chart, with results being recorded in terms of trace, 1+, 2+, or 3+; trace, small, moderate, or large; or negative or positive. Qualitative tests are useful for screening purposes in the medical office because they are easy to perform and can be used to screen large numbers of individuals, a procedure that otherwise might be too expensive and time consuming.

Quantitative tests indicate the exact amount of a chemical substance that is present; the results are reported in measurable units (e.g., milligrams per deciliter, grams per 100 milliliters). Quantitative urine tests usually involve the use of more complex equipment and testing procedures than are found in the medical office; they are also more time-consuming to run.

Chemical tests that are routinely performed during a urinalysis include testing for pH, glucose, protein, and ketone bodies. Other chemical tests that may be performed include testing for blood, bilirubin, urobilinogen, and nitrite.

Commercially prepared diagnostic kits are most frequently used in the medical office for the chemical testing of urine. These kits are usually preferred because they contain premeasured reagents, the procedure is easy to follow, and they provide an immediate answer. Most of these tests are qualitative, and a positive reading may indicate the need for further testing. The majority of the tests are manufactured in the form of reagent strips, reagent tablets, or reagent tape and rely on a color change for interpretation of results. A color chart is provided with the kit for making a visual comparison.

The medical assistant should carefully read the instructions that accompany each kit. For example, test strips containing more than one reagent may require different time intervals for reading. Certain medications that the patient is taking may also interfere with the test results; these medications will be listed in the instructions. Before a test is used, its expiration date must be checked. Test material must not be used if a color change has occurred or if the *tested* strip gives off a color that does not match the shades on the color chart. Light, heat, and moisture can alter the effectiveness of the strips or tablets; therefore, care must be taken to store the test materials in a cool, dry area; most test materials are packaged in light-resistant containers to protect them from light. The test materials must never be transferred from their original container to another, because the other container may harbor traces of moisture, dirt, or chemicals that could affect the test results. When results are recorded, the type of test that was used should be specified. A list of commercially available diagnostic kits for performing chemical tests on urine is presented in Table 10–1. Chemicals tested in an analysis of urine are described below in more detail.

pH

The pH (potency of hydrogen) is the unit that indicates the acidity or alkalinity of a solution. The pH scale ranges from 0.0 to 14.0. The lower the number, the greater the acidity; the higher the number, the greater the alkalinity. A pH reading of 7.0 is neutral; a reading below 7.0 indicates acidity, and a reading above 7.0 indicates

TABLE 10-1. Diagnostic Kits Used for Chemical Testing of Urine

BRAND NAME	FUNCTION
Products of Ames Corporation	
Acetest	Reagent strip to detect ketone bodies.
Albustix	Reagent strip to detect protein.
Bili-Labstix	Reagent strip to detect pH, protein, glucose, ketone bodies, bilirubin, and blood.
Bili-Labstix SG	Reagent strip to detect pH, protein, glucose, ketone bodes, bilirubin, blood, and specific gravity.
Clinistix	Reagent strip to detect glucose.
Clinitest	Reagent tablet to detect glucose.
Combistix	Reagent strip to detect pH, protein, and glucose.
Diastix	Reagent strip to detect glucose.
Hema-Combistix	Reagent strip to detect pH, protein, glucose, and blood.
Hemastix	Reagent strip to detect blood.
Ictotest	Reagent tablet to detect bilirubin.
Keto-Diastix	Reagent strip to detect glucose and ketone bodies.
Ketostix	Reagent strip to detect ketone bodies.
Labstix	Reagent strip to detect pH, protein, glucose, ketone bodies, and bilirubin.
Multistix	Reagent strip to detect pH, protein, glucose, ketone bodies, urobilinogen, bilirubin, and blood.
Multistix SG	Reagent strip to detect pH, protein, glucose, ketone bodies, urobilinogen, bilirubin, blood, and specific gravity.
Multistix 2	Reagent strip to detect leukocytes and nitrite.
Multistix 7	Reagent strip to detect pH, protein, glucose, ketone bodies, blood, leukocytes, and nitrite.
Multistix 8	Reagent strip to detect pH, protein, glucose, ketone bodies, bilirubin, blood, leukocytes, and nitrite.
Multistix 8 SG	Reagent strip to detect pH, protein, glucose, ketone bodies, blood, leukocytes, nitrite, and specific gravity.
Multistix 9	Reagent strip to detect pH, protein, glucose, ketone bodies, urobilinogen, bilirubin, blood, leukocytes, and nitrite.
Multistix 9 SG	Reagent strip to detect pH, protein, glucose, ketone bodies, bilirubin, blood, leukocytes, nitrite, and specific gravity.
Multistix 10 SG	Reagent strip to detect pH, protein, glucose, ketone bodies, urobilinogen, bilirubin, blood, leukocytes, nitrite, and specific gravity.
N-Multistix	Reagent strip to detect pH, protein, glucose, ketone bodies, urobilinogen, bilirubin, blood, and nitrite.
N-Multistix SG	Reagent strip to detect pH, protein, glucose, ketone bodies, urobilinogen, bilirubin, blood, nitrite, and specific gravity.
Uristix	Reagent strip to detect protein and glucose.
Uristix 4	Reagent strip to detect protein, glucose, leukocytes, and nitrite.
Products of Boehringer Mannheim Diagnostics	
Chemstrip 5L	Reagent strip to detect pH, protein, glucose, ketone bodies, blood, and leukocytes.
Chemstrip 6L	Reagent strip to detect pH, protein, glucose, ketone bodies, bilirubin, blood, and leukocytes.
Chemstrip 7L	Reagent strip to detect pH, protein, glucose, ketone bodies, urobilinogen, bilirubin, blood, and leukocytes.
Chemstrip 9	Reagent strip to detect pH, protein, glucose, ketone bodies, urobilinogen, bilirubin, blood, leukocytes, and nitrite.
Chemstrip GP	Reagent strip to detect protein and glucose.
Chemstrip LN	Reagent strip to detect leukocytes and nitrite.
Product of Eli Lilly and Company	
Tes-Tape	Reagent tape to detect glucose.

alkalinity. The kidneys help to regulate the acid-base balance of the body. To obtain an accurate pH reading of the urine, the measurement should be done on freshly voided urine. If the urine is allowed to remain standing, it becomes more alkaline as urea is converted to ammonia by bacterial action.

The pH of the urine of patients on normal diets is generally acidic and ranges from pH 5.0 to pH 7.0, with an average of 6.0. A high pH reading on a fresh specimen (that is, an alkaline urine) may indicate a bacterial infection of the urinary tract.

Glucose

Normally, there should be no glucose detectable in the urine. Glucose in the blood is filtered through the nephrons and is reabsorbed into the body. If the glucose concentration in the blood becomes too high, the kidney is unable to reabsorb all of it back into the blood, the renal threshold is exceeded, and glucose is spilled into the urine—a condition known as *glycosuria.* (The *renal threshold* is the concentration at which a substance in the blood that is not normally excreted by the kidney begins to appear in the urine.) The renal threshold for glucose is generally between 160 and 180 mg/dl (100 ml of blood), but this figure may vary among individuals. Diabetes mellitus is the most common cause of glycosuria. Some individuals have a low renal threshold, and glucose may appear in their urine after the consumption of a large quantity of foods containing sugar. This condition is known as *alimentary glycosuria.* If glucose appears in a patient's urine, the physician may request that the medical assistant check several specimens at different times of the day to rule out alimentary glycosuria.

Common tests used to check for glycosuria include Clinitest, Clinistix, Tes-Tape (Fig. 10–6), and Diastix. Other tests for glucose are included in Table 10–1.

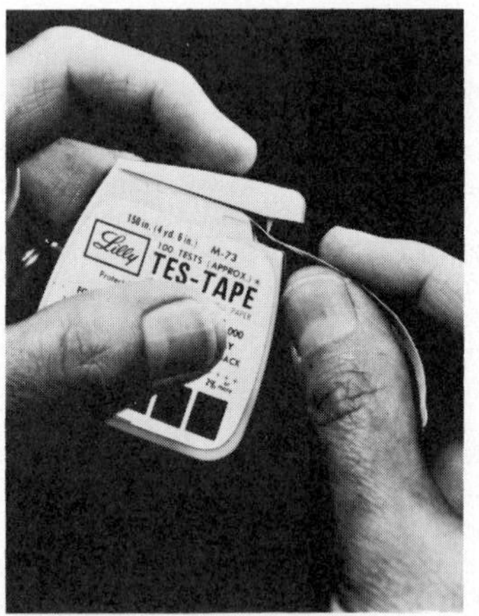

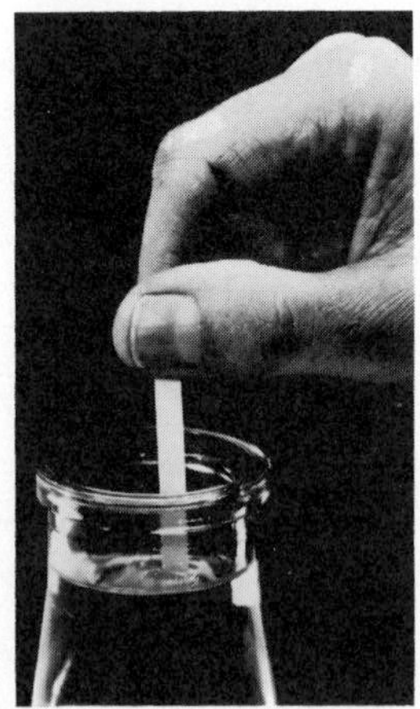

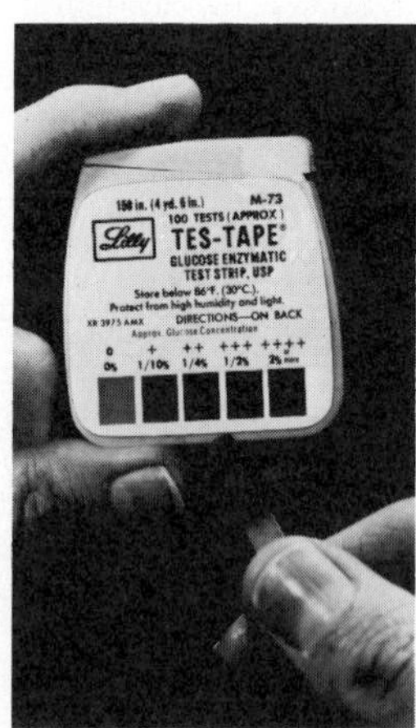

FIGURE 10–6. Tes-Tape can be used to test for the presence of sugar in the urine as follows: *A*, Tear off 1½ inches of Tes-Tape from the dispenser. *B*, Dip ¼ inch of one end of the tape into the specimen, making sure it is moistened uniformly. Remove the tape immediately. *C*, Wait 1 minute and compare the darkest area on the tape with the color chart on the dispenser. (Courtesy of Eli Lilly and Company, Indianapolis, Indiana.)

Protein

An abnormally high amount of protein in the urine is known as *proteinuria.* Some of the conditions that may cause proteinuria to occur include glomerular filtration problems, renal diseases, and bacterial infections of the urinary tract. If proteinuria occurs, the physician usually requests an examination of the sediment to aid in the determination of the patient's condition. Commercially prepared diagnostic kits that test for protein in the urine include Albustix, Combistix (includes tests for protein, glucose, and pH), and Uristix (includes tests for protein and glucose). Other tests are listed in Table 10–1.

Ketone Bodies

There are three types of ketone bodies, including beta-hydroxybutyric acid, acetoacetic acid, and acetone. Ketone bodies are the normal products of fat metabolism and can be used by muscle tissue as a source of energy. When more than normal amounts of fat are used, the muscles cannot handle all of the ketone bodies that result. Large amounts of ketone bodies therefore accumulate in the tissues and body fluids; this condition is known as *ketosis.* When excessive amounts of ketone bodies also begin appearing in the urine, this is known as *ketonuria.* Conditions that may lead to ketonuria include uncontrolled diabetes mellitus, starvation, and a diet composed almost entirely of fat. Commercially prepared diagnostic kits that test for the presence of ketone bodies in the urine include Acetest and Ketostix. Others are listed in Table 10–1.

Bilirubin

The average life span of a red blood cell is 120 days. When a red blood cell breaks down, one of the substances released from the breakdown of hemoglobin is a vivid yellow pigment known as bilirubin. Normally, bilirubin is transported to the liver and excreted into the bile, leaving the body through the intestines. Certain liver conditions such as biliary obstruction, hepatitis, and cirrhosis may result in the presence of bilirubin in the urine, or *bilirubinuria.* The urine becomes yellow-brown or greenish and a yellow foam appears when the urine is shaken. A commercially prepared diagnostic kit for detecting bilirubinuria is Ictotest. Others are listed in Table 10–1.

Urobilinogen

Normally, bilirubin is excreted by the liver into the intestinal tract. Bacteria present in the intestines convert it to urobilinogen. Approximately 50 per cent of the urobilinogen is then reabsorbed into the body to be re-excreted by the liver. Small amounts may appear in the urine, but most of the urobilinogen is excreted in the feces. An increase in the production of bilirubin in turn increases the amount of urobilinogen excreted in the urine. Conditions such as excessive hemolysis of red blood cells, infectious hepatitis, cirrhosis, congestive heart failure, and infectious mononucleosis may increase the level of urobilinogen in the urine.

Blood

Blood is considered an abnormal constituent of urine, unless it is present as a vaginal contaminant during menstruation. The condition in which blood is found in the urine is termed ***hematuria.*** It may be due to an injury, or to disorders such as cystitis, tumors of the bladder, urethritis, kidney stones, and certain kidney disorders. A commercially prepared diagnostic kit for detecting hematuria is Hemastix. Others are listed in Table 10–1.

Nitrite

Nitrite in the urine indicates the presence of a pathogen in the (normally sterile) urinary tract, which results in a UTI. The pathogen possesses the ability to convert nitrate, which normally occurs in the urine, to nitrites, which are normally absent. The nitrite test must be performed using urine that has been in the bladder for at least 4 to 6 hours to ensure that bacteria have converted nitrate to nitrite. Therefore, it is recommended that first-voided morning specimen be used. The test should *not* be performed on specimens that have been left standing out, because a false-positive result may occur owing to bacterial contamination from the atmosphere. Nitrite tests are only to be considered as screening tests and must be followed by a quantitative culture and identification of the invading organism.

Leukocytes

The presence of leukocytes in the urine is known as *leukocyturia* and accompanies inflammation of the kidneys and the lower urinary tract. Examples of specific conditions include acute and chronic pyelonephritis, cystitis, and urethritis. Reagent strips are available containing a reagent area that permits the chemical detection of both intact and lysed leukocytes in the urine. The advantage of detecting lysed leukocytes is that these cells cannot be observed during a microscopic examination of urine sediment and would otherwise remain undetected. The recommended urine specimen, particularly for women, is a clean-catch midstream collection, to prevent contamination of the specimen with leukocytes from vaginal secretions leading to false-positive test results.

Reagent Strips

In the medical office, reagent strips are the most commonly used diagnostic urine testing kit. Reagent strips consist of disposable plastic strips on which are affixed separated reagent areas for testing specific chemical constituents that may be present in the urine during pathologic conditions. The results provide the physician with information relating to the status of the patient's carbohydrate metabolism, kidney and liver function, acid-base balance, and bacteriuria. Reagent strips are considered qualitative tests and a positive result requires further testing. (Refer to Table 10–2 for an outline of reagent strip parameters and the diagnoses in which they assist.)

The number and type of reagent areas included on the reagent strip depend on the particular brand of reagent strips. Multistix 10 SG, for example, contains ten reagent areas for testing the following: pH, protein, glucose, ketone bodies, bilirubin, blood, urobilinogen, nitrite, specific gravity, and leukocytes. Other brands and the tests included for each are listed in Table 10–1.

Testing urine with reagent strips is a relatively easy procedure to perform; however, quality control measures must be employed to obtain accurate test results. Of particular importance is the comparison of the reagent strip with the color chart. The reagent strip must be compared with the color chart in good lighting to obtain a good visual match of the color reactions with the color chart provided with the test kit.

The reagent strips are sensitive to light, heat, and moisture, and the bottle containing the strips must therefore be stored in a cool, dry area with the cap tightly closed to maintain reactivity of the reagent. The bottle may contain a desiccant, which should not be removed because its purpose is to promote dryness by absorbing moisture. The bottle of reagent strips must be stored at a temperature under 30°C (86°F) but should not be stored in the refrigerator or freezer. A tan-to-brown discoloration or darkening on the reagent areas indicates deterioration of the chemical reagent strips, which should not be used because the test results would be inaccurate.

The specimen container used must be thoroughly clean and free from any detergent or disinfectant residue, because cleansing agents contain oxidants that react with the chemicals on the reagent strip, leading to inaccurate test results. The best results are obtained by using a freshly voided urine specimen; most reagent strips are designed to be used with a random specimen collection; however, clean-catch midstream, first-voided morning, and postprandial specimens are suggested for specific tests. For example, the nitrite test results are optimized by using a first-voided morning specimen, whereas a clean-catch midstream collection is recommended for the leukocyte test.

The reagent strip procedure in this chapter is specifically for Multistix 10 SG; however, it can be followed for the chemical testing of urine with most reagent strips. In all instances, the medical assistant should read the manufacturer's instructions before performing the test.

TABLE 10-2. Urine Test Strip Parameters and the Diagnoses They Assist*

SYSTEM/SOURCE	LEUKOCYTES	NITRITE	URINE pH		PROTEIN
Genitourinary	Renal infection/ inflammation • Acute/chronic pyelonephritis • Glomerulonephritis • Urolithiasis • Tumors • Lower urinary tract infection (cystitis, urethritis, prostatitis)	Bacteriuria • Urinary tract infection (cystitis, urethritis, prostatitis, pyelonephritis)	Up (>pH 6) in: • Renal failure • Bacterial infection (e.g., *Proteus* bacteriuria) • Renal tubular acidosis		Renal/glomerular/ tubular disease • Glomerulonephritis • Glomerulosclerosis (e.g., in diabetes) • Nephrotic syndrome • Pyelonephritis • Renal tuberculosis
Hepatobiliary					
Gastrointestinal			Up in • Pyloric obstruction • Vomiting	Down in • Diarrhea • Malabsorption	
Cardiovascular					Congestive heart failure
Hormonal, Metabolic, and Other Systems			Up in • Alkalosis (metabolic, respiratory)	Down in • Acidosis (metabolic, respiratory, diabetic) • Pulmonary emphysema • Dehydration	Gout Hypokalemia Pre-eclampsia Severe febrile infection
Environmental (Diet, Drugs, Stress)	Phenacetin-induced nephritis		Up in • Diet high in vegetables, citrus fruits • Alkalizing drug use (sodium bicarbonate, acetazolamide)	Down in • Diet high in meats or other protein, cranberries • Starvation • Acidifying drug use (ammonium chloride, methenamine mandelate therapy)	Nephrotoxic drugs

* Reagent-strip detection of an abnormal urine constituent or concentration characteristic of disease (e.g., glycosuria in diabetes mellitus) may provide a useful screen or monitor but requires confirmation by other laboratory and clinical evidence.

Modified from: 1. Conn, H.F., and Conn, R.B. (eds.): *Current Diagnosis 5,* W.B. Saunders Co., Philadelphia, 1977. 2. Davidson, I., and Henry, J.B. (eds.): *Todd-Sanford Clinical Diagnosis by Laboratory Methods,* ed. 15, W.B. Saunders Co., Philadelphia, 1974. 3. Raphael, S.S., et al.: *Lynch's Medical Laboratory Technology,* ed. 3, W.B. Saunders Co., Philadelphia, 1976. 4. Wallach, J.: *Interpretation of Diagnostic Tests,* ed. 2, Little, Brown & Co., Boston, 1974. 5. Widmann, F.K.: *Goodale's Clinical Interpretation of Laboratory Tests,* ed. 7, F.A. Davis Co., Philadelphia, 1973. Courtesy of Boehringer Mannheim Diagnostics, Indianapolis, Indiana.

GLUCOSE	KETONES	UROBILINOGEN	BILIRUBIN	BLOOD ERYTHROCYTES (HEMATURIA)	HEMOGLOBIN
Renal glycosuria (e.g., during pregnancy) Renal tubular disease (e.g., in Fanconi syndrome) Decreased renal glucose threshold (e.g., in old age)				Renal infection/ inflammation/ injury • Renal tuberculosis • Renal infarction • Calculi (urethral, renal) • Polycystic kidneys • Tumors (bladder, renal pelvis, prostate) • Salpingitis • Cystitis	Renal intravascular Hemolysis Acute glomerulonephritis
		Liver cell damage Chronic liver stasis Cirrhosis Dubin-Johnson syndrome Note: May be 0 or down in biliary obstruction	Biliary dysfunction • Gallstones Obstructive jaundice Hepatitis (viral toxic) Dubin-Johnson syndrome	Cirrhosis	
	Vomiting Diarrhea	Note: May be negative with inhibition of intestinal flora by antimicrobial agents.		Colon tumor Diverticulitis	
Myocardial infarction				Bacterial endocarditis	
Diabetes mellitus Hemochromatosis Hyperthyroidism Cushing's syndrome Pheochromocytomas	Diabetic ketosis Glycogen-storage disease Eclampsia Acute fever	Sickle cell anemia Hemolytic disease • Pernicious anemia Leptospirosis	Hemolytic disease Leptospirosis	Blood dyscrasias • Hemophilia • Thrombocytopenia • Sickle cell anemia Disseminated lupus erythematosus Malignant hypertension	Hemolytic disease Plasmodium (malaria) Clostridia (tetanus) infection
Sudden shock or pain Steroid therapy	Weight reducing diet Ketogenic diet (e.g., in anti-convulsant therapy) Starvation			Hemorrhagenic drugs (e.g., anticoagulant, salicylates) Nephrotoxic agents Internal injury or foreign body Vitamin C or K deficiency	Overexertion Exposure to cold Incompatible blood transfusion Drug-induced hemolysis

PROCEDURE 10-3

CHEMICAL TESTING OF URINE USING THE MULTISTIX 10 SG REAGENT STRIP

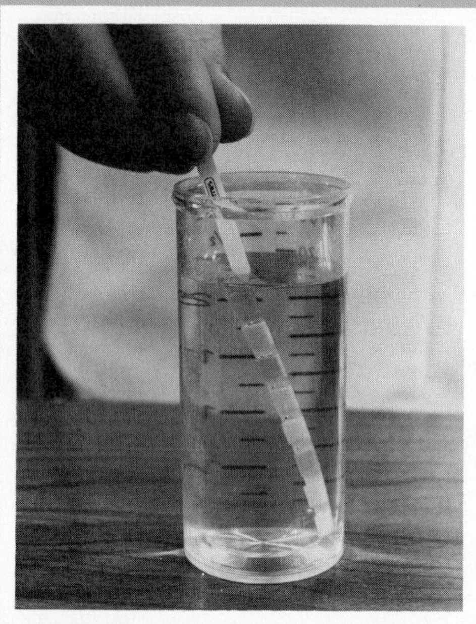

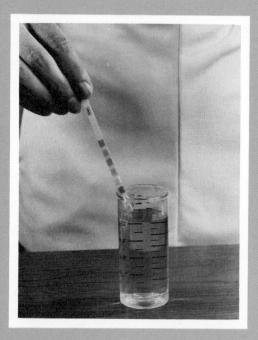

1. **PROCEDURAL STEP.** Obtain a freshly voided urine specimen from the patient, using a clean container. The specimen should be well mixed, uncentrifuged, and at room temperature.
   PRINCIPLE. The best results are obtained by using a freshly voided specimen. The container should be clean, because contaminants could affect the results. Well-mixed, uncentrifuged specimens assure a homogeneous sample.

2. **PROCEDURAL STEP.** Wash the hands.

3. **PROCEDURAL STEP.** Assemble the equipment. The equipment needed includes the **urine specimen** and the **container of Multistix 10 SG reagent strips,** including the Multistix color chart. Check the expiration date of the reagent strips.
   PRINCIPLE. Outdated reagent strips may lead to inaccurate test results.

4. **PROCEDURAL STEP.** Remove a reagent strip from the bottle and recap immediately. Do not touch the test areas with your fingers or lay the strip on the table. However, it is permissible to lay the reagent strip on a clean, dry paper towel.
   PRINCIPLE. Recapping the bottle is necessary to prevent exposing the strips to environmental moisture, light, and heat, which cause altered reagent reactivity. Contamination of the test areas by the hands or table surface may affect the accuracy of the test results.

5. **PROCEDURAL STEP.** Completely immerse the reagent strip in the urine specimen. Remove immediately, and gently tap the edge of the strip against the rim of the urine container to remove excess urine.
   PRINCIPLE. The strip should be completely immersed to ensure that all test areas are moistened for accurate test results. Prolonged immersion of the reagent strip and failure to tap the strip against the urine container may cause the reagents to dissolve and leach onto adjacent test areas, affecting the accuracy of the test results.
   For example, if a drop of urine remains on the strip, it could wash the acid buffer from the adjacent protein chemical reagent block onto the pH reagent block, changing the pH to acid. If the urine specimen was originally neutral or alkaline, a false pH reading would result.

6. **PROCEDURAL STEP.** Hold the reagent strip in a horizontal position and place it adjacent to the corresponding color blocks on the color chart. Read the results carefully and at the exact reading times specified on the color chart and as indicated below.

Glucose	30 seconds
Bilirubin	30 seconds
Ketone bodies	40 seconds
Specific gravity	45 seconds
Blood	50 seconds
pH	60 seconds
Protein	60 seconds
Urobilinogen	60 seconds
Nitrite	60 seconds
Leukocytes	2 minutes

PRINCIPLE. Holding the strip in a horizontal position avoids soiling the hands with urine and prevents reagents from running over into adjacent testing areas, causing inaccurate test results. The strip must be read at the proper time to avoid dissolving out reagents, leading to inaccurate test results.

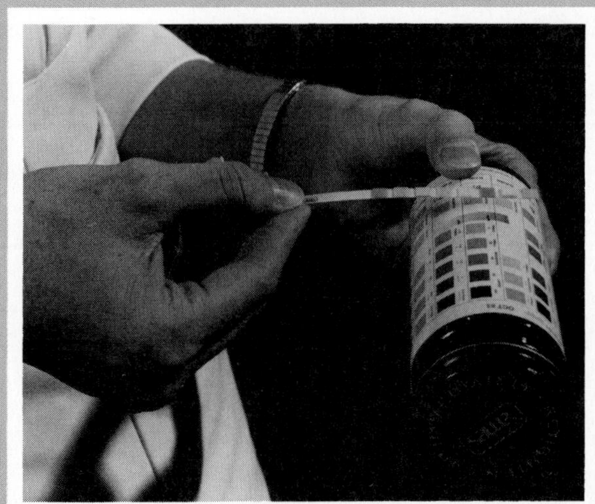

7. **PROCEDURAL STEP.** Record the results. The results should be recorded following the interpretation guide provided above each color block on the color chart. Refer to the front inside cover for the Multistix 10 SG color chart. Be sure to include the patient's name, the date and time, the brand name of the test used (Multistix 10 SG), the results, and your initials.

8. **PROCEDURAL STEP.** Wash the hands and return the equipment.

Record data below.

DATE	TIME	PATIENT'S NAME	RESULTS

PROCEDURE 10-4
MEASURING URINE GLUCOSE USING CLINITEST

The Clinitest procedure is a quantitative test for the determination of reducing sugars in urine. It is performed at home by patients with diabetes mellitus to assess the effectivess of their diet and insulin therapy. It should be noted that the determination of urinary glucose by diabetics at home is gradually being phased out in preference to the more accurate determination of blood glucose using a glucose meter (see Blood Glucose Measurement with a Glucose Meter in Chapter 13). However, until this time, the medical assistant must be able to perform this procedure and thoroughly explain the technique for performing the procedure at home to a diabetic patient.

It is important to use a freshly voided urine specimen. If specimens are allowed to stand, the existing bacteria utilize the glucose as a food source. This reduces the glucose content of the specimen, resulting in inaccurate test results. Care must be taken to protect the Clinitest tablets from light, heat, and moisture by making sure the cap is tightly closed and by storing them in a cool, dry place with a temperature under 30°C (86°F). Moisture causes the tablets to lose their effectiveness, leading to unreliable test results as evidenced by the tablets turning dark blue or blackish; normally, the tablets have a spotted bluish-white color. In addition, if water is allowed to enter the bottle, a chemical reaction occurs that could result in rupture of the bottle. Diabetic patients performing urine testing at home with Clinitest should be told not to store their tablets in the bathroom, to protect them from the high-humidity moisture of showers or baths, and to keep the tablets away from window sills, radiators, and cooking areas to protect them from excessive light and heat. The patient should also be told not to place anything in the container that will hold moisture, such as cotton or tissues.

Patients should be told to keep the tablets out of the reach of children; a tablet put in the mouth or swallowed could cause a chemical burn to the mucous membrane lining the gastrointestinal tract.

The medical assistant must be sure to record medications being taken by the patient. Certain medications, such as cephalosporins, ascorbic acid, nalidixic acid, and probenecid, taken in large quantities may cause a false-positive reaction with Clinitest; therefore, the Tes-Tape procedure must instead be utilized to assess the urine specimen for the presence of glucose.

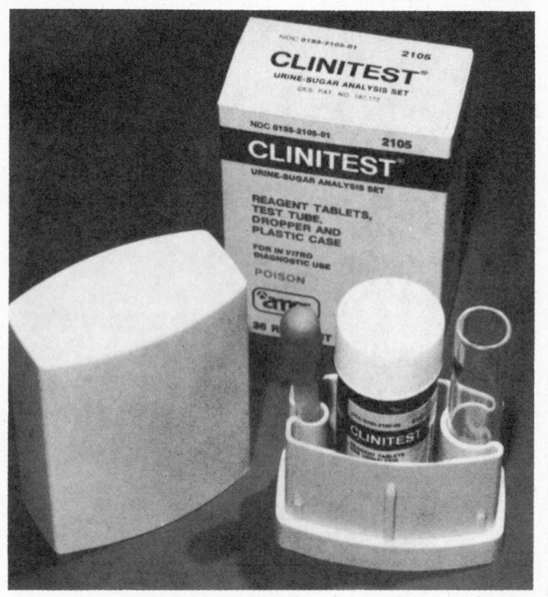

1. **Procedural step.** Obtain a freshly voided urine specimen from the patient, being sure to use a clean container. The specimen should be well mixed and uncentrifuged.

Principle. A freshly voided specimen must be used to prevent bacteria from consuming the glucose, leading to inaccurate test results. The container should be clean, because contaminants may affect the results.

2. **Procedural step.** Wash the hands.

3. **Procedural step.** Assemble the equipment. The equipment needed includes a **glass test tube, a medicine dropper, water,** the **fresh urine,** the **Clinitest tablets,** and the **Clinitest color chart.** Check the expiration date on the tablets.

Principle. Outdated reagent tablets may give inaccurate test results and should not be used.

4. **PROCEDURAL STEP.** Grasp the test tube near the top. Hold the dropper in an upright (vertical) position and place 5 drops of urine in the tube. Be sure the drops hit the bottom of the tube without sliding down the side.

PRINCIPLE. More than 5 drops of urine will give high results, whereas fewer than 5 drops will yield low results.

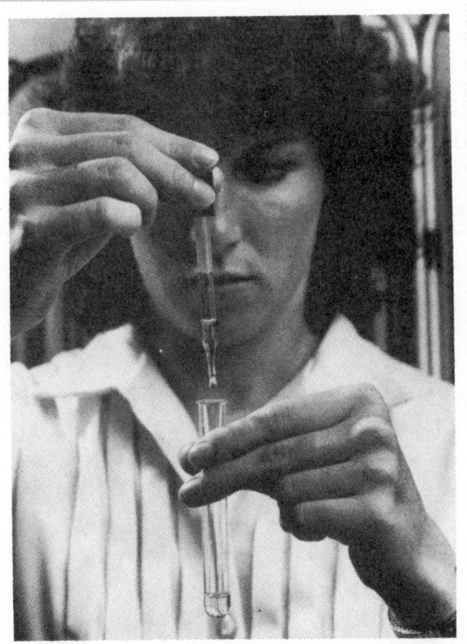

5. **PROCEDURAL STEP.** Discard excess urine that may be in the dropper, and rinse the dropper. Holding the dropper in an upright position, place 10 drops of water in the test tube.

6. **PROCEDURAL STEP.** Gently rotate the test tube to mix the water and urine.

7. **PROCEDURAL STEP.** Remove one tablet from the bottle by pouring it into the lid of the bottle, making sure not to touch the tablet. Hold the test tube at the top and transfer the tablet from the lid into the tube. Do not touch the bottom of the tube during the reaction. Recap the bottle as soon as possible.

PRINCIPLE. Moisture from the fingers could cause a caustic reaction in the tablet to burn the medical assistant's fingers. The reaction generates heat, causing the bottom of the test tube to be hot. Recapping the bottle is necessary to prevent exposing the tablets to environmental light, heat, and moisture.

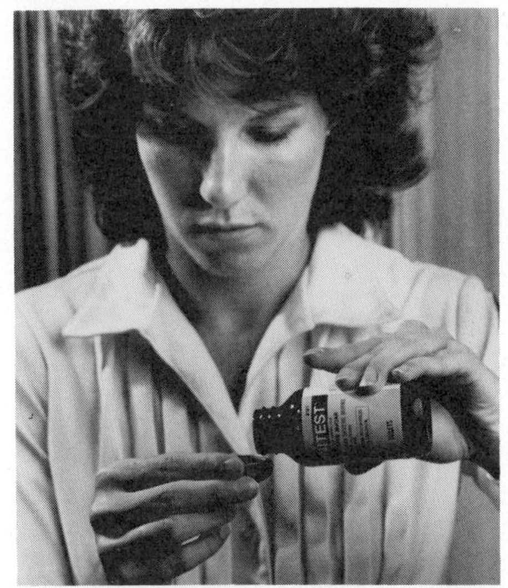

8. **PROCEDURAL STEP.** Observe the test tube as the reaction takes place. Do not shake the test tube during the reaction or for 15 seconds after the boiling in the tube stops.

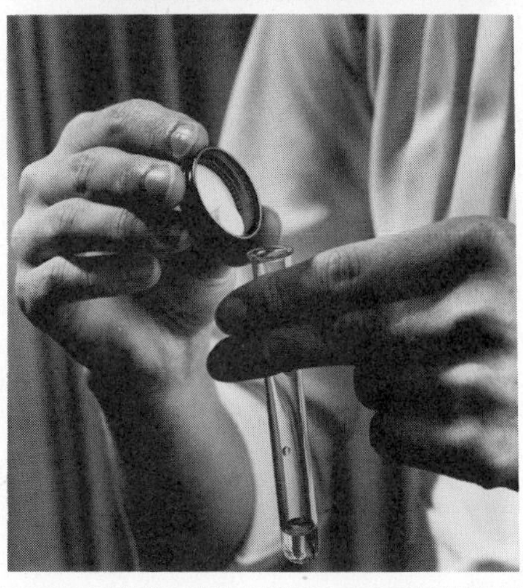

Continued

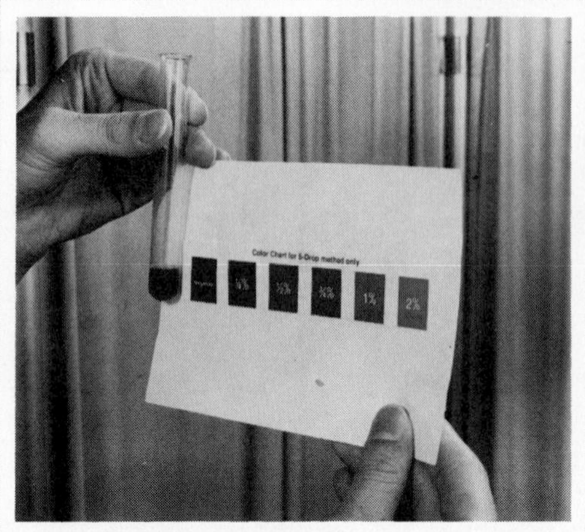

9. **PROCEDURAL STEP.** Fifteen seconds after the boiling has stopped, gently shake the test tube and immediately compare it with the color chart.

PRINCIPLE. If the reading is made immediately after the boiling stops, it may be low. If the reading is made more than 15 seconds after the boiling stops, it may be high.

10. **PROCEDURAL STEP.** Record results. The per cent (%) result that appears on the color block that most closely matches the color of the liquid should be recorded. Be sure to include the patient's name, the date and time, the brand name of the test used (Clinitest), the results, and your initials. The following scale is used to interpret results with Clinitest:

Clinitest Procedure

TEST RESULT	INTERPRETATION	COLOR CHANGE
Negative	No glucose present	Dark blue
.25%	250 mg/dl*	Green
.50%	500 mg/dl	Olive green
.75%	750 mg/dl	Greenish-brown
1%	1000 mg/dl	Tan
2%	2000 mg/dl	Bright orange

* A deciliter (dl) is a unit of measurement of volume that is equal to 0.1 L or 100 ml.

Note: The medical assistant should carefully observe the reaction while it is occurring and also during the 15-second waiting period after the boiling stops. Occasionally, a "pass-through" color change will occur. During pass-through, the color changes rapidly from green to tan to bright orange to a dark brown or greenish-brown. This indicates that the urine has more than a 2 per cent glucose concentration and the regular color chart cannot be used for interpreting results. If the pass-through color change occurs, the medical assistant should consult the physician. He or she may request that the medical assistant record the results as >2 per cent (greater than 2 per cent) or may want to follow up with a 2-drop Clinitest, which is a modification of the regular test.

11. **PROCEDURAL STEP.** Wash the hands and return the equipment.

Record data below.

DATE	TIME	PATIENT'S NAME	RESULTS

Microscopic Examination of Urine

Urine sediment is the solid materials contained in the urine (Fig. 10–7). A microscopic examination of the urine sediment helps to clarify results of the physical and chemical examination. A first-voided morning specimen is generally preferred, because it is more concentrated and contains more dissolved substances; therefore, small amounts of abnormal substances are more likely to be detected. It is important to use a fresh specimen, because changes will take place in a specimen left standing out, as previously discussed. These changes affect the reliability of the test results.

The urine specimen is prepared for microscopic examination by centrifuging approximately 10 to 15 ml of a well-mixed specimen for 3 to 5 minutes. This causes the sediment to settle to the bottom. The supernatant fluid is poured off, and the sediment is resuspended in the remaining liquid by flicking the bottom of the tube with the fingertips. A drop of the material is placed on a clean slide and covered with a coverslip.

CRYSTALS FOUND IN ACID URINE 400 X

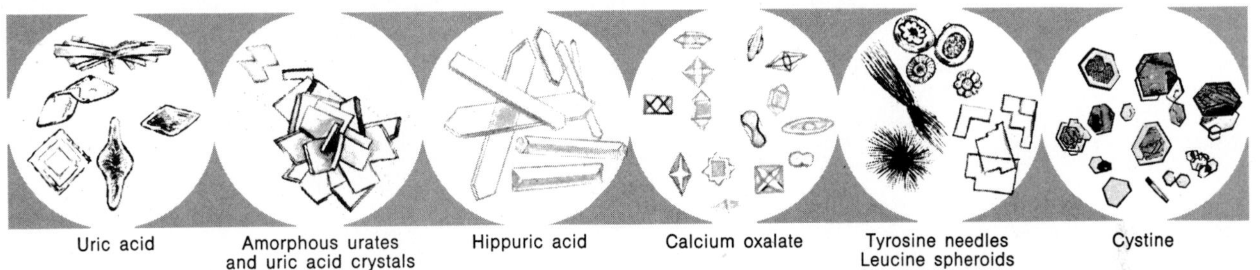

CRYSTALS FOUND IN ALKALINE URINE 400 X

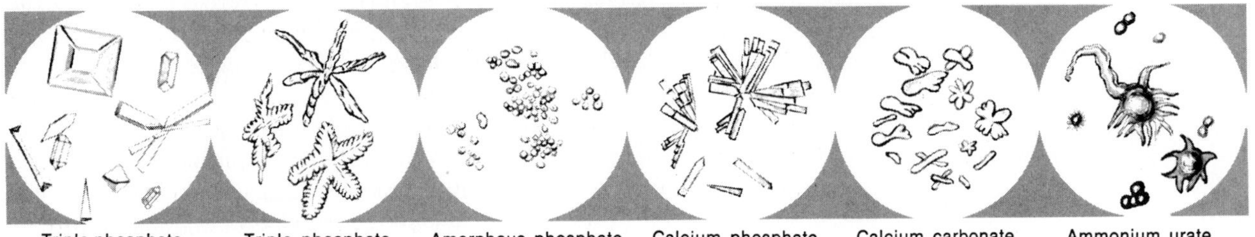

SULFA CRYSTALS

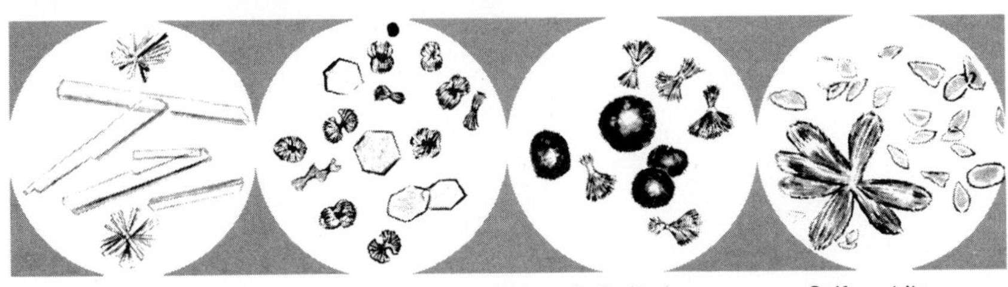

FIGURE 10–7. Ames Atlas of Urine Sediment. (Courtesy of Ames Company, Incorporated, Elkhart, Indiana.)

Illustration continued on following page

CELLS FOUND IN URINE

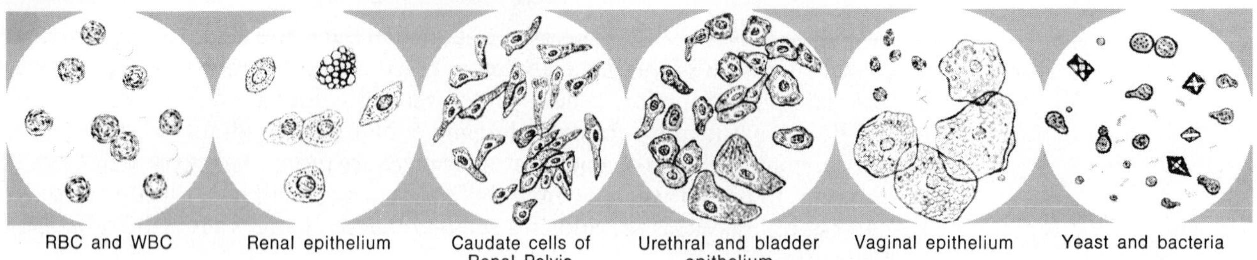

CASTS AND ARTIFACTS FOUND IN URINE 400 X

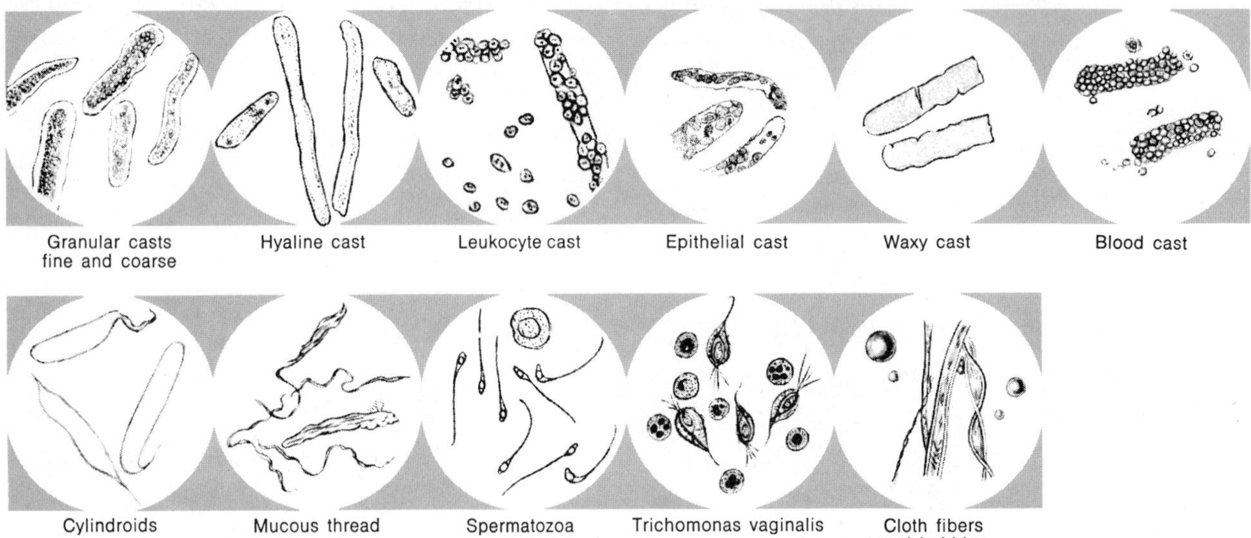

Figure 10-7 *Continued*

The sediment is first examined under low power to scan for the presence of casts. The microscope is changed to the high-power objective to identify the specific type of casts and to examine the sediment for the presence of smaller structures, such as red blood cells, white blood cells, bacteria, or crystals. Ten to fifteen high-power fields should be examined, and an average of these fields recorded. Casts are generally recorded as the average number and type seen per low-power field. Red blood cells, white blood cells, and epithelial cells are recorded as the average number viewed per high-power field. Other structures such as crystals, bacteria, yeast, and spermatozoa are recorded as occasional, frequent, or many.

Structures that may be found in a microscopic examination of urine are described below; Tables 10–3 to 10–6 provide an outline of these structures and of the possible causes of their presence.

TABLE 10–3. Cells in Urine Sediment

TYPE	PRESENCE IN NORMAL URINE	POSSIBLE CAUSES OF ABNORMAL AMOUNTS OF CELLS IN URINE
Red blood cells	0 to 5 cells per high-power field (depending on preparation of urinary sediment)	Inflammatory diseases Acute glomerulonephritis Pyelonephritis Hypertension Renal infarction Trauma Stones Tumor Bleeding diseases Use of anticoagulants
White blood cells	0 to 8 cells per high-power field (depending on preparation of urinary sediment)	Pyelonephritis Cystitis Urethritis Prostatitis Transplant rejection (manifested by lymphocytes in urine) Tissue injury accompanied by severe inflammation (manifested by monocytes in urine) Inflammation, immune mechanisms, and other host defense mechanisms (manifested by histiocytes in urine)
Squamous epithelial cells	Often present, depending upon collection technique	Vaginal contamination
Transitional epithelial cells	Moderate number of cells present	Disease of bladder or renal pelvis Catheterization
Renal tubular epithelial cells	Present in small numbers; higher numbers in infants	Acute tubular necrosis Glomerulonephritis Acute infection Renal toxicity Viral infection
Cytomegalic inclusion bodies	Not normally present in urine	Cytomegalic inclusion disease
Tumor cells	Not normally present in urine	Tumors of • Renal pelvis • Renal parenchyma • Ureters • Bladder

Courtesy of Boehringer Mannheim Diagnostics, Indianapolis, Indiana.

TABLE 10-4. Casts in Urine Sediment

TYPE	DESCRIPTION	POSSIBLE CAUSES
Hyaline casts	Colorless, transparent Low refractive index	Normal urine Strenuous exercise Acute glomerulonephritis Acute pyelonephritis Malignant hypertension Chronic renal disease
Red blood cell casts	Red cells in hyaline matrix Yellow-orange color High refractive index	Acute glomerulonephritis Lupus nephritis Severe nephritis Collagen diseases Renal infarction Malignant hypertension
White blood cell casts	Neutrophils in hyaline matrix High refractive index	Acute pyelonephritis Acute glomerulonephritis Chronic renal disease
Epithelial cell casts	Renal tubular epithelial cells in hyaline matrix High refractive index	Glomerulonephritis Vascular disease Toxin Virus
Granular casts	Opaque granules in matrix	Heavy proteinuria (nephrotic syndrome) Orthostatic proteinuria Congestive heart failure with proteinuria Acute or chronic renal disease
Waxy casts	Sharp, refractile outlines Irregular "broken off" ends Absence of differentiated structures	Severe chronic renal disease Malignant hypertension Kidney disease resulting from diabetes mellitus Acute renal disease
Fatty casts	Fat globules in transparent matrix	Nephrotic syndrome Diabetes mellitus Mercury poisoning Ethylene glycol poisoning
Broad casts	Larger diameter than other casts	Acute tubular necrosis Severe chronic renal disease Urinary tract obstruction
Mixed casts	Combination of any of the above	Any of the above, depending on cellular constituents

Courtesy of Boehringer Mannheim Diagnostics, Indianapolis, Indiana.

TABLE 10-5. Urinary Crystals

TYPE OF URINE	TYPE OF CRYSTALS	DESCRIPTION OF CRYSTALS	SIGNIFICANCE WHEN FOUND IN URINE
Normal acid urine	Amorphous urate	Colorless or yellow-brown granules (pink macroscopically)	Nonpathologic
	Uric acid	Occur in many shapes; may be colorless, yellow-brown, or red-brown; and square, diamond shaped, wedge shaped, or grouped in rosettes	Usually nonpathologic; in lage numbers, may indicate gout
	Calcium oxalate	Octahedral or dumbbell shaped; possess double refractive index	Usually nonpathologic; may be associated with stone formation
Normal alkaline urine	Amorphous phosphates	Small, colorless, granules	Nonpathologic
	Triple phosphates	Colorless prisms with three to six sides ("coffin lids") or feathery, shaped like fern leaves	Usually nonpathologic; may be associated with urine stasis or chronic urinary tract infection
	Ammonium biurate	Yellow-brown "thorny apple" appearance or yellow-brown spheres	Nonpathologic
	Calcium phosphate	Colorless prisms or rosettes	Usually nonpathologic; may be associated with urine stasis or chronic urinary tract infection
	Calcium carbonate	Usually appear colorless and amorphous; may be shaped like dumbbells, rhombi, or needles	Usually nonpathologic; may be associated with inorganic calculi formation
Abnormal urine	Tyrosine	Thin, dark needles, arranged in sheaves or clumps; usually colorless, but may be pale yellow-brown	Liver disease or inherited metabolic disorder
	Leucine	Yellow-brown spheres with radial striations	Liver disease or inherited metabolic disorder
	Cystine	Clear, hexagonal plates	Cystinuria
	Hippuric acid	Star-shaped clusters of needles, rhombic plates, or elongated prisms; may be colorless or yellow-brown	Usually nonpathologic
	Bilirubin	Delicate needles or rhombic plates; red-brown in color; birefringent	Bilirubinuria
	Cholesterol	Colorless, transparent plates with regular or irregular corner notches	Chyluria, urinary tract infections, nephrotic syndrome
	Creatine	Pseudohexagonal plates with positive birefringence	Destruction of muscle tissue due to muscular dystrophies, atrophies, and myositis
	Aspirin	Distinctive prismatic or starlike forms; usually colorless; show positive birefringence	Ingestion of aspirin or other salicylates
	Sulfonamide	Yellow-brown dumbbells, asymmetric sheaves, rosettes, or hexagonal plates	Ingestion of sulfonamide drugs
	Ampicillin	Long, thin, clear crystals	Parenteral administration of ampicillin
	X-ray media	Long, thin rectangles or flat, four-sided, notched plates	X-ray procedure with contrast media

Courtesy of Boehringer Mannheim Diagnostics, Indianapolis, Indiana.

TABLE 10–6. Microorganisms and Artifacts in the Urine

MICROORGANISMS/ARTIFACTS	SIGNIFICANCE WHEN FOUND IN THE URINE
Bacteria	More than 100,000 bacteria per ml indicates urinary tract infection 10,000 to 100,000 bacteria per ml indicates that tests should be repeated Less than 10,000 bacteria per ml may signify urine in which any bacteria are due to urethral organisms or contamination Bacteria accompanied by white blood cells and/or white cell or mixed casts may indicate acute pyelonephritis
Fungi	May indicate contamination by yeasts from skin and hair May indicate diabetes mellitus or urinary tract infection *Candida albicans* may occur in patients with diabetes mellitus or in the contaminated urine of female patients with candidal vaginitis
Parasites and parasitic ova	Usually indicate fecal or vaginal contamination and should be reported *Trichomonas* may be found in patients with urethritis and in the contaminated urine of women with trichomonas vaginitis Pinworm is a common contaminant and should be reported
Spermatozoa	Nonpathologic
Urinary artifacts • Hair • Starch from surgical gloves • Pollen grains • Bubbles • Oil droplets • Fibers • Talc • Dust • Threads • Glass particles	Nonpathologic May result from improper urine collection, improper slide preparation, or outside contamination

Courtesy of Boehringer Mannheim Diagnostics, Indianapolis, Indiana.

Red Blood Cells

Red blood cells appear as round, colorless, biconcave discs that are highly refractile. The presence of 0 to 5 per high-power field is considered normal. More than this amount may indicate bleeding somewhere along the urinary tract. Refer to Table 10–3 for a list of possible causes of an abnormal number of red blood cells in the urine. Concentrated urine causes the red blood cells to become shrunken or *crenated,* whereas dilute urine causes them to swell and become rounded.

White Blood Cells

White blood cells are round and granular and have a nucleus. They are approximately 1.5 times as large as a red blood cell. The presence of 0 to 8 per high-power field is considered normal. More than this amount may indicate inflammation of the genitourinary tract. Refer to Table 10–3 for a list of possible causes of an abnormal number of white blood cells in the urine.

Epithelial Cells

Most structures making up the urinary system are composed of several layers of epithelial cells. The outer layer is constantly being sloughed off and replaced by the cells underneath it. *Squamous epithelial cells* are large, clear, flat cells with an irregular shape. They contain a small nucleus and come from the urethra, bladder, and vagina. Squamous epithelial cells are normally present in small amounts in the urine. *Renal epithelial cells* are round and contain a large nucleus. They come from the deeper layers of the urinary tract, and their presence in the urine is considered abnormal. Refer to Table 10–3 for a list of the types of epithelial cells and possible causes of the presence of abnormal amounts in the urine.

Casts

Casts are cylindrical structures formed in the lumen of the tubules that make up the nephron. Materials in the tubules harden, are flushed out, and appear in the urine in the form of casts. Various types of casts may be present in the urine. Their presence generally indicates a diseased condition.

Casts are named according to what they contain. *Hyaline casts* are pale, colorless cylinders with rounded edges; they vary in size. *Granular casts* are hyaline casts that contain granules. They are described as "coarsely granular" or "finely granular," depending on the size of the granules. *Fatty casts* are hyaline casts that contain fat droplets. *Waxy casts* are light yellowish and have serrated edges. Their name is derived from the fact that they appear to be made of wax. *Cellular casts* contain organized structures and are named according to what they contain. Examples include red blood cell casts, which are hyaline casts containing red blood cells; white blood cell casts, which are hyaline casts containing white blood cells; epithelial casts, which are hyaline casts containing epithelial cells; and bacterial casts, which are hyaline casts containing bacteria. Refer to Table 10–4 for a list of the types of casts and possible causes of their presence in urine.

Crystals

A variety of crystals may be found in the urine. The type and number vary with the pH of the urine. Abnormal crystals found include leucine, tyrosine, cystine, and cholesterol. Crystals that commonly appear in acid urine include amorphous urates, uric acid, and calcium oxalate. Those that commonly appear in alkaline urine include amorphous phosphate, triple phosphate, calcium phosphate, and ammonium urate crystals. Refer to Table 10–5 for a list of the types of urine crystals and their significance when found in urine.

Miscellaneous Structures

Mucous threads are normally present in small amounts in the urine. They appear as long, wavy, threadlike structures with pointed ends.

Bacteria should not normally exist in the urinary tract. The presence of more than a few bacteria may indicate either contamination of the specimen during collection or a UTI. Bacteria are small structures and may be rod shaped or round.

Yeast cells are smooth refractile bodies that have an oval shape. A distinguishing feature of yeast cells is small buds projecting from the cells that are involved with reproduction. Yeast cells in the urine of female patients are usually a vaginal contaminant caused by the yeast *Candida albicans* and produce the vaginal infection known as candidiasis. They may also be present in the urine of patients with diabetes mellitus.

Parasites may be present in the urine sediment as a contaminant from fecal or vaginal material. *Trichomonas vaginalis* is a parasite that causes trichomonas vaginitis.

Spermatozoa may be present in the urine of a male or female after coitus. The spermatozoa have round heads and long, slender, hairlike tails. Refer to Table 10–6 for a list of miscellaneous structures which may be present in the urine and the significance when found.

Urine Pregnancy Testing

Determining whether or not a woman is pregnant can be accomplished in a number of ways. By the eighth week after fertilization, pregnancy can be confirmed through the medical history and physical examination. However, the physician may desire an earlier diagnosis through the use of a pregnancy test to initiate early prenatal care. A pregnancy test may also be required before certain medications are ordered or procedures are performed that may cause injury to a fetus (e.g., insertion of an intrauterine device [IUD]).

In the medical office, immunologic tests are often used for pregnancy testing. These tests are performed on a concentrated urine specimen and rely upon the presence of a hormone known as human chorionic gonadotropin (hCG) for a positive reaction. This hormone is produced by the developing fertilized egg, and small amounts of it are secreted into the urine and blood. Immediately after conception and implantation of the fertilized egg, the plasma level of hCG rises rapidly and can be used to detect pregnancy as early as 5 days after the first missed menstrual period. The highest plasma levels of hCG occur at about the eighth week after conception. After this time, the production of hCG declines and remains at a lower level for the duration of the pregnancy. Within 72 hours of delivery, the level of hCG disappears entirely from the plasma. As a result, these tests are most sensitive during the first trimester and may even show a negative reaction once the level of hCG begins to decline during the second and third trimester. Urine pregnancy testing involves the detection of the presence of hCG using an hCG antiserum reagent. Positive and negative reactions are evidenced by a specific visible reaction that is observed and interpreted by the individual performing the test. Pregnancy tests are commercially available in kits that contain all of the required reagents and supplies to perform the test. Each kit can be used to perform a specific number of tests, ranging between 10 and 100.

The two main types of urine pregnancy tests are the rapid slide agglutination test and the test tube agglutination test. These tests are used in the medical office because they are convenient to perform and provide immediate test results. The manufacturer's instructions must carefully be followed to prevent inaccurate test results. When used properly, these tests are 95 per cent accurate.

The *slide agglutination test* is used most frequently to perform pregnancy testing in the medical office. Positive test results are based upon the inhibition of latex particle agglutination. The test takes place in two steps and can be performed in only 2 minutes. In the first step, a drop of the urine specimen is placed on a specially provided glass slide that comes with the kit. The hCG antiserum reagent (antibody) is then added to the urine specimen. If the patient's urine contains hCG, the antiserum combines with the hCG (antigen) in the urine specimen, resulting in an antigen-antibody reaction. The next step involves the addition of an antigen reagent containing latex particles coated with hCG. If the antigen-antibody reaction has previously occurred in the first step of the procedure, no available hCG antiserum is left in the specimen to react with the latex particles. Therefore, the absence of agglutination of the slide test, known as agglutination inhibition, indicates a positive reaction for pregnancy. On the other hand, if agglutination occurs on the slide, the results are interpreted as negative (Fig. 10–8*A*). Coating the hCG with latex permits visible agglutination that can be observed and interpreted as a negative reaction by the individual performing the test. Without the latex, agglutination would not be visible when the hCG antigen and antibody combine.

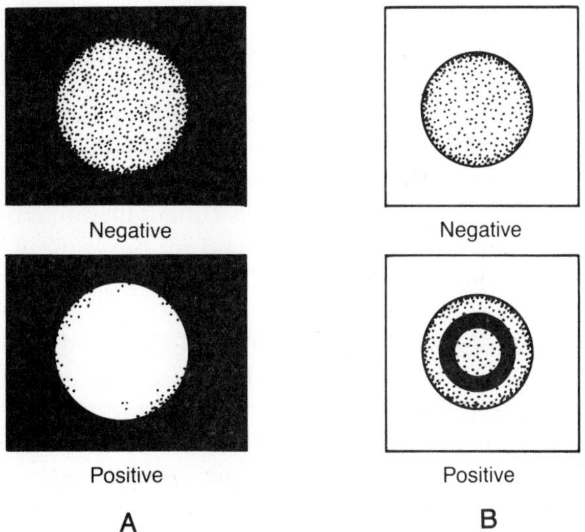

FIGURE 10–8. Urine pregnancy test results. *A*, Slide agglutination pregnancy test results. *B*, Test tube agglutination test results.

The second type of pregnancy test, the *test tube agglutination test* is more sensitive than the slide agglutination test; however, it takes longer to perform. This test method is used in home pregnancy tests. The test tube agglutination test occurs in two steps, requires the use of a small test tube, and takes 2 hours to complete. The first step of the testing procedure is identical to the slide agglutination test. Thus, if the patient's urine contains hCG, it reacts with the hCG antiserum, resulting in an antigen-antibody reaction. In the second step, red cells coated with hCG are added to the test tube. If the antigen-antibody reaction has previously occurred in the first step, no available hCG antiserum is left in the specimen to react with the hCG and the red blood cells settle in a sharp, precise, ring on the bottom of the tube, indicating a positive reaction. If the urine specimen does not contain hCG, the hCG antiserum is available to combine with the hCG antigen bound to the red blood cells. In this case, a small round film of agglutination settles at the bottom of the tube, indicating a negative reaction (Fig. 10–8*B*).

Guidelines

Specific guidelines must be followed in performing a urine pregnancy test to ensure accurate test results. These guidelines are outlined below.

1. Use clean, preferably disposable, urine containers to collect the specimen. Traces of detergent in the specimen container may cause inaccurate test results.
2. Use a first-voided morning specimen, because it contains the highest concentration of hCG.
3. The specific gravity of the urine specimen should be determined before the test is performed. A specific gravity of less than 1.010 is considered too dilute for pregnancy testing as it may lead to a false-negative test result.
4. The urine specimen should be at room temperature before the procedure is performed.
5. The reagents should be stored in the refrigerator and brought to room temperature before use to ensure accurate test results.
6. Test reagents past their expiration dates should not be used. In addition, reagents that have changed color or formed a precipitate should not be used.

7. While the test is performed, care should be taken to avoid contaminating the reagents with one another or with the test specimen. If the urine specimen cannot be tested immediately after voiding it should be preserved in the refrigerator. The patient who collects the specimen at home, should be given instructions on preserving the specimen.

8. When performing the slide agglutination test, a new stirrer must be used for each specimen to prevent cross contamination among specimens.

The slide agglutination method for performing a urine pregnancy test is presented in Procedure 10-5.

Serum Pregnancy Test

The radioimmunoassay (RIA) for hCG is used to detect hCG in the serum of the blood. This test is more sensitive than a urine test and can detect pregnancy at approximately the eighth day after fertilization; therefore, the pregnancy can be detected even before the time of the missed menstrual period. This test uses a radioisotope technique and is capable of detecting minute amounts of hCG in the blood. This test is generally used to diagnose abnormalities such as ectopic pregnancy, to follow the course of early pregnancy when abnormalities of embryonic development are suspected, and to provide an early diagnosis of pregnancy in high-risk individuals such as diabetic patients.

PROCEDURE 10-5

URINE PREGNANCY TEST — *SLIDE AGGLUTINATION METHOD*

1. **PROCEDURAL STEP.** Wash the hands and assemble the equipment, which includes the **antiserum reagent,** the **antigen reagent,** the **glass slide,** a **stirrer,** a **disposable pipet,** a **rubber bulb,** and the **urine specimen.** Make sure the slide is clean.
PRINCIPLE. A dirty slide interferes with adequate interpretation of test results.

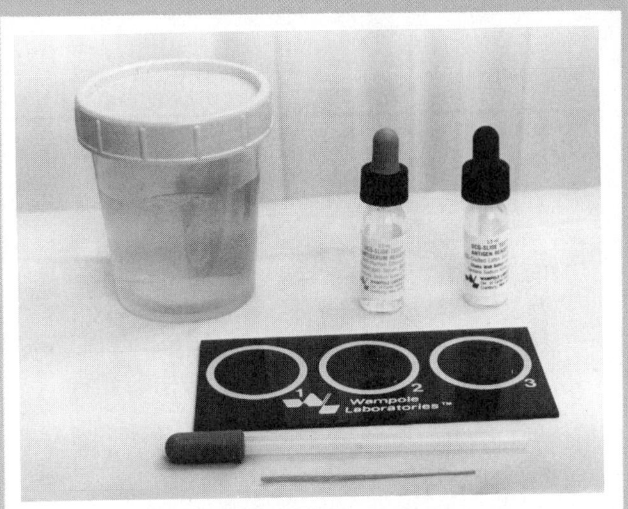

2. **PROCEDURAL STEP.** Check the expiration date on the reagent bottles.
PRINCIPLE. The expiration date usually appears on the label of the reagent container. Outdated reagents may lead to inaccurate test results.

3. **PROCEDURAL STEP.** Allow the reagents to reach room temperature.
PRINCIPLE. Test results are more accurate if the reagents reach room temperature before being used.

4. **PROCEDURAL STEP.** Using a disposable pipet, place 1 drop of the urine within a circle on the slide.

5. **PROCEDURAL STEP.** Holding the reagent dropper in an upright position, add 1 drop of the antiserum reagent to the slide. Do not allow the dropper to touch the urine specimen.
PRINCIPLE. Holding the dropper in a vertical position ensures a standard representative drop. Touching the dropper to the urine specimen contaminates it, affecting the contents of the antiserum reagent.

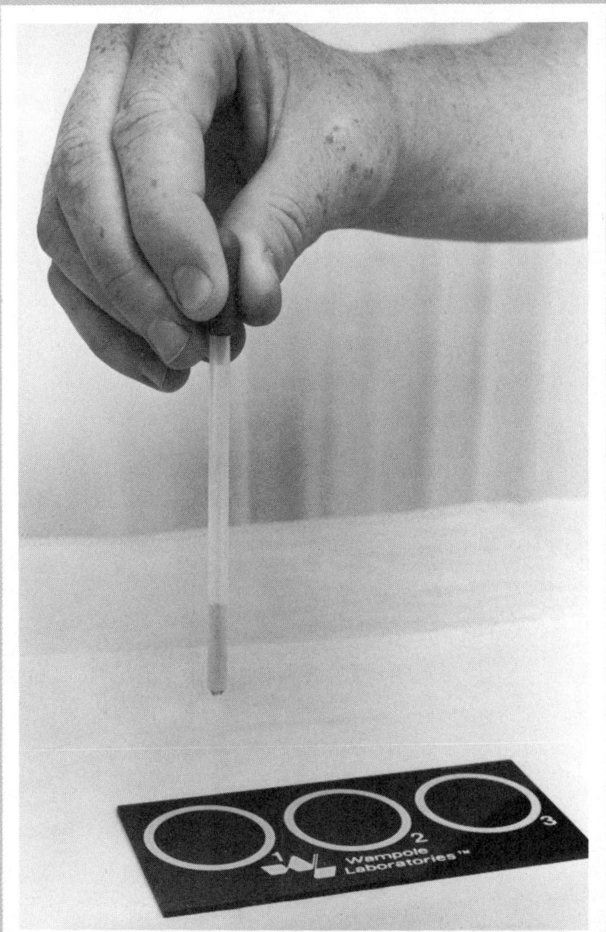

Continued

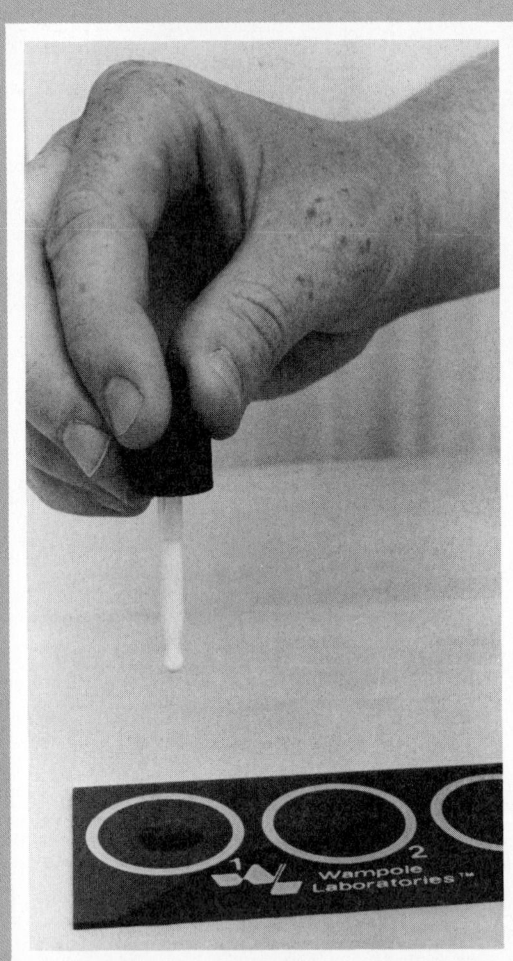

6. **Procedural step.** Thoroughly shake the antigen reagent to resuspend the latex particles. Hold the reagent dropper in an upright position, and add 1 drop of the antigen reagent to the slide. Do not allow the dropper to touch the urine specimen.

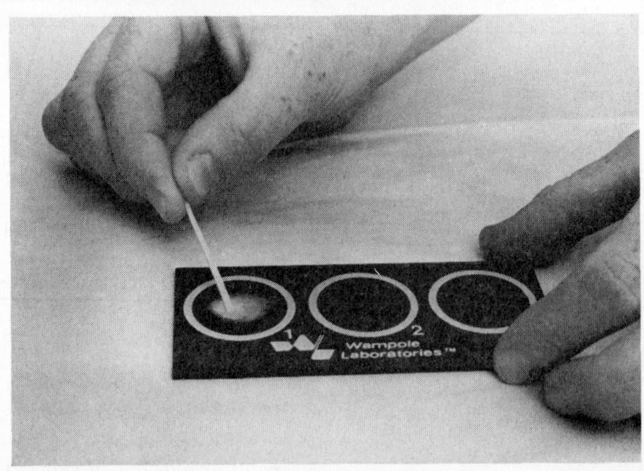

7. **Procedural step.** Mix the reagents with the urine specimen, using a stirrer, by spreading the mixture over the entire circle.

8. **PROCEDURAL STEP.** Rock the slide slowly and gently for 2 minutes and observe it for agglutination. The absence of agglutination (agglutination inhibition) is observed as an opaque suspension on the slide and is interpreted as a ***positive reaction***. The presence of agglutination is interpreted as a ***negative reaction*** (see Fig. 10–8*A*). The slide should not be rocked for longer than 2 minutes.

PRINCIPLE. The slide must be rocked to mix the reagents with the urine specimen and to ensure complete exposure of the latex particles to available antiserum reagent. Rocking the slide for longer than 2 minutes causes evaporation of the reagents, leading to inaccurate test results.

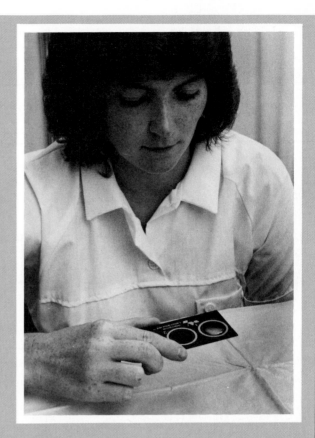

9. **PROCEDURAL STEP.** Wash the hands and record the results. Include the patient's name, the date and time, the date of the patient's last menstrual period (LMP), and the results recorded as either positive or negative. Place your initials next to the recording.

10. **PROCEDURAL STEP.** Thoroughly wash the glass slide, using tap water, to remove all traces of detergent. Wipe the slipe dry using a lint-free tissue to avoid spotting.

Record data below.

DATE	TIME	PATIENT'S NAME	RESULTS

Study Questions

1. What is the purpose of collecting a clean-catch midstream specimen?
2. What changes may occur if urine is allowed to remain standing for more than 1 hour?
3. What may cause the urine to have an unusual color?
4. What may cause the urine to become cloudy?
5. What guidelines must be followed in performing a urine pregnancy test to ensure accurate test results?

11

VENIPUNCTURE

CHAPTER OUTLINE

Venipuncture Methods
Types of Blood Specimens
Separating Serum from Whole Blood
Separating Plasma from Whole Blood

COMPETENCIES

After completing this chapter, you should be able to demonstrate the proper procedure to perform the following:

1. Collect a venous blood specimen, and record the procedure using the vacuum tube venipuncture method.
2. Collect a venous blood specimen, and record the procedure using the syringe venipuncture method.
3. Separate serum from a whole blood specimen.
4. Separate plasma from a whole blood specimen.

LEARNING OBJECTIVES

After completing this chapter, you should be able to do the following:

1. Define the terms listed in the vocabulary.
2. List the layers the blood separates into when an anticoagulant is added to the specimen.
3. List the layers the blood separates into when an anticoagulant is not added to the specimen.
4. Explain how each of the following blood specimens are obtained: clotted blood, serum, whole blood, and plasma.
5. State the additive content of the following vacuum tubes and list the type of blood specimens that can be obtained from each: red, lavender, gray, light blue, green.
6. Explain how the serum separator tube functions in the collection of a serum specimen.
7. List four ways to prevent a blood specimen from becoming hemolyzed.
8. Explain the principle underlying each step in the venipuncture procedure and the procedure for separating serum from whole blood.

• VOCABULARY •

anticoagulant (an" ti-ko-ag' u-lant)—A substance that inhibits blood blotting.

buffy coat (buf' e kōt)—A thin, light-colored layer of white blood cells and platelets that lies between a top layer of plasma and a bottom layer of red blood cells when an anticoagulant has been added to a blood specimen.

hematoma (he" mah-to' mah)—A swelling or mass of coagulated blood caused by a break in a blood vessel.

hemolysis (he-mol' i-sis)—The breakdown of blood cells.

plasma (plaz' mah)—The liquid part of the blood consisting of a clear yellowish fluid that makes up approximately 55 per cent of the total blood volume.

serum (se' rum)—Plasma from which the clotting factor fibrinogen has been removed.

venipuncture (ven" i-pungk' tūr)—Puncturing of a vein.

Venipuncture Methods

The term *venipuncture* means the puncturing of a vein. In the medical office a venipuncture is performed when a large blood specimen is needed for testing. Because it is not legal in every state for medical assistants to perform venipuncture, each is responsible for checking the laws in his or her state before performing this procedure.

The venipuncture may be performed by the *syringe method* or the *vacuum tube method* (Fig. 11–1). With the syringe method, the medical assistant is able to control the withdrawal of blood. This is especially helpful when working with small veins. The vacuum tube method is faster and a greater quantity of blood can be collected at one time when the multiple-draw system is used. The blood is usually obtained from the antecubital veins of the arm (Fig. 11–2). These veins are generally large, easily accessible, and close to the surface of the skin. The medical assistant should not be misled by the presence in some patients of many very blue veins that lie close to the surface of the skin. These are superficial veins and are not suitable for performing a venipuncture. The antecubital veins are beneath these superficial veins.

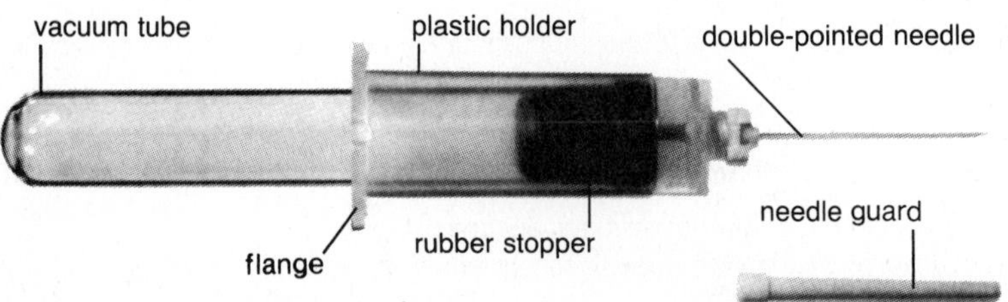

FIGURE 11–1. A Vacutainer system used for the vacuum tube method of performing a venipuncture. The Vacutainer consists of a dry sterile glass vaccum tube with a rubber stopper, a plastic holder used to secure the needle, and a double-pointed needle. (Courtesy of Becton-Dickinson, Rutherford, New Jersey.)

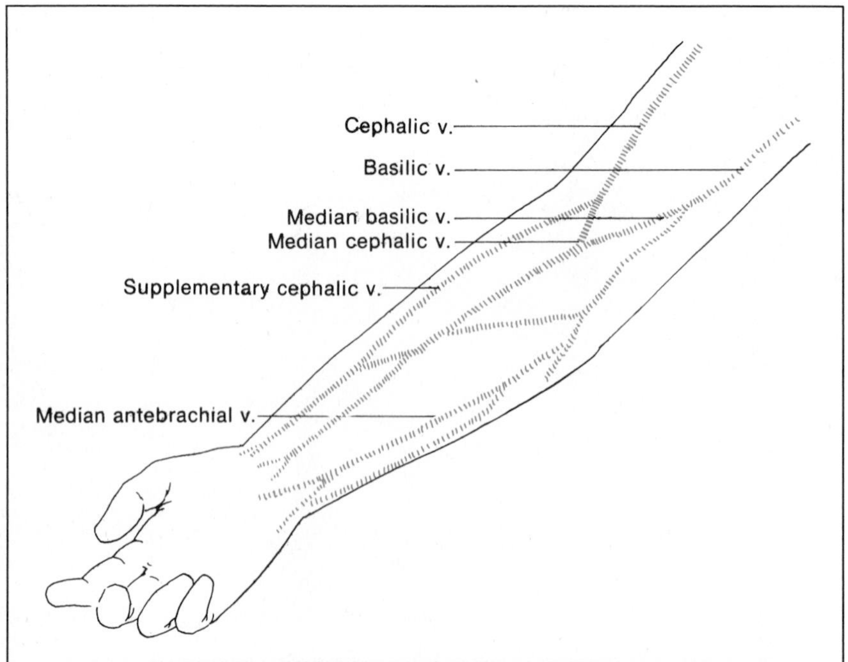

FIGURE 11–2. Representation of the antecubital veins located in the arm. The median cephalic is the vein most often used for venipuncture.

The gauge of the needle used for venipuncture ranges from 20 to 22, and the length of the needle ranges from 1 to 1.5 inches. The size of the syringe or vacuum tube varies according to the amount of blood needed for testing.

The patient should be given appropriate instructions on the preparation for the procedure. Some tests require special preparation such as fasting or the avoidance of certain medications, and other tests require no preparation at all. The medical assistant should consult with the physician to determine the type of preparation that may be required.

The medical assistant should develop skill and confidence in performing venipuncture, to prevent patient discomfort and injury. Some blood specimens may be tested in the medical office, whereas others will be sent to a laboratory for testing. The latter specimens need to be accompanied by a laboratory request so that the laboratory personnel know what type of test the physician desires. The medical assistant may be responsible for filling out the laboratory request form. Included should be the physician's name and address; the patient's name, address, age, and sex; the date and time of collection of the specimen; the type of specimen (e.g., whole blood, serum, plasma); the physician's clinical diagnosis; and a check mark next to the type of tests to be performed (Fig. 11–3).

Prevention of Hemolysis

The blood specimen should be handled carefully at all times. Blood cells are fragile, and rough handling may cause ***hemolysis*** or breakdown of the blood cells. Hemolyzed blood specimens lead to inaccurate test results. To prevent hemolysis, these guidelines should be followed:

1. Store the vacuum tubes at room temperature because chilled tubes can result in hemolysis.
2. Do not use a small gauge needle to collect the specimen; a needle with a gauge between 20 and 22 should be used to collect the specimen.

Physician's Name ______________________

______________________ Date __________

Patient's Name (Please Print) ______________________ Age ______ Sex ______

____

PROFILES ☐ Fasting ☐ Non-Fasting

Thyroid ☐
Liver ☐
Prenatal ☐
Lipid ☐
Coronary Assessment Profile (C.A.P.) ☐
C.A.P. + Lipo ☐
Rheumatoid ☐
Electrolyte ☐
General ☐

☐ **Executive**
☐ **SMAC**
☐ **Routine**
☐ **SMA 12**

Other Tests Desired

Please Mark Boxes Clearly ☒

☐ Complete Blood Count (CBC)
☐ Blood Count (without differential)
☐ T4 RIA ☐ T3 Uptake
☐ Glucose ☐ TSH
☐ VDRL ☐ RH + Type
☐ GC Smear ☐ Urinalysis
☐ GC Culture* ☐ Rubella
☐ Culture ☐ Culture & Sensitivity*
☐ Lipoprotein Electrophoresis If Chol or Trig Elevated
☐ Lipoprotein Electrophoresis (includes Chol, Trig & Phenotype)
☐ HDL Cholesterol
☐ HDL Cholesterol + Total Cholesterol

*Specimen source ______________________

Clinical diagnosis ______________________

MARCUM LABORATORIES

FIGURE 11–3. Laboratory request form.

3. Practice good technique in collecting the specimen; excessive trauma to the blood vessel can result in hemolysis.

4. Always handle the blood specimen carefully; do not shake it or handle it roughly.

Types of Blood Specimens

There are various types of blood specimens that the medical assistant will be required to obtain through the venipuncture procedure. They are as follows:

1. *Clotted Blood.* Clotted blood is obtained from a tube to which an anticoagulant has not been added.
2. *Serum.* Serum is obtained from clotted blood by allowing the specimen to stand and then centrifuging it. This causes the specimen to separate into a top layer of serum and a bottom layer of blood cells.
3. *Whole Blood.* Whole blood is obtained by using a tube containing an anticoagulant to prevent clotting. It is important to mix the anticoagulant with the blood by gently inverting the tube eight to ten times.
4. *Plasma.* Plasma is obtained from whole blood that has been centrifuged. This causes the specimen to separate into a top layer of plasma, a middle layer (termed the buffy coat) that contains white blood cells and platelets, and a bottom layer of red blood cells.

The type of blood specimen required depends on the type of test to be performed. For example, serum is required for most blood chemistries, whereas whole blood is required for a complete blood count.

Whole blood and plasma specimens both require the use of an anticoagulant. There are a number of types of anticoagulants available for laboratory testing. The type of anticoagulant used must not alter the blood components or affect the laboratory test to be performed. The medical assistant must be sure to use the anticoagulant specified by the test ordered. Anticoagulants must not be substituted one for another, because inaccurate test results will occur.

The vacuum tube method utilizes a color-coded system for ease in identifying the additive content of each type of tube (refer to the back inside cover). The most frequently used vacuum tubes are classified here according to the color of the stopper and additive content.

1. *Red.* Red-stoppered tubes do not contain an anticoagulant and are used to obtain clotted blood or serum. Serum is required for serologic tests and most blood chemistries.
2. *Lavender.* Lavender-stoppered tubes contain the anticoagulant ethylenediaminetetra-acetic acid (EDTA) and are used to obtain whole blood or plasma; the most common use is to collect a blood specimen for a complete blood count (CBC).
3. *Gray.* Gray-stoppered tubes contain the anticoagulant potassium oxalate and are used to obtain whole blood or plasma; the most common use is to collect blood specimens to perform a glucose tolerance test.
4. *Light Blue.* Light blue-stoppered tubes contain the anticoagulant sodium citrate and are used to obtain whole blood or plasma; the most common use is for coagulation tests such as the prothrombin time (PT).
5. *Green.* Green-stoppered tubes contain the anticoagulant heparin and are commonly used to collect blood specimens to perform blood gas determinations and pH assays.

Vacuum tubes are available in varying capacities, the most common being the 5-, 7-, 10-, and 15-ml sizes. The capacity of the tube used depends on the amount of the specimen required by the test. Information regarding additive content, expiration date, and tube capacity is found on the label of each box of vacuum tubes.

PROCEDURE 11-1

VENIPUNCTURE USING THE VACUUM TUBE METHOD

This procedure outlines the steps for performing venipuncture using the single-draw needle.

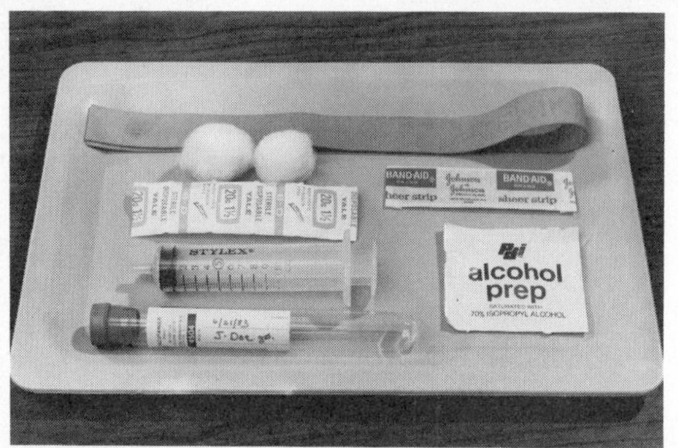

1. **PROCEDURAL STEP.** Wash the hands.

2. **PROCEDURAL STEP.** Assemble the equipment. The equipment needed includes **clean gloves**, a **tourniquet**, an **alcohol prep**, a **sterile glass vacuum tube with a rubber stopper**, a **plastic holder with a guide line**, a **single-draw needle**, **sterile cotton balls**, and an **adhesive bandage**. Be sure to select the proper vacuum tube, according to the test to be performed. For example, a red-stoppered tube is utilized when serum is required. Check the expiration date of the tube, and label the tube with the patient's name, the date, and your initials. If the specimen will be tested at an outside laboratory, complete a laboratory request form.
PRINCIPLE. Outdated tubes may no longer contain a vacuum, and, as a result, they may not be able to draw blood into the tube. Proper labeling of blood specimens avoids mix-up of specimens.

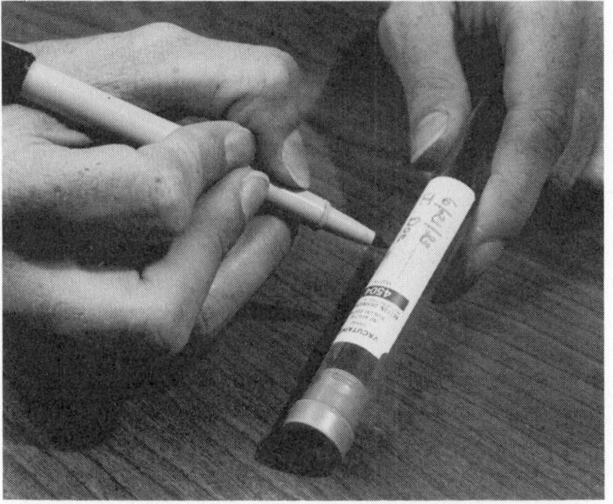

3. **PROCEDURAL STEP.** Prepare the equipment. Screw the needle into the plastic holder and tighten securely. If the vacuum tube contains an anticoagulant, tap the tube just below the stopper to release any anticoagulant adhering to the stopper. Place the glass vacuum tube in the plastic holder with the posterior needle just touching the stopper. Push the tube forward into the posterior needle until the rubber stopper just reaches the guide line. Release the tube. It will fall back slightly below the guide line and should remain in this position.
PRINCIPLE. The tip of the posterior needle is in the rubber stopper, which will cover the opening of the needle and prevent blood loss once the venipuncture has been made. At the same time, the needle has not yet broken the vacuum in the tube, which is needed to draw the blood into the tube.

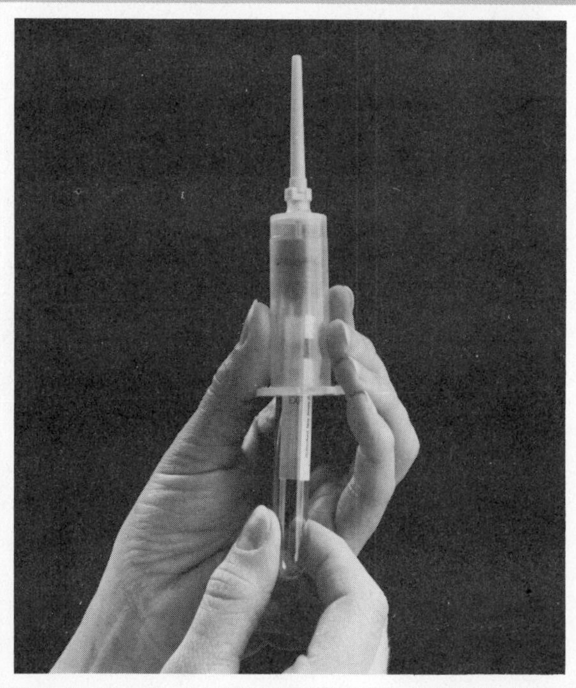

4. **PROCEDURAL STEP.** Identify the patient and explain the procedure.
PRINCIPLE. Venipuncture is often a frightening experience for the patient, and reassurance should be offered to help reduce apprehension.

5. **PROCEDURAL STEP.** Position the patient. The patient should be seated comfortably in a chair with an armrest. Palpate the veins of both arms to determine the best vein to use. It is also helpful to ask the individual which arm has been used in the past to obtain blood. The arm with the vein selected for the venipuncture should be extended and placed on the armrest with the antecubital veins facing anteriorly. The arm should be supported by a rolled towel or by having the patient place the fist of his other hand under the elbow.
PRINCIPLE. This position allows for easy access to the antecubital veins. It is more convenient for the medical assistant to stand in front of the patient during the procedure.

Continued

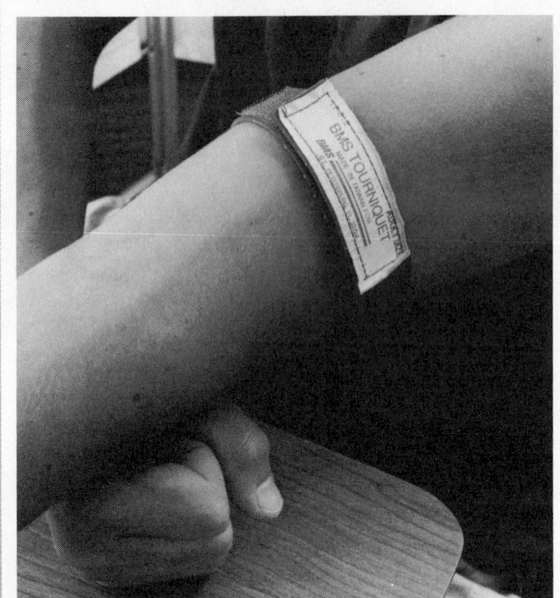

Velcro tourniquet.

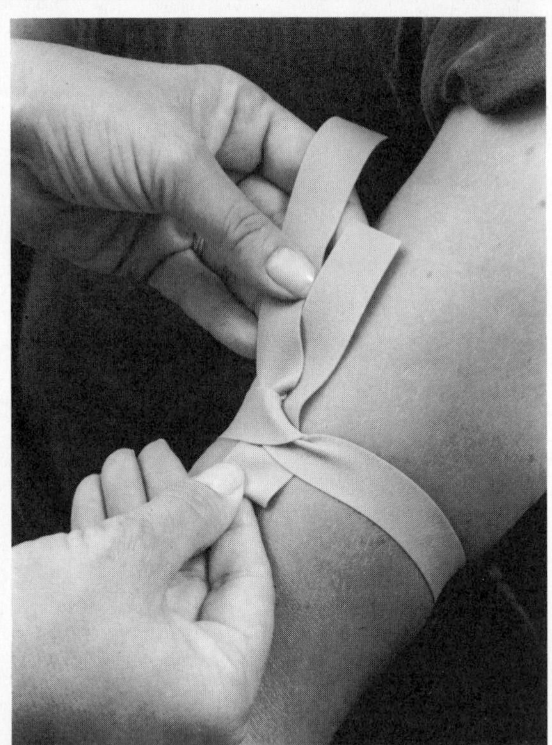
Rubber tourniquet.

6. **PROCEDURAL STEP.** Apply the tourniquet as follows:

Velcro tourniquet. Hold each end of the tourniquet with one hand. Position the tourniquet 2 to 3 inches above the bend in the elbow. Wrap the tourniquet around the arm and secure it with the Velcro fastener.

Rubber tourniquet. Hold each end of the tourniquet with one hand and pull the ends away from each other to create tension. Position the tourniquet 2 to 3 inches above the bend in the elbow while you maintain proper tension. Secure the tourniquet with a half-bow.

The tourniquet should have enough tension to impede the venous flow. Ask the patient to clench the fist of the arm to which the tourniquet has been applied. Never leave the tourniquet on for more than 60 seconds at a time.

PRINCIPLE. Securing the rubber tourniquet with a half-bow allows for easy removal of it with one hand. The correct tourniquet tension must be obtained. A tourniquet that is too loose fails to cause the veins to stand out in order to be palpated. A tourniquet that is too tight obstructs the arterial blood flow as well as the venous flow. Obstructing the arterial flow results in a blood specimen that may produce inaccurate test results.

The combined effect of the pressure of the tourniquet and the clenched fist should cause the antecubital veins to stand out so that accurate selection of a puncture site can be made. Leaving the tourniquet on for more than 60 seconds is uncomfortable for the patient and may alter the test results.

7. **PROCEDURAL STEP.** Palpate the vein again. At times, the medical assistant is not able to see the vein but is able to palpate it. The vein should not be used unless it can be palpated.

PRINCIPLE. The median cephalic vein is generally the best vein to use. The veins on either side of the arm tend to roll and are difficult to stabilize. The vein does not have to be visualized in order to be a good selection.

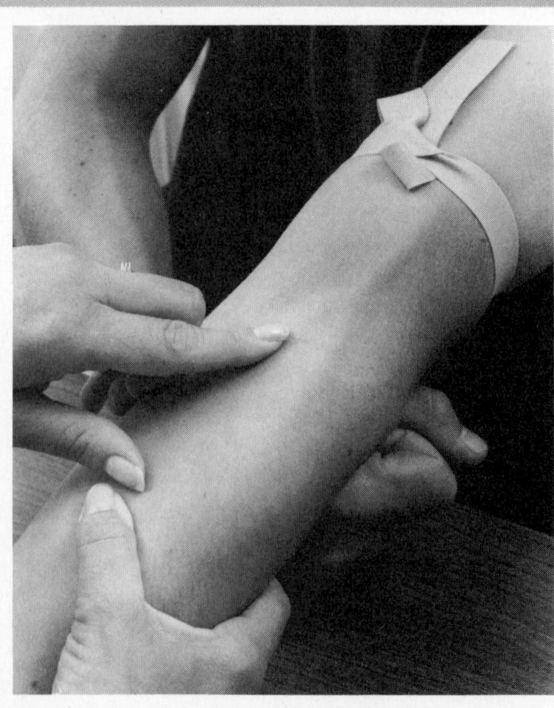

8. **Procedural step.** Cleanse the area with an antiseptic, such as 70 per cent ethyl alcohol. Cleansing should be done in a circular motion, starting from the inside and moving away from the puncture site. Allow the site to dry and do not touch the area after cleansing.
Principle. Using a circular motion helps to carry foreign particles away from the puncture site. The site must be allowed to dry, because alcohol entering the blood specimen contaminates it, leading to inaccurate test results. In addition, the alcohol causes the patient to experience a stinging sensation. Touching the area causes contamination, and the cleansing process has to be repeated.

9. **Procedural step.** Apply gloves and remove the cap from the needle. Hold the venipuncture set-up (plastic holder, needle, and glass vacuum tube) by placing the thumb and index finger of the dominant hand on the plastic holder while supporting the rest of the holder and vacuum tube with the remaining three fingers. The needle should be positioned with bevel facing up. Place the thumb of the nondominant hand approximately 1 to 2 inches below the puncture site.
Principle. Gloves are a precaution that provides a barrier against contaminated blood. The thumb helps to hold the skin taut for easier entry and to stabilize the vein to be punctured.

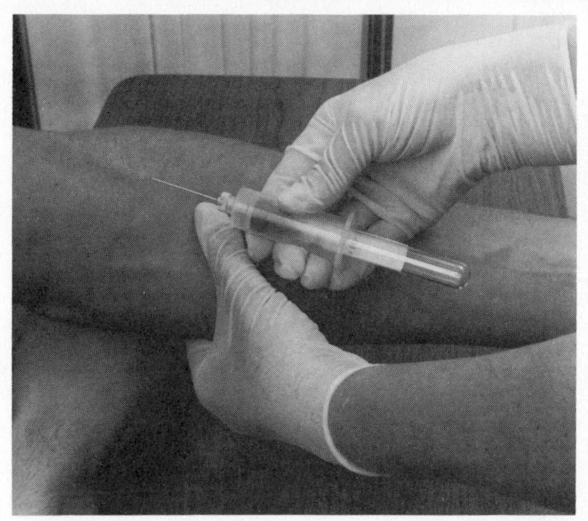

10. **Procedural step.** Position the venipuncture set-up at a 15-degree angle to the arm. Make sure the needle points in the same direction as the vein to be entered.
Principle. An angle of less than 15 degrees may cause the needle to enter above the vein, preventing puncture. An angle of more than 15 degrees may cause the needle to go through the vein by puncturing its posterior wall. This could result in a hematoma.

11. **Procedural step.** With one continuous motion, enter the skin and then the vein. The needle should penetrate the skin approximately ¼ to ½ inch below the place where the vein is to be entered. The patient may need reassurance because this step may be painful. After entering the vein, place two fingers on the flange of the plastic holder and with the thumb push the tube forward to the end of the holder. This allows the posterior needle to puncture the rubber stopper. Blood begins flowing into the tube if the (anterior) needle is in a vein. If the blood is filling the tube at a rapid or moderate rate, remove the tourniquet and ask the patient to unclench the fist. If the blood flow is slow, it is recommended that the tourniquet be left on until the tube is filled. Do not move the needle once the venipuncture has been made.
Principle. Using one continuous motion helps to reduce tissue damage. The medical assistant feels a lack of resistance once the vein has been penetrated. When the vacuum in the tube has been broken, the suction inside the tube draws the blood into it. Moving the needle causes patient discomfort.

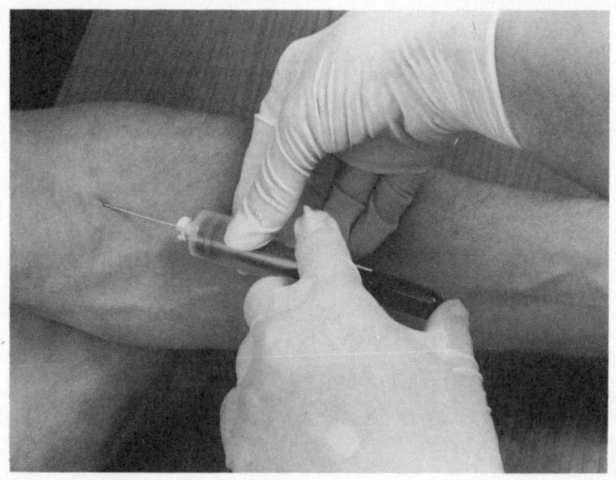

Continued

12. **Procedural Step.** Allow the vacuum tube to fill to the exhaustion of the vacuum as indicated by the cessation of the blood flow into the tube. (The tube will be almost, but not quite, full when the vacuum is exhausted.) The suction action of the vacuum tube automatically draws the blood into the tube.

Principle. If the vacuum tube is removed before the vacuum is exhausted, a rush of air enters the tube, damaging the red blood cells. Also, a tube containing an additive such as an anticoagulant must be filled completely to ensure accurate test results.

13. **Procedural Step.** Remove the tourniquet (if it has not previously been removed in Procedural Step 11) and ask the patient to unclench the fist.

Principle. The tourniquet must be removed before the needle. Otherwise, the pressure on the vein from the tourniquet could cause internal and external bleeding around the puncture site.

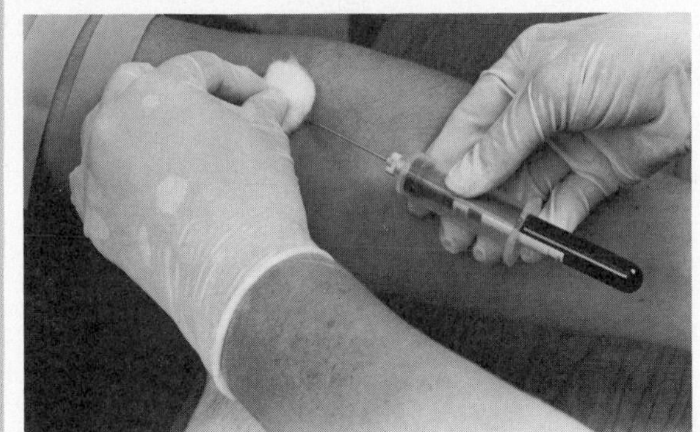

14. **Procedural Step.** Place a dry sterile cotton ball over the site and withdraw the needle slowly and at the same angle as that for penetration. Do not apply any pressure to the puncture site until the needle is completely removed.

Principle. Placing the cotton ball over the puncture site helps to prevent tissue movement as the needle is withdrawn and reduces patient discomfort. Careful withdrawal prevents further tissue damage.

15. **Procedural Step.** Apply pressure with the cotton ball. Elevate the patient's arm or have the patient bend the arm at the elbow until a clot forms. Apply an adhesive bandage if needed. The medical assistant should stay with the patient until the bleeding has stopped.

Principle. Elevating the arm or bending it at the elbow decreases the amount of blood in the arm and reduces its leakage from the puncture site either externally or internally. Internal leakage into the tissues could result in a hematoma.

16. **Procedural Step.** Remove the vacuum tube from the plastic holder. Leave the rubber stopper in place. If the vacuum tube contains an anticoagulant, it must be mixed immediately by gently inverting the tube 8 to 10 times. Do not shake the tube.

Principle. The blood can be stored in the vacuum tube until it is ready to be tested. The tube containing an anticoagulant must be inverted immediately to prevent the blood from clotting. Careful mixing of the blood with the anticoagulant prevents hemolysis.

17. **Procedural Step.** Properly dispose of the equipment.

Principle. Proper disposal of the equipment protects the medical assistant from being pricked by a contaminated needle.

18. **Procedural Step.** Remove gloves and wash the hands.

19. **Procedural Step.** Record the procedure. Include the patient's name, the date and time, which arm and vein were used, and any unusual patient reaction. Be sure to include your initials next to the recording.

20. **PROCEDURAL STEP.** Test, transfer, or store the blood specimen according to the medical office policy. If the specimen is to be transported to an outside laboratory for testing, record this information in the patient's chart, including the types of tests ordered.

Note: Multiple blood specimen tubes may be collected using the vacuum tube method. A specially designated double-pointed needle with a rubber sheath over the posterior needle, known as a multiple-draw needle, is available. The sheath automatically covers the needle opening during switching from one vacuum tube to another. This prevents leakage and loss of blood during changing of tubes. Tubes without additives (e.g., red-stoppered tubes) should be filled first, before those with additives (e.g., lavender, gray, green and light blue stoppered tubes). When the needle is withdrawn from the patient's arm, the last tube should be left attached to the posterior needle and the entire assembly pulled out as a unit.

Record data below.

DATE	TIME	PATIENT'S NAME	RECORDING

PROCEDURE 11-2
VENIPUNCTURE USING THE SYRINGE METHOD

1. **PROCEDURAL STEP.** Wash the hands.

2. **PROCEDURAL STEP.** Assemble the equipment. The equipment needed includes **clean gloves,** a **tourniquet,** an **alcohol prep,** a **sterile syringe and needle of appropriate size, sterile cotton balls,** a **glass vacuum tube,** and an **adhesive bandage.** Label the tube with the patient's name, the date, and your initials. If the specimen will be tested at an outside laboratory, complete a laboratory request form.
PRINCIPLE. Proper labeling of blood specimens avoids mix-up of specimens.

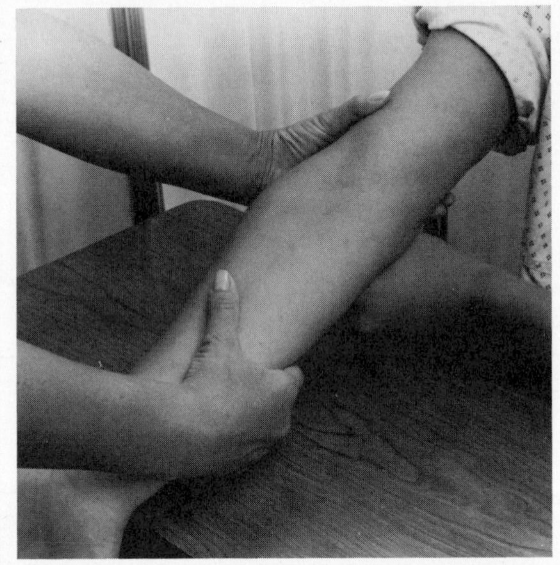

3. **PROCEDURAL STEP.** Prepare the equipment, making sure to keep the needle and inside of the syringe sterile. Break the seal on the syringe by moving the plunger back and forth several times. Loosen the cap on the needle and check to make sure that the hub is screwed tightly into the syringe.

4. **PROCEDURAL STEP.** Identify the patient and explain the procedure.
PRINCIPLE. Venipuncture is often a frightening experience for the patient and reassurance should be offered to help reduce apprehension.

5. **PROCEDURAL STEP.** Position the patient. The patient should be seated comfortably in a chair with an armrest. Palpate the veins of both arms to determine the best vein to use. It is also helpful to ask the patient which arm has been used in the past to obtain blood. The arm with the vein selected for the venipuncture should be extended and placed on the armrest with the antecubital veins facing anteriorly. The arm should be supported by a rolled towel or by having the patient place the fist of his other hand under the elbow.
PRINCIPLE. This position allows for easy access to the antecubital veins. It is more convenient for the medical assistant to stand in front of the patient during the procedure.

6. **PROCEDURAL STEP.** Apply the tourniquet as follows:

Velcro tourniquet. Hold each end of the tourniquet with one hand. Position the tourniquet 2 to 3 inches above the bend in the elbow. Wrap the tourniquet around the arm and secure it with the Velcro fastener.

Rubber tourniquet. Hold each end of the tourniquet with one hand and pull the ends away from each other to create tension. Position the tourniquet 2 to 3 inches above the bend in the elbow while you maintain proper tension. Secure the tourniquet with a half-bow.

The tourniquet should have enough tension to impede the venous flow. Ask the patient to clench the fist of the arm to which the tourniquet has been applied. Never leave the tourniquet on for more than 60 seconds at a time.

PRINCIPLE. Securing the rubber tourniquet with a half-bow allows for easy removal of it with one hand. The correct tourniquet tension must be obtained. A tourniquet that is too loose fails to cause the veins to stand out in order to be palpated. A tourniquet that is too tight obstructs the arterial blood flow as well as the venous flow. Obstructing the arterial flow results in a blood specimen that may produce inaccurate test results.

The combined effect of the pressure of the tourniquet and the clenched fist should cause the antecubital veins to stand out so that accurate selection of a puncture site can be made. Leaving the tourniquet on for more than 60 seconds will be uncomfortable for the patient and may alter the test results.

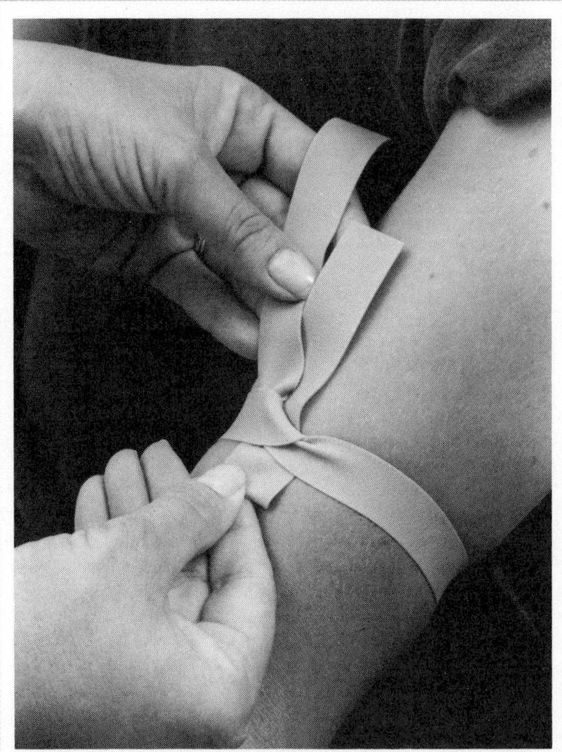

7. **PROCEDURAL STEP.** Palpate the vein again. At times, the medical assistant will not be able to see the vein but will be able to palpate it. The vein should not be used unless it can be palpated.

PRINCIPLE. The median cephalic vein is generally the best vein to use. The veins on either side of the arm tend to roll and are difficult to stabilize. The vein does not have to be visualized in order to be a good selection.

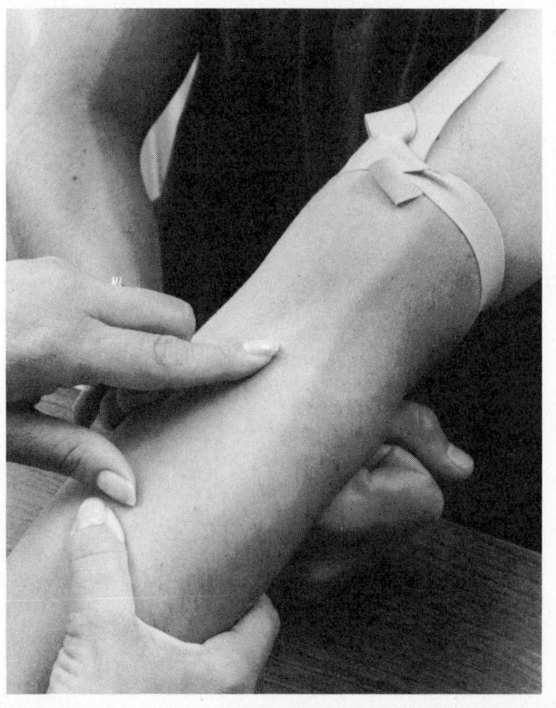

8. **PROCEDURAL STEP.** Cleanse the area with an antiseptic, such as 70 per cent ethyl alcohol. Cleansing should be done in a circular motion starting from the inside and moving away from the puncture site. Allow the site to dry and do not touch the area after cleansing.

PRINCIPLE. Using a circular motion helps to carry foreign particles away from the puncture site. The site must be allowed to dry, because alcohol entering the blood specimen contaminates it and leads to inaccurate test results. In addition, the alcohol causes the patient to experience a stinging sensation. Touching the area causes contamination and the cleansing process has to be repeated.

9. **PROCEDURAL STEP.** Apply gloves and remove the cap from the needle. Hold the syringe by placing the thumb and index finger of the dominant hand near the needle hub while supporting the barrel of the syringe with the three remaining fingers. The needle should be positioned with the bevel facing up. Place the thumb of the nondominant hand approximately 1 to 2 inches below the puncture site.

PRINCIPLE. Gloves are a precaution that provides a barrier against contaminated blood. The thumb helps to hold the skin taut for easier entry and to stabilize the vein to be punctured.

Continued

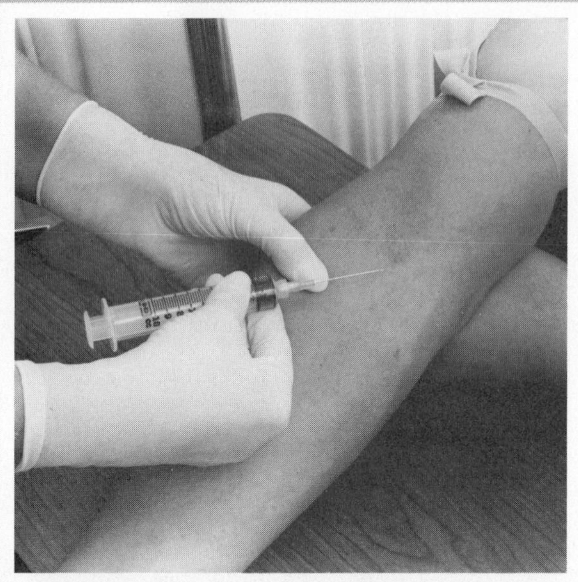

10. **PROCEDURAL STEP.** Position the syringe at a 15-degree angle to the arm. Make sure the needle points in the same direction as the vein to be entered.

PRINCIPLE. An angle of less than 15 degrees may cause the needle to enter above the vein, preventing puncture. An angle of more than 15 degrees may cause the needle to go through the vein by puncturing its posterior wall. This could result in a hematoma.

11. **PROCEDURAL STEP.** With one continuous motion, enter the skin and then the vein. The needle should penetrate the skin approximately ¼ to ½ inch below the place where the vein is to be entered. The patient may need reassurance because this step may be painful. Blood may spontaneously enter the top of the syringe. If not, pull back gently on the plunger until blood begins to enter the syringe. Do not move the needle once the venipuncture has been made.

PRINCIPLE. Using one continuous motion helps to reduce tissue damage. The medical assistant will feel a lack of resistance once the vein has been penetrated. Moving the needle will cause patient discomfort.

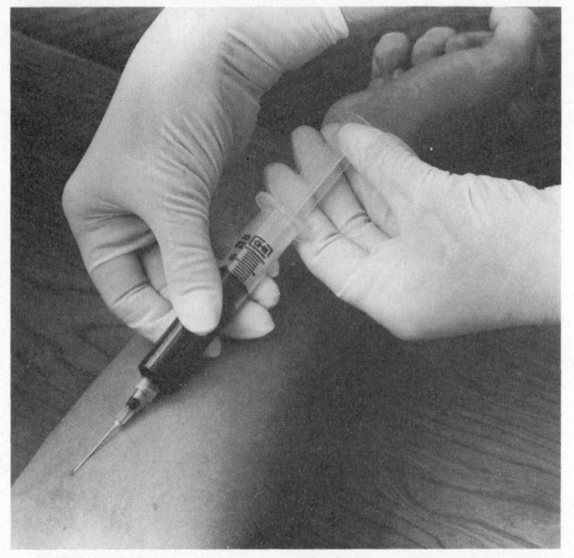

12. **PROCEDURAL STEP.** Remove the desired amount of blood by pulling back slowly and gently on the plunger.

PRINCIPLE. Pulling back on the plunger causes a suction effect, which draws the blood into the syringe. The blood should be withdrawn slowly from the vein to prevent hemolysis.

13. **PROCEDURAL STEP.** Remove the tourniquet and ask the patient to unclench the fist.

PRINCIPLE. The tourniquet must be removed before the needle. Otherwise, the pressure on the vein from the tourniquet could cause internal and external bleeding around the puncture site.

14. **PROCEDURAL STEP.** Place a dry sterile cotton ball over the puncture site and withdraw the needle slowly and at the same angle as that for penetration. Do not apply any pressure to the puncture site until the needle is completely removed.

PRINCIPLE. Placing the cotton ball over the puncture site helps to prevent tissue movement as the needle is withdrawn and reduces patient discomfort. Careful withdrawal prevents further tissue damage.

15. **PROCEDURAL STEP.** Apply pressure to the puncture site with the cotton ball. Elevate the patient's arm or have the patient bend the arm at the elbow until a clot forms. Apply an adhesive bandage if needed. The medical assistant should stay with the patient until the bleeding has stopped.

PRINCIPLE. Elevating the arm or bending it at the elbow decreases the amount of blood in the arm and reduces its leakage from the puncture site either externally or internally. Internal leakage into the tissues could result in a hematoma.

16. **PROCEDURAL STEP.** Transfer the blood to the labeled glass vacuum tube by inserting the needle through the rubber stopper and allowing the vacuum to fill the tube. If the blood is added to a tube containing an anticoagulant, it must be mixed immediately by gently inverting the tube 8 to 10 times. Do not shake the tube.
PRINCIPLE. A delay in transferring the blood to the collection tube, causes clotting of the blood in the syringe. The suction action of the vacuum tube will automatically draw the blood into the tube. The tube containing an anticoagulant must immediately be inverted to prevent the blood from clotting. Shaking the tube causes hemolysis.

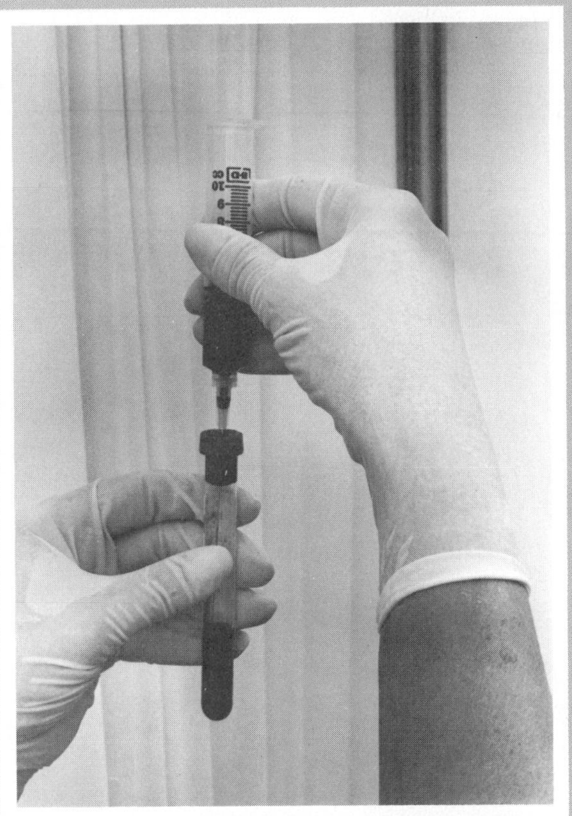

17. **PROCEDURAL STEP.** Properly dispose of the equipment.
PRINCIPLE. Proper disposal of the equipment protects the medical assistant from being pricked by a contaminated needle.

18. **PROCEDURAL STEP.** Remove gloves and wash the hands.

19. **PROCEDURAL STEP.** Record the procedure. Include the patient's name, the date and time, which arm and vein were used, and any unusual patient reaction. Be sure to include your initials next to the recording.

20. **PROCEDURAL STEP.** Test, transfer, or store the blood specimen according to the medical office policy. If the specimen is to be transported to an outside laboratory for testing, indicate this information in the patient's chart, including the types of test ordered.

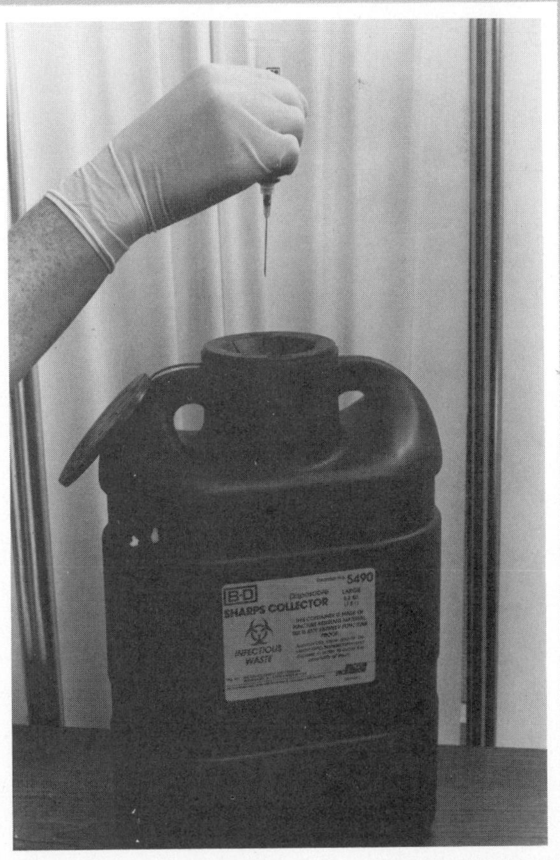

Continued

Record data below.

DATE	TIME	PATIENT'S NAME	RECORDING

Separating Serum From Whole Blood

Serum contains numerous dissolved substances such as glucose, cholesterol, lipids, sodium, potassium, chloride, antibodies, hormones, and enzymes. As a result, many laboratory tests require a serum specimen to determine whether these substances are within normal limits and also to detect the presence of any substances that should not normally be present in the serum and that, if present, indicate a pathologic condition. To perform laboratory tests on serum, it must be separated from the blood specimen, which is usually the responsibility of the medical assistant.

A tube containing no additives (red-stoppered) must be used to collect the blood specimen, to allow the specimen to separate into serum and cells. Since the amount of serum recovered is only a portion of the total specimen collected, a blood specimen must be drawn that is 2½ times the amount required for the test. For example, if 2 ml of serum is required, a 5-ml blood specimen must be collected; if 4 ml of serum is required, a 10-ml tube is collected, and if 6 ml of serum is required, a 15-ml tube is needed.

Once the blood specimen has been collected, the tube must be allowed to stand at room temperature in an upright position for 30 to 45 minutes before being centrifuged. The purpose of this is to allow clot formation, which will yield more serum from the specimen. If the specimen is centrifuged immediately after collection, the clotting factors do not have an opportunity to settle down into the cell layer to form a whole blood clot. The result of this is the formation of a *fibrin clot* in the serum layer consisting of the clotting factors. A fibrin clot is a spongy substance that occupies space, interfering with adequate serum collection. However, the blood specimen should not be allowed to stand for longer than 1 hour, because changes will take place in the specimen that will lead to inaccurate test results. Once clot formation has occurred, the specimen is centrifuged and the serum is then removed from the cells and placed in a separate transfer tube. It is important that proper technique be employed in removing the serum, to avoid disturbing the cell layer and drawing red blood cells into the serum. If cells do enter the pipet, the entire specimen must be recentrifuged.

Once the serum has been removed from the blood specimen, the medical assistant should hold the specimen up to good light to inspect it for the presence of intact red blood cells or hemolyzed blood; in both cases, the specimen has a reddish appearance. Any specimen having a reddish appearance must be recentrifuged. If the specimen contains intact red blood cells, they settle to the bottom of the tube and the serum can be removed. If the blood is hemolyzed, recentrifugation will not make the red color disappear because the red blood cells have ruptured and released hemoglobin into the serum. Hemolyzed serum is unsuitable for laboratory tests because the results will be inaccurate; therefore, another blood specimen must be collected. Procedure 11-3 presents the method for separating serum from whole blood using a conventional vacuum tube.

Serum Separator Vacuum Tubes

A serum separator tube is a specially designed glass vacuum tube used to facilitate the collection of a serum specimen. This type of tube is identified by its red and slate-gray stopper and is used for both the collection and separation of blood. The serum separator tube contains a thixotropic gel, which is in a solid state in the bottom of the unused tube (Fig. 11–4*A*). The blood specimen is collected and processed following Procedure 11-1, Venipuncture Using the Vacuum Tube Method. The specimen must be allowed to stand in an upright position for means of proper clot formation and then centrifuged as previously described. During centrifugation, the gel temporarily becomes fluid and moves to the dividing point between the serum and cells, where it re-forms into a solid gel, thus serving as a physical and chemical barrier between the serum and cells (Fig. 11–4*B*). The serum can be transported or stored in the separator tube; however, the medical assistant must carefully inspect the tube to ensure that the gel barrier is firmly attached to the glass wall. If a complete barrier has not formed, the serum specimen must be placed in a transfer tube to prevent leaching of substances from the cell layer into the serum, thereby affecting the accuracy of the test results.

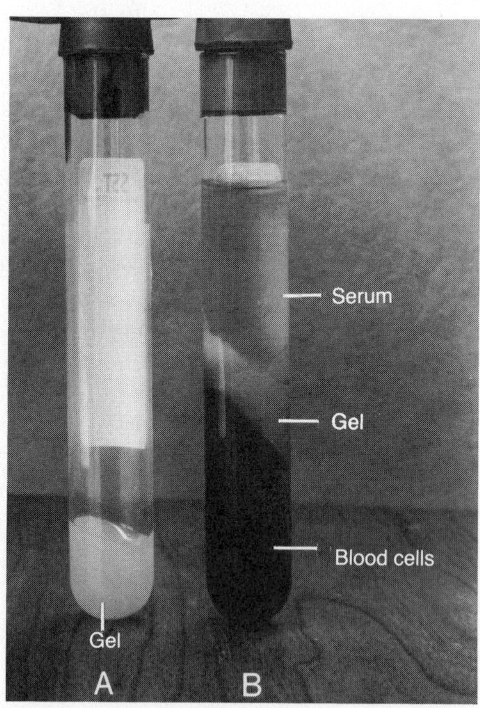

FIGURE 11–4. Serum separator tubes. *A*, A tube containing the thixotropic gel in the bottom of the unused tube. *B*, A tube that has been used to collect a venous blood specimen. During centrifugation the gel temporarily becomes fluid and moves to the dividing point between the serum and cells.

PROCEDURE 11-3

SEPARATING SERUM FROM WHOLE BLOOD

1. **PROCEDURAL STEP.** Collect the blood specimen following the venipuncture procedure. A tube containing no additives (red-stoppered) should be used to collect the specimen. The size tube selected should have a capacity of 2½ times the amount of serum required. Be sure to label *both* the red-stoppered tube and the transfer tube with the patient's name, the date, and your initials. In addition, the transfer tube should bear the word *serum*. Allow the tube to fill until the vaccum is exhausted.
   PRINCIPLE. In order to obtain serum, a tube containing no additives must be used. The tube must be allowed to fill completely in order to obtain the proper amount of serum. Several different types of specimens such as serum, plasma, and urine are straw colored; therefore, the transfer tube containing serum must be labeled as such to avoid confusion and mix-up among these specimens.

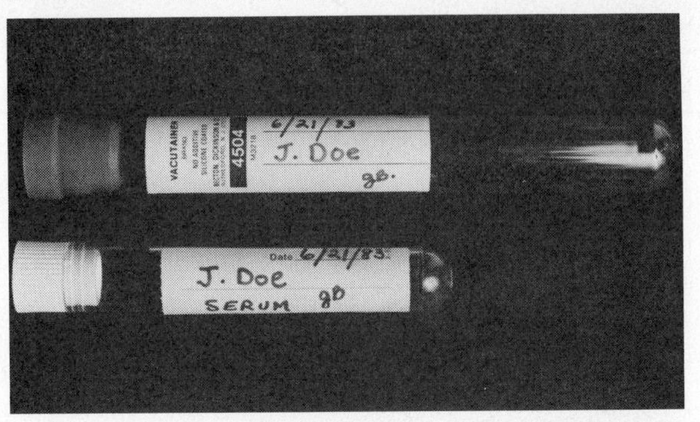

2. **PROCEDURAL STEP.** Place the blood specimen tube in an upright position for 30 to 45 minutes at room temperature. Do not remove the stopper from the tube, to prevent evaporation of the serum sample.
   PRINCIPLE. Specimens must be placed in an upright position and allowed to stand to permit clot formation, which will yield more serum from the specimen. Evaporation of the sample will lead to falsely elevated test results.

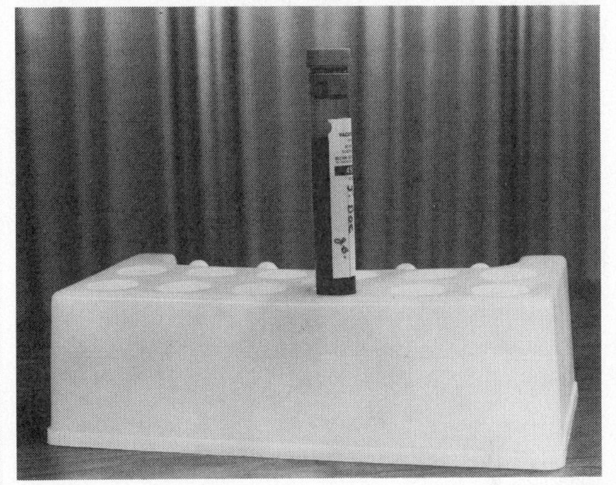

3. **PROCEDURAL STEP.** Place the specimen in the centrifuge, stopper end up. Balance the specimen with the same type and weight of tube or another specimen tube. Make sure the tube is stoppered to prevent evaporation of the sample during centrifugation. Centrifuge the specimen for 10 to 15 minutes.
   PRINCIPLE. Centrifuging packs the cells and causes them to settle to the bottom of the tube, thereby yielding more serum. If the centrifuge is not balanced, it may vibrate and move across the table top. An unbalanced centrifuge may also cause the specimen tube to break.

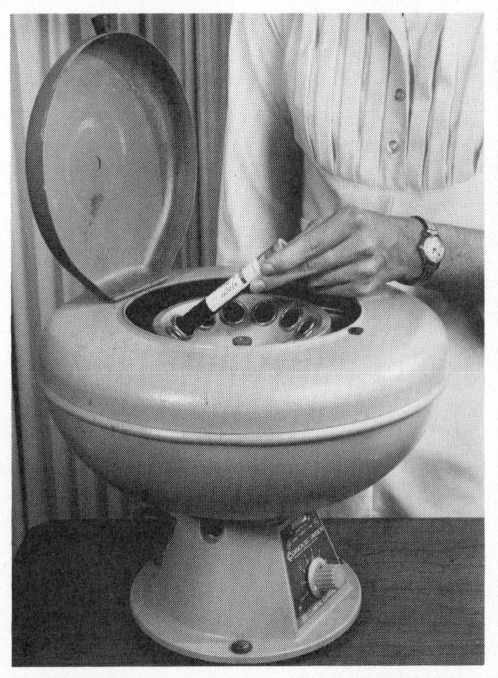

Continued

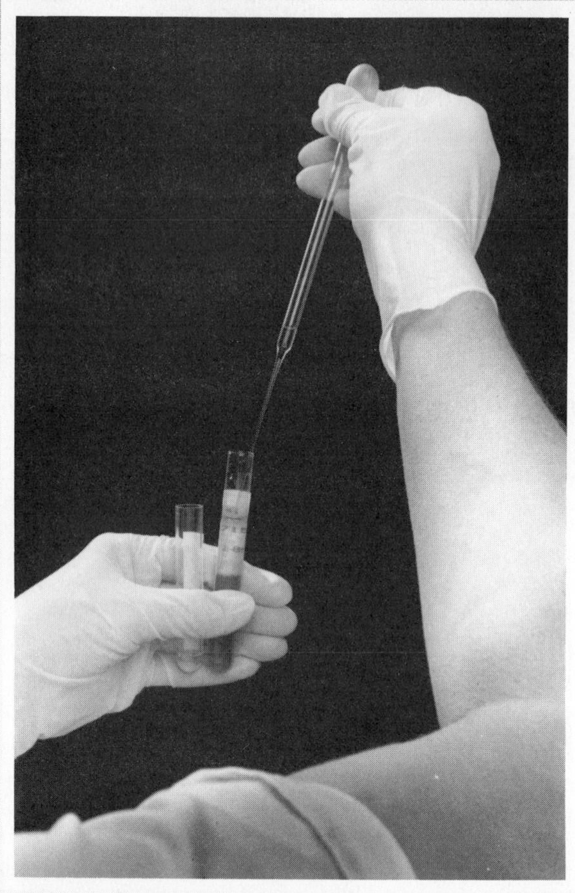

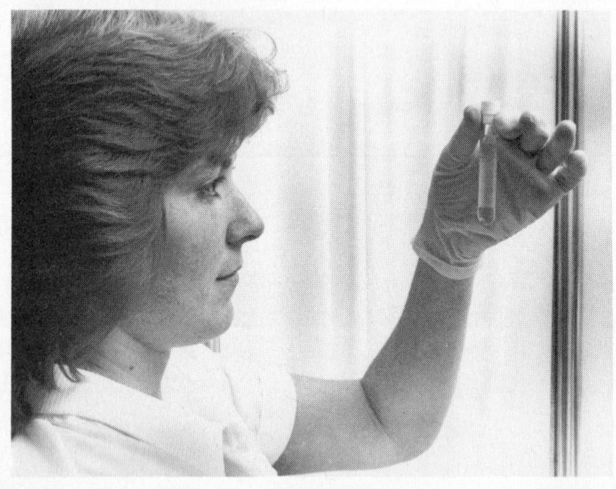

4. **Procedural step.** Carefully remove the tube from the centrifuge without disturbing the contents.

Principle. Disturbing the contents may cause the cells to enter the serum, and the specimen will need to be recentrifuged.

5. **Procedural step.** Apply gloves and carefully remove the stopper from the tube pointing the stopper away from you. Squeeze the rubber bulb of the pipet to push the air out; then insert it into the serum. Place the tip of the pipet against the side of the tube approximately ¼ inch above the cell layer. Using mechanical suction, pipet serum from the cells. Do not allow the tip of the pipet to touch the cell layer.

Principle. The air should be removed from the bulb before inserting the pipet into the serum to prevent disturbance of the cell layer. If the cell layer is disturbed, red blood cells will enter the serum and the specimen will need to be recentrifuged. Pointing the stopper away prevents accidental spraying or splashing of the specimen on the medical assistant.

6. **Procedural step.** Transfer the serum in the pipet to the transfer tube. Continue pipetting until as much serum as possible is removed without disturbing the cell layer. Tightly cap the transfer tube to prevent sample evaporation.

7. **Procedural step.** Hold the specimen up to the light and examine it for the presence of hemolysis. Make sure the proper amount of serum has been obtained.

Principle. Hemolyzed serum is unsuitable for laboratory testing.

8. **Procedural step.** Properly dispose of equipment, remove gloves, and wash hands.

9. **Procedural step.** Test, transfer, or store the specimen according to the medical office policy.

Record data below.

DATE	TIME	PATIENT'S NAME	RECORDING

Separating Plasma From Whole Blood

At times a plasma specimen may be required for the performance of a laboratory test. The procedure for separating plasma from whole blood is essentially the same as that for separating serum from whole blood with minor variances, which are described here.

A tube containing an anticoagulant must be used to obtain plasma. The medical assistant should check the laboratory directory or the medical office laboratory procedures manual to determine the type of anticoagulant to be used; it is usually specified by the color of the tube stopper. The tube used to collect the specimen *and* the transfer tube should be properly labeled with the patient's name, the date, and the medical assistant's initials. In addition, the transfer tube should bear the word *plasma.*

As with serum, a blood specimen must be collected that is 2½ times the amount required for the test. Before collecting the specimen, the vacuum tube should be tapped just below the stopper to release any of the anticoagulant that may have adhered to the stopper. It is important to allow the specimen to fill to the exhaustion of the vacuum to ensure the proper ratio of anticoagulant to blood, which, in turn, will ensure accurate test results. Immediately after drawing the specimen, invert the tube 8 to 10 times to mix the anticoagulant with the blood specimen. The specimen is then placed in a centrifuge with the stopper on for 10 to 15 minutes. (The specimen does not need to stand before it is centrifuged.) Centrifuging the specimen packs the blood cells and causes it to separate into three layers: a top layer of plasma, a middle layer termed the buffy coat, and a bottom layer of red blood cells. The plasma is then separated from the blood specimen using the same procedure as that outlined in the separation of serum from whole blood. On the laboratory request form, the medical assistant should indicate the color of the tube stopper (e.g., lavender, gray, green, and light blue) into which the specimen was originally drawn.

Study Questions

1. What layers does blood separate into when an anticoagulant is added to the specimen?
2. What layers does blood separate into when an anticoagulant has *not* been added to the specimen?
3. How are each of the following specimens obtained: clotted blood, serum, whole blood, and plasma?
4. What guidelines should be followed to prevent hemolysis of a blood specimen?

12

Blood Banking

CHAPTER OUTLINE

The Components and Function of Blood
Blood Antigens
Blood Antibodies
The Rh Blood Group System
Antigen and Antibody Reactions
Agglutination and Blood Typing

COMPETENCIES

After completing this chapter, you should be able to demonstrate the proper procedure to perform the following:

1. Determine the ABO blood type of a blood specimen and record the results.
2. Determine the Rh blood type of a blood specimen and record the results.

LEARNING OBJECTIVES

After completing this chapter, you should be able to do the following:

1. Define the terms listed in the vocabulary.
2. Name the two parts of the blood and what is contained in each.
3. State the functions of the three types of blood cells.
4. Explain why the ABO and Rh blood grouping systems are the ones most commonly tested for in the medical laboratory.
5. Explain why the body will not produce a blood antibody against its own type of antigen.
6. Identify the location of the blood antigens and antibodies.
7. Explain what occurs during the antigen-antibody reaction and how it can be a threat to life.
8. Tell how the blood antigen-antibody reaction is used as the basis for blood typing in vitro.
9. List the antigens and antibodies that are present in each of the following blood types: A, B, AB, and O.
10. Explain the difference between Rh+ and Rh− blood.
11. Explain the principles underlying each step in the blood typing procedure.

• VOCABULARY •

agglutination (ah-gloo" ti-na' shun)—Clumping of blood cells.

antiserum (an" ti-se' rum) (pl. antisera)—A serum that contains antibodies.

blood antibody (blud an' ti-bode)—A protein present in the blood plasma that is capable of combining with its corresponding blood antigen to produce an antigen-antibody reaction.

blood antigen (blud an' ti-jen)—A protein present on the surface of red blood cells that determines the blood type of an individual.

donor (do' ner)—One who furnishes something such as blood, tissue, or organs to be used in another person.

erythrocyte (ĕ-rith' ro-sīt)—Red blood cell.

gene (jēn)—A unit of heredity.

in vitro (in ve' tro)—Occurring in glass. Refers to tests performed under artificial conditions, as in the laboratory.

in vivo (in ve' vo)—Occurring in the living body or organism.

leukocyte (loo' ko-sīt)—White blood cell.

recipient (re-sip' e-ent)—One who receives something, such as a blood transfusion, from a donor.

thrombocyte (throm' bo-sīt)—Platelet.

The medical assistant may be involved in recording a patient's blood type in the chart. She should have a basic knowledge of blood types and an appreciation of the importance of this area, which can be utilized for patient education.

The Components and Function of Blood

Blood consists of two parts: liquid and solid. The liquid portion of the blood, consisting of a clear yellowish fluid, is known as the *plasma* and makes up approximately 55 per cent of the total blood volume. The function of the plasma is to transport nutrients to the tissues of the body to nourish and sustain them. The plasma picks up wastes from the tissues, which are eliminated through the kidneys. The plasma also transports antibodies, enzymes, and hormones to help regulate normal body functioning.

The solid portion of the blood consists of three different types of cells. Red blood cells, or *erythrocytes,* function in transporting oxygen to the tissues of the body. The oxygen is picked up in the lungs and transported in the erythrocytes by a compound known as hemoglobin. Carbon dioxide is removed from the tissues and transported by the erythrocytes to the lungs to be eliminated. White blood cells, or *leukocytes,* function in defense of the body. Leukocytes help to fight off invading pathogens that could cause disease. Platelets, or *thrombocytes,* function in the blood-clotting mechanism of the body. The solid portion of the blood accounts for 45 per cent of the total blood volume. The average adult body contains 5 to 6 L (10 to 12 pints) of blood.

Blood Antigens

Each individual has a blood type. Blood type depends upon the presence of certain factors, or *antigens,* on the surface of the red blood cells. Antigens consist of protein and are inherited through genes, which program the body to produce a particular antigen. If a blood antigen is present, it will appear on the surface of all the red blood cells in the body.

There are many different types of antigens that can appear in the blood. These antigens can be grouped into categories known as blood group systems. The blood group systems that are most likely to cause problems in blood transfusions and in

Type A blood:
A antigen is present

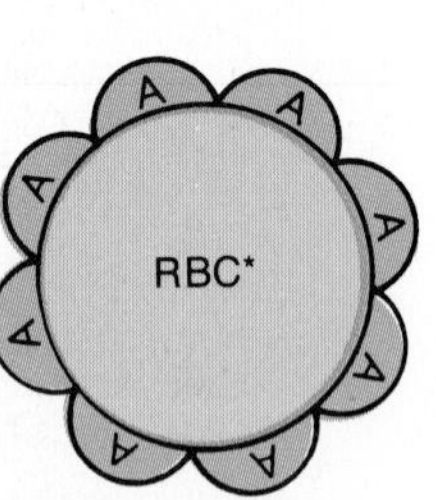

Type B blood:
B antigen is present

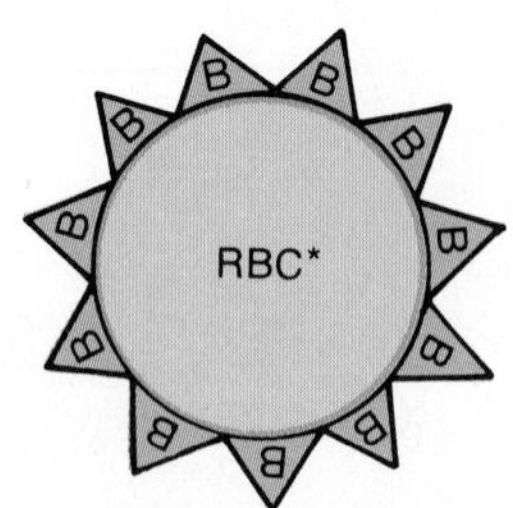

Type AB blood:
A and B antigens are both present

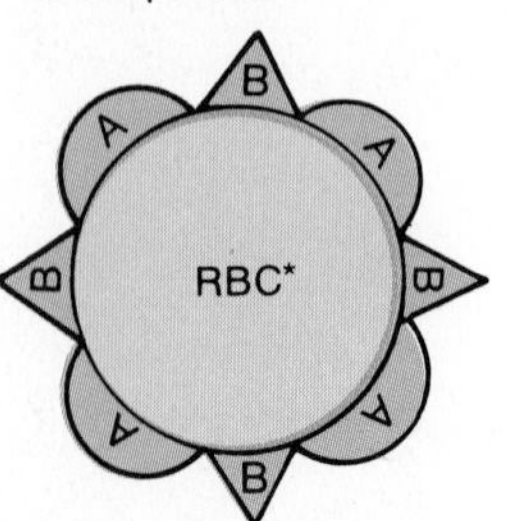

Type O blood:
Neither A nor B antigen is present

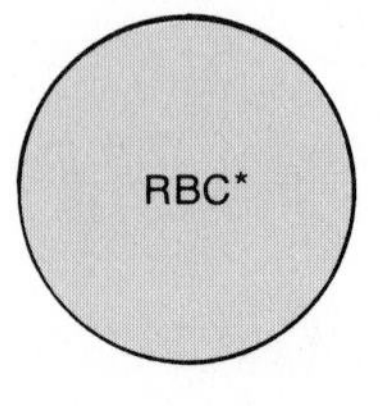

*red blood cell

FIGURE 12–1. Blood type depends upon which antigens are present on the surface of the red blood cells.

Rh disease of the newborn are the ABO and Rh blood group systems. Therefore, these are the blood group systems most commonly tested for in the medical laboratory.

Within the ABO blood group system, there are four main blood types: A, B, AB, and O. The blood type depends on which antigens are present on the surface of the red blood cells.

If the A antigen is present, the blood type is A.

If the B antigen is present, the blood type is B.

If both the A and B antigens are present, the blood type is AB.

If neither the A nor the B antigen is present, the blood type is O. Figure 12–1 helps to illustrate this principle.

Blood Antibodies

Blood antibodies are proteins that are naturally present in the plasma of the blood. An antibody is a substance that is capable of combining with an antigen. The body never produces an antibody to combine with its own blood antigen. For example, if the blood type is A, the plasma does not contain the A antibody. However, the B antibody naturally occurs in that plasma. The B antibody cannot combine with the A antigen. If a blood antigen and its corresponding antibody combine (in this case, the A antigen combining with the A antibody), a serious antigen-antibody reaction will take place that could pose a threat to life.

If the blood type is A, the plasma contains the B antibody.

If the blood type is B, the plasma contains the A antibody.

If the blood type is AB, neither the A nor the B antibody appears in the plasma.

If the blood type is O, both the A and B antibodies appear in the plasma. Remember, Type O blood has neither the A nor the B antigen on the surface of its red blood cells. The A and B antibodies appearing in the plasma would not have an A or B antigen to combine with them (Table 12–1).

Table 12–2 shows the percentage of the United States population with each blood type.

TABLE 12–1. ABO Blood Group System

BLOOD TYPE	ANTIGEN PRESENT ON THE RED BLOOD CELL	ANTIBODY PRESENT IN THE PLASMA
A	A	B
B	B	A
AB	A, B	Neither A nor B
O	Neither A or B	A, B

TABLE 12–2. Distribution of Blood Type in the United States

BLOOD TYPE	PERCENTAGE (%) OF THE POPULATION HAVING THIS BLOOD TYPE
O+	36
O−	6
A+	38
A−	6
B+	8
B−	2
AB+	3–4
AB−	0.5

The Rh Blood Group System

In 1940, Landsteiner and Wiener discovered the Rh blood group system while working with rhesus monkeys. Approximately 85 per cent of the white population has the Rh antigen present on the red blood cells and therefore has Type Rh+ blood. The remaining 15 per cent of the population does not have the Rh antigen present on the red blood cells and thus has Type Rh− blood. The Rh antibodies do not normally occur in the plasma as do the A and B antibodies.

Antigen and Antibody Reactions

When an antigen and its corresponding antibody unite, the result is the clumping, or *agglutination,* of red blood cells. Agglutination of red blood cells can be serious and even fatal if it occurs in vivo (in the living body). The clumped red blood cells cannot pass through the small tubules of the kidneys, and this may lead to kidney failure. Also, the clumping of the red blood cells eventually leads to *hemolysis,* or breakdown of the red blood cells.

Blood antigen-antibody reactions can occur if the wrong blood type is administered to an individual during a blood transfusion. If an individual with Type A blood is given a transfusion of Type B blood, the B antibody of the recipient (person receiving the blood) would combine with the B antigen of the donor (person donating the blood), and an antigen-antibody reaction would occur, resulting in agglutination of red blood cells. Therefore, we say that Type A blood is incompatible with Type B blood.

Agglutination and Blood Typing

Agglutination of red blood cells is the basis for the ABO and Rh blood typing procedure. The antigen-antibody reaction occurs in vitro, or "in glass" in the laboratory, so there is no threat to life.

To test for the ABO blood group system, a commercially prepared antiserum is used. An antiserum is a serum containing antibodies. An antiserum containing the A antibody is added to an unknown blood specimen. If the A antigen is present, it combines with the A antibody, resulting in agglutination. An antiserum containing the B antibody is added to another sample of the unknown blood. If the B antigen

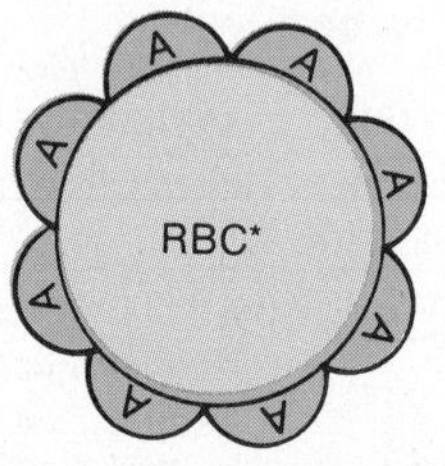
Unknown blood sample containing Type A blood:
RBC*
A

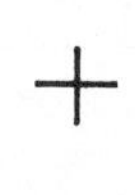

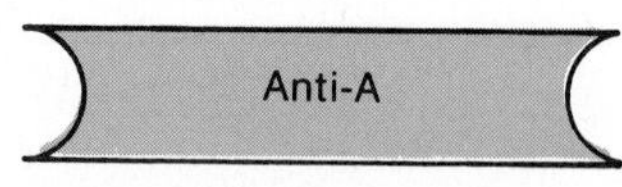
The antiserum containing the A antibody:
Anti-A

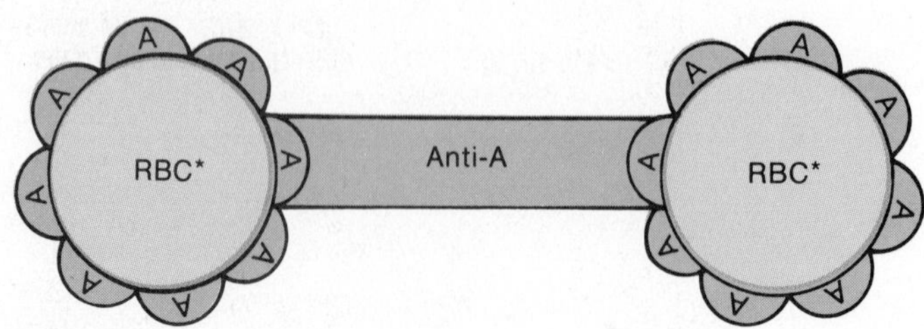
The bridge forming between the antigen and antibody represents the antigen-antibody reaction. This reaction leads to agglutination of red blood cells, which is visible to the naked eye.
RBC*
Anti-A
RBC*
A
*red blood cell

FIGURE 12–2. The antigen-antibody reaction that occurs in vitro when the unknown blood sample is Type A.

is present, it will combine with the B antibody, resulting in agglutination. If agglutination occurs in both instances, the sample is Type AB. If no agglutination occurs, this indicates the absence of blood antigens, or Type O blood. Agglutination that occurs in vitro is visible to the naked eye.

The antigen-antibody reaction that occurs when the unknown blood sample is Type A is diagrammed in Figure 12–2.

PROCEDURE 12-1
BLOOD TYPING (SLIDE TEST METHOD)

In the medical laboratory, the test tube method is the preferred method for blood typing. The medical assistant can use the slide test method to learn the relationship between blood antigens and antibodies.

The blood typing procedure may vary, depending on the particular brand of antiserum used. Be sure to read the directions that accompany the commercially prepared antiserum in case the manufacturer's procedure varies from the one shown here.

1. **PROCEDURAL STEP.** Wash the hands.
PRINCIPLE. The hands should be clean and free from contamination during blood typing.

2. **PROCEDURAL STEP.** Assemble the equipment. The equipment and supplies needed for blood typing include an **unknown blood specimen, wooden applicator sticks, clean gloves, two clean glass slides, a colored wax pencil, a rocker board (optional),** and **commercially prepared Anti-A, Anti-B, and Anti-Rh blood grouping antisera.**

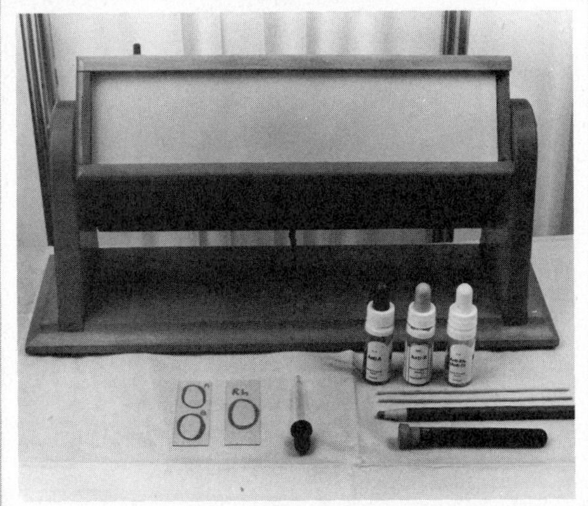

3. **PROCEDURAL STEP.** Check the expiration date of the antisera.
PRINCIPLE. The expiration date usually appears on the label of the antiserum container. Outdated antiserum may produce inaccurate test results.

4. **PROCEDURAL STEP.** Allow the antisera to reach room temperature.
PRINCIPLE. Test results are more accurate if the antisera reach room temperature before being used. *Note:* The antisera should be stored in the refrigerator at a temperature of 35 to 46°F (2 to 8°C).

5. **PROCEDURAL STEP.** Prepare the slides. The slides should be clean and free of lint or dirt. With the colored wax pencil, label the slides with the patient's name for identification. Make two large circles on one of the slides and one large circle on the other slide with the colored wax pencil. Make sure that the outline of the circles is thick enough that the blood will not be able to break through the circle. Mark the circles with the letters A, B, and Rh as indicated.
PRINCIPLE. Lint or dirt on the slides may falsely be mistaken for agglutination.

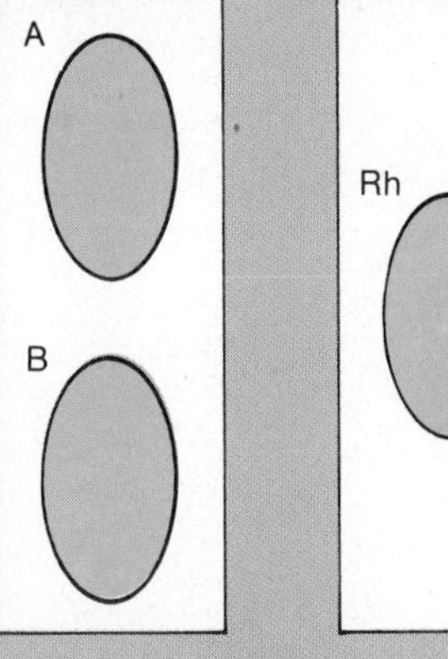

Continued

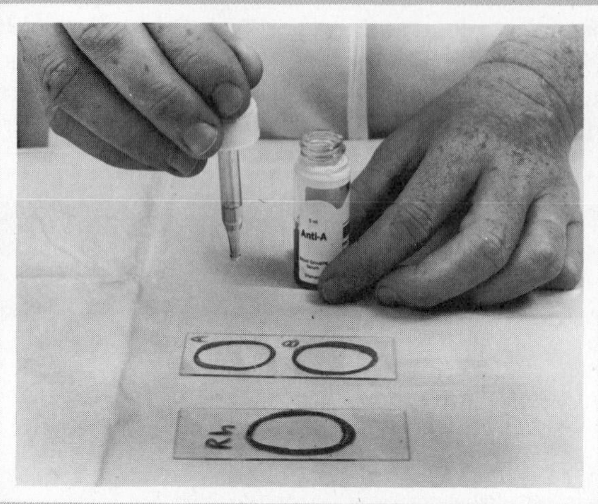

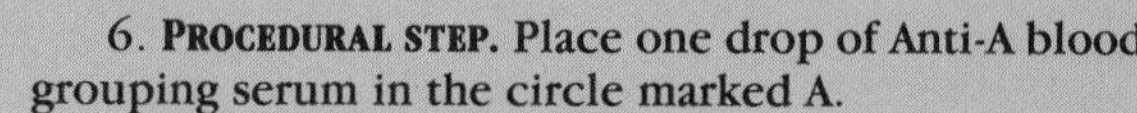

6. **Procedural step.** Place one drop of Anti-A blood grouping serum in the circle marked A.

Principle. The Anti-A blood grouping serum contains the A antibody, and internationally its code is blue.

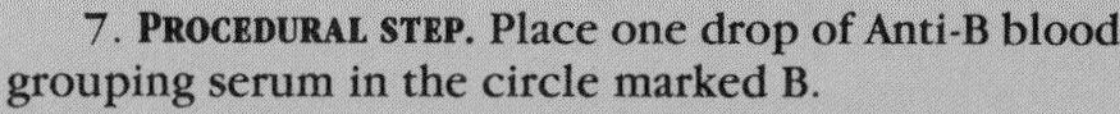

7. **Procedural step.** Place one drop of Anti-B blood grouping serum in the circle marked B.

Principle. The Anti-B blood grouping serum contains the B antibody, and internationally its code is yellow.

8. **Procedural step.** Place one drop of the Anti-Rh blood grouping serum in the circle marked Rh.

Principle. The Anti-Rh blood grouping serum contains the Rh antibody.

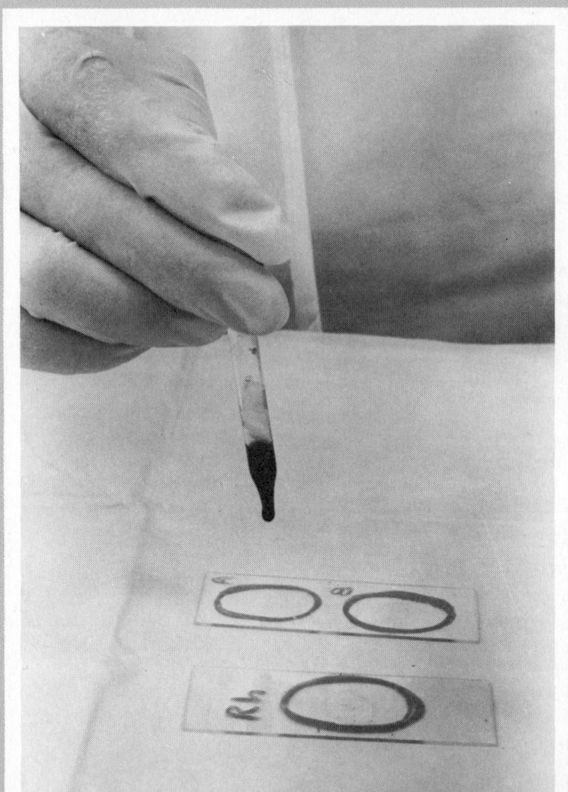

9. **Procedural step.** Apply gloves and place one drop of the unknown blood specimen beside the drop of antiserum in each circle.

Principle. Gloves are a precaution that provides a barrier against contaminated blood. It is preferable to use freshly drawn blood. All blood specimens from patients should be treated with care, because they may be potentially hazardous.

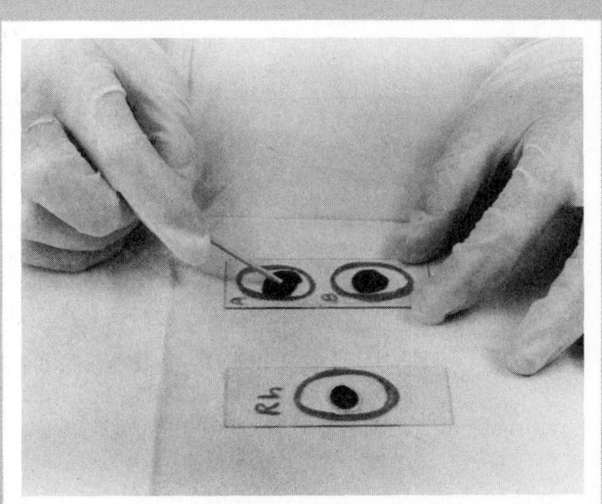

10. **PROCEDURAL STEP.** Quickly mix each drop of blood and antiserum together with an applicator stick. A separate stick should be used to mix the blood and antiserum in each circle. Mix the blood over an area about ¾ inch in diameter, keeping within the confines of the wax circle. It may be difficult to interpret the test results if a smaller area is used. Properly dispose of the applicator sticks.

PRINCIPLE. Separate applicator sticks should be used to prevent the blood and antiserum of one circle from being transferred to another circle, leading to inaccurate test results. It is permissible to use opposite ends of the applicator stick for stirring.

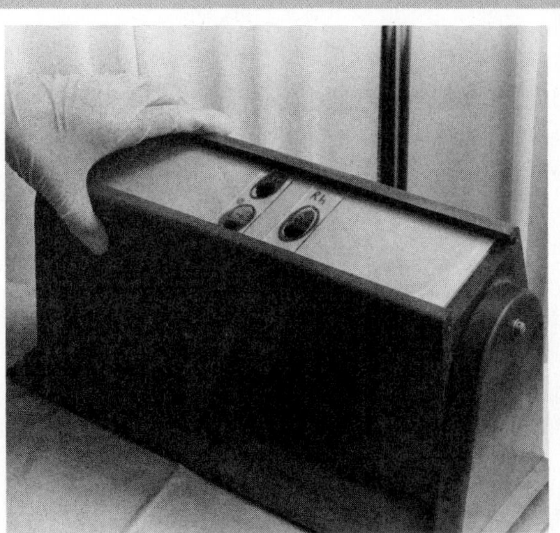

11. **PROCEDURAL STEP.** Rock the slides, on the rocker board or by hand, for 1 minute. The test results should not be read until the slides have been rocked for 1 minute but must be read before 2 minutes have elapsed.

PRINCIPLE. The slides must be rocked for 1 minute to give any antigens present on the red blood cells a chance to combine with the appropriate A, B, or Rh antibody contained in the antisera. The test results must be read before 2 minutes have elapsed because the antiserum and blood mixture will begin to dry up and resemble agglutination, which could result in a false-positive reaction.

Continued

12. **PROCEDURAL STEP.** Observe the slides for agglutination after 1 minute has elapsed.

PRINCIPLE. Agglutination indicates that an antigen-antibody reaction has taken place and a particular antigen is on the surface of the red blood cells. The absence of agglutination indicates that the antibody contained in the commercially prepared antiserum did not find an antigen to combine with, indicating the absence of the antigen on the surface of the red blood cells. Use the slide diagram to help interpret results and to determine the correct blood type of the unknown blood specimen.

13. **PROCEDURAL STEP.** Properly dispose of the slides. Remove gloves and wash hands.

14. **PROCEDURAL STEP.** Record the results. Include the patient's name, the date and time, and the blood type of the specimen. Include your initials next to the recording.

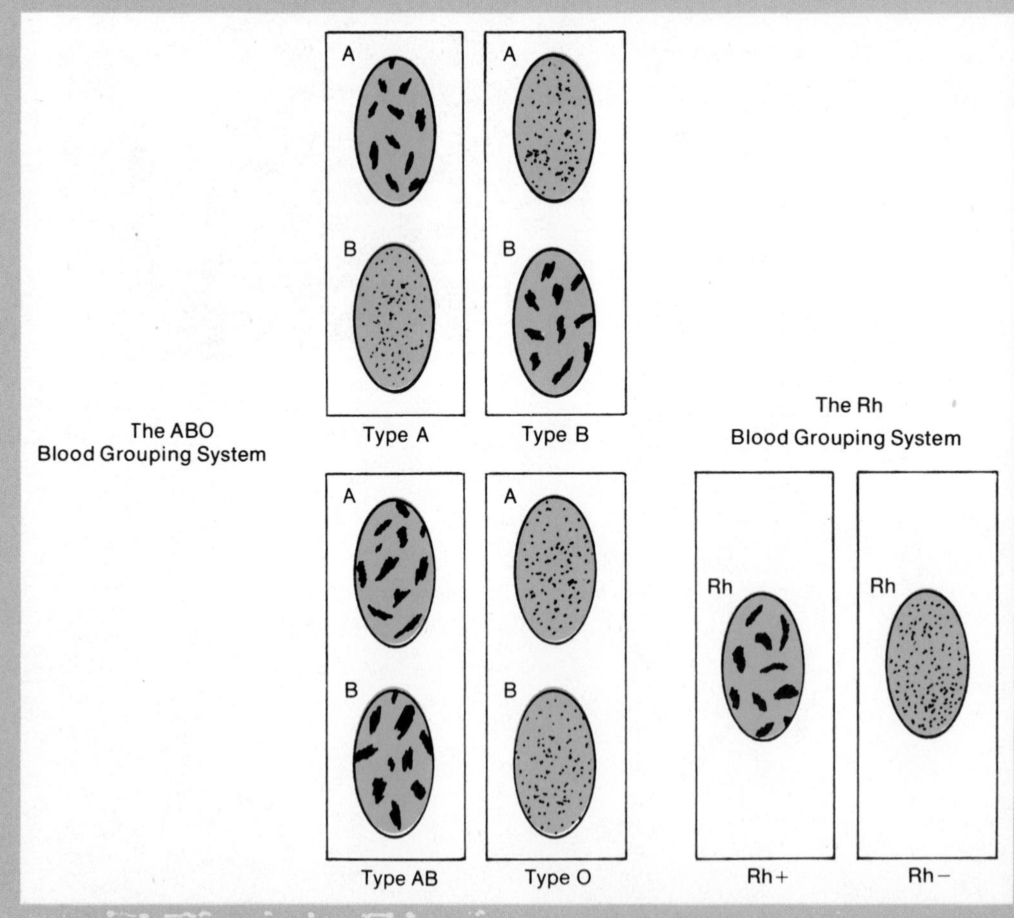

Record data below.

DATE	TIME	PATIENT'S NAME	BLOOD TYPE

Study Questions

1. What is the function of each of the three types of blood cells (erythrocytes, leukocytes, and thrombocytes)?
2. Where are the blood antigens located?
3. Where are the blood antibodies located?
4. What antigens and antibodies are present in each of the following blood types: A, B, AB, and O?

13

HEMATOLOGY AND BLOOD CHEMISTRY

CHAPTER OUTLINE

HEMATOLOGIC LABORATORY TESTS

Hematology
Erythrocytes
Leukocytes
Thrombocytes
Plasma
Capillary Blood Specimen
Hematocrit
White Blood Cell Count
Red Blood Cell Count
White Blood Cell Differential Count
Hemoglobin

BLOOD CHEMISTRY TESTS

Blood Chemistry
Cholesterol
Blood Urea Nitrogen (BUN)
Blood Glucose
Fasting Blood Sugar (FBS)
Two-Hour Postprandial Blood Sugar
Glucose Tolerance Test
Blood Glucose Measurement with a Glucose Meter
Self Monitoring of Blood Glucose

INTRODUCTION

Hematologic and blood chemistry laboratory tests are often performed in the medical office. Over the past decade, advances in automated analyzers specially designed for use in the medical office have made this possible. Automated analyzers perform laboratory tests in a very short period of time with accurate test results. Each automated analyzer is accompanied by a detailed instruction manual explaining its operation, test parameters, care, and maintenance.

The procedure for most of the tests in this chapter are presented using the manual method because each step in the procedure requires a physical manipulation and the application of clinical laboratory theory. If the medical assistant understands the manual procedure, he or she will also understand what is occurring when an automated analyzer is operating. The material presented in this chapter on blood testing is intended only to serve as a basic guide for the medical assistant and should be supplemented by much well-supervised practice in a classroom laboratory and/or the medical office.

This chapter is divided into two units: The first presents hematologic laboratory tests, and the second presents blood chemistry tests. Each unit has separate competencies, learning objectives, vocabulary lists, procedures, and study questions.

• VOCABULARY •

ameboid movement (ah-me'boid moov'ment)—Movement used by leukocytes that permits them to propel themselves from the capillaries out into the tissues.

anemia (ah-ne'me-ah)—A condition in which there is a decrease in the number of erythrocytes or in the amount of hemoglobin in the blood.

bilirubin (bil"i-roo'bin)—An orange-colored bile pigment produced by the breakdown of heme from the hemoglobin molecule.

diapedesis (di"ah-pĕ-de'sis)—The ameboid movement of blood cells (especially leukocytes) through the wall of a capillary and out into the tissues.

hematology (he"mah-tol'o-je)—The study of blood and blood-forming tissues.

hemocytometer (he"mo-si-tom'ĕ-ter)—An instrument used to count blood cells.

hemoglobin (he"mo-glo'bin)—The iron-containing pigment of erythrocytes that transports oxygen in the body.

hemolysis (he-mol'i-sis)—The breakdown of erythrocytes with the release of hemoglobin into the plasma.

leukocytosis (loo"ko-si-to'sis)—An abnormal increase in the number of white blood cells (above 10,000 per cubic millimeter of blood).

leukopenia (loo"ko-pe'ne-ah)—An abnormal decrease in the number of white blood cells (below 5,000 per cubic millimeter of blood).

oxyhemoglobin (ok"si-he"mo-glo'bin)—Hemoglobin that has combined with oxygen.

phagocytosis (fag"o-si-to'sis)—The engulfing and destruction of foreign particles, such as bacteria, by special cells called phagocytes.

pipet (pi-pet')—A glass tube used to measure and/or transfer small quantities of a liquid by drawing it into the tube through mechanical suction (can also be spelled pipette).

polycythemia (pol"e-si-the'me-ah)—A disorder in which there is an increase in the red cell mass.

COMPETENCIES

After completing this unit, you should be able to demonstrate the proper procedure to perform the following:

1. Obtain a capillary blood specimen using a lancet.
2. Obtain a capillary blood specimen using an automatic lancet device.
3. Perform a hematocrit determination, and record the results using the microhematocrit method.
4. Perform a manual white blood cell count, and record the results.
5. Perform a differential cell count and record the results.
6. Perform a hemoglobin determination, and record the results using an automated reflectance photometer and instruction manual.

LEARNING OBJECTIVES

After completing the unit, you should be able to do the following:

1. Define the terms listed in the vocabulary.
2. List the tests included in a complete blood count (CBC).
3. Describe the shape of an erythrocyte and explain how it acquires this shape.
4. Describe the composition of hemoglobin and explain its function.
5. Describe the normal appearance of leukocytes and explain how they work to fight infection in the body.
6. Explain the function of plasma and list the solutes found in the plasma.
7. State the normal value or range for each of the following hematologic tests: hematocrit, hemoglobin, red and white blood cell counts, and the differential cell count.
8. State the purpose of the hematocrit, and list the layers the blood separates into after it has been centrifuged to obtain a hematocrit reading.
9. Explain the purpose of the differential cell count, and list and describe the appearance of each of the five types of white blood cells.
10. List two methods used to measure hemoglobin concentration.
11. Explain the principle underlying each step in the hematologic testing procedures.

Hematologic Laboratory Tests

Hematology

Hematology involves the study of blood, including the morphologic appearance, function, and diseases of the blood and blood-forming tissues. As discussed in Chapter 12, the blood is made up of two main components—plasma and cells (erythrocytes, leukocytes, and thrombocytes).

Laboratory analysis in hematology concerns the examination of blood for the purpose of detecting pathologic conditions. It includes performing blood cell counts, evaluating the clotting ability of the blood, and identifying cell types. These tests are valuable tools that allow the physician to determine whether each of the blood components falls within its normal value or range. Examples of hematologic tests include the white blood cell count, red blood cell count, differential white blood cell count, hemoglobin, hematocrit, prothrombin time, erythrocyte sedimentation rate, and the platelet count. Refer to Table 13-1 for a summary of common hematologic tests, including specimen requirements, normal values, and conditions leading to abnormal test results.

The most frequently performed hematologic laboratory test is the *complete blood count (CBC)*. A CBC is routinely performed on new patients and on patients with a pathologic condition. The test results provide valuable information to assist the physician in making a diagnosis, evaluating the patient's progress, and regulating treatment. Although the tests included in a CBC may vary somewhat depending on the laboratory, they generally include the hematocrit, hemoglobin, white blood cell count, red blood cell count, differential cell count, and red blood cell indices. This unit includes an overview of hematology as well as the theory and manual testing procedure for each test included in the CBC. Automated hematology analyzers such as the QBC II by Becton Dickinson (Fig. 13-1) are available

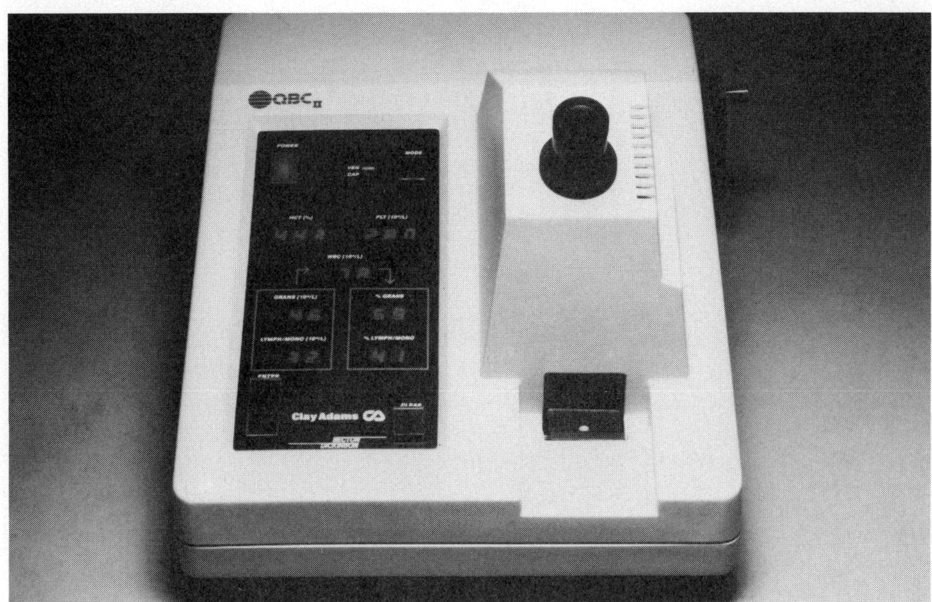

FIGURE 13-1. The QBC II is an example of an automated hematology analyzer. It performs the following tests: hematocrit, platelet count, total white blood cell count, total granulocyte count, percentage of granulocytes, total lymphocyte/monocyte count and percentage of lymphocytes/monocytes. (Courtesy of Becton Dickinson, New Jersey.)

TABLE 13-1. Common Hematologic Tests

NAME OF TEST AND SPECIMEN REQUIREMENT	ABBREVIATION	PURPOSE	NORMAL RANGE	INCREASED WITH	DECREASED WITH
White blood cell count (whole blood)	WBC	Used to assist in the diagnosis and prognosis of disease.	5000–10,000/cu mm	**Leukocytosis** Acute infections (appendicitis, chickenpox, diphtheria, infectious mononucleosis, meningitis, pneumonia, rheumatic fever, smallpox, tonsillitis) Hemorrhaging Trauma Malignant disease Leukemia Polycythemia vera	**Leukopenia** Viral infections Hypersplenism Bone marrow depression Infectious hepatitis Cirrhosis
Red blood cell count (whole blood)	RBC	Used to assist in the diagnosis of anemia and polycythemia.	Male: 5–6 million/cu mm Female: 4–5 million/cu mm MCV 81–99 μm^3 MCH 27.0–31.0 pg MCHC 32.0–36.0%	Polycythemia vera Secondary polycythemia Severe diarrhea Dehydration Acute poisoning Pulmonary fibrosis Severe burns	Anemia Hodgkin's disease Multiple myeloma Leukemia Hemolytic anemia Pernicious anemia Lupus erythematosus Addison's disease
Differential white blood cell count (fresh whole blood)	Diff	Used to assist in the diagnosis and prognosis of disease.	Neutrophils 50–70% Eosinophils 1–4% Basophils 0–1% Lymphocytes 20–35% Monocytes 3–8%	**Neutrophilia** Acute bacterial infections Parasitic infections Liver disease	**Neutropenia** Acute viral infections Blood diseases Hormone diseases
				Eosinophilia Allergic conditions Parasitic infections Addison's disease Lung and bone cancer	**Eosinopenia** Infectious mononucleosis Hypersplenism Congestive heart failure Aplastic and pernicious anemia
				Basophilia Leukemia Chronic inflammation Polycythemia vera Hemolytic anemia Hodgkin's disease	**Basopenia** Acute allergic reactions Hyperthyroidism Steroid therapy
				Lymphocytosis Acute and chronic infections Hemopoietic disorders Addison's disease Carcinoma Hyperthyroidism	**Lymphopenia** Cardiac failure Cushing disease Hodgkin's disease Leukemia

TABLE 13-1. Common Hematologic Tests *(Continued)*

NAME OF TEST AND SPECIMEN REQUIREMENT	ABBREVIATION	PURPOSE	NORMAL RANGE	INCREASED WITH	DECREASED WITH
				Monocytosis Viral infections Bacterial and parasitic infections Collagen diseases Cirrhosis Polycythemia vera	**Monocytopenia** Prednisone treatment Hairy cell leukemia
Hemoglobin (whole blood)	Hgb	Used to screen for the presence and severity of anemia and to monitor the patient's response to treatment for anemia.	Male: 14–18 g/100 ml Female: 12–16 g/100 ml	Polycythemia Severe burns Chronic obstructive pulmonary disease Congestive heart failure	Anemia Hyperthyroidism Cirrhosis Severe hemorrhage Hemolytic reactions Hodgkin's disease Leukemia
Hematocrit (whole blood)	Hct, HCT	Assists in the diagnosis and evaluation of anemia.	Male: 37–47% Female: 40–54%	Polycythemia vera Severe dehydration Shock Severe burns	Anemia Leukemia Hyperthyroidism Cirrhosis Acute blood loss Hemolytic reactions
Prothrombin time (whole blood)	PT	Used to screen for the presence of coagulation disorders and to regulate treatment of patients on oral anticoagulant therapy with warfarin sodium (Coumadin).	11–16 sec	**Thrombocytosis** Prothrombin deficiency Vitamin K deficiency Hemorrhagic disease of the newborn Liver disease Anticoagulant therapy Biliary obstruction Acute leukemia Polycythemia vera	**Thrombocytopenia** Acute thrombophlebitis Diuretics Multiple myeloma Pulmonary embolism Vitamin K therapy
Erythrocyte sedimentation rate (whole blood)	ESR	Used as a nonspecific test for connective tissue diseases, malignancy, and infectious diseases. Also used to evaluate the progress of inflammatory diseases. (Elevated test results warrant further testing.)	Westergren method Male: <50 yr 0–15 mm/hr ≥ 50 yr 0–20 mm/hr Female: <50 yr 0–20 mm/hr ≥ 50 yr 0–30 mm/hr	Collagen diseases Infections Inflammatory diseases Carcinoma Cell or tissue destruction Rheumatoid arthritis	Polycythemia vera Sickle cell anemia Congestive heart failure
Platelet count (whole blood)		Assists in the evaluation of bleeding disorders that occur with liver disease, thrombocytopenia, uremia, and anticoagulant therapy.	200,000–400,000/cu mm	**Thrombocytosis** Cancer Leukemia Polycythemia vera Splenectomy Acute blood loss Rheumatoid arthritis Trauma (fractures, surgery)	**Thrombocytopenia** Pernicious anemia Aplastic anemia Hemolytic anemia Pneumonia Allergic conditions Infection Bone marrow–depressant drugs

and automatically perform each step of the testing procedure. The accompanying manual should carefully be reviewed before the analyzer is used, to ensure accurate and reliable test results.

Erythrocytes

In the adult, *erythrocytes,* or red blood cells, are formed in the red bone marrow of the ribs, sternum, skull, and pelvic bone and in the ends of the long bones of the limbs. The immature form of an erythrocyte contains a nucleus. As the cell develops and matures, however, it loses its nucleus and therefore acquires the shape of a biconcave disc, thicker at the rim than at the center. This shape provides the erythrocyte with a greater surface area for the exchange of substances. An erythrocyte is approximately 7 to 8 microns in diameter. The average number of erythrocytes in the adult female ranges from 4 to 5 million per cubic millimeter of blood and in the adult male from 5 to 6 million per cubic millimeter of blood.

A major portion of the erythrocyte consists of a complex compound called hemoglobin (abbreviated Hgb or Hb), which functions to transport oxygen and is also responsible for the red color of the erythrocyte. The amount of hemoglobin in the blood averages 12 to 16 g per 100 ml for the adult female and 14 to 18 g per 100 ml for the adult male. A hemoglobin molecule consists of a globin or protein part and an iron-containing pigment called heme. One hemoglobin molecule loosely combines with four oxygen molecules in the lungs to form a substance called *oxyhemoglobin.* Oxyhemoglobin is transported and distributed to the tissues, where the oxygen is easily released from the hemoglobin. The blood then picks up carbon dioxide, a waste product, and transports it back to the lungs to be expelled. When oxygen combines with hemoglobin, a bright red color results that is characteristic of arterial blood. Venous blood has a darker red color, owing to its lower oxygen content.

The average life span of a red blood cell is 120 days. Toward the end of this time, it becomes more and more fragile and eventually ruptures and breaks down; this process is known as *hemolysis.* Hemoglobin, liberated from the red blood cell, also breaks down. The iron is stored and later reused to form new hemoglobin, and the protein is metabolized by the body. *Bilirubin* is formed from metabolism of the heme units and transported to the liver, where it is eventually excreted as a waste product in the bile.

Leukocytes

Leukocytes, or white blood cells, are clear, colorless cells that contain a nucleus. The average number of leukocytes in the adult ranges from 5000 to 10,000 per cubic millimeters of blood. *Leukocytosis* is the name given to the condition of an abnormal increase in the number of leukocytes (above 10,000), and the term *leukopenia* is used to describe an abnormal decrease in the number (below 5000). Leukocytosis may occur when an infection exists in the body, and certain acute and chronic diseases may cause leukopenia.

The function of leukocytes is to defend the body against infection. Pathogens may gain entrance to the body in a variety of ways (review the Infection Process Cycle in Chapter 1). Leukocytes attempt to destroy the invading pathogens and remove them from the body. Unlike erythrocytes, leukocytes do their work in the tissues; they are transported to the site of infection by the circulatory system. During inflammation, the blood vessels in the infected area dilate, resulting in an increased blood supply. More oxygen, nutrients, and white blood cells can then be delivered to the infected area to aid in the healing process. The cells making up the wall of the capillaries spread apart, enlarging the pores between the cells. White blood cells squeeze through the pores by ameboid movement and move out into the tissues to fight the infection. This movement of the leukocytes through the pores of the capillaries is known as *diapedesis.* Leukocytes (especially the granular forms) are phagocytic, and once they arrive at the site of infection they begin engulfing and destroying the pathogens and damaged cells through a process known as *phagocytosis.* In some conditions pus may form in the infected area (suppuration), which contains dead leukocytes, dead bacteria, and dead tissue cells.

Thrombocytes

Platelets, also known as *thrombocytes,* are small and clear and shaped like discs. They lack a nucleus and are formed in the red bone marrow from giant cells known as megakaryocytes. Platelets function by participating in the blood-clotting mechanism. The average number of platelets in the adult is 200,000 to 400,000 per cubic millimeter of blood.

Plasma

Plasma is the straw-colored liquid portion of the blood. It serves as a transportation medium in which various substances are dissolved and blood cells are suspended for circulation through the body. Approximately 92 per cent of plasma consists of water; the remaining 8 per cent is dissolved solid substances (solutes) that are carried by the blood to and from the tissues. The solutes present in greatest amounts are the *plasma proteins,* which include serum albumin, globulins, fibrinogen, and prothrombin. Serum albumin is synthesized in the liver and functions in regulating the volume of plasma within the blood vessels. Globulins play an important role in the immunity mechanism of the body, and fibrinogen and prothrombin are essential for proper blood clotting. Various *electrolytes* are carried by the plasma and are needed for normal cell functioning and the maintenance of the normal fluid and acid-base balance of the body. Some of these electrolytes are sodium, chloride, potassium, calcium, phosphate, bicarbonate, and magnesium. *Nutrients* derived from the breakdown of food substances are carried by the plasma to nourish the tissues of the body and include glucose, amino acids, and lipids. *Waste products* formed as the by-products of metabolism and carried by the plasma to be excreted include urea, uric acid, lactic acid, and creatinine. *Respiratory gases* dissolved in and carried by the plasma include carbon dioxide and a small amount of oxygen. Substances present in the plasma that help to *regulate and control the functions of the body* include hormones, antibodies, enzymes, and vitamins.

Capillary Blood Specimen

Capillary blood can be used when a test requires a small blood specimen. A venipuncture must be performed for those tests requiring a large specimen (refer to Chapter 11). Capillary blood is obtained from either the finger or the earlobe of an adult; in an infant, it is taken from the plantar surface of the heel. Both the amount of blood needed and the technique and equipment used to obtain it from the skin puncture depend on the test being performed. Blood taken for a manual white blood cell count involves drawing the specimen into a pipet. The tip of the pipet should be held in a horizontal position, touching only the blood and not the patient's finger. The sample of blood for a hematocrit reading is obtained by holding a capillary tube in a horizontal position and allowing the blood to flow into the tube by capillary action. When a blood specimen for a differential cell count is taken, a slide is touched to a drop of blood flowing from the patient's finger. The medical assistant must carefully observe aseptic technique during this procedure.

The capillary blood specimen is obtained using either a lancet or an automatic lancet device such as an Autolet, Glucolet, or Autoclix. The automatic lancet device is gaining popularity; most consist of a spring-loaded instrument containing a platform and a lancet (Fig. 13–2). The platform controls the tissue penetration, resulting in a puncture that is of a specified tissue depth based on the type of platform utilized. This causes a smaller wound to occur, which results in less pain for the patient than the lancet method. There are usually two platforms available for use with the automatic lancet device. The standard platform is used for infants, children, and most adults; it produces a puncture to a maximum penetration of 2.4 mm. The super-puncture platform is used for patients with thick or calloused skin; it produces a puncture to a maximum penetration of 3.0 mm. The lancet method is used when an automatic lancet device is not available or when the patient's skin is so thick or calloused that a good puncture cannot be obtained with the automatic lancet device. The procedures for obtaining a blood specimen using the lancet and Autolet methods are outlined on the following pages.

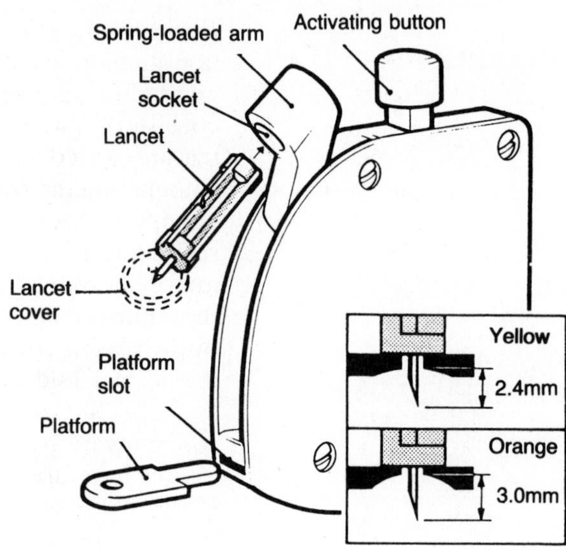

FIGURE 13–2. Components of the Autolet. The smaller box (lower right) shows the depth of penetration of the standard (yellow) platform and the super-puncture (orange) platform.

PROCEDURE 13-1

LANCET METHOD TO OBTAIN A CAPILLARY BLOOD SPECIMEN

1. **PROCEDURAL STEP.** Wash the hands.

2. **PROCEDURAL STEP.** Assemble the equipment. The equipment includes an **alcohol pledget,** a **sterile lancet, cotton balls,** and **clean gloves.**

3. **PROCEDURAL STEP.** Select an appropriate puncture site. The lateral part of the tip of the middle or ring finger is most often used to obtain the specimen. If the patient's finger is cold, it can be warmed by rubbing it or placing it in warm water. Cleanse the puncture site with the alcohol pledget and allow it to dry.
PRINCIPLE. The middle and ring fingers are less calloused than the thumb and index fingers. The lateral part of the tip is the least sensitive part of the finger.

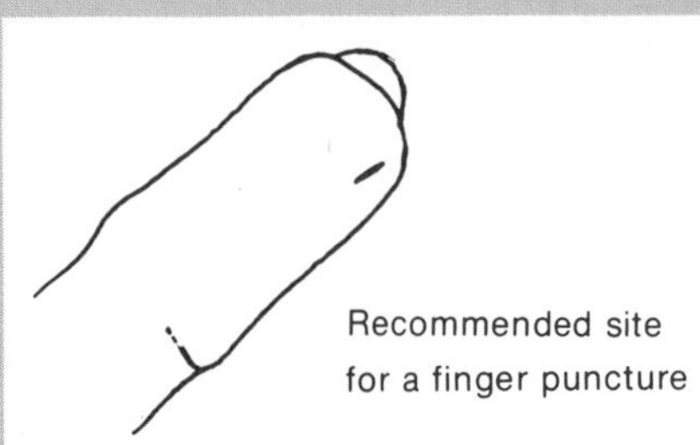

4. **PROCEDURAL STEP.** Open the sterile lancet without contaminating the tip. If the tip becomes contaminated, a new one must be obtained.
PRINCIPLE. A contaminated lancet may harbor pathogens.

5. **PROCEDURAL STEP.** Apply gloves. Without touching the puncture site, firmly grasp the patient's finger and make a puncture with the sterile lancet, using a quick jabbing motion. The puncture should be made at a right angle to the lines of the skin and be approximately 2 to 3 mm deep.
PRINCIPLE. Gloves provide a barrier precaution against contaminated blood. Touching the site after cleansing contaminates it, and the cleansing process has to be repeated. A well-made puncture results in a free-flowing wound for which only slight pressure is needed to make it bleed.

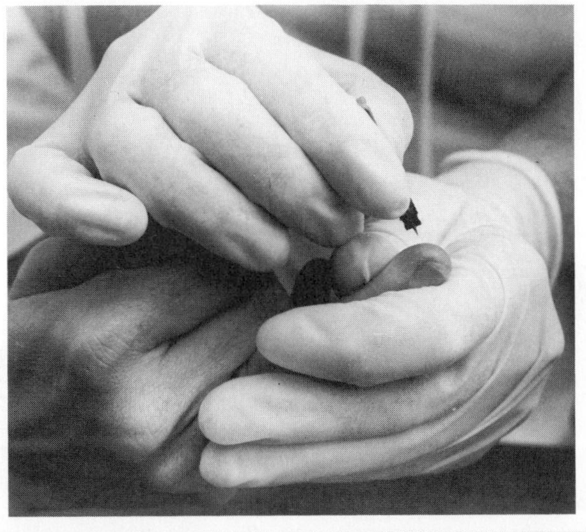

6. **PROCEDURAL STEP.** Wipe away the first drop of blood with a piece of gauze or a cotton ball.
PRINCIPLE. The first drop of blood is diluted with alcohol and tissue fluid and is not a suitable specimen.

7. **PROCEDURAL STEP.** Use the second drop of blood for the test. Exert gentle pressure without squeezing the finger to obtain the blood specimen.
PRINCIPLE. Squeezing the finger causes dilution of the blood sample with tissue fluid; inaccurate test readings result.

8. **PROCEDURAL STEP.** Obtain the blood specimen as required by the test.

9. **PROCEDURAL STEP.** Have the patient hold a piece of gauze or cotton over the puncture site and apply pressure until the bleeding stops. Remain with the patient until the bleeding stops for safety precautions.

10. **PROCEDURAL STEP.** Properly dispose of the lancet. Remove gloves and wash the hands.
Note: This procedure can be adapted for obtaining a blood specimen from the earlobe of an adult or the heel of an infant.

PROCEDURE 13-2

AUTOLET METHOD TO OBTAIN A CAPILLARY BLOOD SPECIMEN

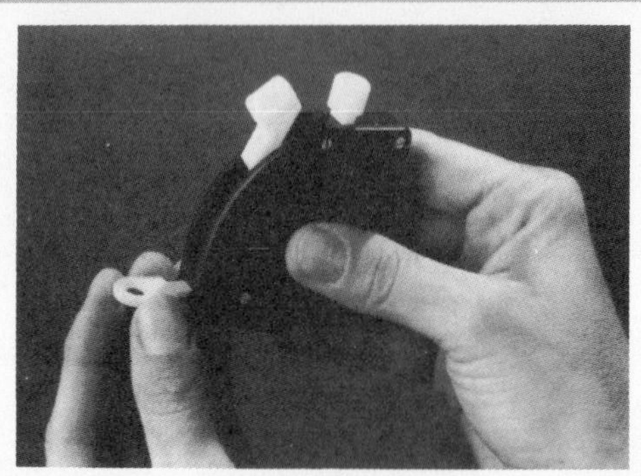

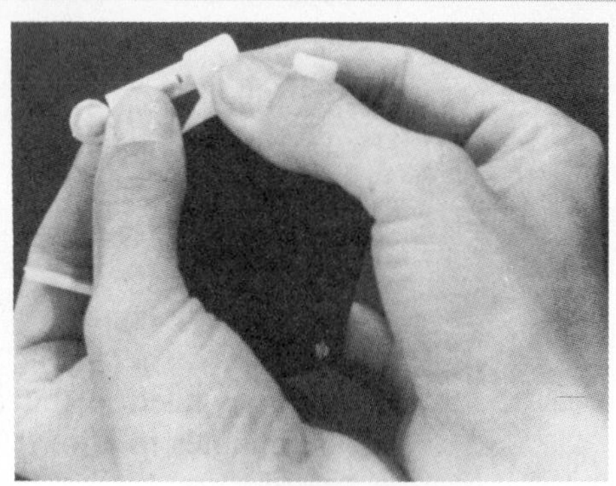

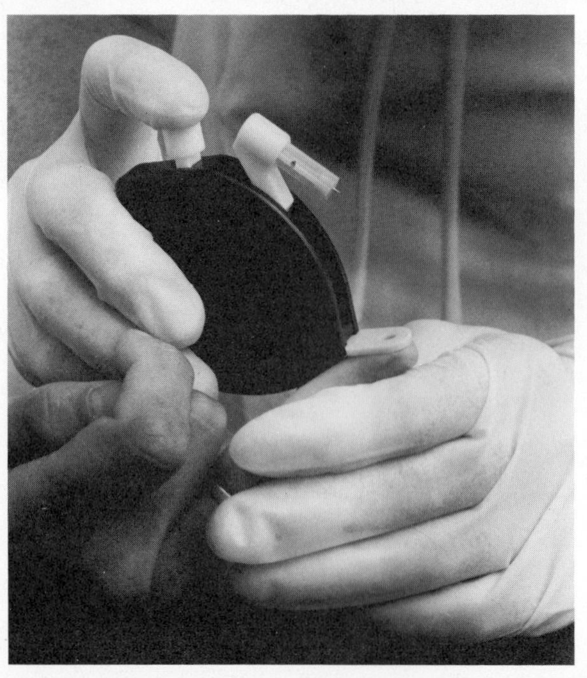

1. **PROCEDURAL STEP.** Wash the hands.

2. **PROCEDURAL STEP.** Assemble the equipment. The equipment includes the **Autolet instrument,** a **disposable platform and lancet,** an **alcohol pledget, cotton balls,** and **clean gloves.**

3. **PROCEDURAL STEP.** Pull the spring-loaded arm of the Autolet back toward the activating button until it clicks into position. Once the arm clicks into place, it will be held stationary until the activating button is pressed.

4. **PROCEDURAL STEP.** Insert the appropriate platform into the proper slot of the Autolet. The standard (yellow) platform is used for infants, children, and most adults, and the super-puncture (orange) platform is used for patients with thick or calloused skin.

5. **PROCEDURAL STEP.** Insert the lancet into the lancet socket located at the end of the arm. Push it firmly into place. If the lancet is not firmly anchored, it can be moved into place by twisting it about a quarter of a turn.

6. **PROCEDURAL STEP.** Select an appropriate puncture site. The lateral part of the tip of the middle or ring finger is most often used to obtain the specimen. If the patient's finger is cold, it can be warmed by rubbing it or placing it in warm water. Cleanse the puncture site with the alcohol pledget and allow it to dry. Apply gloves.
PRINCIPLE. The middle and ring fingers are less calloused than the thumb and index fingers. The lateral part of the tip is the least sensitive part of the finger. Gloves are a precaution that provides a barrier against contaminated blood.

7. **PROCEDURAL STEP.** Remove the plastic cover from the end of the lancet using a twisting motion; this exposes its sterile point. Firmly place the platform against the puncture site so that the tissue protrudes into the hole in the center of the platform.

8. **PROCEDURAL STEP.** Press the release button with a slight pressure, which permits the lancet to puncture the skin. Wait a few seconds to allow blood flow to begin. The tissue surrounding the puncture site can be massaged firmly but gently to initiate the blood flow. To obtain the blood specimen, follow Steps 6 through 9 in the lancet method procedure.

9. **PROCEDURAL STEP.** Remove the platform and lancet from the Autolet and properly dispose of them. The Autolet should be stored with the arm in its resting position to prolong its lifespan. Remove gloves and wash hands.

Hematocrit

The *hematocrit* (abbreviated Hct) is a simple, reliable, and informative test that is frequently performed in the medical office. The word hematocrit means "to separate blood." The solid or cellular elements are separated from the plasma by centrifuging an anticoagulated blood specimen. The heavier red blood cells become packed and settle to the bottom of a tube. The top layer contains the clear straw-colored plasma. Between the plasma and the packed red blood cells is a small, thin, yellowish-gray layer known as the buffy coat, which contains the platelets and white blood cells.

The purpose of the hematocrit is to measure the percentage volume of packed red blood cells in whole blood. The normal hematocrit range for the adult female is 37 to 47 per cent and for the adult male 40 to 54 per cent. A low hematocrit reading may indicate *anemia,* whereas a high reading may indicate *polycythemia.* The hematocrit, used in conjunction with other hematologic tests, is useful as an aid to the physician in the diagnosis of a patient's condition. The hematocrit is also used as a screening measure for the early detection of anemia and therefore is often included as part of a general physical examination.

There are two methods for determining the hematocrit—the microhematocrit method and the Wintrobe method. The microhematocrit method is most often utilized in the medical office. It requires less centrifugation time, less preparatory work, and a smaller blood specimen than the Wintrobe method. Through capillary action, blood is drawn directly from a free-flowing skin puncture into a disposable capillary tube lined with an anticoagulant. An anticoagulated blood specimen collected by other means such as venipuncture can also be used. The microhematocrit centrifuge spins the blood at an extremely high speed and requires only 3 to 5 minutes (as designated by the manufacturer) to pack the red blood cells.

Occasionally, the Wintrobe method is used to determine the hematocrit. This method utilizes a Wintrobe hematocrit tube, which is calibrated from 0 to 10 cm. The tube is filled to the 10-cm mark with anticoagulated blood and centrifuged for 30 minutes to allow the heavier red blood cells to settle at the bottom of the tube. The results are read on the graduations on the side of the tube, and the hematocrit reading is obtained by multiplying the figure indicated by 10.

PROCEDURE 13-3
HEMATOCRIT (MICROHEMATOCRIT METHOD)

1. **PROCEDURAL STEP.** Assemble the equipment. The equipment needed includes an **automatic lancet device or a sterile lancet**, an **alcohol pledget, clean gloves, capillary tubes, sealing compound**, and a **microhematocrit centrifuge.**

2. **PROCEDURAL STEP.** Apply gloves and perform a finger or earlobe puncture.
PRINCIPLE. Gloves provide a barrier precaution against contaminated blood.

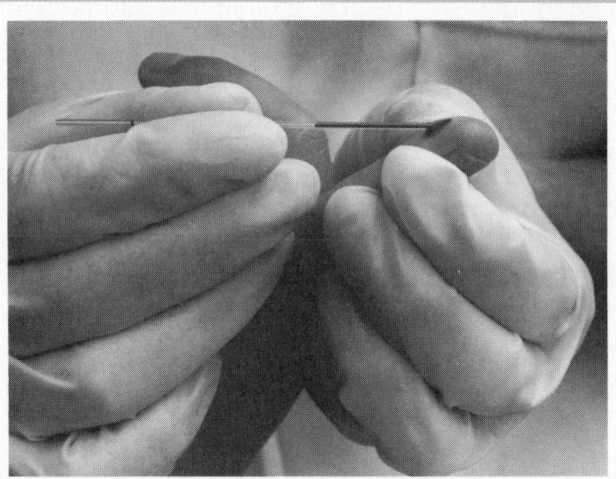

3. **PROCEDURAL STEP.** Fill the capillary tube by holding one end of it horizontally next to the free-flowing puncture. Calibrated tubes are filled to the calibration line, whereas uncalibrated tubes are filled to approximately three-quarters (within 10 to 20 mm of the end of the tube). The blood will be drawn into the tube through capillary action. Fill a second tube using the method just described.
PRINCIPLE. The type of tube used (calibrated or uncalibrated) is based on the method used to read the test results. The hematocrit should be performed in duplicate to ensure accuracy and to provide test results in case one tube breaks during centrifuging.

4. **PROCEDURAL STEP.** Seal one end of each tube with a small amount of putty or a commercially prepared sealing compound (e.g., Critoseal, Sealease).
PRINCIPLE. The capillary tubes must be properly sealed to prevent leakage of the blood specimen during centrifugation.

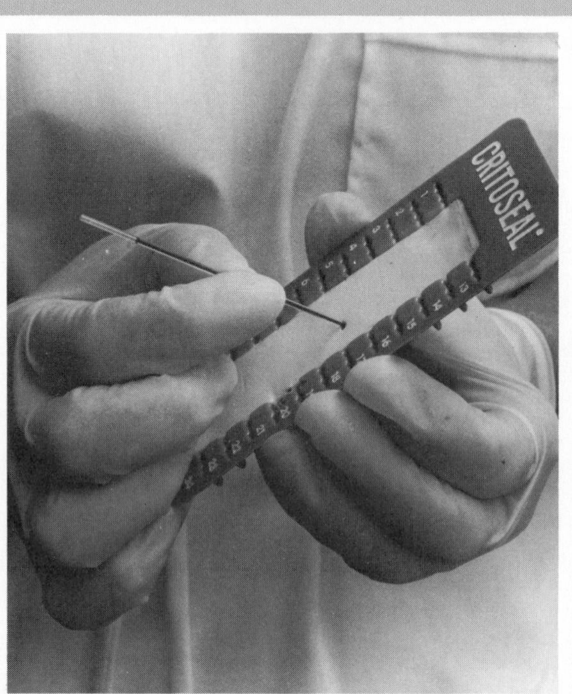

5. **PROCEDURAL STEP.** Place the capillary tubes in the microhematocrit centrifuge with the sealed end facing the outside. Balance one tube with the other capillary tube placed on the opposite side of the centrifuge.
PRINCIPLE. Placing the sealed end toward the outside prevents the blood specimen from spinning out of the capillary tube when the centrifuge is in operation.

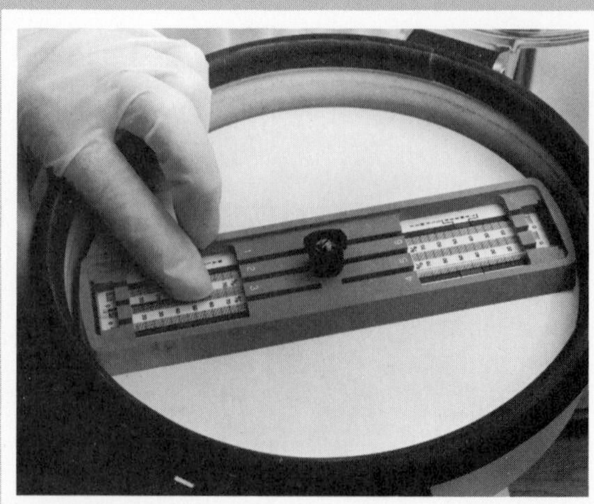

6. **PROCEDURAL STEP.** Place the cover on the centrifuge and lock it securely. Centrifuge the blood specimen for 3 to 5 minutes at a speed of 10,000 rpm.

PRINCIPLE. Centrifuging the blood specimen causes the red blood cells to become packed and to settle on the bottom of the tube.

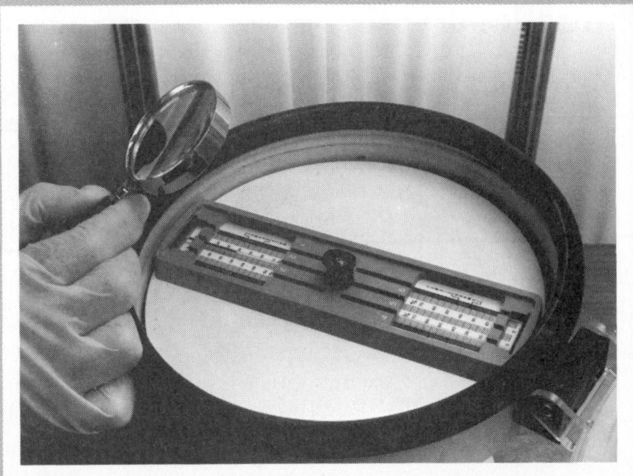

7. **PROCEDURAL STEP.** Allow the centrifuge to come to a complete stop. Read the results. If a capillary tube with a calibration line was used, the results are read using the special graphic reading device that is contained as part of the centrifuge. Adjust the capillary tube so that the bottom of the cell column (just above the sealing compound) is placed on the 0 line. The results are read at the top of the packed cell column using a magnifying glass and are read directly as a percentage on the reading device.

If an uncalibrated tube was used, a microhematocrit reader card must be used to determine the results; the top of the plasma column is placed on the 100 per cent mark and the bottom on the cell column is placed on the 0 line. The results are read on the scale, which corresponds to the top of the packed cell column.

In both cases, the buffy coat should not be included in the reading. The answer represents the percentage of the total volume of blood occupied by the red blood cells. (The hematocrit determination on this reading device is 42.)

PRINCIPLE. Stopping the centrifuge by using the hands may injure the medical assistant and may also damage the machine.

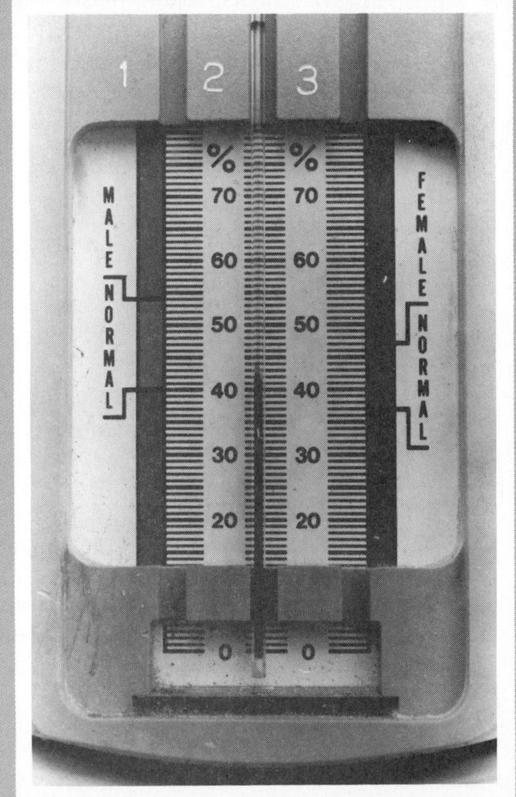

8. **PROCEDURAL STEP.** Read the second tube in the manner just described; the results of the tubes should agree within 4 percentage points. If not, the hematocrit procedure must be repeated. If they are within 4 percentage points, the two values are averaged together to derive the test results.

9. **PROCEDURAL STEP.** Properly dispose of the capillary tubes. Remove gloves and wash the hands. Record the results. Include the patient's name, the date and time, and hematocrit results. Place your initials next to the recording.

10. **PROCEDURAL STEP.** Return the equipment.

Record data below.

DATE	TIME	PATIENT'S NAME	RESULTS

White Blood Cell Count

In the medical office, the *white blood cell count* (WBC) is performed using the manual method or using an automated blood analyzer. The manual method is described here to provide the knowledge and skill for performing the individual steps in this procedure. A counting chamber (also called a *hemocytometer*) is used, which is a thick, rectangular glass slide with a ruled counting area (Fig. 13–3) on its surface for counting the white blood cells. A specially designed coverglass must be used and is placed over the ruled area of the counting chamber. The chamber and coverglass must be clean and free from lint so that a piece of dirt is not mistaken for a cell during the counting procedure. The white blood cells contained in the blood specimen must be spread out for ease in counting. This is accomplished with a diluting fluid; 2 per cent acetic acid is commonly used. It also hemolyzes the numerous red blood cells, leaving only the desired white blood cells for counting. A white blood cell diluting pipet (Fig. 13–4) is used to obtain the correct dilution of the blood and diluting fluid. If a pipet is broken or chipped, it must be discarded because it may cause inaccurate test results. The Unopette system can also be used to collect and dilute the blood specimen. It consists of a disposable plastic pipet and a reservoir that holds the premeasured white blood count diluting fluid. The blood specimen is drawn into the plastic pipet using mechanical suction and is then placed in the diluent. The blood and diluent are thoroughly mixed following the manufacturer's instructions. The diluted blood specimen is then used to fill the chamber of the hemocytometer. Capillary blood, obtained directly from a skin puncture, or an anticoagulated blood specimen, obtained from a venipuncture, can be used for the white blood cell count.

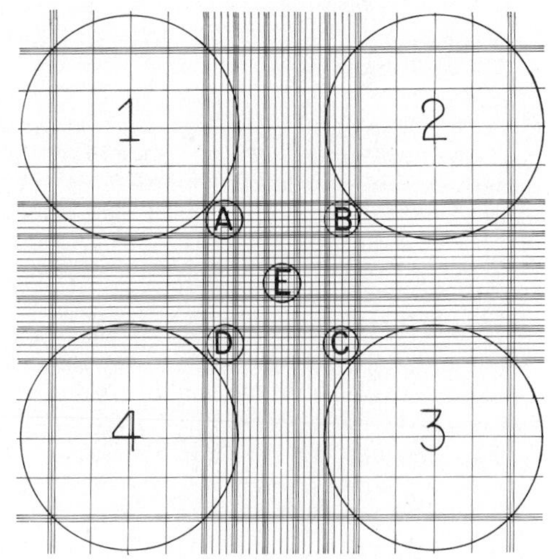

FIGURE 13–3. The ruled counting area on the surface of the counting chamber (hemocytometer). White blood cells are counted in the four large outside corner squares (labeled 1, 2, 3, and 4). Red blood cells are counted in the five smaller squares (labeled A, B, C, D, and E) contained in the middle square of the ruled counting area.

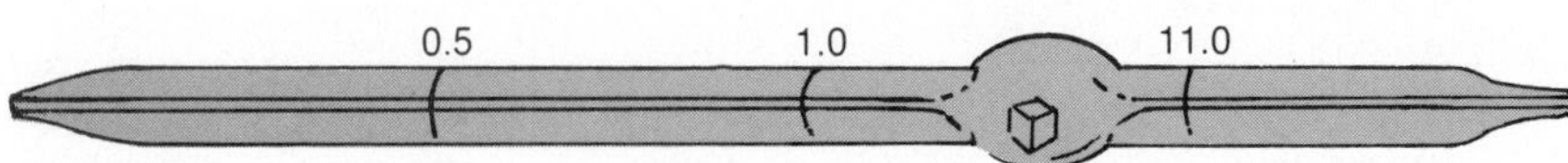

FIGURE 13–4. White blood cell diluting pipet.

PROCEDURE 13-4

WHITE BLOOD CELL COUNT (MANUAL METHOD)

1. **PROCEDURAL STEP.** Assemble the equipment. The equipment needed includes **clean gloves, a white blood pipet** (containing a white bead in the bulb), **rubber tubing with a mechanical suction device,** a **counting chamber (hemocytometer)** and a **coverglass, diluting fluid** to which gentian violet may be added, a **microscope with a mechanical stage,** a **white blood cell counter,** and a **mechanical shaker (optional).**

Note: If the Unopette system is used to collect and dilute the blood specimen, follow the procedure outlined in the manufacturer's directions in lieu of Steps 3 through 7.

PRINCIPLE. The gentian violet lightly stains the white blood cells, making them easier to identify.

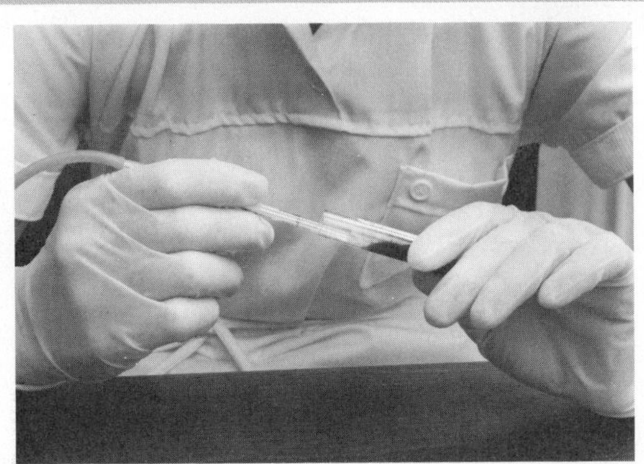

2. **PROCEDURAL STEP.** Apply gloves and perform a finger puncture (if required).

3. **PROCEDURAL STEP.** Draw the blood up to the 0.5-ml mark on the white blood cell pipet using mechanical suction.

4. **PROCEDURAL STEP.** Wipe the blood off the outside of the tip of the pipet with a piece of clean gauze without touching the opening.

PRINCIPLE. If the gauze touches the opening of the pipet, plasma is drawn out, leaving a higher concentration of cells and erroneously changing the white blood cell count.

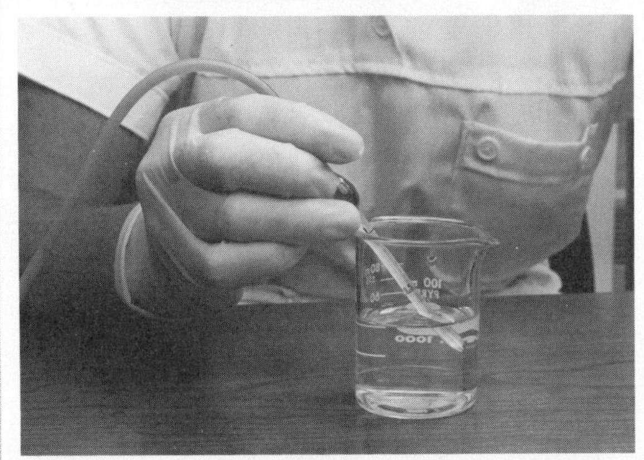

5. **PROCEDURAL STEP.** Using mechanical suction, immediately draw the diluting fluid into the pipet up to the 11.0-ml mark to make a 1 : 20 dilution. Make sure the tip of the pipet remains completely immersed in the diluting fluid. Rotate the pipet between your fingers as you fill it. When the solution enters the bulb, tap the bulb with your finger to keep the bead below the solution level.

PRINCIPLE. Filling the pipet quickly prevents the blood from clotting. Rotating it also keeps the blood from clotting and helps to mix it with the diluent. Keeping the tip of the pipet immersed in the diluting fluid and tapping the bulb prevent air bubbles from entering and changing the dilution factor.

6. **PROCEDURAL STEP.** Remove the tubing and hold the pipet in a horizontal position with one finger placed over the end (the end closest to the bulb) to prevent the solution from flowing out of the pipet. Mix the blood and diluting fluid by placing the pipet on a mechanical shaker, or mix them manually by holding the pipet between the thumb and index finger and vigorously shaking it with a figure-eight motion for 3 minutes.

PRINCIPLE. Mixing distributes the cells equally through the diluting fluid so that they will be spread out evenly when placed on the ruled area of the counting chamber. The bead in the bulb aids in mixing the solution.

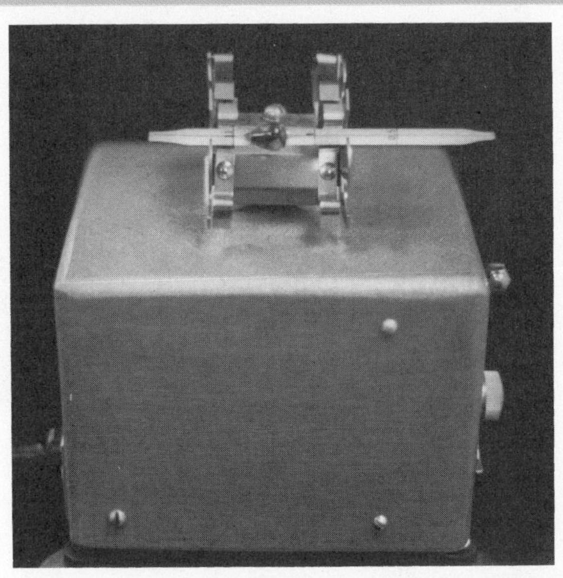

Continued

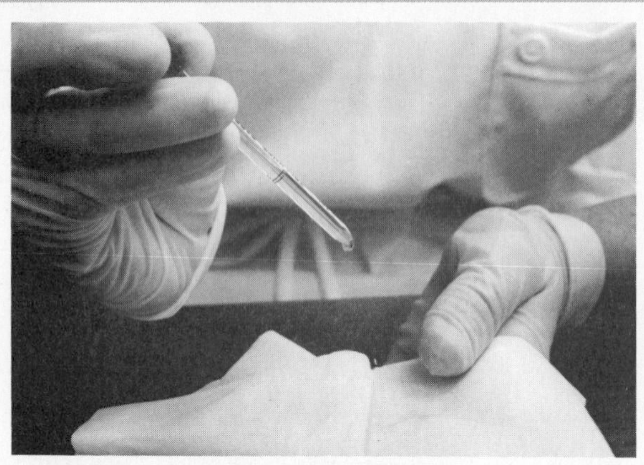

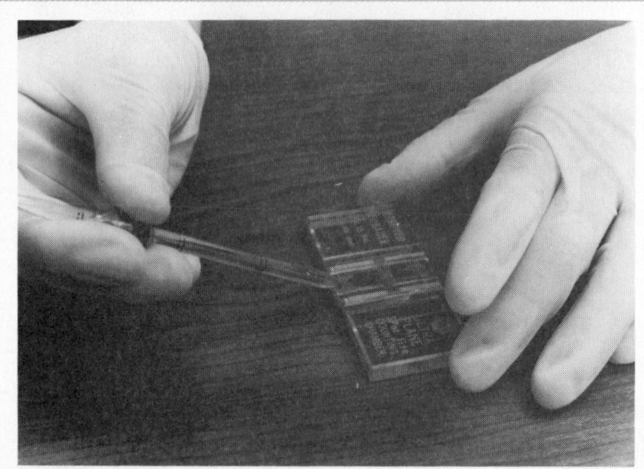

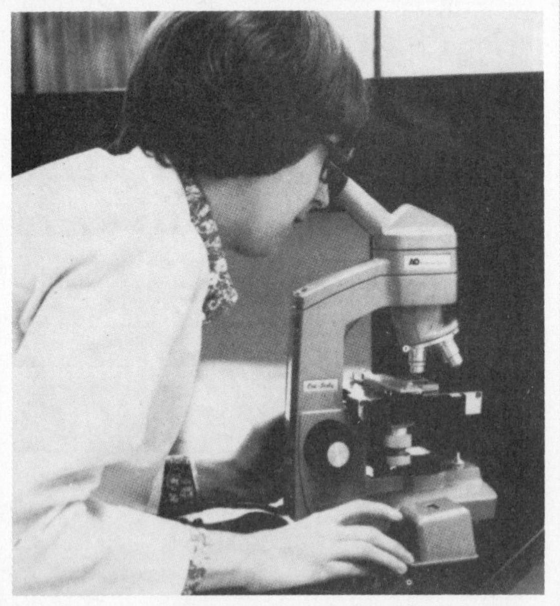

7. **PROCEDURAL STEP.** Control the flow of the solution by placing your finger over the end of the pipet (the end closest to the bulb). Expel 3 drops from the pipet to rid the stem of diluting fluid and to allow the cell suspension to move into the stem.

8. **PROCEDURAL STEP.** Place a clean coverglass on the counting chamber. Fill the chamber by touching the tip of the pipet, held at an angle, to the junction of the coverglass and counting chamber. Control the flow of the solution by placing your index finger over the end of the pipet. Allow the solution to flow into the chamber between the ruled area and the coverglass. The solution will be drawn up under the coverglass by capillary action. Fill both sides of the chamber. If the chamber has been filled properly, the solution will amply cover the ruled area. Overfilling is indicated by fluid spilling into the moats, whereas underfilling is indicated by a flattened air bubble and incomplete filling of the ruled area. In both instances, the medical assistant should clean the counting chamber and begin again.

PRINCIPLE. Overfilling or underfilling the chamber leads to inaccurate results.

9. **PROCEDURAL STEP.** Allow the cells to settle for 2 to 3 minutes in the counting chamber placed on a flat surface.

PRINCIPLE. This allows the cells to settle in one plane.

10. **PROCEDURAL STEP.** Place the counting chamber on the mechanical stage microscope. Using the low-power objective, focus the microscope until you can see the ruled counting area (see Fig. 13–3). Scan the area to make sure the cells are evenly distributed. The white blood cells appear as slightly iridescent round bodies. They are counted in the 16 small squares contained in the 4 large outside corner squares using a definite pattern (see Fig. 13–5). Only those cells touching the upper and left boundary lines of each of the 16 smaller squares should be counted. The cells touching the lower and right boundary lines are not counted. The cells counted in each of the four corner squares should not vary from one another by more than 10. Performing the count in duplicate, using both sides of the chamber, assures greater accuracy, especially while the medical assistant is first learning and acquiring skill in the procedure.

PRINCIPLE. Counting the cells in the manner described prevents omitting or counting a cell twice.

11. **PROCEDURAL STEP.** Calculate the number of white blood cells per cubic millimeter of blood by multiplying the total number of cells counted by 50. The normal range for a white blood cell count for an adult is 5000 to 10,000 per cubic millimeter of blood. Record the results. Include the patient's name, the date and time, and the white blood cell count. Place your initials next to the recording.

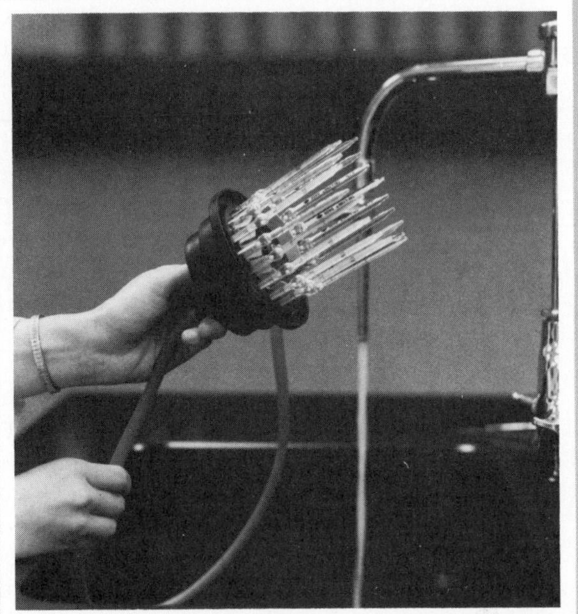

12. **PROCEDURAL STEP.** Clean the equipment. The pipets are washed with a suction pump-pipet washing device. The pipets are inserted into the head of the washer. A cleaning solution (such as soap or a low-sudsing detergent), water, and a drying liquid such as acetone are siphoned through the pipets, in that order. (Each of these liquids is contained in a separate beaker or jar.) The cleaning solution should be permitted to flow through the pipets for several minutes or until they appear to be free from all blood or contamination. The water is used to rinse the cleaning solution from the pipets. A small amount of acetone is then drawn through them, followed by warm air to completely dry the inside. When the bead moves freely and does not stick to the side of the bulb, the pipet is dry.

The counting chamber is cleaned with water or mild soap and dried with a soft, lintless cloth or paper tissue to prevent scratching it.

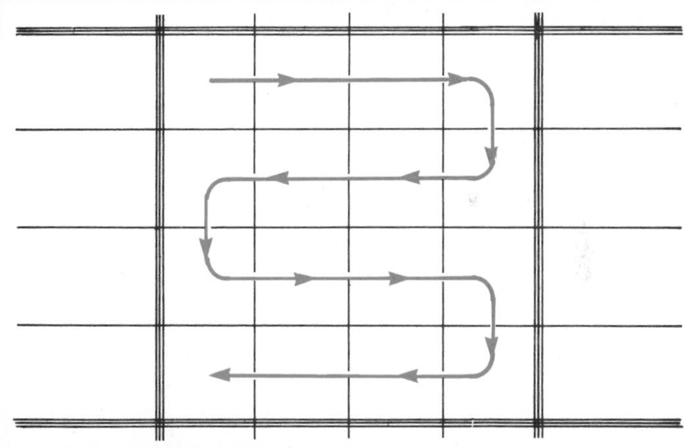

FIGURE 13–5. Pattern for counting white blood cells in a representative corner square.

Record data below.

DATE	TIME	PATIENT'S NAME	RESULTS

Red Blood Cell Count

Red blood cell counts (RBC) are performed in a manner similar to that for white cell counts, using a red blood cell pipet that has a bigger bulb and different calibrations than the white cell pipet. The pipet has a red bead in the bulb. The blood is drawn up to the 0.5-ml mark, and the diluting fluid to the 101-ml mark, to make a 1 : 200 dilution. Five squares (consisting of 16 smaller squares) contained in the middle square of the ruled counting area of the hemocytometer (see Fig. 13–3) are used for counting the red blood cells. The red count is performed under high-dry magnification. The total number of cells counted is multiplied by 10,000 to obtain the number of red blood cells per cubic millimeter of blood. Performing a red blood cell count using the manual method produces results that are not highly accurate, and it is therefore recommended that this test be performed using an automated analyzer.

White Blood Cell Differential Count

There are five types of white blood cells, each having a certain size, shape, appearance, and function (see Fig. 13–6 and the front inside cover). The purpose of the differential cell count (Diff) is to microscopically identify the five types of white blood cells present in a representative blood sample. An increase or decrease in one or more types may occur in pathologic conditions, which assists the physician in making a diagnosis. Because white blood cells are clear and colorless, they must be stained with an appropriate dye (usually Wright's stain). The nucleus, cytoplasm, and any granules present in the cytoplasm take on the characteristic color of their cell type, which aids in proper identification. The number of each type of leukocyte is recorded as a percentage and reflects the overall distribution of the white blood cells present in the patient's bloodstream.

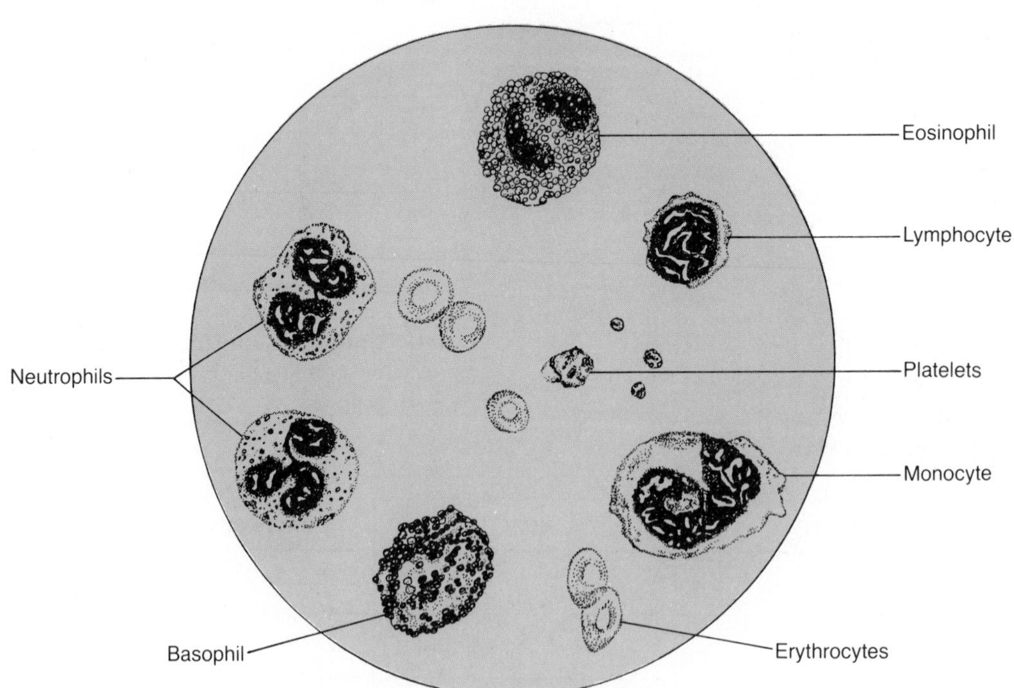

FIGURE 13–6. Microscopic view of a blood film.

Leukocytes are classified into two major categories — granular and nongranular. *Granular leukocytes* contain distinct granules in the cytoplasm and include neutrophils, eosinophils, and basophils. *Nongranular leukocytes* contain few or no granules in the cytoplasm and include lymphocytes and monocytes. The *neutrophils* are the most numerous of the white blood cells. They have a purple multilobed nucleus that may contain from three to five lobes or segments; therefore, they are also known as "segs." The cytoplasm of a neutrophil stains a faint pink and contains many fine granules that stain a violet-pink. Neutrophils exhibit a high degree of ameboid movement and are actively phagocytic. Immature forms of leukocytes are known as *stabs* or *bands* and can be identified by their curved, nonsegmented nucleus. Normally, from zero to five of the neutrophils present will be in the immature band form. An increase in the number of neutrophils, including band forms, is generally seen during an acute infection. *Eosinophils* contain a segmented nucleus, generally of no more than two lobes. Large granules are found in the cytoplasm; these stain a bright red. An increase in eosinophils is often seen in allergic conditions and parasitic infestations. *Basophils* are the least numerous of the white blood cells and contain an S-shaped nucleus. The cytoplasm contains large, coarse, dark bluish-black granules that almost completely obscure the details of the nucleus. *Lymphocytes* have a round or slightly indented nucleus that almost completely fills the cell and stains a deep purplish blue. There is a small rim of sky-blue cytoplasm around the nucleus that contains few or no granules. Lymphocytes are involved with the immune system and the production of antibodies. An increase in lymphocytes generally occurs with certain viral diseases, including infectious mononucleosis, mumps, chickenpox, rubella, and viral hepatitis. *Monocytes* are the largest of the white blood cells and have a large nucleus that is usually kidney- or horseshoe-shaped but may be round or oval. They contain abundant cytoplasm that stains grayish blue.

The normal adult range for each type of white blood cell making up the total number of leukocytes is listed here:

Neutrophils	50 to 70 per cent
Eosinophils	1 to 4 per cent
Basophils	0 to 1 per cent
Lymphocytes	20 to 35 per cent
Monocytes	3 to 8 per cent

The size and shape of the nucleus, the structures present in the cytoplasm, and the staining reaction help to identify the five types of white blood cells. The medical assistant should practice and acquire skill in recognizing the normal-appearing white blood cells. However, he or she is not trained or qualified to make an assessment of abnormal cells and should always seek assistance if a question arises or if a white blood cell cannot be identified.

PROCEDURE 13-5

DIFFERENTIAL CELL COUNT

The differential cell count involves making a blood film (preferably with fresh blood), staining it, and examining it under the microscope. A minimum of 100 white blood cells is identified, and each is assigned to its appropriate category (neutrophil, eosinophil, basophil, lymphocyte, and monocyte). Before performing a differential cell count, the physician may want the medical assistant to examine the blood film to observe the morphologic appearance of the red blood cells to make sure they are normal and to estimate the number of platelets. There should be 7 to 20 platelets in every field when the film is examined with the oil-immersion objective, and the results can be reported as adequate, increased, or decreased. The medical assistant should be able to recognize normal-appearing red blood cells and normal numbers of platelets present on the blood film but should always ask for assistance if any abnormalities are noticed.

1. **PROCEDURAL STEP.** Assemble the equipment. The equipment needed includes an **alcohol pledget,** an **automatic lancet device or a sterile lancet, clean gloves,** a **staining rack, Wright's stain,** a **buffer solution, clean glass slides,** a **microscope with a mechanical stage, immersion oil,** and a **mechanical differential cell counter.** Using a pencil, label the slide on the frosted edge with the patient's name and the date.

2. **PROCEDURAL STEP.** Apply gloves and perform a finger puncture to obtain a capillary blood specimen.

3. **PROCEDURAL STEP.** Place a drop of blood from the patient's finger in the middle of one end of the slide (approximately ¼ inch from the edge of the slide) by touching the slide to the drop of blood. Do not allow the patient's finger to touch the slide.
   PRINCIPLE. If the patient's finger touches the slide, it will cause the blood specimen to spread out, producing an uneven smear. In addition, the patient's finger may contain moisture or oil that would interfere with the smear.
   (*Note:* The blood specimen can also be obtained after performing a venipuncture from the fresh whole blood left in the needle as follows: After withdrawing the needle from the patient's arm, deposit a drop of blood remaining in the needle onto the middle of the slide.)

4. **PROCEDURAL STEP.** Hold a second "spreader" slide in front of the drop of blood and at a 30-degree angle to the first slide. Move the spreader slide until it touches the drop of blood. The blood distributes itself along the edge of the spreader by capillary action. Using a smooth, continuous motion, spread the blood thinly and evenly across the surface of the first slide. The length of the smear should be approximately 1½ inches. The blood smear is thickest at the beginning and gradually thins out to a very fine "feathered" edge. If the blood film has been prepared correctly, it exhibits the following characteristics: (1) it is smooth and even, (2) it is not too thick or too thin, (3) there is a feathered edge at the thin end of the smear, and (4) there is a margin on all sides of the smear.

PRINCIPLE. An angle of more than 30 degrees causes the smear to be too thick and the cells overlap, do not stain well, and are smaller than normal, making them difficult to count. If the angle is less than 30 degrees, the smear will be too thin and the cells will be spread out, increasing the time needed to count them.

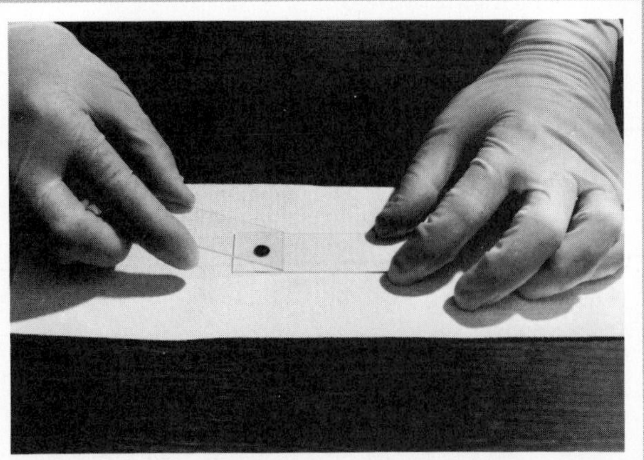

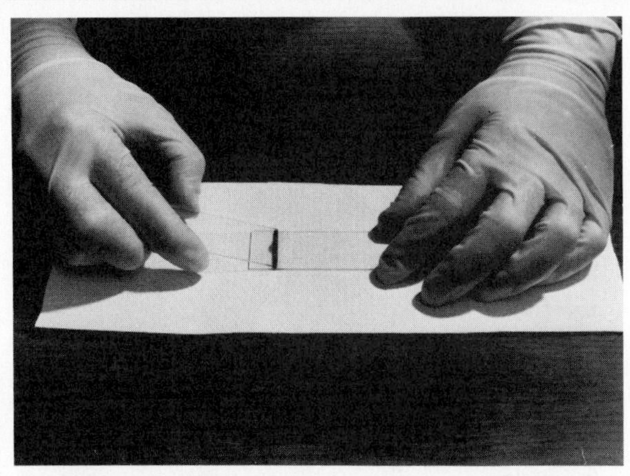

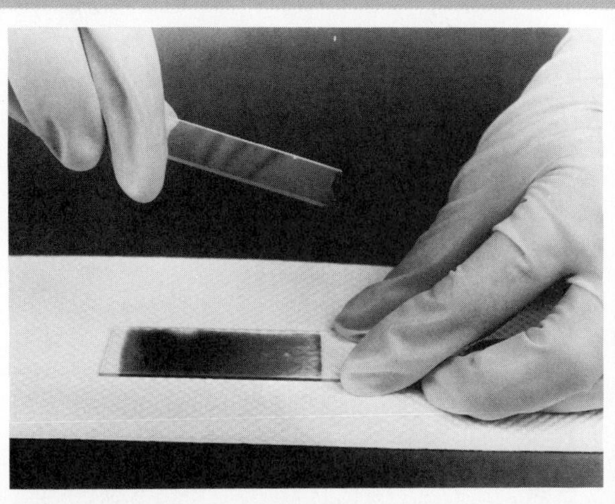

Continued

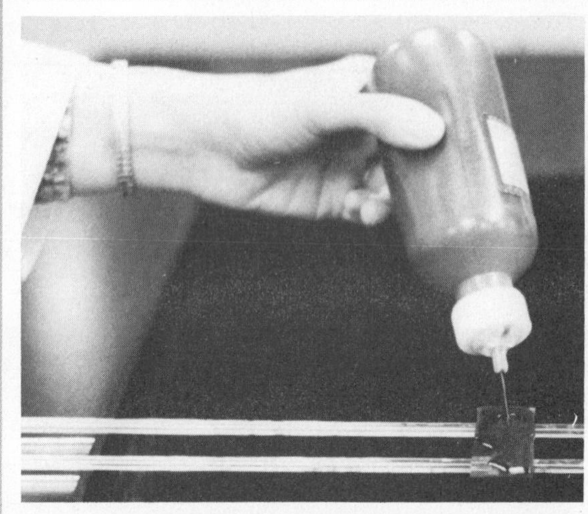

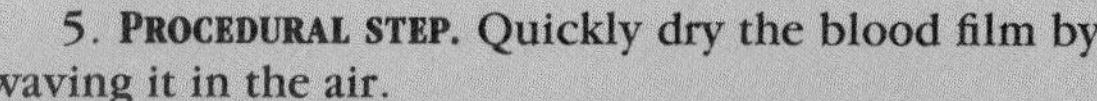

5. **PROCEDURAL STEP.** Quickly dry the blood film by waving it in the air.

PRINCIPLE. The blood film must be dried immediately to prevent shrinkage of the blood cells, which makes them difficult to identify.

6. **PROCEDURAL STEP.** Stain the blood film by placing the slide face up on a staining rack and flooding it with Wright's stain. Allow the stain to remain on the slide for 3 to 5 minutes, depending on the batch of stain. (Do not wash off the stain.)

PRINCIPLE. The timing for each batch of stain varies. There should be a preliminary test of each batch to determine the timing for the best staining reaction.

7. **PROCEDURAL STEP.** Add an equal amount of the buffer solution with a dropper. Mix the stain and buffer by gently blowing on the surface of the slide until a metallic sheen appears. Allow the stain and buffer solution to remain on the slide for 5 to 15 minutes, depending on the batch of stain. Do not understain or overstain the smear.

PRINCIPLE. The white blood cells in an understained or overstained smear are difficult to identify.

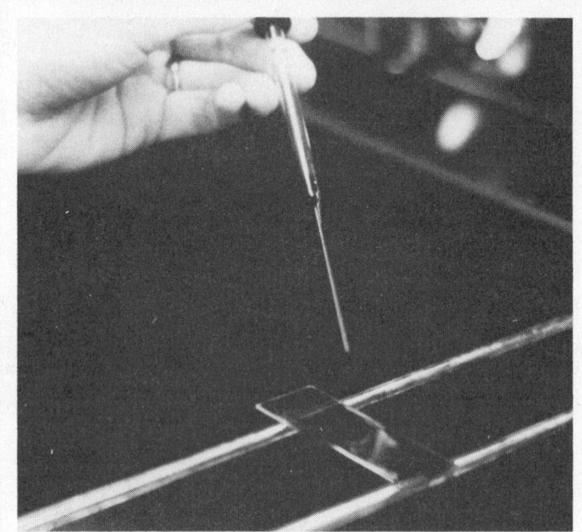

8. **PROCEDURAL STEP.** Wash the stain and buffer solution off with distilled water, starting at the thick end of the smear. Stand the blood film in a vertical position to dry, with the thick end of the smear facing downward. Once it is dry, wipe off the underside of the slide using an alcohol wipe to remove any stain present on this part of the slide.

9. **PROCEDURAL STEP.** First examine the blood film using the low-power objective, to assess the quality of the smear and to determine the best area in which to count the white blood cells. They should be counted in an area where the red blood cells do not overlap but are just touching each other. Generally, the center half of a well-made smear can be used for counting.

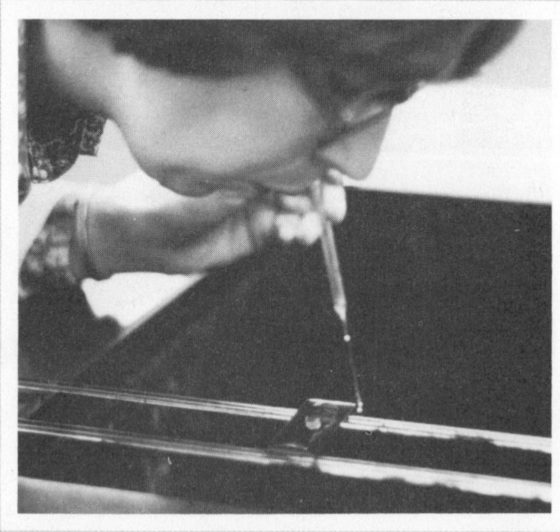

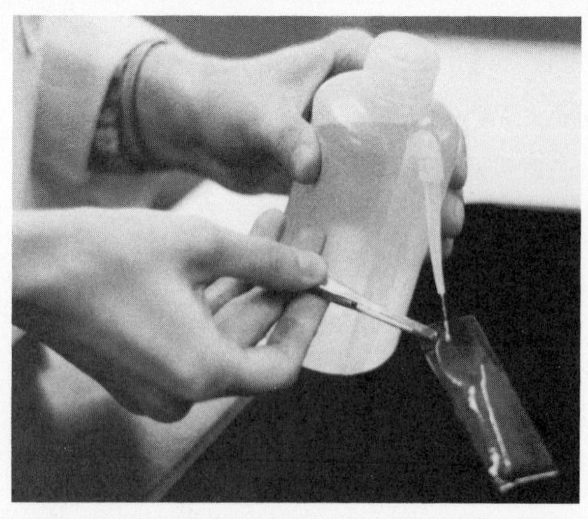

10. **PROCEDURAL STEP.** Place a drop of oil on the appropriate counting area, focus, and examine the smear with the oil-immersion objective of the microscope. Because the blood contains more red than white blood cells, the red cells will be more numerous on the slide, with the white cells scattered among them. In a well-stained smear, the red blood cells appear as small, round, pink- or buff-colored structures. The edges of the cell are darker, whereas the center is paler because the hemoglobin concentration is lower there. The platelets should be purplish-blue ovoid bodies. The nuclei of the white blood cells should stain purplish blue, and the cytoplasm and any granules present will take on various colors, as described on pages 380 and 381.

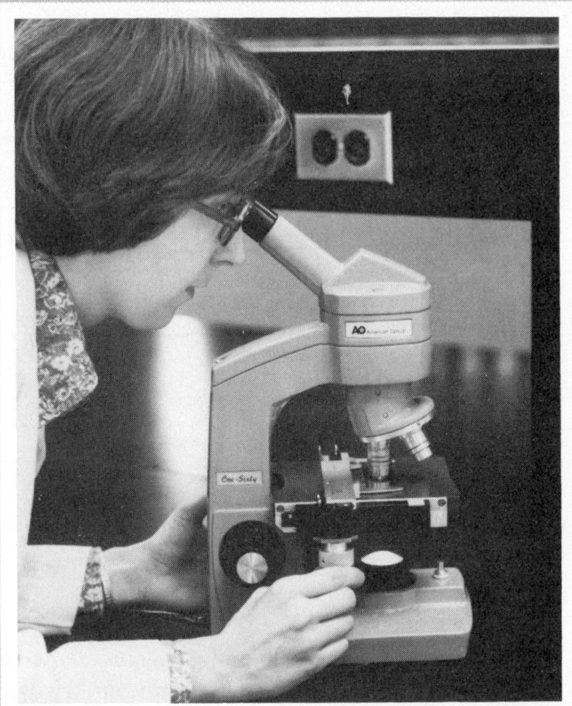

11. **PROCEDURAL STEP.** Count 100 consecutive white blood cells by following a definite pattern to avoid going over the same area more than once. Do not skip a cell if you cannot identify it; ask for assistance. Assign each cell to its specific category by pressing the appropriate button on the mechanical differential cell counter. (As the medical assistant registers each cell in its specific category, the counter keeps a running total of all the cells that have been tabulated.)

Note: One should count 100 cells when the WBC is within normal range of 5000 to 10,000 per cubic millimeter. In excess of 10,000, one should count 200 cells to obtain a better sample.

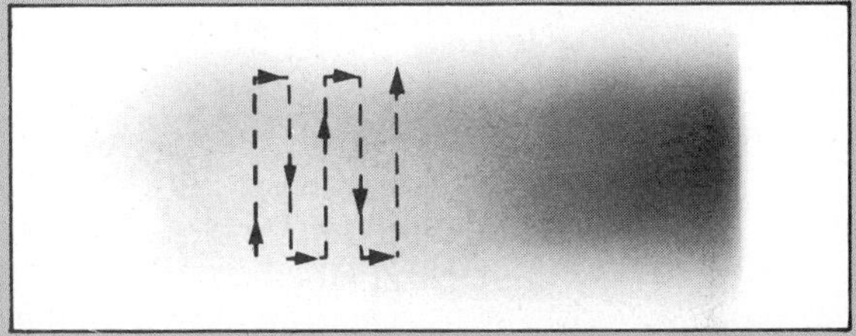

12. **PROCEDURAL STEP.** Convert the number of each of the five types of white blood cells counted to a percentage and record the results. Include the patient's name, the date and time, and the results of the differential cell count. Place your initials next to the recording.

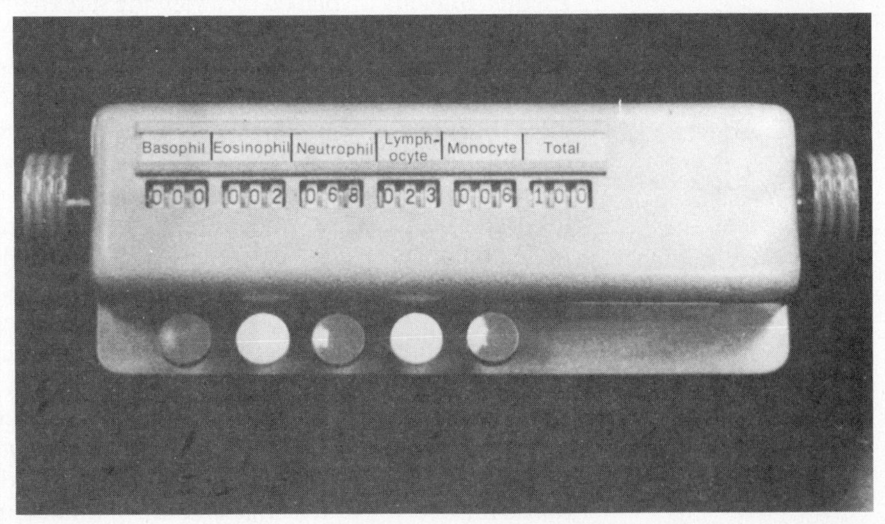

A mechanical differential cell counter. Note that 100 white blood cells have been identified and assigned to their appropriate categories.

Continued

13. **Procedural Step.** Wash your hands and return the equipment.

Record data below.

DATE	TIME	PATIENT'S NAME	RESULTS

Hemoglobin

The most accurate and reliable method for measuring *hemoglobin* concentration involves photometry using a reflectance photometer. A *reflectance photometer* is an instrument that measures light intensity to determine the exact amount of a substance present in a specimen. This instrument permits the processing of specimens in a short period of time, allowing the physician to evaluate the patient's test results while he or she is still in the office.

Examples of reflectance photometers used in the medical office include the Reflotron by Boehringer Mannheim (Fig. 13–7) and the Seralyzer by the Ames Corporation. The Reflotron and Seralyzer are both dry chemistry analyzers, meaning that dry rather than liquid chemicals are used as reagents to perform the tests. Disposable plastic reagent strips are used, on each of which is affixed a dry chemical reagent area for testing a specific chemical constituent in the blood. The blood specimen is pipetted onto the reagent area, and the strip is placed in the reflectance photometer according to the manufacturer's instructions. The test results are then digitally displayed on a viewing screen in less than 2 minutes. In the case of the hemoglobin determination, the normal range should fall between 12 to 16 g per 100 ml for the adult female and 14 to 18 g per 100 ml for the adult male. A decreased hemoglobin level occurs with anemia (especially iron-deficiency anemia), hyperthyroidism, cirrhosis of the liver, severe hemorrhaging, hemolytic reactions, and certain systemic diseases such as leukemia and Hodgkin's disease. Increased levels of hemoglobin are present with polycythemia, chronic obstructive pulmonary disease, and congestive heart failure.

Hemoglobin can also be measured using a visual *color comparison method* such as the Sahli, Talliquist, or Dare method. The Sahli method involves converting hemoglobin to acid hematin, which is visually matched with a standard containing a known amount of hemoglobin. Hydrochloric acid is used to hemolyze the red blood cells to release hemoglobin, which is then converted to the acid hematin. The color of the acid hematin solution is compared with the color of the standard and diluted until its color matches that of the standard. If the color matches the standard after only a small amount of diluent is added, the hemoglobin concentration is relatively low. If a large amount of diluent must be added, the hemoglobin concentration is fairly high. The hemoglobin determination is based on the volume of diluent that must be added. The amount of hemoglobin present is read directly from the calibrations on the tube containing the acid hematin solution and recorded as grams of hemoglobin per 100 ml of blood. The color comparison method is not a highly reliable method, because it is subject to human error; it is

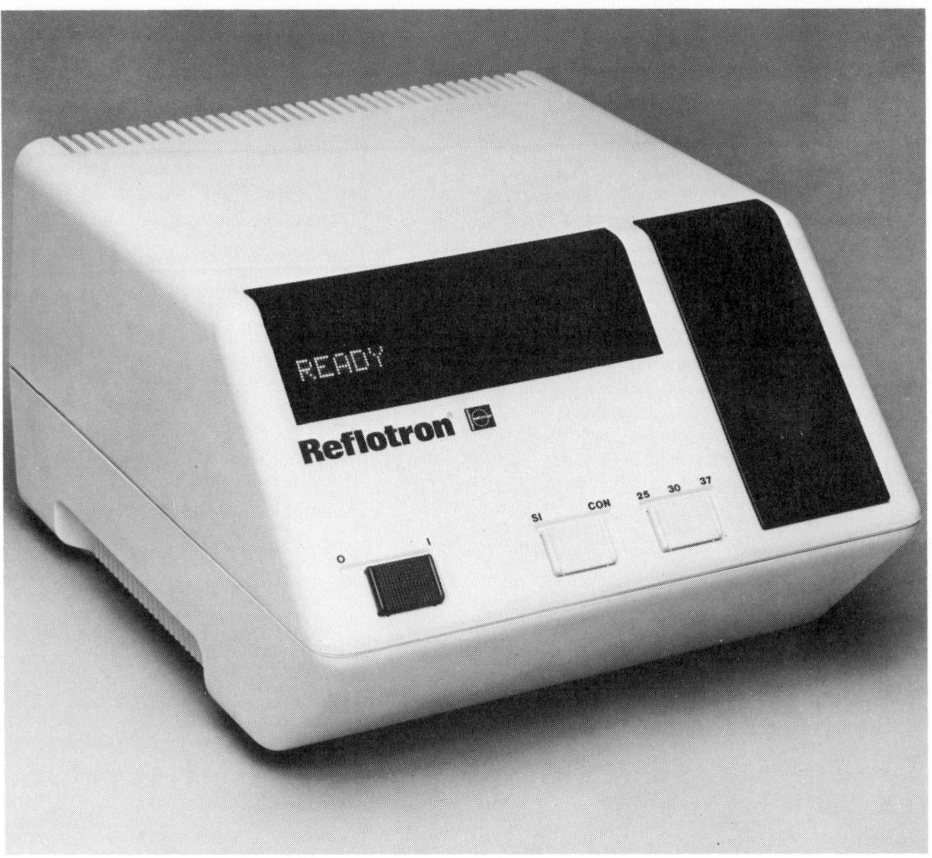

FIGURE 13–7. The Reflotron is an example of an automated reflectance photometer. It performs the following tests: glucose, hemoglobin, BUN, uric acid, bilirubin, cholesterol triglycerides, gamma-GT, SGOT(AST), and SGPT(ALT). (Courtesy of Boehringer Mannheim Diagnostics, Indianapolis, Indiana.)

difficult for the eye to accurately estimate color intensity. Therefore, this method is not used as much today as it was in the past.

Study Questions

1. What tests are included in a complete blood count?
2. What is the function of plasma?
3. What is the normal value or range for each of the following hematologic tests: hemoglobin, red and white blood cell counts, and the differential cell count?
4. What is the purpose of the hematocrit?

• VOCABULARY •

glycogen (gli'ko-jen)—The form in which carbohydrate is stored in the body.

high-density lipoprotein (HDL) (hi den'si-te lip"o-pro'tēn)—A lipoprotein consisting of protein and cholesterol, which removes excess cholesterol from the cells.

hyperglycemia (hi"per-gli-se'me-ah)—An abnormal increase in the glucose level in the blood.

hypoglycemia (hi"po-gli-se'me-ah)—An abnormally low level of glucose in the blood.

low-density lipoprotein (LDL) (lo den'si-te lip"o-pro'tēn)—A lipoprotein consisting of protein and cholesterol, which picks up cholesterol and delivers it to the cells.

lipoprotein (lip"o-pro'tēn)—A complex molecule consisting of protein and a lipid fraction such as cholesterol. Lipoproteins function in transporting lipids in the blood.

COMPETENCIES

After completing this unit, you should be able to demonstrate the proper procedure to do the following:

1. Perform a serum cholesterol test and record results using an automated reflectance photometer and instruction manual.
2. Perform an FBS using a glucose meter and record the results.
3. Demonstrate the proper care and maintenance of the glucose meter.
4. Instruct a patient in the procedure for obtaining and testing a capillary blood specimen for glucose.

LEARNING OBJECTIVES

After completing this unit, you should be able to do the following:

1. Define the terms listed in the vocabulary.
2. Explain the purpose of performing a blood chemistry test.
3. Describe the function of low-density lipoprotein (LDL) and high-density lipoprotein (HDL) in the body.
4. State the patient preparation required for a serum cholesterol test.
5. Identify the primary use of the serum cholesterol test.
6. Explain the use of the blood urea nitrogen test.
7. Explain the function of glucose in the body.
8. Explain the function of insulin in the body.
9. State the patient preparation required for a fasting blood sugar.
10. Identify the normal range for a fasting blood sugar.
11. State the purpose of the fasting blood sugar.
12. Describe the procedure for performing a 2-hour postprandial glucose test.
13. State the purpose for performing a 2-hour postprandial glucose test.
14. Identify the patient preparation required for a glucose tolerance test.
15. State the restrictions that must be followed by the patient during the glucose tolerance test.
16. State the purpose for performing a glucose tolerance test.
17. List and explain the storage requirements for the blood glucose reagent strips.
18. List three advantages of self-monitoring of blood glucose by diabetic patients at home.
19. Explain the principle underlying each step in the procedure for the measurement of blood glucose.

Blood Chemistry Tests

Blood Chemistry

Blood chemistry testing involves the quantitative measurement of chemical substances present in the blood. These chemicals are dissolved in the liquid portion of the blood; therefore, most blood chemistry tests require a serum specimen for analysis. In the medical office, automated reflectance photometers are often used to perform blood chemistry testing; examples include the Seralyzer and the Reflotron (see Fig. 13–7). There are numerous types of blood chemistry tests; the type of test (or tests) ordered depends upon the physician's clinical diagnosis. Table 13–2 provides a listing of common blood chemistry tests, including specimen requirements, normal values, and conditions resulting in abnormal test results. The blood chemistry tests that are most frequently performed are described in more detail below.

Cholesterol

Cholesterol is a fat-soluble steroid (lipid) found in animal fats and oils, organ meats (e.g., liver and brains), egg yolk, whole milk, and other foods of animal origin. Cholesterol is widely distributed in the body, particularly in blood, bile, brain tissue, myelin sheaths of nerve fibers, liver, kidneys, and the adrenal glands. Most of the cholesterol found in the body is synthesized by the liver; however, a portion is obtained from food of animal origin (as plants do not contain cholesterol). Cholesterol is transported in the blood as a complex molecule known as a *lipoprotein.* A lipoprotein consists of protein and a lipid fraction such as cholesterol. Lipoproteins are classified according to their composition and density. Two types of lipoproteins containing cholesterol are termed low-density lipoproteins (LDL) and high-density lipoproteins (HDL). *Low-density lipoprotein* picks up cholesterol from ingested fats and from the liver and delivers it to blood vessels and muscles, where it is deposited in the cells. *High-density lipoprotein* collects excess cholesterol from the cells and carries it to the liver to be excreted. Therefore, LDL and HDL have a combined function in the body; LDL brings cholesterol to the cell, whereas HDL removes it from the cell.

Current research shows that high levels of total serum cholesterol are associated with atherosclerosis and, in turn, an increased risk of coronary artery disease. Further research indicates that the levels of LDL and HDL may be of more significance in detecting coronary artery disease than the total concentration of cholesterol in the blood. The risk of coronary heart disease appears to increase as the level of LDL increases and the level of HDL decreases. Because HDL removes excess cholesterol, it is thought to be protective or beneficial to the body, rather than harmful to it.

The medical assistant needs to provide the patient with instructions for the proper preparation for the serum cholesterol test. Since food and fluids may affect the cholesterol level, the patient must not eat or drink anything except water for 12 hours before the test. The patient should be told to follow a normal diet for 7 days before the test. In addition, the patient is not permitted to consume alcohol or lipid-lowering medications, such as estrogen, salicylates, and oral contraceptives, for 24 hours prior to the test. Before collecting the blood specimen, the medical assistant should ask the patient if the proper food and medication restrictions have been followed to avoid inaccurate test results, which may warrant having to repeat the test.

The normal values for total blood cholesterol vary according to age, diet, and nationality. Most physicians agree, however, that a cholesterol level above 200 mg/dl indicates a need for further testing and efforts to reduce the blood cholesterol level through reduction of the dietary intake of cholesterol. Although the

TABLE 13–2. Common Blood Chemistry Tests

NAME OF TEST AND SPECIMEN REQUIREMENT	ABBREVIATION	PURPOSE	NORMAL RANGE	INCREASED WITH	DECREASED WITH
Alkaline phosphate (serum)	ALP	Assists in the diagnosis of liver and bone diseases.	30–115 mU/ml	Liver disease Bone disease Hyperparathyroidism Infectious mononucleosis	Hypophosphatasia Malnutrition Hypothyroidism Chronic nephritis
Blood urea nitrogen (serum)	BUN	Used as a screening test to detect renal disease, especially glomerular functioning.	8–25 mg/dl	Kidney disease Urinary obstruction Dehydration Gastrointestinal bleeding	Liver failure Malnutrition Impaired absorption
Calcium (serum)	Ca	Used to assess parathyroid functioning and calcium metabolism, and to evaluate malignancies.	8.5–10.5 mg/dl	**Hypercalcemia** Hyperparathyroidism Bone metastases Multiple myeloma Hodgkin's disease Addison's disease Hyperthyroidism	**Hypocalcemia** Hypoparathyroidism Acute pancreatitis Renal failure
Chloride (serum)	Cl	Assists in diagnosing disorders of acid-base and water balance.	96–110 mEq/L	Dehydration Cushing's syndrome Hyperventilation Eclampsia Anemia	Severe vomiting Severe diarrhea Ulcerative colitis Pyloric obstruction Severe burns Heat exhaustion
Cholesterol (serum)	CH Chol	Used to screen for the presence of atherosclerosis related to coronary artery disease. Also used as a secondary aid in the study of thyroid and liver functioning.	**Total cholesterol** 120–200 mg/dl (An upper range of 200 mg/dl is usually now preferred by most physicians to reduce the risk of coronary artery disease.) **LDL cholesterol** 0–19 yr 50–170 mg/dl 20–29 yr 60–170 mg/dl 30–39 yr 70–190 mg/dl 40–49 yr 80–190 mg/dl 50–59 yr 80–210 mg/dl **HDL cholesterol** **Male** 0–19 yr 30–65 mg/dl 20–29 yr 35–70 mg/dl 30–39 yr 30–65 mg/dl 40–49 yr 30–65 mg/dl 50–59 hr 30–65 mg/dl **Female** 0–19 yr 30–70 mg/dl 20–29 yr 35–75 mg/dl 30–39 yr 35–85 mg/dl 40–49 yr 40–95 mg/dl 50–59 yr 35–85 mg/dl	Atherosclerosis Cardiovascular disease Obstructive jaundice Hypothyroidism Nephrosis	Malabsorption Liver disease Hyperthyroidism Anemia
Creatinine (serum)	creat	Used as a screening test of renal functioning.	0.4–1.5 mg/dl	Impaired renal function Chronic nephritis Obstruction of the urinary tract Muscle disease	Muscular dystrophy

TABLE 13-2. Common Blood Chemistry Tests *(Continued)*

NAME OF TEST AND SPECIMEN REQUIREMENT	ABBREVIATION	PURPOSE	NORMAL RANGE	INCREASED WITH	DECREASED WITH
Globulin (serum)	glob	Used to identify abnormalities in the rate of protein synthesis and removal.	1.0–3.5 g/dl	Brucellosis Chronic infections Rheumatoid arthritis Dehydration Hepatic carcinoma Hodgkin's disease	Agammaglobulinemia Severe burns
Glucose Fasting blood sugar Two-hour postprandial Glucose Tolerance Test (serum)	 FBS 2-hr PPBS GTT	Used to detect disorders of glucose metabolism.	FBS: 70–110 mg/100 ml 2-hr PPBS: <140 mg/dl **GTT (mg/100 ml)** **Normal / Diabetic** FBS 70–110 / >120 30 min 120–170 / >200 1 hr 120–170 / >200 2 hr 100–140 / >140 3 hr <125 / >140	**Hyperglycemia** Diabetes mellitus Hepatic disease Brain damage Cushing's syndrome	**Hypoglycemia** Excess insulin Addison's disease Bacterial sepsis Carcinoma of the pancreas Hepatic necrosis Hypothyroidism
Lactic Acid Dehydrogenase (serum)	LDH LD	Used to assist in confirming a myocardial or pulmonary infarction. Also used in the differential diagnosis of muscular dystrophy and pernicious anemia.	100–225 mU/ml	Acute myocardial infarction Acute leukemia Muscular dystrophy Pernicious anemia Hemolytic anemia Hepatic disease Extensive cancer	
Phosphorus (serum)	P	Assists in the proper evaluation and interpretation of calcium levels. Used to detect disorders of the endocrine system, bone diseases, and kidney dysfunction.	2.5–4.5 mg/dl	**Hyperphosphatemia** Renal insufficiency Severe nephritis Hypoparathyroidism Hypocalcemia Addison's disease	**Hypophosphatemia** Hyperparathyroidism Rickets and osteomalacia Diabetic coma Hyperinsulinism
Potassium (serum)	K	Used to diagnose disorders of acid-base and water balance in the body.	3.5–5.5 mEq/L	**Hyperkalemia** Renal failure Cell damage Acidosis Addison's disease Internal bleeding	**Hypokalemia** Diarrhea Pyloric obstruction Starvation Malabsorption Severe vomiting Severe burns Diuretic administration Chronic stress Liver disease with ascites
Serum glutamic–oxaloacetic transaminase (serum)	SGOT (AST)	Used to detect tissue damage.	0–41 mU/ml	Myocardial infarction Liver disease Acute pancreatitis Acute hemolytic anemia	Beriberi Uncontrolled diabetes mellitus with acidosis

Continued

TABLE 13–2. Common Blood Chemistry Tests *(Continued)*

NAME OF TEST AND SPECIMEN REQUIREMENT	ABBREVIATION	PURPOSE	NORMAL RANGE	INCREASED WITH	DECREASED WITH
Serum glutamic–pyruvic transaminase (serum)	SGPT (ALT)	Used to detect liver disease.	0–45 mU/ml	Hepatocellular disease Active cirrhosis Metastatic liver tumor Obstructive jaundice Pancreatitis	
Sodium (serum)	Na	Used to detect changes in water and salt balance in the body.	135–145 mEq/L	**Hypernatremia** Dehydration Conn's syndrome Primary aldosteronism Coma Cushing's disease Diabetes insipidus	**Hyponatremia** Severe burns Severe diarrhea Vomiting Addison's disease Severe nephritis Pyloric obstruction
Free Thyroxine T_4 (serum)	FT_4	Used to assess thyroid functioning and to evaluate thyroid replacement therapy.	1–2.3 mg/dl	Hyperthyroidism Grave's disease Thyrotoxicosis Thyroiditis	Hypothyroidism Cretinism Goiter Myxedema Hypoproteinemia
Total bilirubin (serum)	TB	Used to evaluate liver functioning and hemolytic anemia.	0.1–1.2 mg/dl	Liver disease Obstruction of the common bile or hepatic duct Hemolytic anemia	
Total protein (serum)	TP	Used as a screening test for diseases which alter the protein balance and to assess the state of body hydration.	6.0–8.0 g/dl	Dehydration (vomiting, diarrhea) Chronic infections Acute liver disease Multiple myeloma Lupus erythematosus	Severe hemorrhaging Hodgkin's disease Severe liver disease Malabsorption
Triglycerides (serum)	Trig	Used to evaluate patients with suspected atherosclerosis. (Elevated triglycerides along with elevated cholesterol are risk factors for atherosclerosis.)	40–170 mg/dl	Risk factor for atherosclerosis Liver disease Nephrotic syndrome Hypothyroidism Poorly controlled diabetes Pancreatitis	Malnutrition Congenital lipoproteinemia
Uric acid (serum)	UA	Used to evaluate renal failure, gout and leukemia.	2.2–9.0 mg/dl	Renal failure Gout Leukemia Severe eclampsia Lymphomas	Patients undergoing treatment with uricosuric drugs

primary use of cholesterol testing is to screen for the presence of atherosclerosis related to coronary artery disease, this test is also used as a secondary aid in the study of thyroid and liver function. Refer to Table 13–2 for a list of specific conditions causing abnormal cholesterol test results.

Blood Urea Nitrogen

The blood urea nitrogen BUN is a kidney function test. Urea is the end product of protein metabolism and is normally present in the blood. However, certain kidney diseases may interfere with the ability of the body to excrete the urea properly, causing an increased level of urea in the blood. Refer to Table 13–2 for a list of specific conditions causing abnormal BUN test results.

Blood Glucose

Glucose is the end product of carbohydrate metabolism; its function is to serve as the chief source of energy to carry out normal body functions and to assist in maintaining body temperature. The body maintains a constant blood glucose level to ensure a continuous source of energy for the body. Glucose taken in that is not needed for energy can be stored in the form of *glycogen* in muscle and liver tissue for later use. When no more tissue storage is possible, excess glucose is converted to fat and stored as adipose tissue.

Insulin is a hormone secreted by the beta cells of the pancreas and is required for normal utilization of glucose in the body. Insulin enables glucose to enter the body's cells and be converted to energy. Insulin is also needed for the proper storage of glycogen in liver and muscle cells.

Measuring the amount of glucose present in a blood specimen is one of the most commonly performed blood chemistry tests. It is used to detect abnormalities in carbohydrate metabolism such as occur in diabetes mellitus, hypoglycemia, and liver and adrenocortical dysfunction. Blood glucose measurement is performed using several different testing methods, which include the fasting blood sugar, the 2-hour postprandial glucose test, and the glucose tolerance test. Each of these methods serves a specific role in diagnosing and evaluating abnormalities in carbohydrate metabolism and is described in more detail below.

Fasting Blood Sugar

Blood glucose is usually measured when the patient is in a fasting state. This type of test is termed a *fasting blood sugar (FBS),* which involves collecting a fasting blood sample and measuring the amount of glucose in it. The patient should not have anything to eat or drink, except water, for 12 hours preceding the test. Certain medications, such as oral contraceptives, salicylates, diuretics, and steroids, may affect the test results; therefore, the physician may also place the patient on medication restrictions for a specific period of time before the test—usually for 3 days. The patient should be scheduled for the test in the morning to minimize the inconvenience of abstaining from food and fluid. The normal (fasting) range varies among laboratories and with the specific type of test utilized, but it usually falls between 70 and 110 mg of glucose per 100 ml of blood. An FBS is often performed on diagnosed diabetics in order to evaluate their progress and regulate treatment and as a routine screening procedure to detect diabetes mellitus. An FBS above 120 mg/100 ml is considered the dividing point between normal and hyperglycemic values and is indicative of diabetes mellitus. An elevated test result warrants further testing with the glucose tolerance test.

Two-Hour Postprandial Blood Sugar

The 2-hour postprandial blood sugar test (2-hour PPBS) is used to screen for the presence of diabetes mellitus and to monitor the effects of insulin dosage in diagnosed diabetics. The patient is required to fast, beginning at midnight preceding the test and continuing until breakfast. For breakfast, the patient must consume a prescribed meal containing 100 g of carbohydrate consisting of orange juice, cereal with sugar, toast, and milk. An alternative to this is the consumption of a 100-g test-load glucose solution. A blood specimen is collected from the patient exactly 2 hours after consumption of the meal or glucose solution. In the nondiabetic patient, the glucose level returns to the fasting level within 1½ to 2 hours from the time of glucose consumption, whereas the glucose level in the diabetic patient does not return to the fasting level. A postprandial glucose level of 140 g/100 ml or higher is suggestive of diabetes mellitus and warrants further testing such as the glucose tolerance test.

Glucose Tolerance Test

The *glucose tolerance test (GTT)* provides more detailed information about the ability of the body to metabolize glucose by assessing the insulin response to a glucose load. The GTT is used to assist in the diagnosis of diabetes mellitus, hypoglycemia, and liver and adrenocortical dysfunction. It provides a more thorough analysis of glucose utilization than either the FBS or the 2-hour PPBS.

The patient is usually required to consume a high-carbohydrate diet for 3 days before the test, consisting of 150 g of carbohydrate per day. The patient must be in a fasting state when the test begins. On the morning of the test, a blood specimen is drawn from the patient (FBS) and a urine specimen is taken to measure the amount of glucose in each of these samples. If the FBS indicates hyperglycemia, the physician should be notified, because this situation contradicts the administration of a large test load of glucose. After the FBS has been performed, the patient is instructed to drink a measured amount of a glucose solution (1.75 g of glucose per kilogram of body weight or the standard adult dose of 100 g). Thereafter, at regular intervals (generally 30, 60, 120, and 180 minutes), blood and urine are taken to determine the patient's ability to handle the increased amount of glucose. Each blood and urine specimen must carefully be labeled with the exact time of collection. The patient is permitted to eat and drink normally at the completion of the test.

It is important that the patient adhere to certain restrictions during the test to ensure accurate results. Since food and fluid affect blood glucose levels, the patient must not eat or drink anything during the test, except water. In fact, consumption of water should be encouraged to make it easier for the patient to obtain a urine specimen. Smoking is not permitted during the test because it acts as a stimulant that increases the blood glucose level. The patient should remain at the testing site so that he or she is present when needed for the collection of the blood and urine specimens and to minimize activity. Activity affects the test results by utilizing glucose; therefore, the patient should remain relatively inactive during the test. Sitting and reading, for example, is an activity that would be recommended.

The patient may experience some normal side effects, particularly during the second and third hours of the test, including weakness, a feeling of faintness, and perspiration. These are considered normal reactions of the body to a fall in the glucose level as insulin is secreted in response to the glucose load. The patient should be reassured that this is a temporary condition that will go away. Serious symptoms indicative of hypoglycemic shock should immediately be reported to the physician and include headache, irrational speech or behavior, fainting, and profuse perspiration.

The test results are interpreted by evaluating the data obtained for each collection period. If the glucose level is abnormally increased compared with established norms for the various blood collection times, a disorder of glucose metabolism such as diabetes mellitus may be present. Individuals with diabetes are unable to remove glucose from the bloodstream at the same rate as a nondiabetic individual.

As glucose is absorbed into the bloodstream, the blood glucose level of a nondiabetic rises to a peak level between 160 to 180 mg/100 ml approximately 30 to 60 minutes after the glucose solution is consumed. The pancreas secretes insulin to compensate for this rise, and the blood glucose returns to the fasting level within 2 to 3 hours from the time of ingestion of the glucose solution. In addition, the urine specimens exhibit negative test results for glucose. The individual with diabetes does not exhibit the normal utilization of glucose described above. Rather, the blood glucose level peaks at a much higher level, and glucose is present in the urine. In addition, glucose levels are above normal throughout the test because of the lack of insulin. Refer to Table 13–2 for normal and diabetic glucose values. The glucose tolerance test is generally not used for diagnostic purposes in patients with an FBS above 140 mg/100 ml or a 2-hour postprandial test result above 180 mg/100 ml, because results greater than these values would qualify for the diagnosis of diabetes mellitus and the GTT would not be required.

Hypoglycemia is a condition in which the glucose in the blood is abnormally low. During the GTT, patients with this condition exhibit an abnormally low blood glucose level beginning at the 2-hour interval and continuing up to 4 or 5 hours. Hypoglycemia results from glucose removal from the blood at an excessive rate or from a decreased secretion of glucose into the blood, which may be caused by an overdose of insulin, Addison's disease, bacterial sepsis, carcinoma of the pancreas, hepatic necrosis, or hypothyroidism.

Blood Glucose Measurement with a Glucose Meter

In the medical office, the glucose reflectance photometer (glucose meter) is often used to quantitatively measure the blood glucose level. The specific test most frequently performed using the glucose meter is the FBS, although a significant number of offices also perform the GTT. Glucose meters are commercially available with brand names that include the Accu-Chek (Boehringer Mannheim), Glucometer (Ames), and the Glucoscan (Lifescan). By measuring the blood glucose concentration in the medical office, better patient care can be provided. On-site testing eliminates the time required for an outside laboratory to provide the results, thus allowing the physician to make decisions immediately, regarding patient diagnosis, treatment, and follow-up care.

A reagent strip must be used with the glucose meter; it consists of a plastic strip with a reaction pad at one end. The pad contains chemicals that react with the glucose in whole blood to produce a blue color. The higher the level of glucose, the darker will be the color. After a reaction timing period, the reagent strip is inserted into the glucose meter, which measures color intensity. Through an electronic signal, the glucose results are displayed as a digital read-out. The manufacturer's instructions accompanying the glucose meter must be followed exactly to ensure accurate and reliable test results.

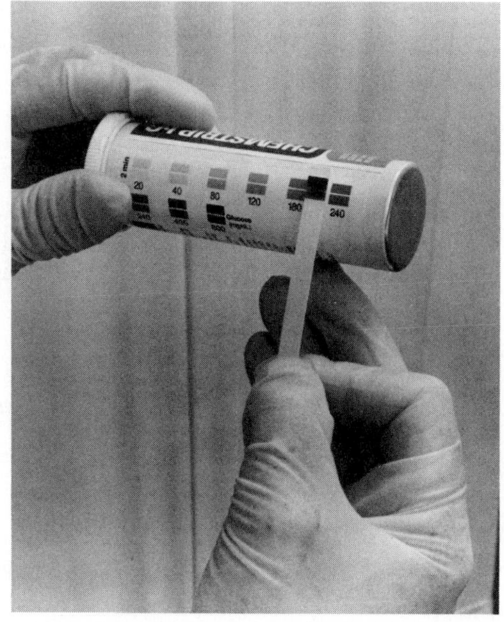

FIGURE 13–8. Blood glucose testing using the reagent strip color comparison method. The resulting color change is visually compared with the color chart to interpret the test results.

Blood glucose measurement using a reagent strip can also be performed by the color comparison method (Fig. 13–8). Using this method, the resulting color change is interpreted by visually comparing the reacted pad with a color chart located on the test strip container. Most physicians prefer to use the glucose meter to interpret the test results, however, because it is more accurate. The color comparison method is subject to human error because of individual differences in the visual interpretation of color intensity.

It is important to properly store the container of reagent strips to prevent their deterioration, which affects the test results. The reagents on the strips are sensitive to heat, light, and moisture and must therefore be stored in a cool, dry area at room temperature (under 86°F) with the cap tightly closed. Strips that are discolored or have darkened should be discarded to prevent inaccurate test results. The container of test strips includes a desiccant, which should not be removed because its purpose is to promote dryness by absorbing moisture.

The glucose meter should be handled carefully. It is a delicate instrument, and a severe physical jar could result in a malfunction. The glucose meter should not be placed in an area of high humidity, such as a bathroom. Exposing the instrument to severe variations in environmental temperature, such as leaving it in a closed vehicle on a hot or cold day, should be avoided. Proper cleaning of the glucose meter is essential for ensuring its accurate and reliable operation. On a regular basis, the exterior of the glucose meter, including the display screen, should be cleaned with a soft, clean cloth moistened with a mild cleaning agent, and it should be dried thoroughly. Do not allow water or detergent to run into the glucose meter, which could damage the internal components. To prolong the life of the instrument, the slot into which the reagent strip is inserted must be cleaned according to the instructions in the operating manual. Because glucose meters are battery operated, periodic replacement of the battery is required. Most glucose meters alert the user to low battery voltage by displaying a special notation on the screen. The type of battery required is specified in the operator's manual along with directions for installation.

PROCEDURE 13-6

BLOOD GLUCOSE MEASUREMENT USING THE ACCU-CHEK II GLUCOSE METER

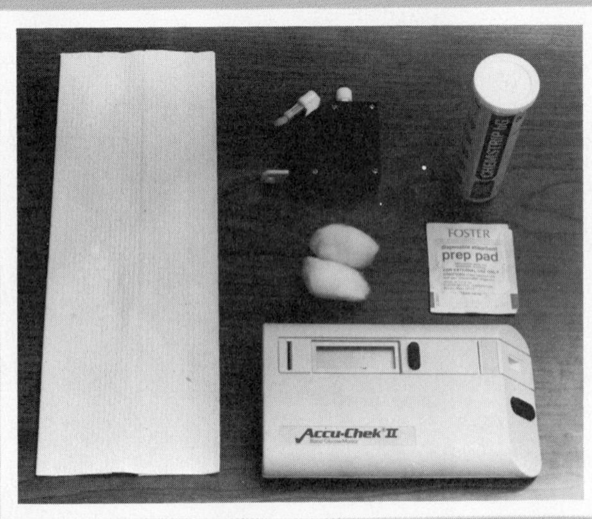

1. **PROCEDURAL STEP.** Assemble the equipment. The equipment includes an **Accu-Chek II glucose meter,** the **container of blood glucose reagent strips (Chemstrip bG reagent strips),** an **automatic lancet device or a sterile lancet,** an **alcohol pledget, cotton balls,** a **paper towel** and **clean gloves.** Check the expiration date on the container of reagent strips.

   PRINCIPLE. Outdated reagent strips can cause falsely low test results.

2. **PROCEDURAL STEP.** Wash the hands to remove any sugar residue that may be present. Sugar remains on the hands after the consumption of certain foods, such as a piece of fruit.

   PRINCIPLE. If sugar residue comes in contact with the reagent pad, a falsely high blood glucose reading results.

3. **PROCEDURAL STEP.** Place the glucose meter on a flat surface and turn it on by pressing the ON/OFF button.

4. **PROCEDURAL STEP.** Ensure that the glucose meter is properly calibrated by viewing the liquid crystal display (LCD) screen. A properly calibrated glucose meter exhibits information as follows: the digits 888 appear on the display screen followed by a three-digit code that corresponds to the code on the container of test strips currently in use. If the meter is not calibrated, perform this operation as outlined at the end of the procedure (see Accu-Chek Calibration Procedure).
PRINCIPLE. The glucose meter must be properly calibrated to ensure accurate and reliable test results.

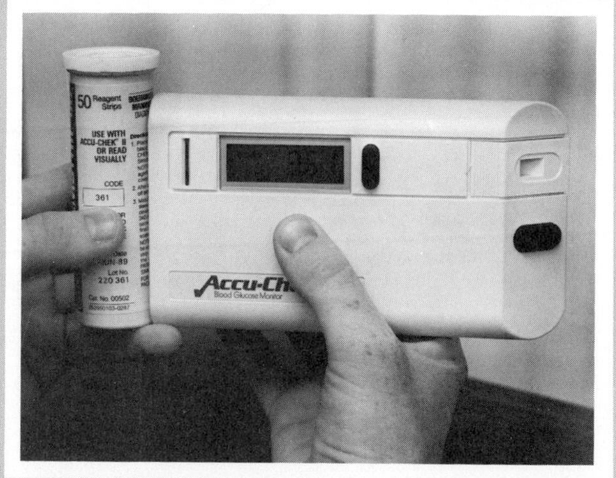

5. **PROCEDURAL STEP.** Remove a Chemstrip bG reagent strip from the container and place it on a paper towel or other clean, dry surface with the reagent pad facing up. Do not touch the reagent pad with the fingers. Promptly replace the lid of the container.
PRINCIPLE. The reagent pads are moisture sensitive and could be affected by environmental moisture or moisture present on the fingers leading to inaccurate test results. In addition, oil from the skin may clog the reagent coating, interfering with a proper chemical reaction.

6. **PROCEDURAL STEP.** Identify the patient and explain the procedure. If a fasting blood specimen is required, ask the patient if he or she has had anything to eat or drink (besides water) for the past 12 hours.
PRINCIPLE. Consumption of food or fluid increases the blood glucose level, leading to inaccurate interpretation of FBS test results.

7. **PROCEDURAL STEP.** Ask the patient to wash his or her hands in warm water and thoroughly dry them.
PRINCIPLE. Washing the hands cleans the fingers and stimulates the flow of blood. The hands must be completely dry to encourage the formation of a hanging drop of blood, which assists in the transfer of the blood to the reagent pad.

8. **PROCEDURAL STEP.** Cleanse the puncture site with an alcohol pledget and allow it to dry. Apply gloves and perform a finger puncture.
PRINCIPLE. The alcohol must be allowed to dry to prevent it from reacting with the chemicals on the reagent pad and leading to inaccurate test results. Gloves are a precaution that provides a barrier against contaminated blood.

9. **PROCEDURAL STEP.** Once the puncture has been made, wipe away the first drop of blood with a cotton ball. Place the hand in a dependent position (palm facing down), and gently squeeze the finger around the puncture site until a large drop of blood forms.
PRINCIPLE. The first drop of blood contains a large amount of serum, which dilutes the specimen and leads to inaccurate test results. A large drop of blood is needed to completely cover the reagent pad.

Continued

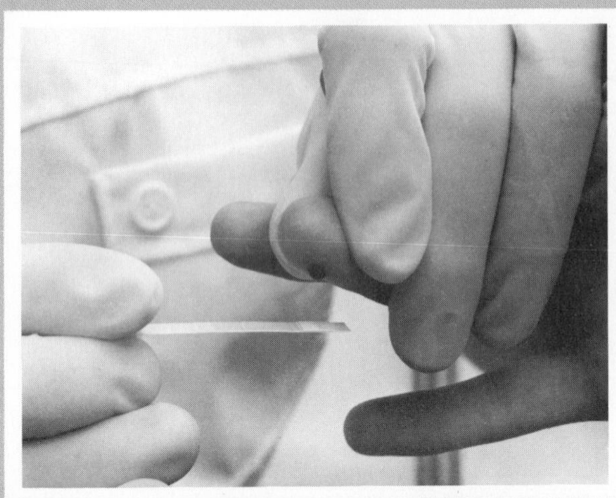

10. **PROCEDURAL STEP.** Hold the plastic strip in a horizontal position with the reagent pad facing upward. Bring the test strip to the finger, and allow the reagent pad to contact the drop of blood. Completely cover both test zones of the reagent area with the blood specimen.

PRINCIPLE. If the reagent pad is not completely covered with blood, test results may be falsely low. The strip must be held in a horizontal position to prevent the blood from spilling off the reagent pad.

11. **PROCEDURAL STEP.** Immediately press the TIME button on the glucose meter, until a beep is heard. The timing button activates and monitors a 60-second reaction period. The LCD screen counts off and displays elapsed seconds (i.e., "1, 2, 3 . . ." up to 60). Be sure to maintain the strip in a horizontal position during the timing period.

PRINCIPLE. The timing period allows the blood to react with the chemicals on the reagent pad, resulting in the development of a blue color.

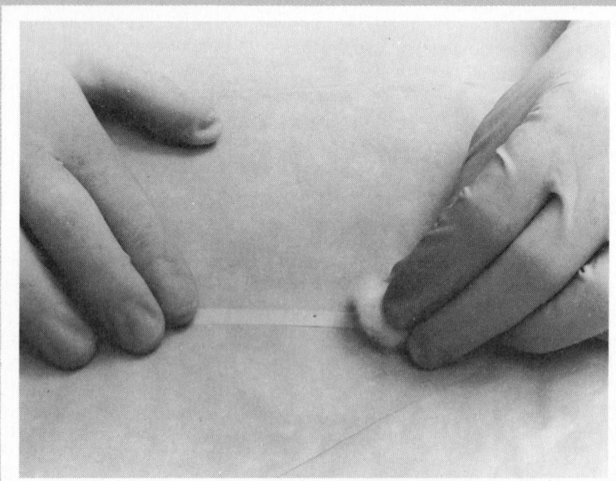

12. **PROCEDURAL STEP.** Apply pressure to the patient's finger with a cotton ball to control blood flow.

13. **PROCEDURAL STEP.** When the screen displays 57, 58, 59, and 60 (seconds), the glucose meter emits three high beeping sounds and one low sound, respectively. The high beeping sounds are emitted to provide advance notice to prepare for the blotting procedure. As soon as the monitor displays 60 and emits the low beep, remove the excess blood from the reagent pad as indicated below.

a. Lay the reacted reagent strip on a firm, clean, dry surface, such as a paper towel placed on a laboratory work table.
b. Using moderate pressure, blot the reagent pad with a clean, dry cotton ball. Blot the pad two more times with a clean part of the cotton ball. All of the excess blood residue must be wiped from the reagent pad. Do not overblot or smear the reagent pad.

Note. During this time, the glucose meter continues to monitor elapsed seconds for another 60 seconds (starting with 60 and continuing to 120).

PRINCIPLE. The excess blood must be removed at the proper time to avoid falsely high test results. Overblotting can lead to falsely low test results. Smearing the reagent pad unevenly distributes the blood on the pad, leading to inaccurate test results.

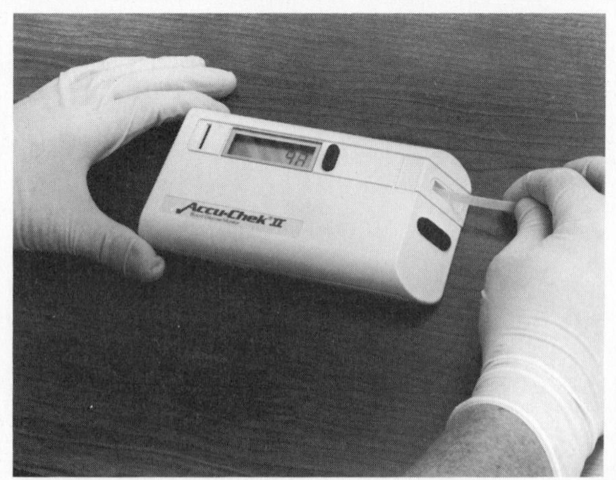

14. **PROCEDURAL STEP.** Turn the reagent strip on its side with the reagent pad facing the ON/OFF button. Insert the reacted reagent pad into the strip adapter located on the side of the glucose meter. The reagent pad must be inserted before the LCD screen displays 120 (seconds).

15. **Procedural step.** When the display reads 120, a high beep automatically sounds and the glucose value is displayed in milligrams per deciliter. If the glucose value is higher or lower than expected or if the screen displays something other than the glucose value, refer to the Troubleshooting Guide section of the Accu-Chek operator's manual to obtain instructions for correcting the problem. (The glucose result indicated on this glucose meter is 105 mg/dl.)

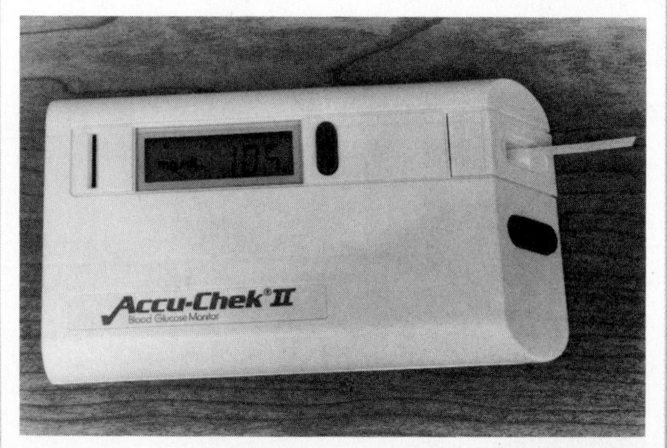

16. **Procedural step.** Remove the reacted reagent pad from the glucose meter and properly dispose of it according to medical office policy.

17. **Procedural step.** Remove the gloves and wash hands. Record the results. Include the patient's name, the date and time, when the patient last ate, the type of test (e.g., FBS, random), and the glucose test result recorded in milligrams per deciliters. If the patient has diabetes mellitus, also record the time of his or her last insulin injection or last consumption of oral hypoglycemic medication. Be sure to place your initials next to the recording.

18. **Procedural step.** Turn off the instrument and properly store it according to the medical office policy.

Record data below.

DATE	TIME	PATIENT'S NAME	RESULTS

Continued

ACCU-CHEK II GLUCOSE METER CALIBRATION PROCEDURE

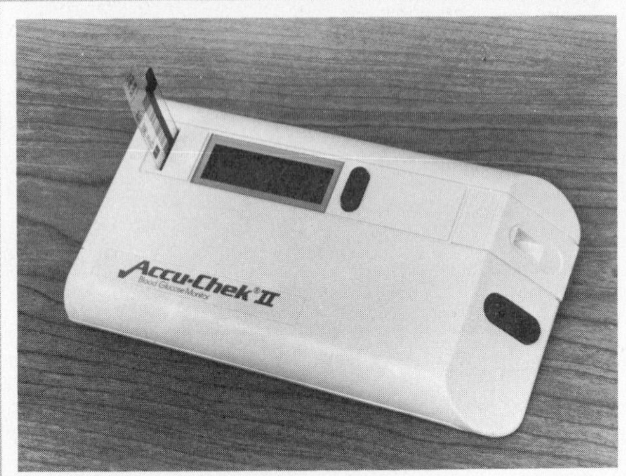

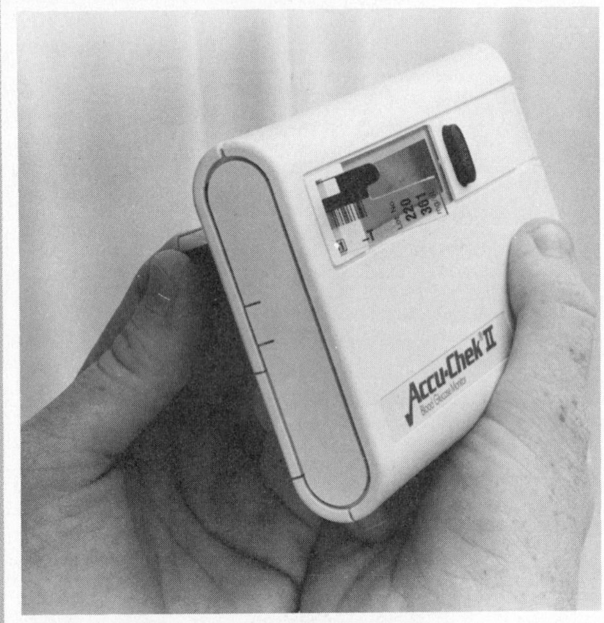

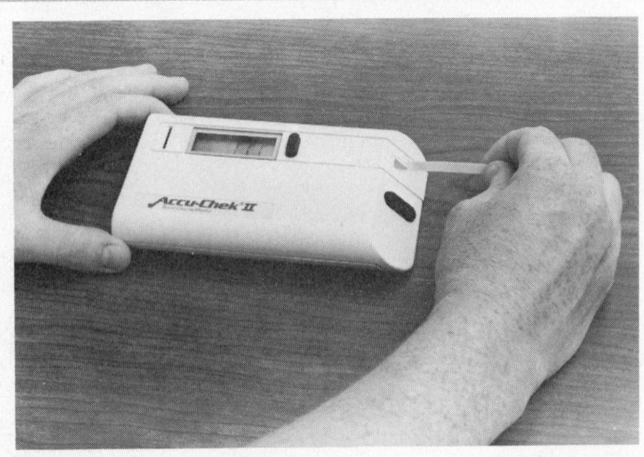

The purpose of calibrating the glucose meter is to ensure accurate and reliable test results by compensating for variables that exist in the manufacturing process of each container of reagent strips. Calibration programs the electronics of the glucose meter to match the reactivity of the container of strips that are in current use. The calibration procedure is performed using a coated strip of plastic that accompanies each container of fifty Chemstrips. Accu-Chek requires lot-specific calibration, meaning that the calibration procedure needs to be performed only once per container of test strips. This is possible because the Accu-Chek glucose meter has a built-in memory system that enables it to retain a point of reference, once it has been calibrated. This reference point is retained until the glucose meter is reprogrammed for a new container of test strips. Once the glucose meter has been calibrated, the calibration strip should be stored in the Chemstrip container until all the reagent strips have been used.

The calibration procedure delineated below should be followed when a new container of test strips is opened.

1. Place the glucose meter on a flat surface.

2. Insert the pointed end of the calibration strip into the calibration compartment located to the left of the display screen.

3. Continue inserting the strip until it touches the flat surface on which it sits.

4. Press the ON/OFF button to turn on the glucose meter.

5. The following symbol will appear on the LCD screen: ı|ı|ı|

6. Pick up the glucose meter and grasp the end of the calibration strip, which extends from the back of the calibration compartment.

7. Using a slow and steady motion, pull the calibration strip through the compartment.

8. Proper calibration of the glucose meter results in a beeping sound and a display of CCC on the LCD screen.

9. Position an unused Chemstrip bG reagent strip on its side with the reagent pad facing away from the ON/OFF button. (The strip is inserted in this position for calibration only.)

10. Insert the reagent strip into the test strip adapter until it reaches the end of the chamber.

11. Press the TIME button until a beep is heard. The numbers 888 will appear on the display screen followed by a three-digit code, which corresponds to the code printed on the label of the Chemstrip vial.

12. Remove the test strip from the test strip adapter and turn off the glucose meter.

PROCEDURE 13-7

BLOOD GLUCOSE MEASUREMENT USING THE GLUCOMETER II GLUCOSE METER

Measurement of blood glucose using the Glucometer II glucose meter is performed in a manner similar to the procedure outlined for Accu-Chek II. Variations to this procedure are identified and described below. The Glucometer II requires a programming procedure to calibrate the glucose meter for each bottle of test strips. A control test is also required and should be run on a daily basis. The programming and control procedures are outlined in the operator's manual accompanying the glucose meter.

1. The equipment required includes a **Glucometer II glucose meter,** the **container of blood glucose reagent strips (Glucostix reagent strips),** an **automatic lancet device or a sterile lancet,** an **alcohol pledget,** a **tissue** and **clean gloves.** Prepare the tissue for the blotting procedure by folding it in half, and then in quarters. Place the tissue on a firm surface in preparation for blotting.

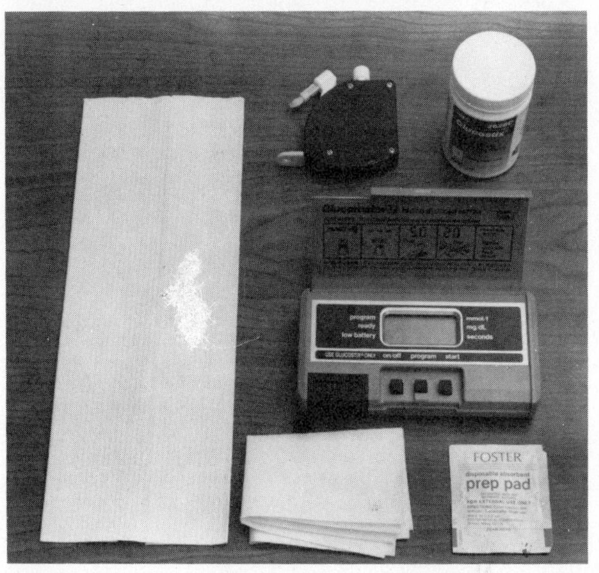

2. Lift the lid of the Glucometer II and press the ON/OFF button. The last entered program number should appear on the display screen. If this number does not match the program number on the reagent strip container, repeatedly press the program button until the numbers match. (Refer to the Glucometer II operator's manual for more detailed information regarding this procedure.)

3. Apply gloves and perform the finger puncture. Form a large drop of blood at the end of the patient's finger and proceed as follows:

   a. Press the START TEST button.
   b. When a beeping sound occurs, quickly apply the drop of blood to the reagent pad. (The screen of the glucose meter displays 50 (seconds) when the beep is emitted). Make sure both of the yellow reagent pads are completely covered with blood. Be sure to maintain the reagent strip in a horizontal position.

4. Two short beeps sound at 22 and 21 (seconds). When the screen displays 20 (seconds), the glucose meter emits a long beep. At this time, lay the reacted reagent strip on the folded tissue and immediately blot the reagent pads two times with a different fold of the tissue. Do not overblot or smear the reagent pad. Overblotting is evidenced by the tissue sticking to the surface of the reagent pads.

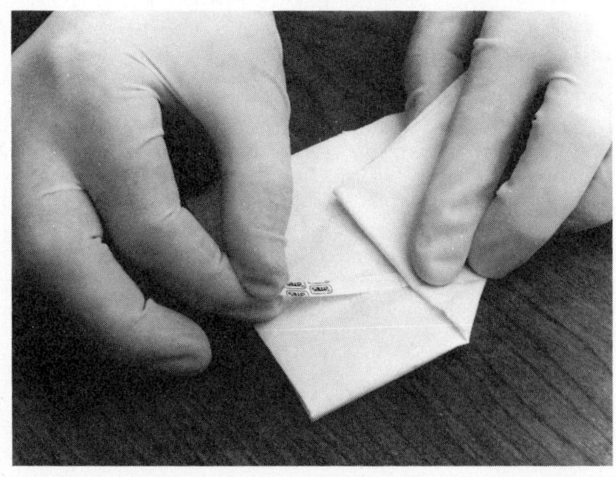

Continued

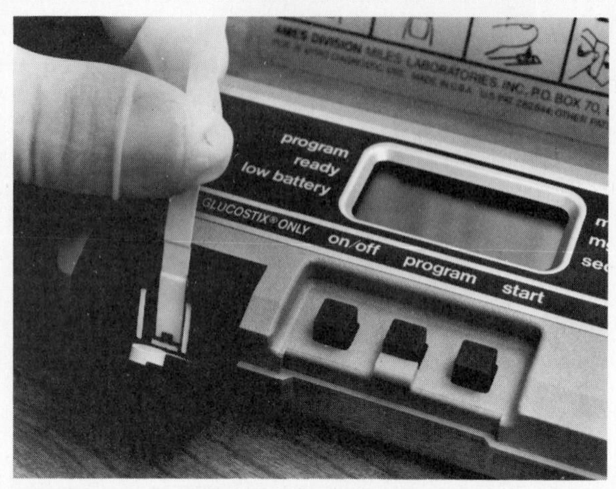

5. Immediately open the test door of the glucose meter and insert the reagent strip into the strip guide with the reacted reagent pad facing the test window. Make sure the end of the strip is positioned behind the strip guide tab.

6. Close the door as soon as possible.

7. A countdown period occurs. At the end of this period five short beeps sound as the screen displays 1 (second) followed briefly by a display of three bars (– – –) on the screen. The test results are then displayed on the screen in milligrams per deciliters, along with a final beep. If the glucose value is higher or lower than expected or if the screen displays something other than the glucose value, refer to the Problem Solving section of the Glucometer operator's manual to obtain instructions on correcting the problem. (The glucose result indicated on this glucose meter is 135 mg/dl.)

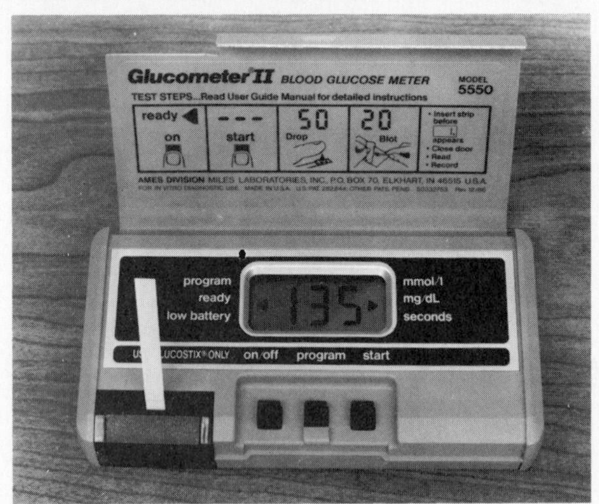

8. **Procedural step.** Remove the reacted reagent pad from the glucose meter and properly dispose of it according to medical office policy.

9. **Procedural step.** Remove the gloves and wash hands. Record the results. Include the patient's name, the date and time, when the patient last ate, the type of test (e.g., FBS, random), and the glucose test result recorded in milligrams per deciliters. If the patient has diabetes mellitus, also record the time of his or her last insulin injection or last consumption of oral hypoglycemic medication. Be sure to place your initials next to the recording.

10. **Procedural step.** Turn off the instrument and properly store it according to the medical office policy.

Record data below.

DATE	TIME	PATIENT'S NAME	RESULTS

Self Monitoring of Blood Glucose

Diabetic patients taking insulin must monitor blood glucose levels at home to provide for effective management of their condition. Based upon the results, decisions can be made regarding insulin and dietary adjustments that may be necessary to maintain normal glucose levels and to avoid the extremes of hypoglycemia or hyperglycemia. Satisfactory control of the blood glucose level reduces symptoms of the disease and helps to decrease or delay long-term complications that can occur with diabetes mellitus, such as retinopathy and peripheral vascular disease. Several methods are available to assess glucose levels, including urine testing and capillary blood testing.

Before the development of the glucose meter, urine testing was used most frequently by diabetics to monitor their glucose levels. The tests most often employed include Clinitest, Tes-Tape and Diastix. Although urine testing is still being done because it is the least expensive method and does not require a painful finger puncture, it does not provide test results as accurate as those from blood glucose testing.

Glucose levels determined by urine testing are not as accurate for several reasons. There are significant variations among individuals in the renal threshold for glucose (i.e., the concentration above which glucose cannot be reabsorped by the kidneys and spills into the urine). In particular, the very young tend to have a low renal threshold, whereas the elderly have a high renal threshold. Therefore, a diabetic with a low renal threshold may test positive for urine glucose, even though the blood glucose is not elevated. On the other hand, a patient with a high renal threshold may produce a negative urine glucose test result when the actual blood glucose level is elevated, leading to a false impression of good control. In both of the cases described above, the patient would not have accurate information for determining proper insulin dosage. Another factor affecting urine testing is the lag time between the actual production of the urine by the kidneys and its analysis. The urine that is being tested may have been filtered through the kidney several hours before being tested and, as a result, would not reflect the current blood glucose level.

Blood glucose monitoring at home provides the diabetic patient with a direct measurement of the glucose level, rather than the less reliable measurement of urinary glucose excretion, and results in a program of tighter control for most patients. Because of the necessity of performing a finger puncture and the fact that the patient must assume more responsibility in self-management decisions, the medical assistant may need to reinforce some of the advantages of home blood glucose monitoring, which are discussed below.

1. *Convenience of testing.* The patient is able to test his or her blood at any time of the day without a physician's order. Before the development of blood glucose reagent strips and glucose meters, patients could obtain a blood glucose test only through a laboratory order from the physician. Because of the cost and inconvenience involved in this process, most patients did not comply with the testing requirements needed to achieve and maintain satisfactory control. In addition, the patient was unable to obtain the test when the office or laboratory was closed. With some patients, the lowest blood glucose level occurs from 3:00 to 5:00 AM when most laboratory facilities are closed. Testing at home also lets the patient check his or her blood glucose when a side effect common to diabetes mellitus occurs, such as hypoglycemia.

2. *More involvement in self-management decisions.* The patient is able to become more involved in self-management decisions regarding insulin dosage, meal planning, and physical activity. Initially some patients may lack confidence in making insulin and dietary adjustments based upon the blood glucose test results. The medical assistant should provide encouragement and stress the benefits to be derived in terms of improved regulation of the blood glucose level.

3. *Reliable decisions regarding insulin dosage.* More reliable decisions regarding insulin needs can be made during situations that affect the blood glucose level, such as illness, emotional stress, increased physical activity, or suspected hypoglycemia.

4. *Decrease or delay in long-term complications.* Diabetic patients maintaining good blood glucose control generally experience fewer symptoms, and they decrease or delay long-term complications of the disease; these results can lead to a longer life expectancy. Having a record of the patient's daily blood glucose values also assists the physician in making decisions regarding treatment and follow-up care.

Patient Teaching

The medical assistant may need to instruct the patient in the procedure for obtaining and testing a capillary blood specimen for blood glucose measurement. Properly educating the patient to perform the procedure is the most important factor in obtaining accurate test results. Although the blood glucose procedure has already been presented in this chapter, certain aspects denote special emphasis for effective patient teaching. These areas are listed and described below.

1. *Obtaining the capillary blood specimen.* The medical assistant should inform the patient of the sites available for obtaining the blood specimen. These include the fingers, the earlobes, and the side of the hand where there are no callouses. Most patients prefer to use an automatic lancet device to perform the finger puncture. Using such a device makes the puncture less painful, and the preset puncture depth generally assures a successful stick. For a finger puncture, instruct the patient to obtain the blood specimen from the lateral side of the tip of the finger, because this area contains fewer nerve endings and less pain results. If the patient's hands are cold, tell him or her to rub them together or place them in warm water, which improves the blood flow to the area. Instruct the patient in the proper procedure for obtaining a large drop of blood to ensure accurate test results.

2. *Performing the blood glucose test.* The patient performs the test with a reagent strip, using either the color comparison method or the glucose meter to interpret the results. Instruct the patient in the proper procedure for performing the test, making sure he or she understands that accurate test results assist in greater glucose control. Patients using a glucose meter should also be given detailed instructions on the proper care and maintenance of the instrument.

3. *Proper blotting procedures.* This aspect of the testing procedure warrants special emphasis because a false low or false high test result is likely if it is not performed properly. False high or low results can lead to an improper insulin dosage adjustment, resulting in poor regulation of the blood glucose level.

4. *Recording results.* The patient should record each test result in a log book to provide a permanent record between office visits. Some glucose meters (e.g., Glucometer II with Memory) are equipped with a memory system that stores test results for later retrieval. Information that should be included with each recording is listed below:

a. Date and time.
b. Number of hours since the patient last ate.
c. Time of the last insulin injection or oral hypoglycemic medication.
d. Any feeling of physical or emotional stress.
e. How much exercise the patient has undergone.

Keeping track of the factors listed above helps to explain a shift in the blood glucose level and provides the basis for sound self-management decisions.

The frequency of the blood glucose testing depends upon a number of factors, including the severity of the diabetes, the presence of special conditions such as pregnancy, and variations in activity level. Ideally, the blood glucose level should be monitored four times a day as follows: in the morning (after an 8-hour fast), before lunch and dinner, and at bedtime. The FBS test result (obtained in the morning) is the best overall indicator of control, while the other determinations provide guidance for adjusting insulin dosage, diet, and exercise. Some physicians may periodically recommend a 2-hour postprandial specimen to further assist in maintaining good control by detecting hyperglycemia that might otherwise be missed. Overall, self monitoring of the blood glucose level at home provides an important feedback mechanism to maintain normal blood glucose levels and to assist the diabetic patient in anticipating and treating fluctuations in glucose levels brought on by food, exercise, stress, and infection.

Study Questions

1. What is the function of LDL and HDL?
2. What is the primary use of the serum cholesterol test?
3. What patient preparation is required for a fasting blood sugar?
4. What is the purpose of performing a glucose tolerance test?
5. What are the advantages of self monitoring of blood glucose by diabetic patients at home?

14

MICROBIOLOGY AND DISEASE

CHAPTER OUTLINE

The Normal Flora
Infection
Microorganisms and Disease
The Microscope
Microbiologic Specimen Collection
Cultures
Streptococcus Testing
Sensitivity Testing
Microscopic Examination of Microorganisms
Prevention and Control of Infectious Diseases

COMPETENCIES

After completing this chapter, you should be able to demonstrate the proper procedures to perform the following:

1. Use a compound microscope.
2. Properly handle and care for a microscope.
3. Obtain a specimen for a throat culture, and record the procedure.
4. Obtain a microbiologic specimen using a collection and transport system.
5. Perform a streptococcus test, using a rapid strep test and record results.
6. Perform a streptococcus test, using the bacitracin susceptibility test, and record results.
7. Prepare a wet mount.
8. Prepare a hanging drop slide.
9. Prepare a microbiologic smear.
10. Prepare a gram-stained smear.

LEARNING OBJECTIVES

After completing this chapter, you should be able to do the following:

1. Define the words listed in the vocabulary.
2. List and explain the stages in the course of an infectious disease.
3. List and describe the three classifications of bacteria based on shape.
4. Give examples of infectious diseases caused by the following types of cocci: staphylococci, streptococci, and diplococci.
5. State examples of infectious diseases caused by bacilli, spirilla, and viruses.
6. Explain the function of the following parts of a compound microscope: base, arm, stage, light source, substage condenser, iris diaphragm, body tube, coarse adjustment, and fine adjustment.
7. Describe the function of the ocular lens of a microscope.
8. Explain the difference between a monocular and a binocular microscope.
9. Identify the function of each of the following microscope lenses: low power, high power, and oil immersion.
10. Calculate the total magnification of an objective lens of a microscope.
11. Explain the purpose of using oil with the oil immersion microscope objective.
12. List five guidelines that should be followed for proper care of the microscope.
13. Explain the purpose of obtaining a specimen, and identify five body areas from which a specimen may be taken for microbiologic examination.
14. List two ways to prevent contamination of a specimen by extraneous microorganisms.
15. Explain what types of precautions a medical assistant should take to prevent infection from a pathogenic specimen.
16. Describe the proper method for handling and transporting microbiologic specimens.
17. Explain the purpose and describe the procedure for culturing a microbiologic specimen.

Continued

• VOCABULARY •

bacilli (bah-sil'i) (singular, bacillus)—Bacteria that have a rod shape.

cocci (kok'si) (singular, coccus)—Bacteria that have a round shape.

colony (kol'o-ne)—A mass of bacteria growing on a solid culture medium that have arisen from the multiplication of a single bacterium.

contagious (kon-ta'jus)—Capable of being transmitted directly or indirectly from one person to another.

culture (kul'tūr)—The propagation of a mass of microorganisms in a laboratory culture medium.

culture medium (kul'tūr me'de-um)—A mixture of nutrients on which microorganisms are grown in the laboratory.

false negative (fôls neg'ah-tiv)—A test result denoting that a condition is absent when, in actuality, it is present.

false positive (fôls poz'i-tiv)—A test result denoting that a condition is present when, in actuality, it is absent.

fastidious (fas-tid'e-us)—Extremely delicate; difficult to culture, therefore involving specialized growth requirements.

immunization (im"u-ni-za'shun)—The process of becoming protected from a disease through vaccination.

incubate (in'ku-bāt)—In microbiology, the act of placing a culture in a chamber (incubator), which provides optimal growth requirements for the multiplication of the organism, such as the proper temperature, humidity, and darkness.

incubation period (in"ku-ba'shun pir'ē-ud)—The interval of time between the invasion by a pathogenic microorganism and the appearance of first symptoms of the disease.

infectious disease (in-fek'shus di-zēz')—A disease caused by a pathogen that produces harmful effects on its host.

inoculate (i-nok'u-lāt)—The introduction of microorganisms into a culture medium for means of growth and multiplication.

inoculum (i-nok'u-lum)—The specimen used to inoculate a medium.

microbiology (mi"kro-bi-ol'o-je)—The scientific study of microorganisms and their activities.

mordant (mor'dant)—A substance that fixes a stain or dye.

mucous membrane (mu'kus mem'brān)—A membrane lining body passages or cavities that open to the outside.

normal flora (nor'mal flo'rah)—Harmless, nonpathogenic microorganisms that normally reside in many parts of the body but do not cause disease.

prodrome (pro'drōm)—A symptom indicating an approaching disease.

resistance (re-zis'tans)—The natural ability of an organism to remain unaffected by harmful substances in its environment.

sequela (se-kwel'lah)—A morbid (secondary) condition occurring as a result of a less serious primary infection.

smear (smēr)—Material spread on a slide for microscopic examination.

specimen (spes'i-men)—A small sample or part taken from the body to show the nature of the whole.

spirilla (spi-ril'ah) (singular, spirillum)—Bacteria that have a spiral shape.

streaking (strēk'ing)—In microbiology, the process of inoculating a culture to provide for the growth of colonies on the surface of a solid medium. Streaking is accomplished by skimming a wire inoculating loop containing the specimen across the surface of the medium, using a back-and-forth motion.

streptolysin (strep-tol'i-sin)—An exotoxin produced by beta hemolytic streptococci which completely hemolyzes red blood cells.

susceptible (sū-sep'ti-b'l)—Easily affected; lacking resistance.

18. Explain the importance of the early diagnosis of streptococcal pharyngitis.
19. Explain how to differentiate between alpha, beta, and gamma streptococci.
20. Explain the purpose and describe the procedure for performing a sensitivity test.
21. Explain why some microorganisms must be examined in the living state.
22. Explain the purpose for making a microbiologic smear.
23. Explain the purpose of gram staining.
24. Identify four infectious diseases caused by gram-positive bacteria and four caused by gram-negative bacteria.
25. Give examples of methods to prevent and control infectious diseases in the community.
26. Explain the principle underlying each step in the microbiologic procedures.

Introduction

Microbiology is the scientific study of microorganisms and their activities. As described in Chapter 1, microorganisms are tiny living plants and animals that cannot be seen by the naked eye but must be viewed under the microscope. Antony van Leeuwenhoek (1632–1723) designed a magnifying glass strong enough for viewing microorganisms. He was the first individual to observe and describe protozoa and bacteria (Fig. 14–1). Leeuwenhoek's magnifying glass was the precursor of the modern microscopes used today for studying microorganisms. A microscope allows the observer to see individual microbial cells and thereby to differentiate and identify microorganisms.

For the most part, microbiology deals with unicellular, or one-celled, microscopic organisms. All the life processes needed to sustain the microbe are performed by one cell. Among them are the ingestion of food substances and their utilization for energy, growth, reproduction, and excretion.

Microorganisms are *ubiquitous;* they are found almost everywhere — in the air, in food and water, in the soil, and in association with plant, animal, and human life. Although there are vast numbers of microorganisms, only a relatively small minority are pathogenic and able to cause disease. When a pathogen infects a host, it often produces a specific set of symptoms peculiar to that disease only. For example, scarlet fever is frequently characterized by a sore throat, swelling of the lymph nodes of the neck, a red and swollen tongue, and a bright red rash covering the body. These symptoms aid the physician in diagnosing the disease. The medical assistant must be alert to any symptoms described by the patient and relay this information to the physician. Microbiologic laboratory tests are also used to help the physician identify the pathogen causing the disease. Identification of the pathogen leads to the proper treatment of the disease.

Although most microbiologic tests are performed in the hospital or the medical laboratory, the medical assistant is frequently responsible for the collection of specimens. This chapter provides an introduction to the field of microbiology, including a description of those techniques that may be performed in the medical

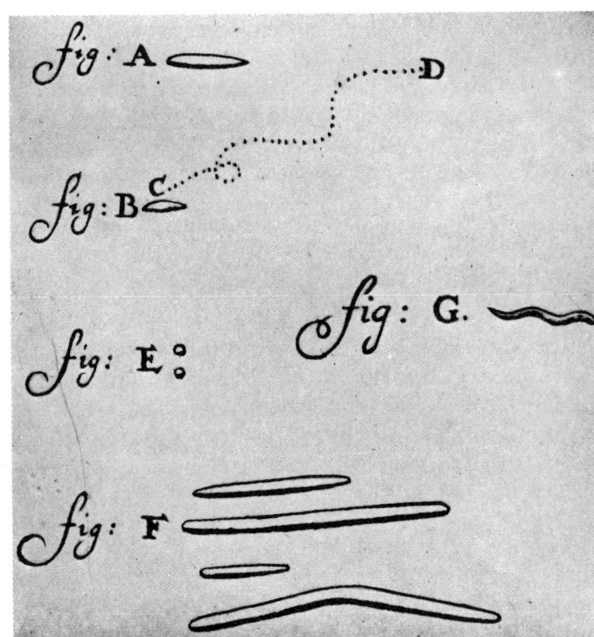

FIGURE 14–1. Drawings of bacteria made by van Leeuwenhoek in 1684. (From Frobisher, M., and Fuerst, R.: *Microbiology in Health and Disease.* 13th edition, Philadelphia, W. B. Saunders Company, 1983.)

office. Before undertaking this study, the medical assistant should review Chapter 1, which discusses introductory concepts that are basic to this chapter. There are numerous microbiology textbooks available (some are listed in the Suggestions for Further Reading at the end of this book) for those desiring additional information about this field.

The Normal Flora

Each individual has a *normal flora,* which consists of the harmless, nonpathogenic microorganisms that normally reside in many parts of the body but do not cause disease. The surface of the skin, the mucous membrane of the gastrointestinal tract, and parts of the respiratory and genitourinary tracts all have an abundant normal flora. The microorganisms making up the normal flora may sometimes be beneficial to the body, such as those contained in the intestinal tract that feed on other potentially harmful microscopic organisms. Another example is those microorganisms found in the intestinal tract that synthesize vitamin K, an essential vitamin needed by the body for proper blood clotting. In rare instances, if the opportunity arises, such as in a condition of lowered body resistance, certain microorganisms making up the normal flora are capable of becoming pathogenic and causing disease.

Infection

The invasion of the body by pathogenic microorganisms is known as *infection.* Under conditions favorable to the pathogens, they grow and multiply, resulting in an *infectious disease* that produces harmful effects on the host. However, not all pathogens that enter a host are able to cause disease. When a pathogen enters the body, it attempts to invade the tissues so it can grow and multiply. The body, in turn, tries to stop the invasion with its second line of natural defense mechanisms,* which includes inflammation, phagocytosis by white blood cells, the production of antibodies, and others. These defense mechanisms work to destroy the pathogen and remove it from the body. If the body is successful, the pathogens are destroyed and the individual suffers no adverse effects. If the pathogen is able to overcome the body's natural defense mechanisms, an infectious disease results.

Many infectious diseases are *contagious,* meaning the pathogen causing the disease can be spread from one person to another either directly or indirectly. Frequently, *droplet infection* is the mode of transmission of pathogens. This is the inhalation of pathogens from a fine spray emitted by a person already infected with the disease. When the infected individual exhales, as during breathing, talking, coughing, or sneezing, the pathogens are dispersed into the air on minute liquid particles. Therefore, infected individuals should cover their mouths or noses while coughing or sneezing. Refer to Figure 1–1, the Infection Process Cycle, for examples of other means of pathogen transmission.

Stages of an Infectious Disease

Once a pathogen becomes established in the host, a series of stages generally ensues. The stages of an infectious disease are as follows:

1. The *infection* is the invasion and multiplication of pathogenic microorganisms in the body.

2. The *incubation period* is the interval of time between the invasion by a pathogenic microorganism and the appearance of the first symptoms of the disease. Depending on the type of disease, the incubation period may range in duration from only a few days to several months.

3. The *prodromal period* is a short period in which the first symptoms that indicate an approaching disease occur. Headache and a feeling of illness are common prodromal symptoms.

---

* The first line of natural defense mechanisms that works to *prevent* the entrance of pathogens into the body (e.g., coughing and sneezing) has already been described in Chapter 1.

4. The *acute period* is when the disease is at its peak and symptoms are fully developed. Fever is a common symptom of many infectious diseases.
5. The *decline period* is when the symptoms of the disease begin to subside.
6. The *convalescent period* is the stage in which the patient regains strength and returns to a state of health.

Microorganisms and Disease

The groups of microorganisms known to contain species capable of causing human disease include bacteria, viruses, protozoa, fungi (including yeasts), and animal parasites. Bacteria and viruses are most frequently responsible for causing disease in humans and are discussed below in more detail.

Bacteria

Bacteria are small plantlike organisms. Of the 1700 species known to humans, approximately only 100 produce human disease. The discovery of antibiotics has helped immensely in combating and controlling infections caused by bacteria. It must be remembered, however, that antibiotics are not effective against viral infections.

Bacteria can be classified into three basic groups, according to their shape (Fig. 14-2). Bacteria having a round shape are known as *cocci.* The cocci can be further divided into diplococci, streptococci, and staphylococci, depending on their pattern of growth. Bacteria having a rod shape are termed *bacilli;* those having a spiral shape are known as *spirilla,* and they include spirochetes and vibrios.

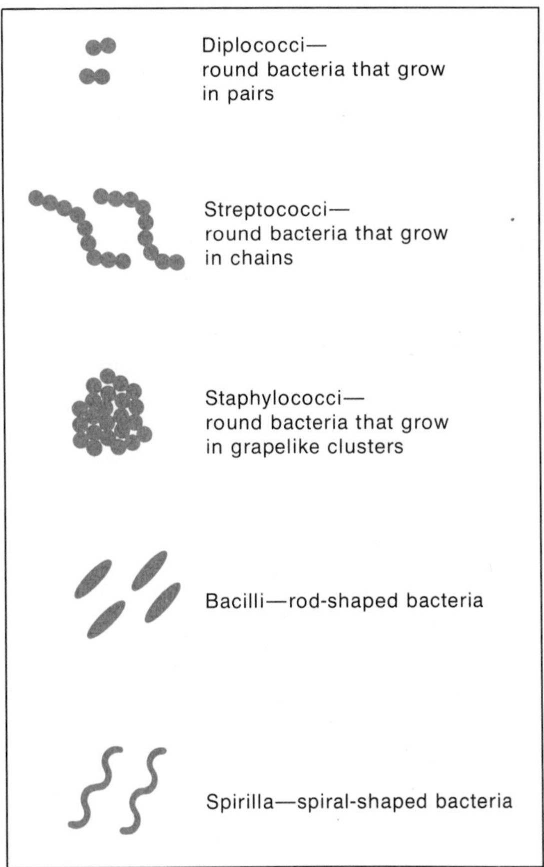

FIGURE 14-2. Classification of bacteria based on shape.

The Cocci

Staphylococci are round bacteria that grow in grapelike clusters. The species *Staphylococcus epidermidis* is widely distributed and is normally present on the surface of the skin and the mucous membranes of the mouth, nose, throat, and intestines. *S. epidermidis* is usually nonpathogenic; however, a cut, abrasion, or other break in the skin may result in the invasion of the tissues by the organism, resulting in a mild infection.

Staphylococcus aureus is the species commonly associated with pathologic conditions such as boils, carbuncles, pimples, impetigo, abscesses, staphylococcus food poisoning, and wound infections. Infections caused by staphylococci usually cause much pus formation (suppuration) and are termed pyogenic infections. Medical asepsis should be exercised when removing a dressing from a wound containing a staphylococcal infection to prevent transfer of this pathogen. The contaminated dressing should be wrapped in a plastic bag and fastened securely before it is disposed of in a waste container.

Streptococci are round bacteria that grow in chains. Before the advent of antibiotics, streptococcal infections were one of the major causes of death in humans. Some of the diseases caused by different types of streptococci include streptococcal sore throat ("strep throat"), scarlet fever, rheumatic fever, pneumonia, puerperal sepsis, erysipelas, and skin conditions such as carbuncles and impetigo.

Diplococci are round bacteria that grow in pairs. Pneumonia, gonorrhea, and meningitis are examples of infectious diseases caused by different types of diplococci.

The Bacilli

Bacilli are rod-shaped bacteria that are frequently found in the soil and air. Some bacilli are able to form spores, a characteristic that enables them to resist adverse conditions such as heat and disinfectants. Some of the diseases caused by different types of bacilli include botulism, tetanus, gas gangrene, gastroenteritis produced by *Salmonella* food poisoning, typhoid fever, pertussis (whooping cough), bacillary dysentery, diphtheria, tuberculosis, leprosy, and the plague.

Escherichia coli is the name of one type of bacillus that is found among the normal flora of the intestinal tract in enormous numbers. It is normally a harmless bacterium; however, if it enters the urinary tract as a result of lowered resistance or poor hygienic practices or both, it may cause a urinary tract infection.

The Spirilla

Spirilla are spiral bacteria. *Treponema pallidum,* a spirochete, is the causative agent of syphilis. This microorganism cannot be grown in commonly available culture media; therefore, diagnosis of syphilis is generally made using serologic tests. A serologic test is made on the serum of the blood. Cholera is caused by another type of spirillum, *Vibrio cholerae.* Immunization and proper methods of sanitation and water purification have all but eliminated cholera epidemics in the United States.

Viruses

Viruses are the smallest living organisms. They are so small that an electron microscope must be used to view them. Viruses infect plants and animals as well as humans and utilize nutrients inside the host's cells for their metabolic and reproductive needs. Some of the human infectious diseases caused by different types of viruses include influenza, chickenpox, rubeola (measles), rubella (German measles), mumps, poliomyelitis, smallpox, rabies, herpes simplex, herpes zoster, yellow fever, hepatitis, and the majority of infectious diseases of the upper respiratory tract, including the common cold.

The Microscope

There are many kinds of microscopes available, but the type used most often for office laboratory work is the *compound microscope.* The compound microscope consists of a two-lens system and the magnification of one system is increased by the other. A source of bright light is required for proper illumination of the object to be viewed. This combination of lenses and light permits visualization of structures that cannot be seen with the unaided eye, such as microorganisms and cellular forms. The compound microscope consists of two main components: the support system and the optical system, each of which includes a number of parts that are discussed below. The medical assistant should be able to identify the parts of a microscope (Fig. 14–3) and be able to properly use and care for it.

Support System

The working parts of the microscope are supported by a sturdy frame consisting of a *base* for support and an *arm* for carrying it without damaging the delicate parts. The arm is also needed to support the magnifying and adjusting systems. The *stage*

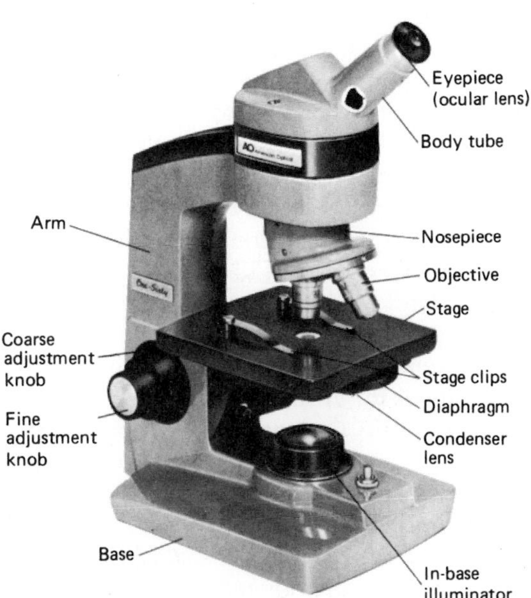

FIGURE 14–3. Parts of the microscope. (Courtesy of the American Optical Corporation.)

of a microscope is the flat, horizontal platform on which the microscope slide is placed. It is located directly over the condenser and beneath the objective lenses. The stage has a small round opening in the center that permits light from below to pass through the object being viewed and up into the lenses above. The slide should be placed on the stage so that the object to be viewed is positioned over this opening so that it is satisfactorily illuminated by the light source below. Most microscopes have metal clips attached to the stage to hold the glass slide securely in place. With this type of stage, the slide must be moved by hand to examine various areas on it. Other types of microscopes have a *mechanical stage* that allows movement of the slide in a vertical or horizontal position by using adjustment knobs. The mechanical stage provides smoothness and control in moving the slide, which is essential for performing certain procedures such as differential white blood counts and inspection of gram-stained smears.

The *light source* is located at the base of the microscope and consists of a built-in illuminator (or bulb), along with a switch for turning it on. The light is directed to the condenser above it and then through the object to be viewed.

Compound microscopes have a lens system between the light source and object, known as the *substage condenser.* A commonly used condenser is the *Abbe condenser,* which consists of two lenses used to illuminate objects with transmitted light. The condenser collects and concentrates the light rays and directs them up, bringing them to a focus on the object so that it is well illuminated. The condenser can be lowered or raised by means of an adjustment knob. Lowering the condenser reduces the amount of light that reaches the object, whereas raising it admits more light. When the substage condenser is properly positioned, the visual field should be evenly lit.

The amount of light focused on the object can also be controlled by the *iris diaphragm,* located in the lower part of the condenser. The diaphragm consists of a series of horizontally arranged interlocking plates with a central opening or aperture. The iris diaphragm has a lever that is used to increase or decrease the amount of light admitted by increasing or decreasing the size of the aperture. The diaphragm aperture opening is combined with the movement of the substage condenser to control the light intensity. Appropriate adjustment of the light intensity is essential for properly viewing the specimens, especially at a higher magnification. A general rule is that, as the desired magnification increases, the more intense the light must be. For example, increased light intensity is required for good visualization of a specimen with the oil-immersion objective. On the other hand, when using the low-power objective, the light must be somewhat diminished in order to produce the appropriate contrast for specimen detail and to reduce glare. The degree of illumination is also influenced by the density of the object; therefore, stained structures (e.g., a gram-stained smear of bacteria) usually require more light than do unstained ones.

The *body tube* holds the magnifying lenses through which the object is viewed. The body tube is raised and lowered by means of the coarse and fine adjustment knobs on the arm. On some microscope models, the adjustment knobs are mounted as two separate knobs; on others, they may be placed together with the smaller fine adjustment knob extending from a larger coarse adjustment wheel. The *coarse adjustment* is used to quickly move the low-power objective down into position over the slide on the stage to obtain an approximate focus. The *fine adjustment* moves the body tube very slowly and is used to achieve the precise focusing necessary to obtain a sharp, clear image. Refer to Figure 14–3 to locate the parts of the microscope described above.

Optical System

Compound microscopes have a two-lens magnification system. *Magnification* is defined as the ratio of apparent size of an object when viewed through the microscope to the actual size of the object. The first lens system is the *eyepiece* or *ocular* lens located at the top of the body tube and marked with 10×, meaning that it magnifies 10 times. Microscopes that have one eyepiece only are called *monocular* microscopes, and those with two eyepieces are called *binocular.* A binocular microscope is recommended for medical office laboratory work because it causes less eye fatigue than the monocular type. The binocular eyepieces can be adjusted to each individual by moving the eyepieces apart or together as needed.

The second lens system consists of three *objective* lenses located on the revolving *nosepiece,* each with a different degree of magnification. The metal shaft of each objective lens differs in length and is identified with its power of magnification. The short objective is known as the *low-power* objective and has a magnification of 10×. The *high-power objective* is also known as the high-dry objective because it does not require the use of immersion oil and has a magnification of 40×. The *oil-immersion* objective has the highest power of magnification, which is 100×. Some microscope manufacturers identify the objective lenses by variously colored rings. For example, green is used for low power, yellow for high power, and red or black for oil immersion. If the objective is not color coded, it can be identified by the length of the metal shaft; the low-power objective is the shortest, whereas the oil-immersion objective is the longest.

The objective lens magnifies the specimen, and the ocular lens magnifies the image produced by the objective lens. The *total magnification* of each objective is determined by multiplying the ocular magnification by the objective magnification. The total magnification of the low-power objective is 100 times the actual size of the object being viewed (10 × 10). The total magnification of the high-power objective is 400× (10 × 40), and the oil-immersion magnification is 1000 (10 × 100).

The low-power objective is used for the initial focusing and light adjustment of the microscope. The low-power objective is also used for the initial observation and scanning requirements needed for most microscopic work. For example, urine sediment is first examined using the low-power objective to scan the specimen for the presence of casts. The high-power objective is used for a more thorough study such as observing cells and urinary sediment in more detail. The *working distance,* defined as the distance between the tip of the lens and the slide, is quite short when using this objective. Because of this, care must be taken in focusing the high-power objective to prevent it from striking and breaking the slide or damaging the lens. Most compound microscopes are *parfocal.* This means that once the specimen is focused with the low-power objective, the nosepiece can be rotated to the high-power objective and focused simply through the use of the fine adjustment knob.

The oil-immersion objective provides the highest magnification and is used to view very small structures, such as microorganisms and blood cells. The oil-immersion objective has a very short working distance and when it is in use, the lens nearly rests on the microscope slide itself. A special grade of oil known as immersion oil must be used with this lens. Oil has the advantage of not drying out when exposed to air for a long period of time. A drop of the oil is placed on the slide and resides between the oil-immersion objective and the slide. The oil provides a path for the light to travel between the slide and the lens and prevents the scattering of light rays, which in turn permits clear viewing of very small structures. The oil also improves the resolution of the objective lens, that is, its ability to provide sharp detail, which is particularly necessary at high magnifications. Examples of procedures requiring oil immersion include differential white blood counts and examination of gram-stained smears.

Care of the Microscope

The microscope is a delicate instrument and must be handled carefully. The guidelines below should be followed to properly care for the microscope.

1. The microscope should always be carried with two hands. One hand should be placed firmly on the arm and the other hand should be placed under the base for support. Place the microscope down gently to prevent jarring it, which could cause damage to its delicate parts.
2. The microscope should always be handled in such a way that the fingers do not touch the lenses, to avoid leaving fingerprints on them. Wearing mascara should be avoided when one is using a microscope, as this substance is difficult to remove from the ocular lens.
3. When not in use, the microscope should be covered with its plastic dust cover and stored in a case or cupboard. The microscope should be stored with the nosepiece rotated to the low-power objective and the body tube adjusted to its lowest position.
4. The microscope should be cleaned periodically by washing the enameled surfaces with mild soap and water, and drying them thoroughly with a soft cloth. Alcohol should never be used on the enameled surfaces because it may remove the finish.
5. The metal stage should be wiped clean after each use with gauze or tissue. If immersion oil comes in contact with the stage, it should be removed with a piece of gauze slightly moistened with xylene.
6. The ocular, objectives, and condenser consist of hand-ground optical lenses, which must be kept spotlessly clean by using clean dry lens paper. Optical glass is softer than ordinary glass, therefore, tissues or gauze should not be used to prevent scratching of the lens. If the lenses are especially dirty, a commercial lens cleaner or xylene should be used in the cleaning process. A small amount of cleaner is applied to the lens paper, followed by thorough drying and polishing with a clean piece of lens paper.
7. The light source should be kept free of dust, lint, and dirt by periodic polishing with lens paper.
8. A malfunctioning microscope should be repaired only by a qualified service person. Attempting to fix the microscope yourself may result in further damage.

PROCEDURE 14-1
USING THE MICROSCOPE

The following steps should be followed for proper use of the microscope.

1. Clean the ocular and objective lenses with lens paper.

2. Turn on the light source. Move the condenser all the way up with the diaphragm completely open.

3. Rotate the nosepiece to the low-power objective (10×), making sure to click it into place. Raise the objective all the way up using the course adjustment knob, to provide sufficient working space for placing the slide on the stage and to avoid damaging the objective lens.

4. Place the slide on the stage, specimen side up, and make sure it is secure.

5. Bring the low-power objective down until it almost touches the slide, using the coarse adjustment knob. Be sure to observe this step to prevent the objective from striking the slide.

6. Look through the ocular. If a monocular microscope is being used, both eyes should be kept open to prevent eye strain. With a binocular microscope, adjust the two oculars to the width between your eyes until a single circular field of vision is obtained.

7. Slowly raise the objective upward, using the coarse adjustment knob. Observe the specimen through the ocular until it comes into coarse focus.

8. Use the fine adjustment knob to bring the specimen into a sharp clear focus.

9. Adjust the light as needed, using the iris diaphragm and condenser adjustment knob to provide maximum focus and contrast.

10. Rotate the nosepiece to the high-power objective, making sure it clicks into place. Proper focusing with the low-power objective ensures that the objective does not hit the slide during this operation. Use the fine adjustment knob to bring the specimen into a precise focus. Do not use the coarse adjustment to focus the high-power objective, in order to prevent the objective from moving too far and striking the slide.

11. Examine the specimen as required by the test or procedure being performed.

12. Turn off the light after use and remove the slide from the stage.

13. Clean the stage with a tissue or gauze.

14. Properly care for and store the microscope as described on page 416.

Continued

USING THE OIL-IMMERSION OBJECTIVE

The following steps should be followed for proper utilization of the oil-immersion objective. (*Note:* The procedure outlined on the previous page should first be completed before rotating the nosepiece to the oil-immersion objective).

1. Rotate the nosepiece to the oil-immersion objective. Do not click it into place, but move it to one side.

2. Place a drop of immersion oil on the slide directly over the center opening in the stage.

3. Move the oil-immersion objective into place until a click is heard. Make sure that the objective does not touch the stage or slide.

4. Using the coarse adjustment, slowly bring down the oil-immersion objective until the tip of the lens touches the oil but does not come in contact with the slide. A "pop" of light will be observed. Be sure to observe carefully this step of the procedure.

5. Look through the eyepiece and focus slowly upward, until the object is visible.

6. Use the fine adjustment to bring the object into sharp focus to view fine details.

7. Adjust the light as needed, using the iris diaphragm and condenser adjustment knob to provide maximum focus and contrast. Increased light intensity is required for good visualization of the specimen with the oil-immersion objective.

8. Examine the specimen as required by the test or procedure being performed.

9. Turn off the light after use. Remove the slide from the stage, being careful not to get oil on the high-power objective or the stage.

10. Using a piece of clean dry lens paper, gently clean the oil-immersion objective. The lens must be immediately cleaned after use to prevent oil from drying on the lens surface. In addition, the oil may seep into the lens and perhaps loosen it.

11. Clean the oil from the slide by immersing it in xylene and wiping it off with a soft cloth.

Microbiologic Specimen Collection

If the physician suspects that a particular disease is caused by a pathogen, he or she may want to obtain a specimen for microbiologic examination. This will identify the specific pathogen causing the disease and aid in the diagnosis. For example, if a urinary tract infection is suspected, a urine specimen is obtained for bacterial examination. In this instance, a clean-catch midstream collection is required to obtain a specimen that excludes those microorganisms making up the normal flora of the urethra and urinary meatus.

A *specimen* is a small sample or part taken from the body to represent the nature of the whole. The medical assistant is often responsible for collecting specimens from certain areas of the body, such as the throat, nose, or wound areas. He or she may also be responsible for assisting the physician in the collection of specimens from other areas, such as the eye, ear, cervix, vagina, urethra, or rectum. In most instances, a *swab* is used to collect the specimen. A swab is a small piece of cotton gauze wrapped around the end of a slender wooden stick. It is passed across a suspected area to obtain a specimen from a body surface or opening for microbiologic analysis.

Good techniques of medical and surgical asepsis must be practiced when a specimen is obtained, to prevent inaccurate test results. The medical assistant must be careful not to contaminate the specimen with extraneous microorganisms. These are undesirable microorganisms that may enter the specimen in various ways; they grow and multiply and possibly obscure and prevent identification of any pathogens that may be present. To prevent extraneous organisms from contaminating the specimen, all supplies used to obtain the specimen, such as swabs and specimen containers, must be sterile. In addition, the specimen should not contain any microorganisms from areas surrounding the collection site. For example, when obtaining a throat specimen, the swab should not be allowed to touch the inside of the mouth.

Medical assistants must be very careful not to infect themselves with the specimen. Eating, drinking, and smoking are strictly forbidden when one is working with microorganisms, because dangerous pathogens can be transmitted to the medical assistant through this type of hand-to-mouth contact. In addition, labels for specimen containers should not be licked, and any break in the skin, such as a cut or scratch, should be covered with a bandage. If the medical assistant accidentally touches some of the material contained in the specimen, the area of contact should be washed immediately and thoroughly with soap containing an antiseptic. If the material happens to come in contact with a break in the skin, in addition to cleansing, tincture of iodine or another suitable antiseptic should be applied to the area. If the specimen comes in contact with the worktable, it should be cleansed immediately with a suitable disinfectant such as phenol or cresol. The worktable should also be cleaned with a disinfectant at the end of each day.

After collection, the specimen must be placed in its proper container with the lid securely fastened. The container must be clearly labeled with the patient's name, the date, the source of the specimen, the medical assistant's initials, and any other information that may be required.

Handling and Transporting Microbiologic Specimens

Once the specimen has been collected, care should be taken in handling and transporting it. Delay in processing the specimen may cause the death of any pathogens that may be present or the overgrowth of the specimen by microorganisms that are part of the normal flora usually collected along with the pathogen from the specimen site. If the specimen is to be analyzed in the medical office, it should be examined under the microscope or cultured immediately. Otherwise, it should be preserved (if possible) with the method used by the medical office. Some microorganisms, such as gonococcus, are extremely fastidious outside the host and need to be cultured immediately.

The specimens that are to be transported either to a local medical laboratory through a courier pick-up service or to a more distant laboratory through the mail are usually placed in a transport medium. The transport medium prevents drying of the specimen and preserves it in its original state until it reaches its destination. An example of a commercially available transport medium is the Culturette.

Outside laboratories will provide the medical office with specific instructions on the care and handling of specimens being transported to them. Special precautions must be taken for those specimens that are to be transported through the mail. The specimen container must be securely closed and protective material such as cotton or corrugated cardboard should be wrapped around the container to absorb shock and possible leakage. The specimen container is then placed in a watertight metal container (Fig. 14–4), which is placed in a cardboard mailing container with shock-resistant insulating material. A warning label is put on the outside of the container to identify it as a pathologic specimen (Fig. 14–5).

A laboratory request designating the physician's name and address, the patient's name, age, and sex, the date and time of the collection, the type of microbiologic examination requested, the source of the specimen (e.g., throat, wound, urine), and the physician's clinical diagnosis must accompany all specimens being transported to an outside laboratory (Fig. 14–6). There is usually a space on the form to indicate whether the patient is receiving antibiotic therapy. Antibiotics may suppress the growth of bacteria, a factor that could produce falsely negative results.

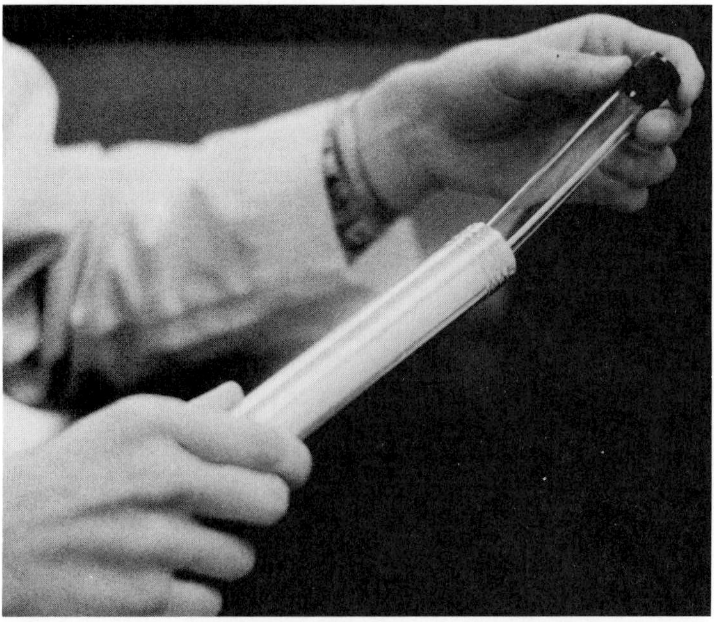

FIGURE 14–4. The medical assistant places the specimen container that will be transported through the mail into a watertight metal container.

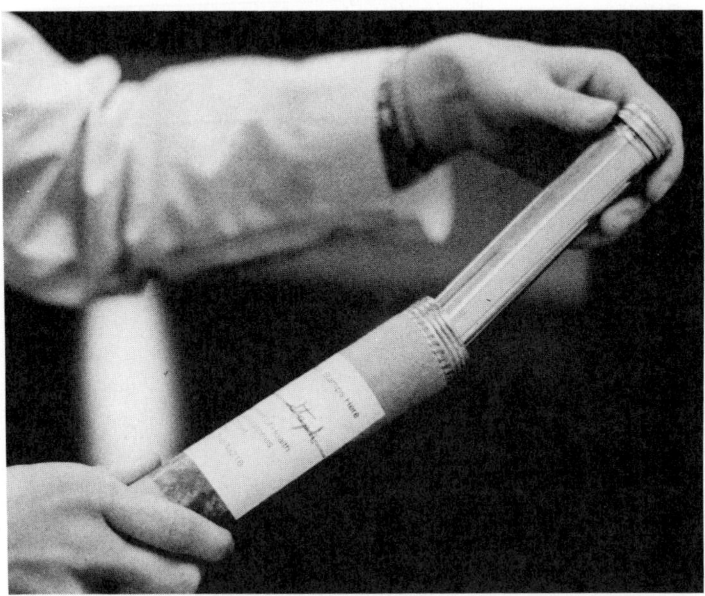

FIGURE 14-5. The medical assistant places the watertight metal container into the cardboard mailing container.

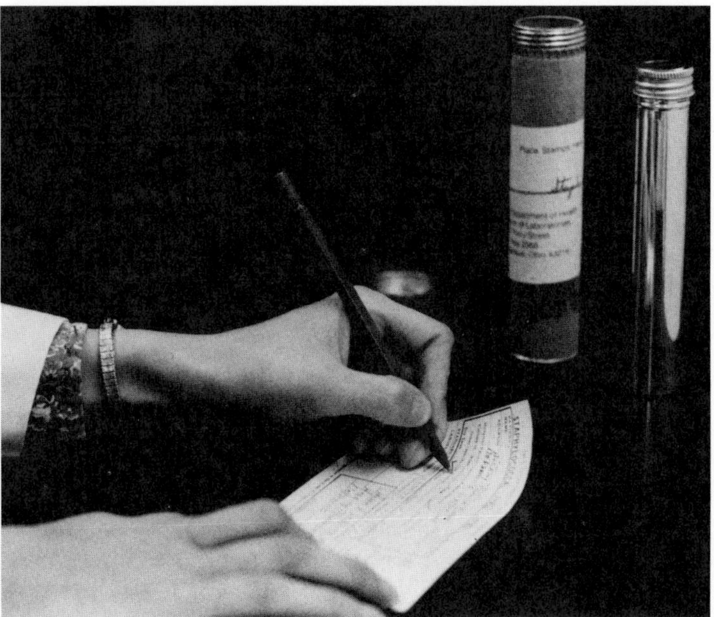

FIGURE 14-6. The medical assistant fills out the laboratory request form that will accompany the specimen being transported to an outside laboratory.

PROCEDURE 14-2
TAKING A SPECIMEN FOR A THROAT CULTURE

A specimen for a throat culture is obtained by using one or more sterile swabs. It is commonly used to aid in the diagnosis of infections such as streptococcal sore throat, pharyngitis, and tonsillitis. Less frequently, it is used to diagnose whooping cough and diphtheria. These latter diseases are not prevalent today because of the availability of immunizations against them.

The following procedure outlines the steps necessary to obtain a throat specimen that will be transported to an outside laboratory for analysis.

1. **PROCEDURAL STEP.** Complete a laboratory request with the physician's name and address, the patient's name, age, and sex, and the date and time of collection. The request should also include the source of the specimen, the physician's clinical diagnosis, the microbiologic examination requested, and any other information that may be required.

2. **PROCEDURAL STEP.** Wash the hands.

3. **PROCEDURAL STEP.** Assemble the equipment. The equipment needed includes a **tongue blade,** a **sterile cotton swab,** and a **sterile specimen container.** Label the container with the patient's name, the date, the source of the specimen (i.e., throat), and your initials.
   PRINCIPLE. The swab and container must be sterile to prevent extraneous microorganisms from contaminating the specimen.

4. **PROCEDURAL STEP.** Identify the patient and explain the procedure.

5. **PROCEDURAL STEP.** Position the patient and adjust the light to provide clear visualization of the throat.
   PRINCIPLE. The throat must be clearly visible so the medical assistant is able to determine the proper area for obtaining the specimen.

6. **PROCEDURAL STEP.** Remove the sterile swab from the specimen container, being careful not to contaminate it.
   PRINCIPLE. Contamination of the swab may lead to inaccurate test results.

7. **PROCEDURAL STEP.** Depress the tongue with the tongue blade.
   PRINCIPLE. The tongue blade holds the tongue down and facilitates access to the throat.

8. **PROCEDURAL STEP.** Place the swab at the back of the throat (posterior pharynx) and firmly rub it over any lesions or white or inflamed areas of the mucous membrane of the tonsillar area and posterior pharyngeal wall. The swab should be rotated constantly as the specimen is obtained, making sure there is good contact with the tonsillar area. Do not allow the swab to touch any areas other than the throat, such as the inside of the mouth.

PRINCIPLE. The swab should be rubbed over suspicious-looking areas where pathogens are likely to be found. A rotating motion is used to deposit the maximum amount of material possible on the swab. Touching it to any areas other than the throat contaminates the specimen with extraneous microorganisms.

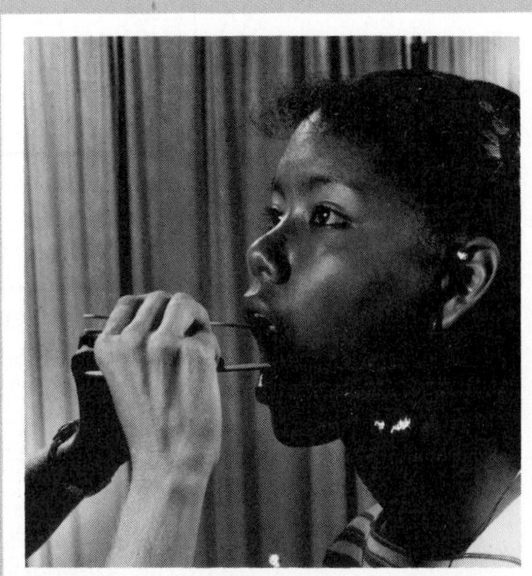

9. **PROCEDURAL STEP.** Keeping the patient's tongue depressed, withdraw the swab and remove the tongue blade from the patient's mouth. Immediately place the swab in the specimen container, and securely fasten the lid.

PRINCIPLE. The swab should be placed in the container as soon as possible to prevent drying of the specimen, which might cause death of the microorganisms contained in it.

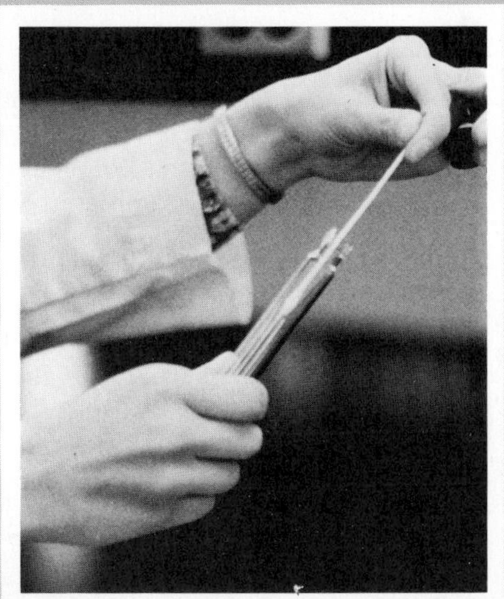

10. **PROCEDURAL STEP.** If two swabs are required, insert another swab and repeat Procedural Steps 6 through 9. *Note:* If two swabs are used, the first swab should be rubbed over one tonsillar area, and the second swab over the opposite tonsillar area.

11. **PROCEDURAL STEP.** Properly dispose of the tongue blade to prevent transmission of microorganisms.

12. **PROCEDURAL STEP.** Wash the hands.

13. **PROCEDURAL STEP.** Record information in the patient's chart, including the date and time of the collection, any unusual patient reaction, the microbiologic examination requested, the source of the specimen, and information indicating its transport to an outside laboratory.

14. **PROCEDURAL STEP.** Process and transport the specimen directly or by mail to the appropriate testing facility. Be sure to include the completed laboratory request.

Record data below.

DATE	TIME	PATIENT'S NAME	RECORDING

Wound Specimens

Wound specimens are collected using many of the techniques described previously. In many cases, two swabs are used to collect the specimen. The specimen is obtained by inserting the swab into the area of the wound that contains the most drainage and gently rotating the swab from side to side to allow it to completely absorb any microorganisms present. The swab is placed in the specimen container and the process is then repeated using a second swab. It is important to collect a specimen from within the wound, rather than from the surface, to obtain accurate and reliable test results.

Collection and Transport Systems

Microbiologic collection and transport systems are commercially available to facilitate the collection of a specimen that is to be transported to an outside laboratory for analysis; examples include Culturette (Marion Scientific Corporation) and Precision Culture CATS (Precision Dynamics Corporation) (Fig. 14–7). These systems consist of a plastic tube containing a sterile swab and transport medium. The medium is effective for 72 hours once the swab has been immersed in it; therefore, it is important that the specimen reach the laboratory within this time frame. The tube comes packaged in a peel-apart envelope and should be stored at room temperature. The procedure for the utilization of a microbiologic collection and transport system is outlined here.

1. Complete a laboratory request form.
2. Wash the hands.
3. Check the expiration date on the peel-apart envelope.
4. Peel open approximately one-third of the length of the envelope.
5. Remove the plastic collection tube from the envelope and label it with the patient's name, the date, the source of the specimen (e.g., throat, wound), and your initials.

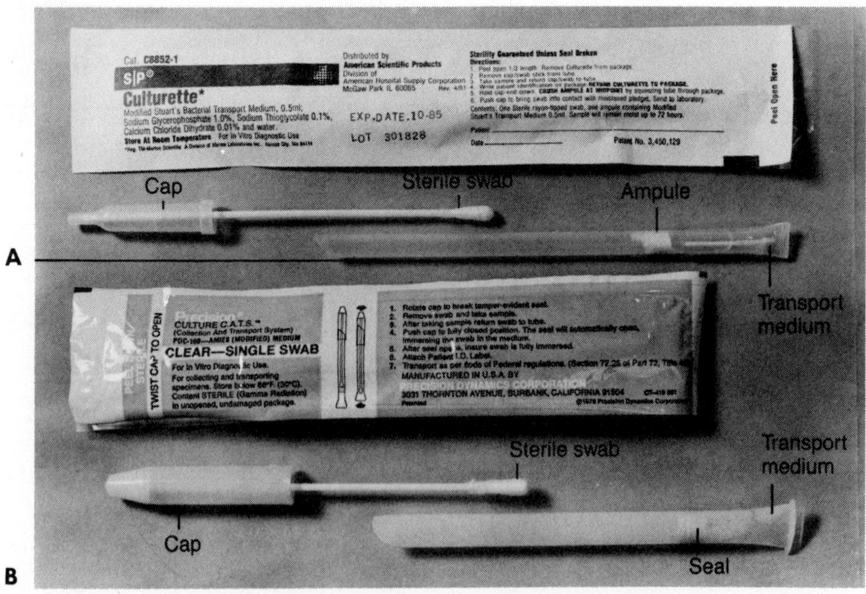

FIGURE 14–7. Two examples of collection and transport systems. *A,* Culterette and *B,* Precision Culture CATS. A collection and transport system is packaged in a peel-apart envelope and consists of a plastic tube containing a sterile swab and transport medium. Once the swab has been used to collect the specimen, the cap/swab unit is then placed in the transport medium. This prevents drying of the specimen and preserves it until it reaches the laboratory.

6. Using a twisting motion, remove the cap/swab unit from the tube. The cap is permanently attached to the sterile swab.
7. Collect the specimen using aseptic technique. Do not allow the swab to touch any area other than the collection site.
8. Return the cap/swab unit to the plastic tube.
9. Completely immerse the swab in the transport medium. Using the Culturette system, this is accomplished by squeezing the plastic tube to crush an ampule that separates the transport medium from the rest of the tube. The cap/swab unit is then pushed forward to bring the swab in contact with the moistened pledge). With the Precision system, the swab must be pushed in as far as it will go; this automatically opens a seal separating the transport medium from the rest of the tube.
10. Wash the hands.
11. Record information in the patient's chart.
12. Transport the specimen to the laboratory within 72 hours.

Cultures

Once a microbiologic specimen is taken, it must be examined to determine the type of microorganisms present. Because most specimens generally contain only a small number of pathogens, it is often desirable to induce any pathogens that may be present to grow and multiply. Most microorganisms, especially bacteria, may be grown on a culture medium. A *culture medium* is a mixture of nutrients on which microorganisms are grown in the laboratory. The culture medium and the environment in which it is placed must contain the necessary requirements to support and encourage the growth of the suspected pathogen. These growth requirements include either the presence or the absence of oxygen (depending on the microorganism); proper nutrition, temperature, and pH; and the presence of moisture. The culture medium may be in a solid or a liquid form. Blood agar is one of the most frequently used solid culture media. It is prepared by adding sheep's blood to a substance known as *agar,* which is transparent and colorless. Blood added to the agar provides nutrients that support the growth of a variety of bacteria. When heated, it melts and becomes a liquid. On cooling, agar solidifies, forming a firm surface on which microorganisms can be grown. A liquid culture medium is often referred to as a broth and is usually contained in a tube; an example is nutrient broth. Culture media must be stored in the refrigerator and then warmed to room temperature before using. A cold culture medium must not be used, because the cold temperature results in the death of microorganisms placed on it.

A Petri plate is frequently used to hold solid culture medium. The plate consists of a shallow circular dish made of glass or clear plastic with a cover, the diameter of which is greater than that of the base. Microorganisms can be cultured on the surface of the medium contained in the plate (Fig. 14–8). Petri plates allow for the examination of a culture and at the same time prevent microorganisms from entering or escaping. A *culture* is defined as a mass of microorganisms growing in a laboratory culture medium.

Most medical offices use commercially prepared culture media contained in disposable plastic Petri plates. The plates come packaged in a plastic bag and must be stored in the refrigerator with the medium side facing upward. The plastic bag prevents the medium from drying out; storing the plates medium side upward prevents condensation on the medium surface. The plate will have an expiration date that must be checked before using; plates that are past the expiration date or are dried out or contaminated should not be used. Culture media can also be prepared in the medical office from a commercially available dehydrated form. The manufacturer's instructions for their preparation, use, and storage are listed on the container.

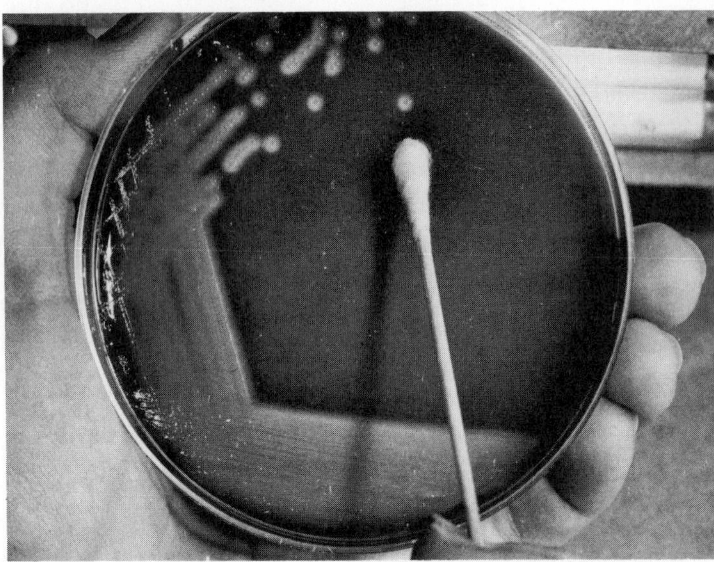

FIGURE 14–8. Streptococcal colonies growing on a blood agar culture medium contained in a Petri plate. (Courtesy of New York State Health Department, Albany, New York.)

The solid culture medium contained in a Petri plate is inoculated by lightly rolling the swab containing the specimen over the surface of the medium; this process is known as *streaking.* The cover of the Petri plate should be removed only when the specimen is being spread on the culture medium. Unnecessary removal of the cover results in contamination of the medium with extraneous microorganisms. The culture is then incubated for 24 to 48 hours, utilizing the proper conditions to encourage the growth of the suspected pathogen. Most specimens taken for analysis contain a mixture of different organisms because of the presence of a normal flora in most parts of the body. When this is the case, the resulting culture is known as a *mixed culture,* or one that contains two or more different types of microorganisms. To analyze most microbiologic specimens, the suspected pathogen must be separated from the mixed culture and permitted to grow alone. This establishes a *pure culture,* or a culture that contains only one type of microorganism. After the culture has sufficiently grown, the appropriate tests are performed to identify the pathogen.

It is not possible to grow viruses by this method; rather, they must be cultured on living tissue or identified using serologic tests.

Streptococcus Testing

The most commonly occurring streptococcal condition is streptococcal sore throat (streptococcal pharyngitis), which primarily affects children and young adults. The causative agent of streptococcal pharyngitis is a Group A beta-hemolytic streptococcus known as *Steptococcus pyogenes.* Streptococcal pharyngitis is a potentially serious condition because some patients develop a poststreptococcal sequela. A *sequela* is a morbid secondary condition that occurs as a result of a less serious primary infection. A small percentage of patients with streptococcal pharyngitis (primary infection) develop rheumatic fever; the rheumatic fever is considered a poststreptococcal sequela. Owing to the risk of sequela, early diagnosis and treatment of streptococcal pharyngitis is important. In the medical office, commercially available tests are often used for identification of Group A beta-hemolytic streptococci. The most frequently used testing methods are presented below and on the next page.

Rapid Streptococcus Tests. Rapid streptococcus tests directly detect Group-A streptococcus from a throat swab in a very short period of time. The most frequently used rapid streptococcus test is the direct antigen identification test, which confirms the presence of Group A streptococcus through an antigen-antibody reaction. The test works by combining particles sensitized to the streptococcus antibody with the throat specimen. If Group A streptococcal antigen is in the specimen, it combines with the antibody-sensitized particles to produce either agglutination or a color change that can be observed with the unaided eye. The advantage of the direct antigen identification test is that it provides the physician with immediate test results rather than requiring an overnight culture. Specific instructions are included with each commercially available antigen identification test; examples of these tests include Ventrescreen (Fig. 14–9), Access Icon Strep A, and TestPack Strep A.

Hemolytic Reaction and Bacitracin Susceptibility Test. Streptococci are classified into three types, according to their hemolytic properties exhibited on a blood agar medium: *alpha, beta,* and *gamma.* They are further divided according to their antigenic properties into 15 subgroups designated by the letters "A" through "O." The hemolytic reaction and bacitracin susceptibility test is a biochemical culture test that relies upon these hemolytic and antigenic properties of streptococci for the interpretation of the test results. The testing procedure in-

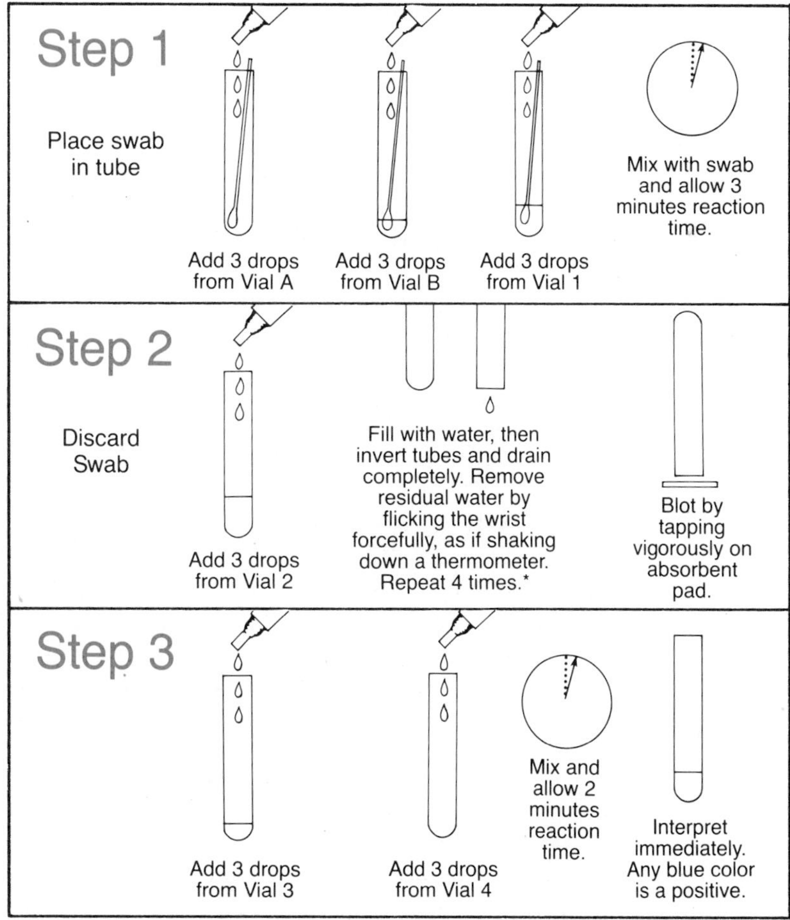

FIGURE 14–9. Procedure for performing the Ventrescreen rapid streptococcus test. Ventrescreen is a type of rapid streptococcus test that relies upon a color change for the interpretation of test results. (Courtesy of Ventrex Laboratories, Portland, Maine.)

volves placing a filter paper disc impregnated with 0.04 U of bacitracin on the surface of a sheep-blood agar medium previously inoculated with the throat specimen. The medium is then incubated for 18 to 24 hours to allow for the growth of the bacteria and also to permit diffusion of the bacitracin into the culture medium surrounding the disc.

After the 18- to 24-hour incubation period, the plate is examined for its hemolytic reaction. As stated above, the causative agent of streptococcal pharyngitis is a (Group A) beta-hemolytic streptococcus. Beta-hemolytic streptococci produce and secrete streptolysin, an exotoxin that completely hemolyzes red blood cells; therefore, a clear, wide, colorless zone of hemolysis (with no intact red blood cells) around the bacterial colonies is indicative of their presence. On the other hand, a greenish halo around the colonies is indicative of the less pathogenic alpha-hemolytic streptococci. The generally nonpathogenic gamma-type streptococci will not cause a reaction on the blood agar medium.

If the hemolytic property exhibited is of the beta type, the area around the bacitracin disc is next inspected for bacitracin susceptibility. Group A streptococci are susceptible or sensitive to bacitracin, whereas Groups B, C, and G (which are also beta hemolytic) are resistant to the bacitracin. If Group A is present, a clear zone of inhibition appears around the disc (Fig. 14–10*A*). Because Groups B, C, and G are resistant to the bacitracin, the bacteria grow right up to the edge of the disc; that is, a zone of inhibition is not present (Fig. 14–10*B*).

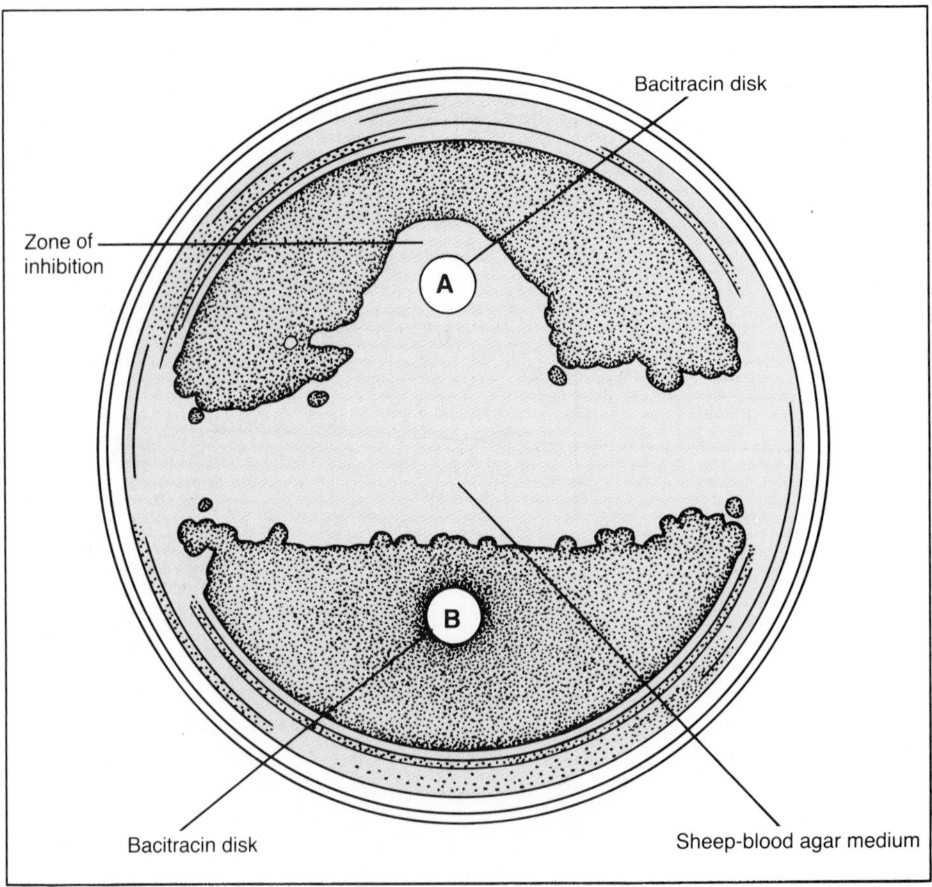

FIGURE 14–10. Hemolytic reaction and bacitracin susceptibility test. *A,* A positive reaction for group A beta hemolytic streptococcus as evidenced by a clear zone of inhibition present around the bacitracin disc. *B,* A negative reaction as evidenced by the bacteria growing right up to the edge of the disc.

Therefore, hemolysis of the blood agar surrounding the bacterial colonies combined with any zone of inhibition around the bacitracin disc is considered presumptive positive for Group A beta-hemolytic streptococci. The test is considered presumptive because a small percentage of bacterial strains included in Groups B, C, and G are sensitive to bacitracin; therefore, a fraction (less than 5 per cent) of the test results obtained will be false positive. A false positive is a test result denoting that a condition is present when, in fact, it is not.

The bacitracin disc test is a convenient, reliable, and cost-effective method used in the medical office to determine the presence of streptococcal pharyngitis. However, it is not used as frequently as it once was, owing to the development of the rapid streptococcus tests.

Sensitivity Testing

The physician may request not only that the laboratory identify the infecting pathogen but also that a sensitivity test be performed on it to determine the best antibiotic to treat the condition. These tests must always be performed on pure cultures rather than on mixed cultures. A sensitivity test determines the susceptibility of pathogenic bacteria to various antibiotics; therefore, only the growth of the infectious pathogen is desired on the culture.

The most commonly used method for sensitivity testing is the disc-plate method (Fig. 14–11). Commercially prepared discs impregnated with known concentrations of various antibiotics are dropped on the surface of a solid culture medium in a Petri plate inoculated with the pathogen. The culture is then incubated, allowing the antibiotics to diffuse out into the culture medium. If the pathogen is susceptible or sensitive to an antibiotic, there is a clear zone without bacterial growth around the disc. This indicates that the antibiotic was effective in destroying the pathogen. If the pathogen is unaffected by or resistant to the antibiotic, there is not a clear zone around the disc, indicating that the antibiotic was unable to kill the pathogen.

CL – Coly-Mycin
AM – Ampicillin
TE – Terramycin
P – Penicillin
C – Chloramphenicol
PB – Polymyxin B
N – Neomycin
Fd – Nitrofurantoin
T – Tetracycline
K – Kanamycin
LR – Cephaloridine
GM – Garamycin
SSS – Triple Sulfa
CB – Carbenicillin
NA – Nalidixic Acid

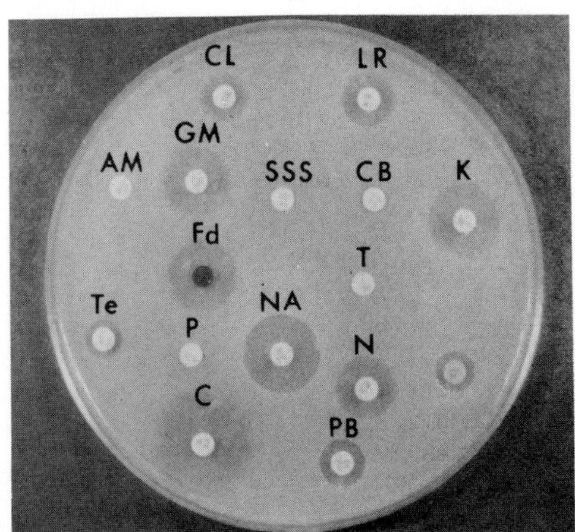

FIGURE 14–11. Testing sensitivity of a bacterium to antibiotics or other chemotherapeutic agents by the "disc-plate method." The entire surface of agar medium in a Petri plate is inoculated with the organism to be tested. Paper discs of uniform thickness containing graded amounts of the agent to be tested (or the same amount of different agents, if a comparison is desired) are then placed on the surface of the agar. The agent diffuses into the agar and prevents growth of the bacterium in a zone around the disc. The width of the zone indicates, roughly, the sensitivity of the organism to the agent or agents being tested, though the *presence* or *absence* of a zone is of greater significance. (About one-half actual size.) (Courtesy of Linda Kaye Hickey; from Frobisher, M., and Fuerst, R.: *Microbiology in Health and Disease.* 13th edition, Philadelphia, W. B. Saunders Company, 1983.)

Sensitivity testing enables the physician to decide which antibiotics will most likely be effective against the infectious disease in question.

Microscopic Examination of Microorganisms

Microorganisms may be examined under a microscope in the fixed state or in the living state. Examination in the fixed state involves the preparation of a smear through heat fixation followed by a staining process such as the Gram stain, which is discussed in more detail later in this chapter. Most microorganisms are examined in the fixed state because it is easier to examine them when they are stained. Some microorganisms require examination in the living state, however, owing to special circumstances such as their inability to be readily stained or difficulty in culturing them. The living state also allows visualization of the movement of motile microorganisms. This is especially helpful in the identification of certain motile microorganisms such as *Trichomonas vaginalis.* To observe the motility of a microorganism, it must first be suspended in a liquid medium so that it is free to move about.

The two most common methods of examining microorganisms in the living state are the *wet mount method* and the *hanging drop preparation,* which are described below.

Wet Mount Method

In the wet mount method, a drop of fluid containing the organism is placed on a glass slide, which is covered with a coverslip (Fig. 14–12). The coverslip may be ringed with petroleum jelly to provide a seal between the slide and coverslip. The purpose is to reduce the rate of evaporation through air currents that lead to drying and possible death of the specimen. The slide is then placed under the microscope for examination using the high-power objective. For satisfactory visualization, the intensity of the light must be diminished by partially closing the diaphragm of the microscope and lowering the condenser. The slide and coverslip should then be properly disposed.

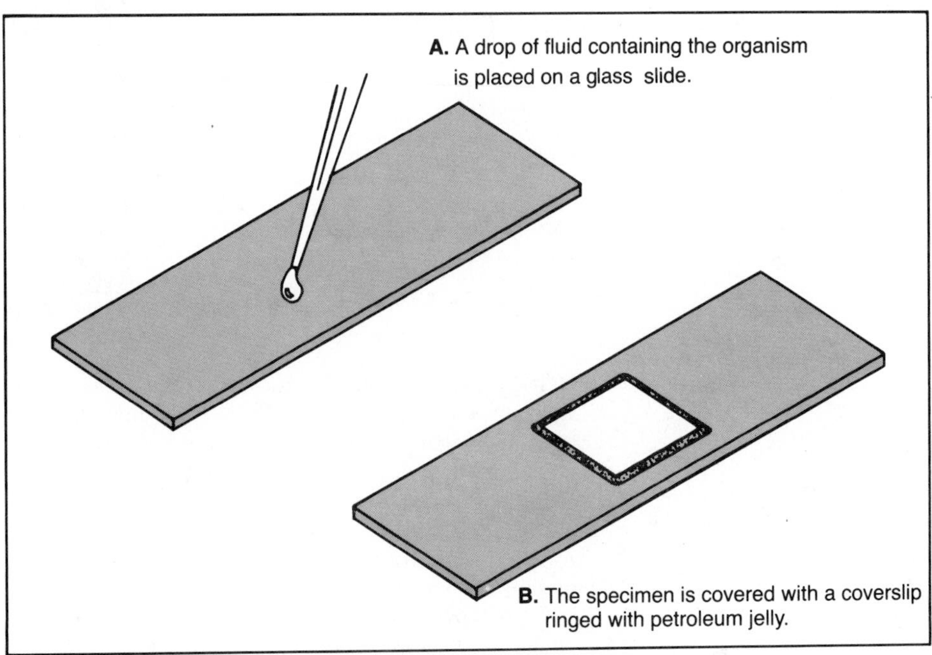

FIGURE 14–12. Wet mount method of slide preparation for means of examining microorganisms in the living state.

PROCEDURE 14-3
PREPARING A HANGING DROP SLIDE

This method is performed using a hanging drop slide, which consists of a thick glass slide with a depression in its center (Fig. 14–13). The hanging drop preparation is made as outlined below.

1. Spread a small amount of petroleum jelly around the edge of the coverslip.

2. Place the coverslip on a clean, dry surface with the petroleum jelly facing up.

3. Transfer a drop of the specimen to the center of the coverslip.

4. Place the hanging drop slide over the coverslip so that the center of the depression lies directly over the drop.

5. Apply slight pressure to the slide to ensure satisfactory contact between the coverslip and slide. The petroleum jelly seals the coverslip to the slide to hold it in place and prevent evaporation through air currents.

6. Invert the slide quickly so that the drop to be examined hangs from the bottom of the coverslip.

7. Place the slide under the microscope.

8. Examine the specimen with the high-power objective. The amount of light must be reduced by partially closing the diaphragm and lowering the condenser.

9. Properly dispose of the slide and coverslip.

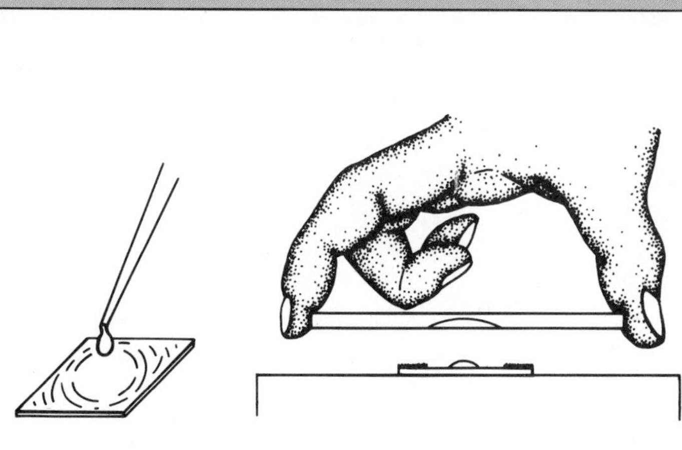

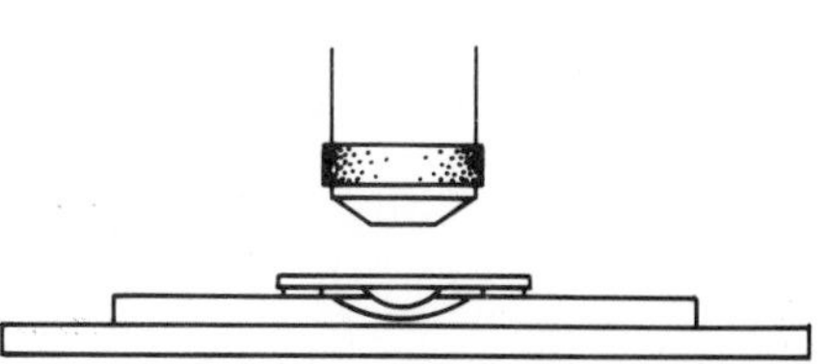

A. A drop of the specimen is placed in the center of the coverslip (ringed with petroleum jelly).

B. The hanging drop slide is placed over the coverslip.

C. The slide is inverted for examination under the microscope.

FIGURE 14–13. Hanging drop slide preparation.

Smears

A smear consists of material spread on a slide for microscopic examination. It may be prepared directly from the specimen collected on the swab, or the specimen may first be grown on a culture medium, and a smear then prepared. Most smears must be stained before they can be viewed under the microscope, using one of a number of available staining techniques. They are often helpful when time is a factor, because a smear can be prepared immediately from the specimen. This gives the physician a preliminary clue to the causative agent while other, more time-consuming tests are being performed.

PROCEDURE 14-4
PREPARING A SMEAR

1. **PROCEDURAL STEP.** Wash the hands.

2. **PROCEDURAL STEP.** Assemble the equipment. The equipment needed includes the **microbiologic specimen, slide forceps,** a **Bunsen burner,** a **sterile swab or inoculating needle,** and **nongreasy slides that are not scratched.** Label the slide with the patient's name and the date.
   PRINCIPLE. Scratches and dirt on the slide may be mistaken for microorganisms. Greasy slides result in an unsatisfactory smear, because the bacteria are harder to spread out.

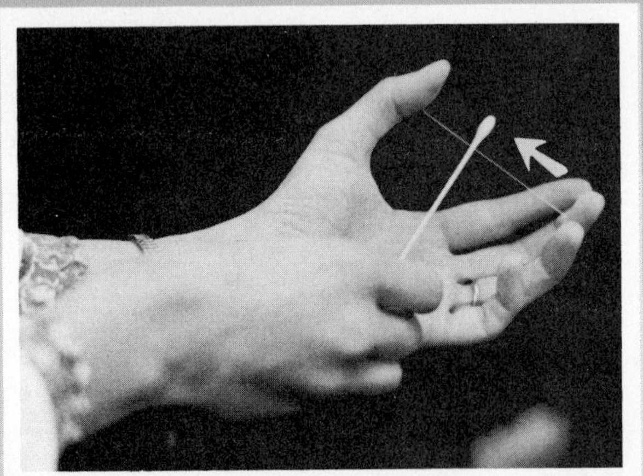

3. **PROCEDURAL STEP.** Hold the edges of the slide between your thumb and index finger. Starting at the right side and using a rolling motion, gently and evenly spread the material from the specimen over the slide. The material should cover approximately one-half to two-thirds of the slide. Do not rub the material vigorously over the slide. Be careful not to allow the material from the specimen to come in contact with your fingers or any other part of your body. Properly dispose of the contaminated swab. Wash your hands once this step is completed.
   PRINCIPLE. A rolling motion is used to deposit the maximum amount of material possible on the slide. Rubbing may disintegrate the cellular structures making up the microorganisms in the specimen. The specimen may contain pathogens that are capable of infecting the medical assistant.

4. **PROCEDURAL STEP.** Allow the smear to air dry in a flat position for at least one-half hour. Heat should not be applied at this time.
   PRINCIPLE. Air drying allows the bacterial cells to dry slowly. Applying heat at this stage would burst the bacterial cells, resulting in an inappropriate smear.

5. **PROCEDURAL STEP.** Holding the slide with the slide forceps, "heat fix" the smear by quickly passing the slide back and forth (approximately three times) through the flame of a Bunsen burner. The slide has been fixed properly if the back of the slide feels uncomfortable (but not too hot) when touched to the back of your hand. Excessive heat should be avoided.

PRINCIPLE. Heat fixing the slide kills the microorganisms and attaches them firmly to the slide so they do not wash off during the staining process. An excessive amount of heat could result in distortion of the bacterial cells.

6. **PROCEDURAL STEP.** Examine the smear under the microscope, or stain it according to your medical office policy.

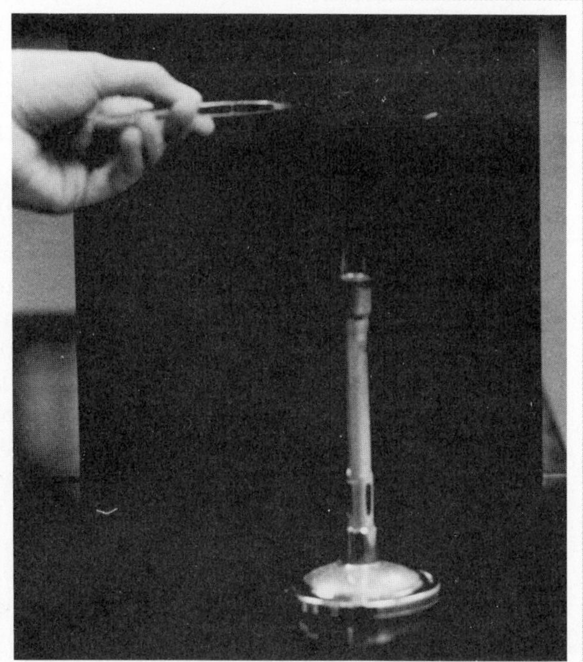

Record data below.

DATE	TIME	PATIENT'S NAME	RESULTS

The Gram Stain

Bacteria contained in a smear are colorless and usually are difficult to identify under the microscope unless some type of staining technique is used. Staining them allows the observer to directly view the size, shape, and growth patterns of the bacteria.

A very commonly employed staining method is the Gram stain. In 1883, Christian Gram, a Danish physician, discovered a way to differentiate bacteria on the basis of their color reactions to various stains. Gram staining is based on the fact that when treated with crystal violet dye, certain bacteria permanently retain this dye after undergoing a decolorization process. These bacteria exhibit a purple color when viewed under the microscope and are known as *gram-positive* bacteria. Other bacteria are unable to retain this dye after being decolorized and become colorless. They must be counterstained with a contrasting hue to become visible under the microscope. These bacteria exhibit a pink or red color and are known as *gram-negative* bacteria. It is theorized that these staining characteristics are due to differences in the chemical composition of the bacterial cell walls.

Gram staining allows for the division of most bacteria into two large groups: gram positive and gram negative. Some of the infectious diseases caused by gram-positive bacteria are streptococcal sore throat, scarlet fever, rheumatic fever, diphtheria, lobar pneumonia, tetanus, and botulism. Infectious diseases caused by gram-negative bacteria include whooping cough, gonorrhea, meningitis, bacillary dysentery, cholera, typhoid fever, and the plague.

Bacteria undergoing Gram staining are also observed for their characteristic shape and fall into one of the following categories: gram-positive rods, gram-negative rods, gram-positive cocci, or gram-negative cocci. For example, the causative agent of gonorrhea is a gram-negative diplococcus.

Gram staining is often used in combination with culture tests to help in the diagnosis and treatment of infectious diseases. The medical assistant may be responsible for preparing a Gram-stained smear for examination by the physician. Proper timing of the various reactions is a critical factor in the preparation of a well-stained smear.

PROCEDURE 14-5
GRAM STAINING

1. **PROCEDURAL STEP.** Wash the hands.

2. **PROCEDURAL STEP.** Assemble the equipment. The equipment needed includes the gram-staining reagents that are commercially available, which include **crystal violet, Gram's iodine solution,** an **alcohol-acetone solution,** and **safranin or another suitable counterstain.** Other supplies include the **microbiologic specimen, clean glass slides,** a **Bunsen burner, slide forceps,** a **staining rack,** a **wash bottle,** an **absorbent paper pad, immersion oil,** and a **microscope.**

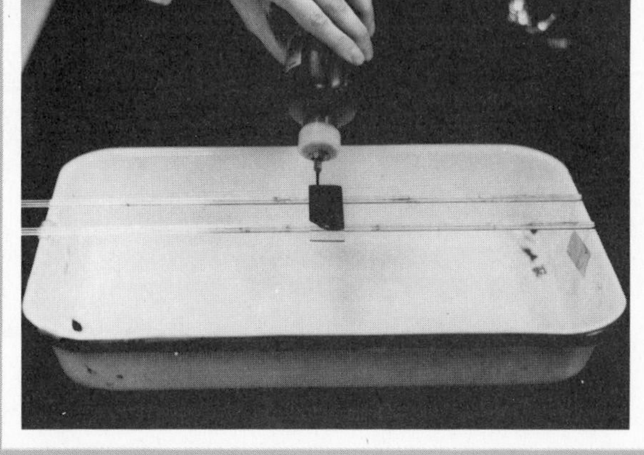

3. **PROCEDURAL STEP.** Make a thin smear, air dry it, and heat fix it with a Bunsen burner flame (refer to the Procedure for the Preparation of a Smear). Allow the slide to cool completely.

4. **PROCEDURAL STEP.** Place the slide on the staining rack with the smear side facing up. Cover the smear with crystal violet and allow it to react for 1 minute.
PRINCIPLE. The crystal violet stains all the bacteria purple.

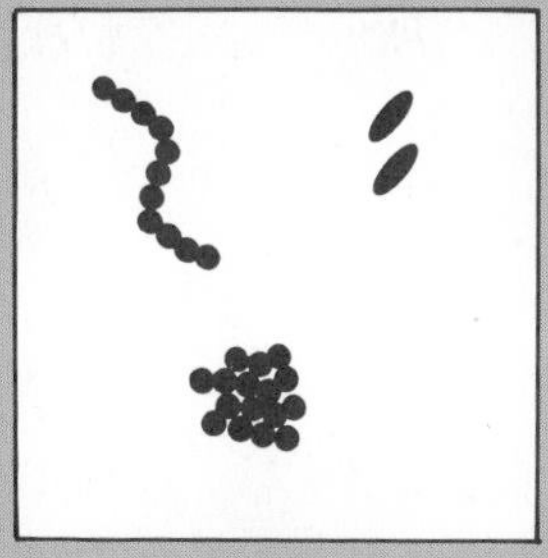

The crystal violet stains all the bacteria purple.

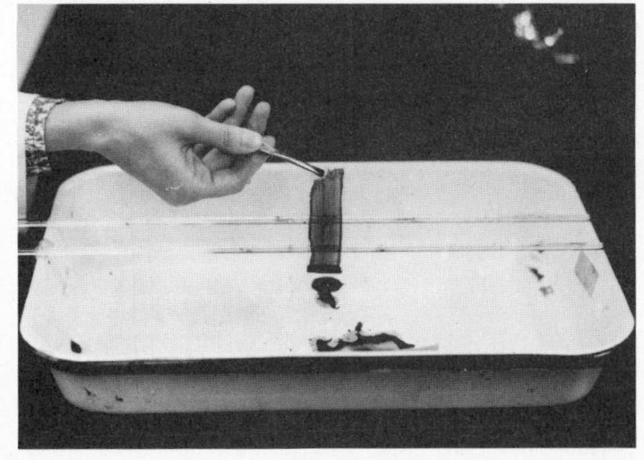

5. **PROCEDURAL STEP.** Handling the slide with slide forceps, tilt it to an angle of approximately 45 degrees to allow the crystal violet to drain off.

Continued

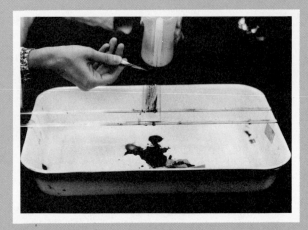

6. **Procedural step.** Continue to hold the slide at an angle and immediately rinse it thoroughly with a gentle stream of water from the wash bottle for approximately 5 seconds.

Principle. Rinsing the slide removes the crystal violet.

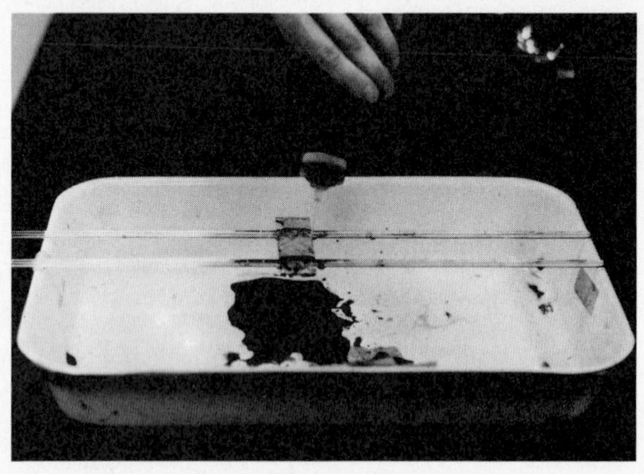

7. **Procedural step.** Replace the slide on the staining rack and cover the smear with the iodine solution. Allow it to react for 1 to 2 minutes.

Principle. The iodine acts as a mordant and causes the crystal violet to become firmly attached to those bacteria that are gram positive. (*Note:* All the bacteria on the smear are still stained purple.)

8. **Procedural step.** With your slide forceps, tilt the slide at a 45-degree angle and allow the iodine solution to drain off.

9. **Procedural step.** Keeping the slide tilted, thoroughly rinse the slide with water from your wash bottle for 5 seconds.

Principle. Rinsing the slide removes the iodine solution.

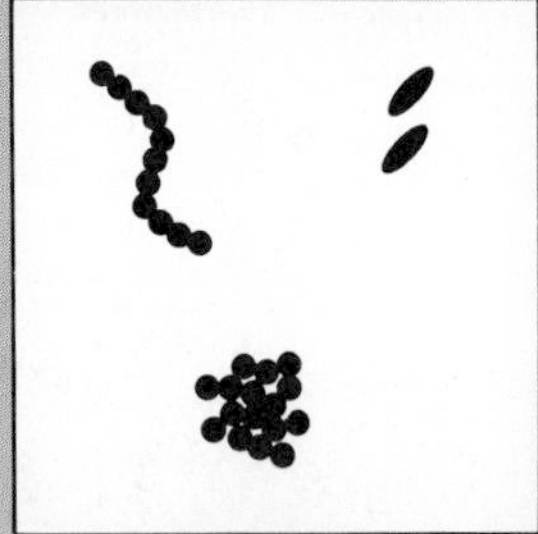

All the bacteria on the smear are still stained purple.

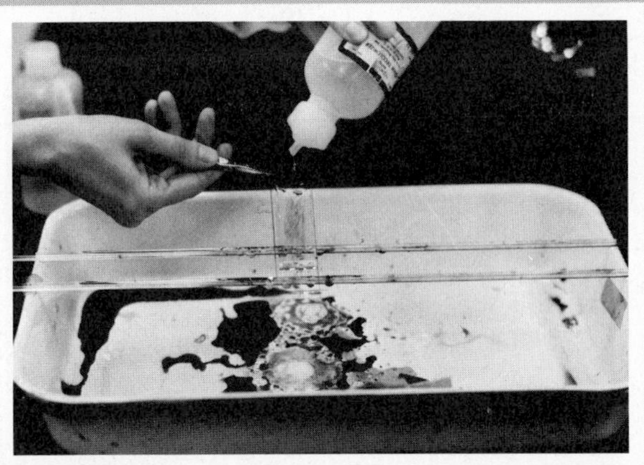

10. **Procedural step.** With the slide still tilted, slowly apply the alcohol-acetone solution. Apply it cautiously until a purple color no longer runs off the smear. Do not overdecolorize (i.e., apply too much of the decolorizer) or underdecolorize (i.e., apply too little of the decolorizer).

Principle. The alcohol-acetone solution is a decolorizer and causes the stain to become washed out of the bacteria to which it was not mordanted (i.e., the gram-negative bacteria); those bacteria then become clear. The gram-negative bacteria are unable to retain the dye and become colorless. The gram-positive bacteria are resistant to decolorization and retain the crystal violet stain, remaining purple. Overdecolorizing of gram-positive bacteria causes them to appear as gram negative. Underdecolorizing of gram-negative bacteria causes them to appear as gram positive.

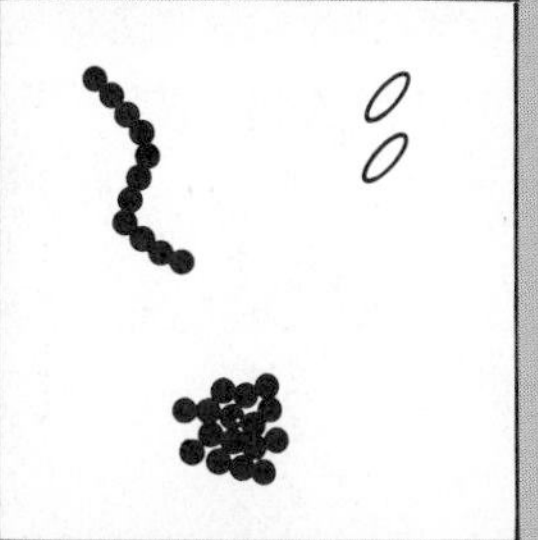

The gram-positive bacteria remain purple, and the gram-negative bacteria become colorless.

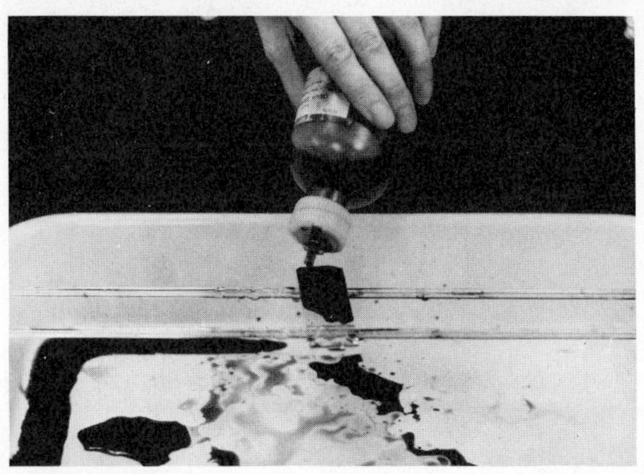

11. **Procedural step.** Immediately rinse the slide with water from your wash bottle for 5 seconds.

Principle. Rinsing the slide stops the decolorization process.

12. **Procedural step.** Replace the slide on the staining rack and cover it with a counterstain, usually safranin. Allow the counterstain to react for 30 to 60 seconds. The gram-negative bacteria must be counterstained with a contrasting dye to become visible under the microscope.

Principle. The safranin stains all of the decolorized or colorless bacteria (i.e., the gram-negative bacteria) pink or red. The gram-positive bacteria remain purple and the gram-negative bacteria now become pink or red.

13. **Procedural step.** Drain the slide by tilting it at a 45-degree angle.

14. **Procedural step.** Thoroughly rinse the slide with water from the wash bottle for 5 seconds.

Principle. Rinsing the smear removes the safranin counterstain.

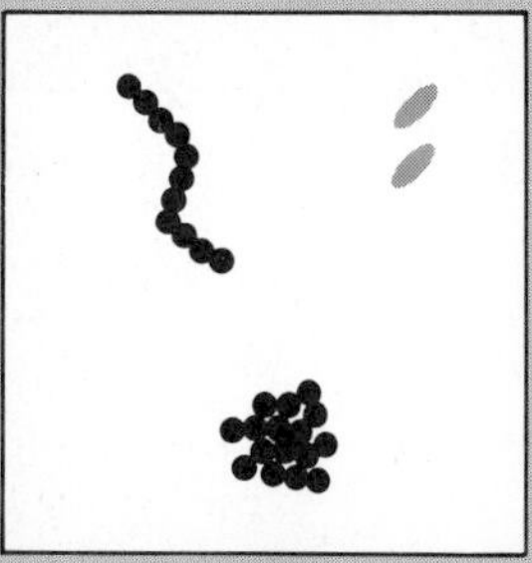

The gram-positive bacteria are still purple, and the gram-negative bacteria become pink or red.

Continued

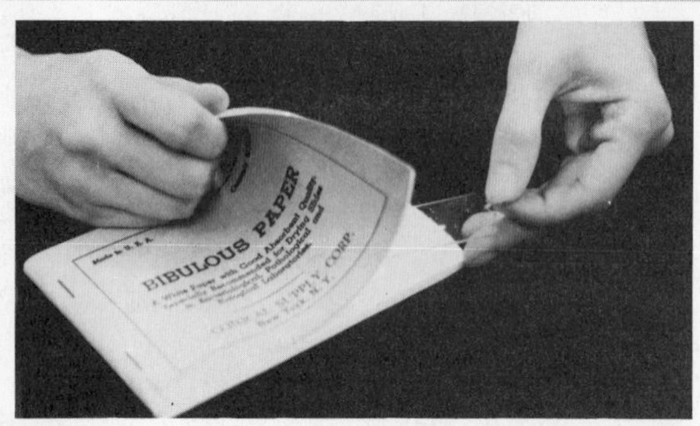

15. **PROCEDURAL STEP.** Blot the smear dry between the pages of an absorbent paper pad (bibulous paper) or on a paper towel with the smear side facing down. *Do not rub,* because this could rub off the very thin smear contained on the slide.

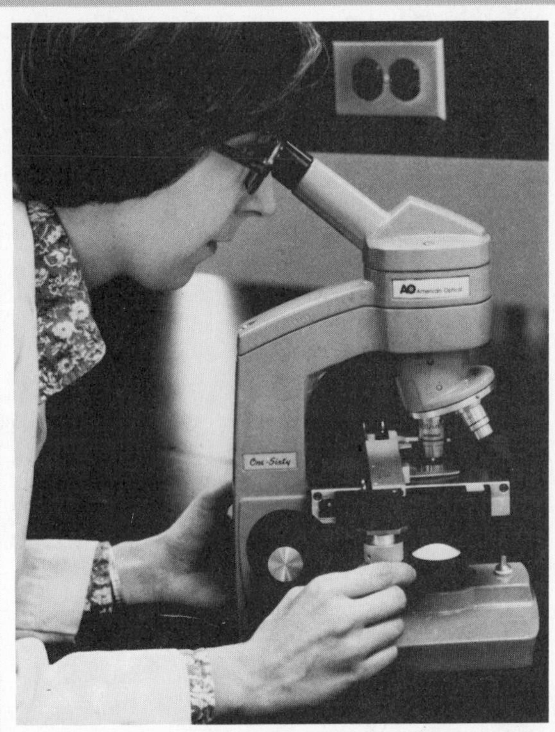

16. **PROCEDURAL STEP.** Observe the smear under the microscope using the oil-immersion objective to make sure it was properly prepared. Notify the physician that the gram-stained smear is ready to be examined.

Record data below.

DATE	TIME	PATIENT'S NAME	RESULTS

Prevention and Control of Infectious Diseases

Individuals in the community can help prevent and control infectious diseases by practicing good techniques of medical asepsis, by obtaining proper nutrition and rest, and by utilizing good hygienic measures. In addition, infected individuals should contact their physicians in an effort to ensure early diagnosis and treatment of the disease. Immunizations are available for a wide range of infectious diseases and function to prevent the disease. The medical assistant has a responsibility to help inform community members in the use of practices that reduce the transmission of pathogens and help control and prevent infectious diseases.

Study Questions

1. What are the stages included in the course of an infectious disease?
2. What are the three classifications of bacteria based on shape?
3. What is the difference between a monocular and binocular microscope?
4. What precautions should the medical assistant take to prevent infection by a pathogenic microorganism?
5. Why is early diagnosis of streptococcal pharyngitis important?

15

ELECTRO-CARDIOGRAPHY

CHAPTER OUTLINE

Structure of the Heart
Conduction System of the Heart
Cardiac Cycle
Electrocardiograph Paper
Standardization of the Electrocardiograph
Electrocardiograph Leads
Electrocardiographic Capabilities
Artifacts
Marking and Mounting the Electrocardiogram
Holter Monitor Electrocardiography
Cardiac Arrhythmias

COMPETENCIES

After completing this chapter, you should be able to demonstrate the proper procedure to perform the following:

1. Prepare the patient and record a standard 12-lead electrocardiogram (ECG). Record the procedure in the patient's chart.
2. Mount and label an ECG.
3. Instruct a patient in the guidelines required for wearing a Holter monitor.
4. Apply a Holter monitor and record the procedure.

LEARNING OBJECTIVES

After completing this chapter, you should be able to do the following:

1. Define the terms listed in the vocabulary.
2. Trace the path the blood takes through the heart, starting with the right atrium.
3. Explain the conduction system of the heart.
4. State the purpose of electrocardiography.
5. Identify the following components on an ECG and state what each represents: P wave, QRS complex, T wave, P-R interval, Q-T interval, P-R segment, S-T segment, and the baseline following the T (or U) wave.
6. State the purpose of standardizing the electrocardiograph. Explain what should be done if the amplitude of the R wave is too large or too small.
7. State the function of the electrodes, electrolyte, amplifier, and galvanometer.
8. List the 12 ECG leads that are recorded and diagram the "picture" of the heart that each lead is taking.
9. Locate the six ECG chest leads on individuals of various body contours.
10. Describe the function served by each of the following electrocardiographic capabilities: single-channel recorder, three-channel recorder, automatic capability, phone transmission, interpretive electrocardiography, and the copy feature.
11. Identify the following types of artifacts and state what may cause each to occur: muscle, wandering baseline, alternating current, and interrupted baseline.
12. Describe Holter monitor electrocardiography.
13. List three reasons for applying a Holter monitor.
14. Explain the use of the patient diary in Holter monitor electrocardiography.
15. Locate the Holter monitor chest leads on individuals of various body contours.
16. Identify the following cardiac arrhythmias and explain what causes each to occur: atrial premature contraction, paroxysmal atrial tachycardia, atrial flutter, atrial fibrillation, premature ventricular contraction, ventricular tachycardia, ventricular flutter, and ventricular fibrillation.

• VOCABULARY •

amplitude (am'pli-tūd)—Refers to amount, extent, size, abundance, or fullness.

artifact (ar'ti-fakt)—Additional electrical activity that is picked up by the electrocardiograph that interferes with the normal appearance of the ECG cycles.

baseline (bās' līn)—The flat horizontal line that separates the various waves of the ECG cycle.

cardiac cycle (kar' de-ak si' k'l)—One complete heart beat.

ECG cycle (ECG si' k'l)—The graphic representation of a cardiac cycle.

electrocardiogram (e-lek" tro-kar' de-o-gram")—The graphic representation of the electrical activity of the heart.

electrocardiograph (e-lek" tro-kar' de-o-graf")—The instrument used to record the electrical activity of the heart.

electrode (e-lek' trōd)—A conductor of electricity, that is used to promote contact between the body and the electrocardiograph (also known as a sensor).

electrolyte (e-lek' tro-līt)—A chemical substance that promotes conduction of an electrical current.

interval (in' ter-val)—The length of a wave or the length of a wave with a segment.

normal sinus rhythm (nor' mal si' nus rith' m)—Refers to an electrocardiogram that is within normal limits.

segment (seg' ment)—The portion of the ECG between two waves.

The *electrocardiograph* is an instrument used to record the electrical activity of the heart. The *electrocardiogram* (abbreviated ECG or EKG) is the graphic representation of this activity. The ECG exhibits the amount of electrical activity produced by the heart and the time required for the impulse to travel through the heart.

Electrocardiography is used for the following purposes: to detect an abnormal cardiac rhythm (arrhythmia); to help diagnose damage to the heart due to a myocardial infarction; to assess the effect on the heart of digitalis or other cardiac drugs; to determine the presence of an electrolyte imbalance; to assess the progress of rheumatic fever; and to determine the presence of hypertrophy of the heart chambers. An ECG is not able to detect the presence of all cardiovascular disorders. In addition, it cannot always detect impending heart disease. The ECG is generally used in combination with other diagnostic and laboratory tests to assess cardiac functioning.

The medical assistant is frequently responsible for recording ECGs in the medical office. They are often included as part of the physical examination. The medical assistant must acquire knowledge and skill in each of the following aspects of electrocardiography: preparation of the patient, operation of the electrocardiograph, identification and elimination of artifacts, mounting and labeling of the completed ECG, and care and maintenance of the electrocardiograph.

Structure of the Heart

The human heart consists of four chambers: the right and left atria are the upper chambers, and the right and left ventricles are the lower chambers (Fig. 15–1). Blood enters the right atrium from two large veins, the superior vena cava and the inferior vena cava, that bring it back from its circulation through the body. The blood entering the right atrium is deoxygenated, meaning it contains very little oxygen and is high in carbon dioxide. From the right atrium, the blood enters the right ventricle. It is pumped from here to the lungs by way of the pulmonary artery.

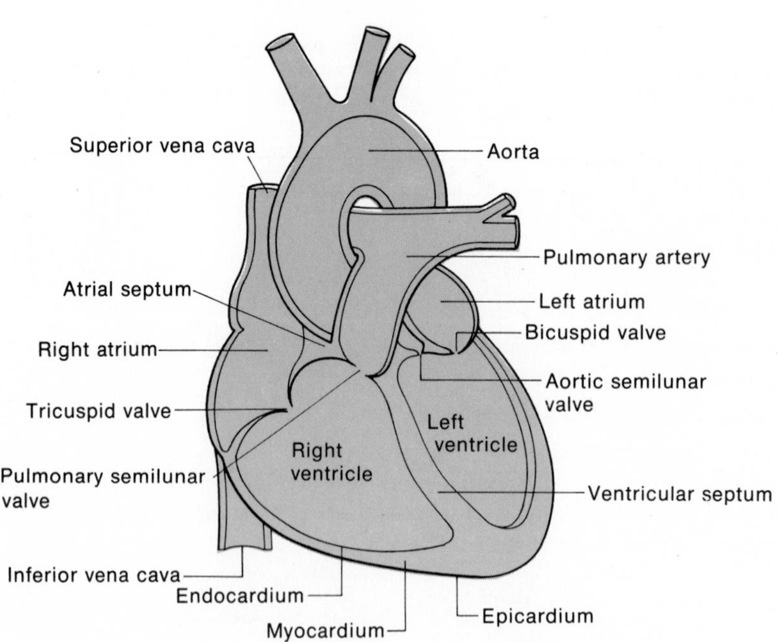

FIGURE 15–1. Diagram of the heart, identifying the structures.

It picks up oxygen in the lungs in exchange for carbon dioxide and returns to the left atrium of the heart by way of the pulmonary veins. From the left atrium, the blood enters the left ventricle. This is the most powerful chamber of the heart and serves to pump blood to the entire body. Blood exits from the left ventricle by way of the aorta, which distributes it to all parts of the body to nourish the tissues with oxygen and nutrients.

Conduction System of the Heart

The *sinoatrial node* (SA node) is located in the upper portion of the right atrium, just below the opening of the superior vena cava. It consists of a knot of modified myocardial cells that have the ability to send out an electrical impulse without an external nerve stimulus. In this way the SA node initiates and regulates the heart beat. Each electrical impulse discharged by the SA node is distributed to the right and left atria and causes them to contract. This contraction forces blood through the open cuspid valves and into the ventricles. The impulse is then picked up by the *atrioventricular node* (AV node), another knot of modified myocardial cells located at the base of the right atrium. Its function is to transmit the electrical impulse to the *bundle of His.* The AV node delays the impulse momentarily to give the ventricles a chance to fill with blood from the atria. The bundle of His divides into right and left branches known as the bundle branches, which then relay the impulse to the *Purkinje fibers.* The Purkinje fibers distribute the impulse evenly to the right and left ventricles, causing them to contract; this forces blood out of the ventricles and into the pulmonary artery and aorta. The entire heart relaxes momentarily. Then a new impulse is initiated by the SA node and the cycle repeats itself (Fig. 15–2).

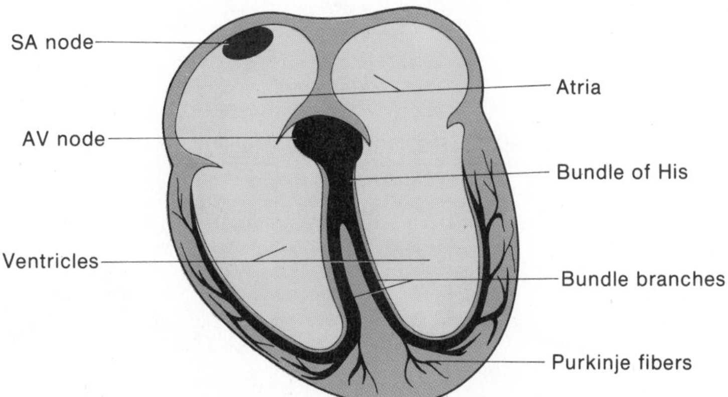

FIGURE 15–2. Diagram of the heart, identifying the structures involved with the conduction of an electrical impulse through the heart.

Cardiac Cycle

The *cardiac cycle* represents one complete heartbeat. It consists of the contraction of the atria, the contraction of the ventricles, and the relaxation of the entire heart (as described previously). The electrocardiograph records the electrical activity that causes these events in the cardiac cycle to occur. The *ECG cycle* is the graphic representation of the cardiac cycle (Fig. 15–3).

The normal ECG cycle consists of a P wave; the Q, R, and S waves (known as the QRS complex); and a T wave. The ECG cycle is recorded from left to right, beginning with the P wave. The impulse initiated by the SA node spreads to the muscle cells of the right and left atria, causing them to contract. The *P wave* represents the electrical activity associated with the contraction of the atria, or *atrial depolarization.* The impulse is picked up by the AV node and distributed to the ventricles by way of the bundle of His and Purkinje fibers, resulting in the contraction of the ventricles. The *QRS complex* represents the electrical activity associated with the contraction of the ventricles, or *ventricular depolarization.* The *T wave* represents the electrical recovery of the ventricles, or *ventricular repolarization.* The muscle cells are recovering in preparation for another impulse. Occasionally, a *U wave* is seen following the T wave. It is a small wave and is associated in some as yet undefined way with repolarization.

The flat, horizontal line that separates the various waves is known as the *baseline.* The waves deflect either upward (positive deflection) or downward (negative deflection) from the baseline. The baseline is divided into segments and intervals for the purpose of interpretation and analysis of the ECG by the physician.

A *segment* is the portion of the ECG between two waves. The *P–R segment* represents the time interval from the end of the atrial depolarization to the beginning of the ventricular depolarization. It is the time needed for the impulse to travel from the AV node through the bundle of His and Purkinje fibers to the ventricles. The *S–T segment* represents the time interval from the end of the ventricular depolarization to the beginning of repolarization of the ventricles.

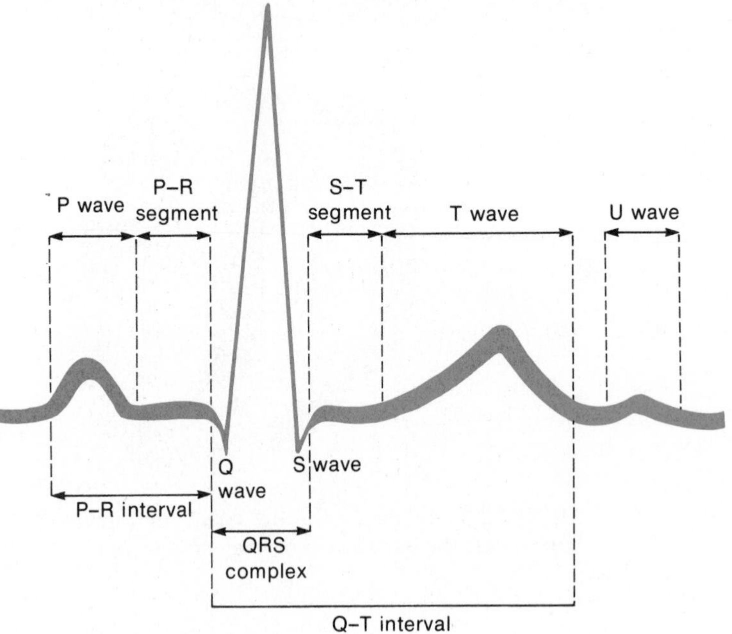

FIGURE 15–3. The ECG cycle.

An *interval* is the length of a wave or the length of a wave with a segment. The *P–R interval* represents the time lapse from the beginning of the atrial depolarization to the beginning of the ventricular depolarization. The *Q–T interval* is the time from the beginning of the ventricular depolarization to the end of repolarization of the ventricles. The baseline occurring after the T wave (or U wave, if present) represents the period when the entire heart returns to its resting, or *polarized,* state.

Electrocardiograph Paper

Electrocardiograph paper is divided into two sets of squares for accurate and convenient measurement of the waves, intervals, and segments by the physician (Fig. 15–4). Each small square is 1 millimeter (mm) high and 1 mm wide. Each large square (made up of 25 small squares) is 5 mm high and 5 mm wide. By measuring the various waves, intervals, and segments of the graph cycle, the physician is able to determine whether the electrical activity of the heart falls within normal limits.

Electrocardiograph paper consists of a black or blue base with a white plastic coating. A black or red graph is printed on top of the plastic coating. A heated stylus moves over the heat-sensitive paper and melts away the plastic coating, resulting in the recording of the ECG cycles. In addition to being heat sensitive, the paper is pressure sensitive and should be handled carefully to avoid making impressions that would interfere with its proper reading.

The stylus heat should be adjusted to obtain a clear and sharp recording. A recording that is too light or too dark is difficult to read. The heat can be adjusted using the Stylus Heat Control. The medical assistant should refer to the instruction manual that accompanies the electrocardiograph to determine how to adjust this control.

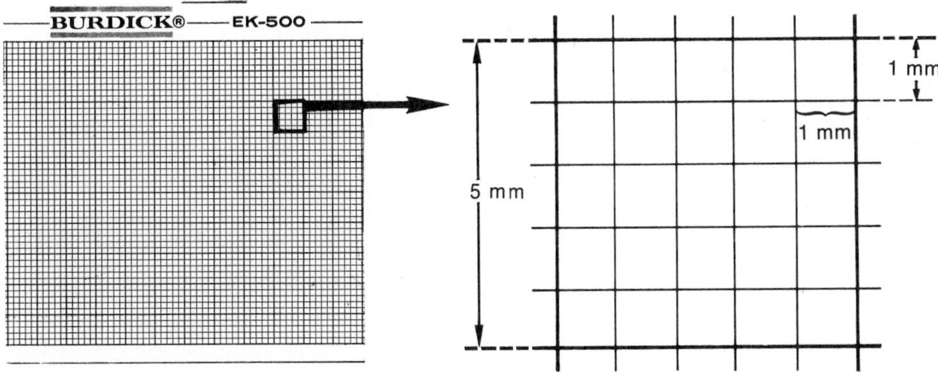

FIGURE 15–4. Diagram of ECG paper with a section enlarged to indicate the size of the large and small squares.

Standardization of the Electrocardiograph

The electrocardiograph machine must always be standardized before an ECG is run. This ensures an accurate and reliable recording. It means that an ECG run on one electrocardiograph will compare with a tracing run on another machine.

By international agreement, 1 millivolt (mV) of electricity should cause the stylus to move 10 mm high in amplitude (10 small squares or 1 centimeter [cm]). Pressing the Standardization Button causes 1 mV to enter the electrocardiograph machine, which should result in an upward deflection of 10 mm. The marking on the ECG paper is known as the *standardization mark* or *reference calibration mark* (Fig. 15–5*A*). The left edge of the top of the standardization mark has a tendency to slant downward toward the right. This is a normal phenomenon. The width of the mark should be approximately 2 mm (two small squares). If it is less or more than 2 mm, the Standardization Button should be depressed for a longer or shorter period of time as required. If the mark is more or less than 10 mm in amplitude, it can be adjusted. The instruction manual must be consulted for proper adjustment information. An electrocardiograph must never be adjusted for the first time without use of the instruction manual.

While an ECG is being run, the R wave may have such a large amplitude that it goes off the graph. This may be corrected by moving the stylus up or down on the graph paper as required, by using the Position Control knob. If the R wave is extremely large and cannot be corrected by adjusting the position of the stylus, it may be shortened by recording the lead at one-half standard. This means that all ECG cycles will be half their normal amplitude.The medical assistant must be sure to include a standardization mark with that particular lead to alert the physician to the change in standard. The mark will be half its normal size, or 5 mm high (Fig. 15–5*B*).

Occasionally, the ECG cycles may be too small on a lead, making it difficult for the physician to interpret. The medical assistant can double the size of the cycles by recording the lead at twice the normal standard. A standardization mark must be included with this lead also, to inform the physician of the change. The mark will be twice its normal amplitude, or 20 mm high (Fig. 15–5*C*). Most ECGs are run at normal standardization; however, the medical assistant should observe the ECG carefully as it is being recorded, to determine whether a change in standard is needed. The machine must be returned to normal standard after it has been changed to prevent accidentally running the next lead at other than normal standard.

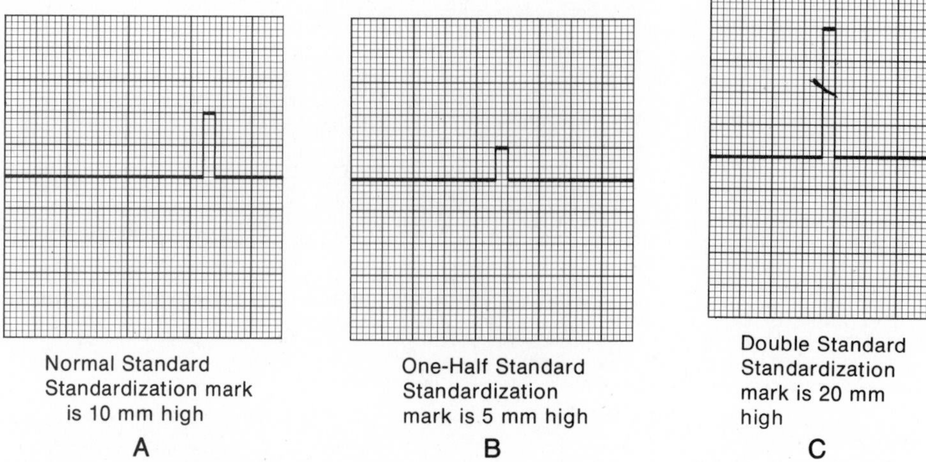

FIGURE 15–5. Standardization marks.

Electrocardiograph Leads

The standard electrocardiogram consists of 12 leads. Each lead records the heart's electrical activity from a different angle. The 12 leads provide an electrical "photograph" of the heart from different angles; this allows for a thorough three-dimensional interpretation of the heart's activity.

The electrical impulses given off by the heart are picked up by electrodes (also known as sensors) and conducted into the machine through lead wires. Electrodes are made of a substance, such as metal, that is a good conductor of electricity. The amount of electrical activity emitted by the body is very small. Therefore, to produce a readable ECG, it must be made larger, or amplified, by a device known as an *amplifier,* located within the electrocardiograph. The amplified voltages are changed into mechanical motion by the *galvanometer* and recorded on the electrocardiograph paper by a heated stylus (Fig. 15–6).

There are four limb electrodes, which include the right arm electrode (RA), the left arm electrode (LA), the right leg electrode (RL), and the left leg electrode (LL). The right leg electrode is known as the ground. It is not used for the actual recording but serves as an electrical reference point. The chest leads are abbreviated V or C and use either one or six chest electrodes, depending upon the type of electrocardiograph being used. This is explained later in more detail.

An *electrolyte* is applied to each electrode to help conduct the electrical current, because skin is a poor conductor of electricity. The electrolyte may be in the form of a paste or gel or it may be flannel or cotton saturated with an electrolyte solution.

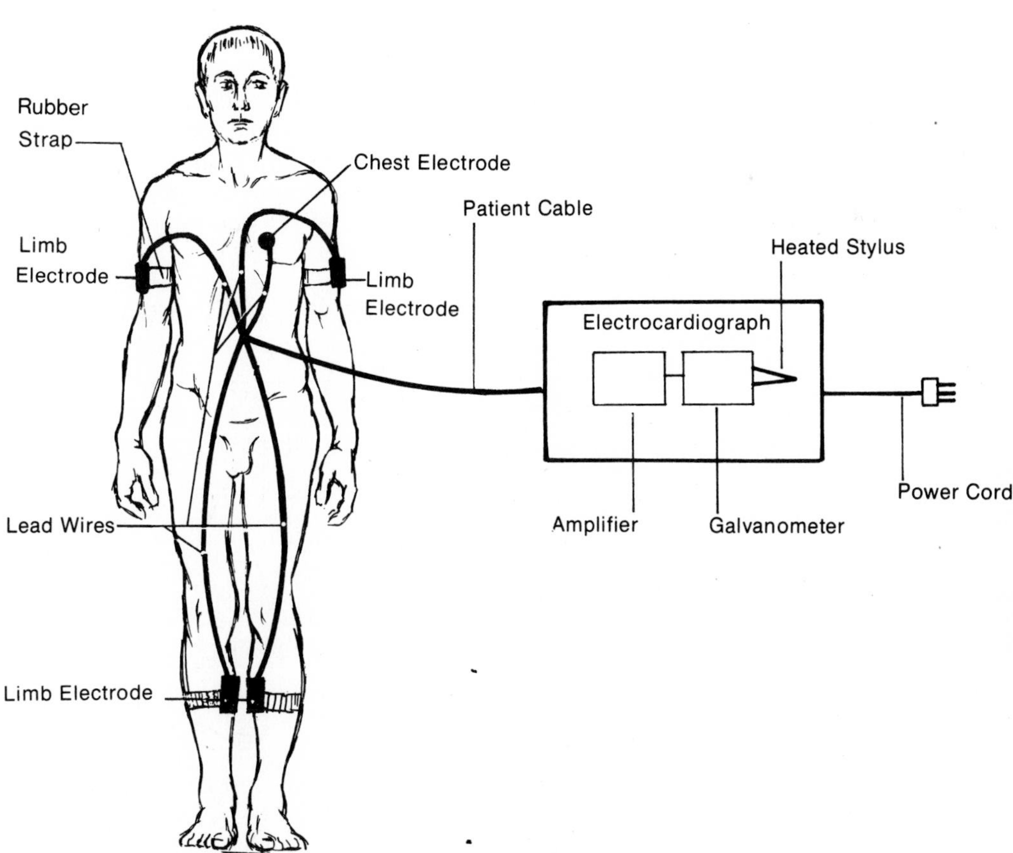

FIGURE 15–6. Diagram of the basic components of the electrocardiograph. The limb electrodes are attached to the fleshy parts of the limbs, and the lead wires are arranged to follow body contour. The patient cable is not dangling, and the power cord points away from the electrocardiograph.

The chest electrode is available in several forms. One type is a metal disc containing a rubber retaining ring. Cotton or flannel saturated in an electrolyte is held in place by the rubber ring. A chest strap with a weighted metal end must be used to hold the metal disc electrode in place on the chest. Another type of chest electrode is the Welsh electrode, or vacuum cup. It consists of a rubber bulb with a metal suction cup. A paste or gel electrolyte is squeezed onto the suction cup before it is placed on the chest.

The first three leads making up the 12-lead ECG are the *standard* or *bipolar* leads; they are leads I, II, and III. The standard limb leads use two of the limb electrodes to record the electrical activity given off by the heart. Lead I records the heart's voltage difference between the right arm and the left arm, lead II records the difference between the right arm and the left leg, and lead III records the difference between the left arm and the left leg (Fig. 15–7).

The next three leads are the *augmented leads.* They include aVR (augmented voltage—right arm), aVL (augmented voltage—left arm), and aVF (augmented voltage—left leg or foot). Lead aVR records the heart's voltage difference between the right arm electrode and a central point between the left arm and left leg. Lead aVL records the heart's voltage difference between the left arm electrode and a central point between the right arm and left leg. Lead aVF records the heart's voltage difference between the left leg electrode and a central point between the right arm and left arm. Leads I, II, III, aVR, aVL, and aVF record the voltage from side to side or from top to bottom of the heart (Fig. 15–7).

The last six leads are the chest leads, or precordial leads. They are V_1, V_2, V_3, V_4, V_5, and V_6. These leads record the heart's voltage from the front to the back of the heart. The voltage is recorded from a central point from "within" the heart to a point on the chest wall at which the electrode is placed. These points are the location of each chest lead. Figure 15–8 shows the proper location of the six chest leads. The medical assistant should accurately be able to locate each one. When first learning to locate the chest leads, it helps to mark their location on the patient's chest with a felt-tipped pen. With a conventional electrocardiograph, the medical assistant must manually move the chest electrode during the recording to

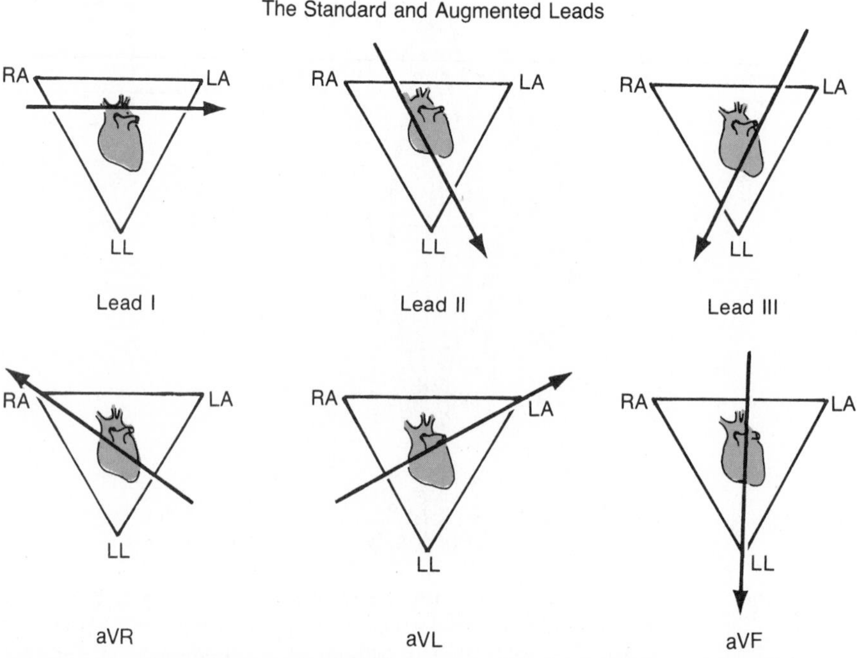

FIGURE 15–7. Diagram of the different "pictures" taken of the heart's voltage for leads I, II, III, aVR, aVL, and aVF.

FIGURE 15–8. Recommended positions for ECG chest leads:

V_1 Fourth intercostal space at right margin of sternum.
V_2 Fourth intercostal space at left margin of sternum.
V_3 Midway between position 2 and position 4.
V_4 Fifth intercostal space at junction of left midclavicular line.
V_5 At horizontal level of position 4 at left anterior axillary line.
V_6 At horizontal level of position 4 at left midaxillary line.

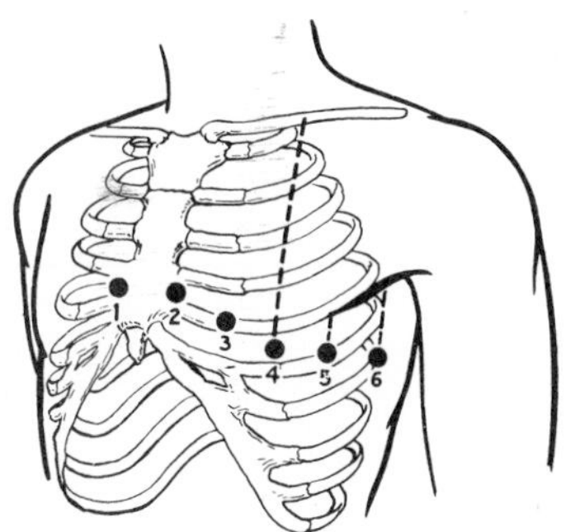

each of the six proper chest lead positions. The chest leads of the newer electrocardiographs are applied all at one time using six chest electrodes (Fig. 15–9). This avoids having to stop the machine to move the chest electrode to each of the chest lead positions.

Normally, the electrocardiogram is recorded with the paper moving at a speed of 25 mm/sec. Occasionally, the ECG cycles may be very close together, making the recording difficult to read. The medical assistant can change the paper speed to 50 mm/sec to help spread the cycles apart. To alert the physician to the change, he or she must make a notation of it by writing it on the mounted recording.

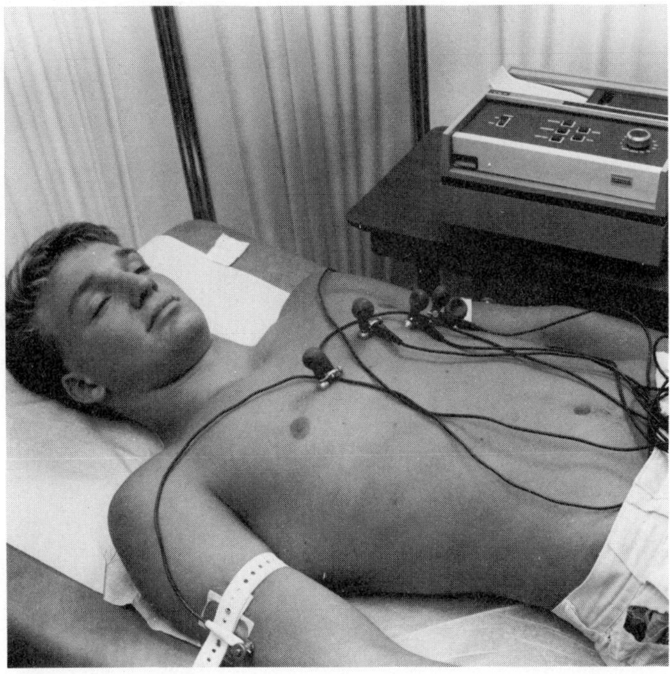

FIGURE 15–9. An example of an electrocardiograph (Burdick EK-8), in which the chest leads are all applied at one time using six chest electrodes.

Electrocardiographic Capabilities

Newer types of electrocardiographs have advanced capabilities allowing for more recording options and fewer manual operating requirements. These capabilities are listed and described below.

Three-Channel Recording Capability

An electrocardiograph with a three-channel recording capability can simultaneously record three different leads. This is in contrast to the conventional single-channel electrocardiograph, which records only one lead at a time (Fig. 15–10). The advantage is that an ECG can be produced in a shorter period of time than would be required if each lead were being recorded separately. The leads that are recorded simultaneously are as follows: Leads 1, 2, and 3, followed by aVR, aVL, and aVF, followed by V_1, V_2, and V_3, followed by V_4, V_5, and V_6. To record three leads at one time, a three-channel recording paper must be used, which is designed in a standard 8½ by 11 format. Refer to Figure 15–11 for an example of a three-channel ECG recording.

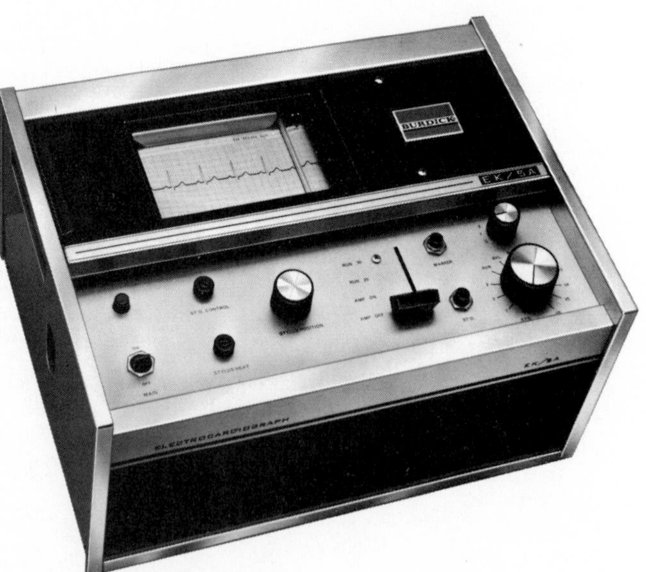

FIGURE 15–10. A single-channel electrocardiograph: Burdick EK/5A. (Courtesy of the Burdick Corporation, Milton, Wisconsin.)

Name JANE DOE
ID 12346
34YR Female

13:57 11/22/88

Vent Rate	Durations			Axes		
	PR	QRS	QT/QTC	P	QRS	T
71	188	68	400/423	42	31	71

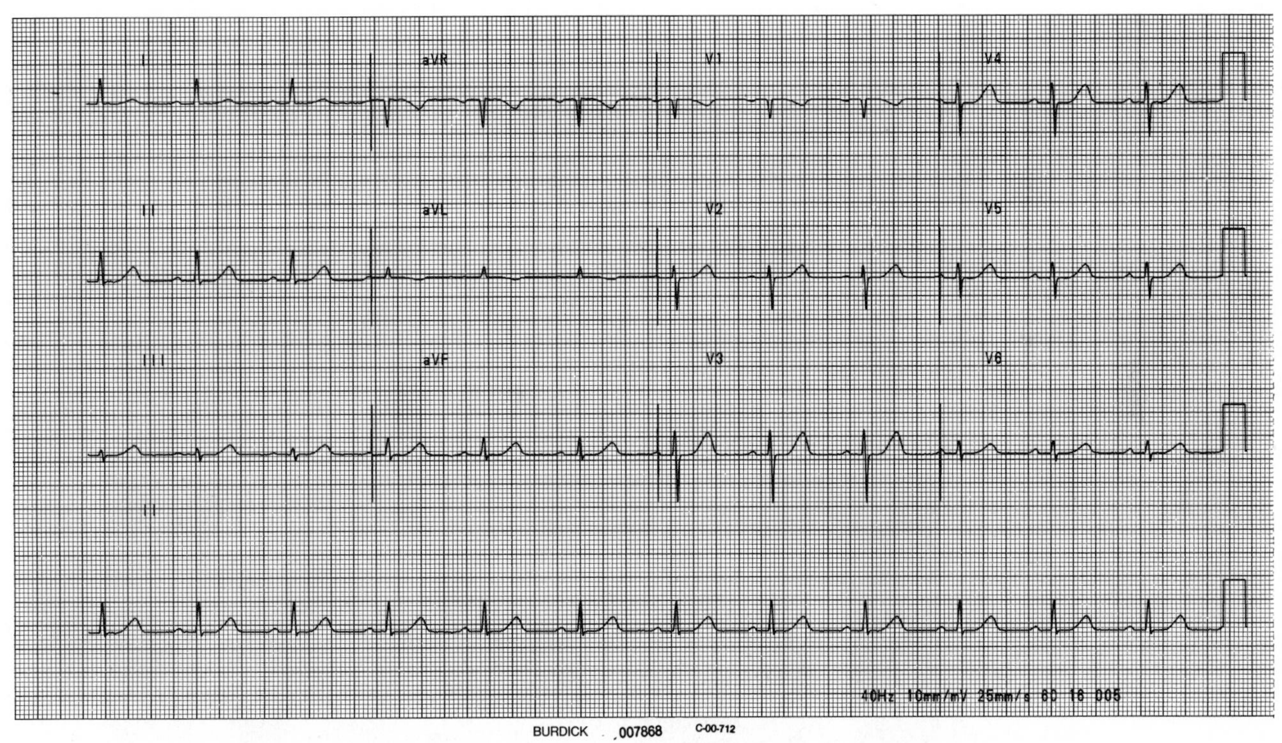

FIGURE 15–11. Example of a three-channel ECG. (Courtesy of the Burdick Corporation, Milton, Wisconsin.)

Automatic Capability

This capability automatically connects the correct electrode combinations without having to advance a control (i.e., the Lead Selector Switch). This capability saves both the time required to run the recording and the paper usage, because lead length and lead switching are automatically controlled. Both single-channel and three-channel electrocardiographs may be equipped with automatic capabilities. With the single-channel electrocardiograph, the 12 leads are automatically sequenced and recorded, one at a time, starting with lead I and progressing to V_6 (Fig. 15–12). In a three-channel electrocardiograph, three leads are automatically recorded at one time until all 12 leads have been recorded (Fig. 15–13). With this capability, a standardization mark is also automatically recorded on the tracing. Most electrocardiographs with automatic capabilities are also equipped with a control to allow manual recording of ECGs when longer tracings are required in order to provide additional data. Some electrocardiographs have a ***copy capability*** that quickly produces an accurate copy of the last ECG recorded.

Telephone Transmission

An electrocardiograph with telephone transmission capabilities can transmit a recording over the telephone line to an ECG data interpretation site. The electrocardiograph is equipped with a connector well interface for the attachment of the telephone headset. The recording is interpreted by a computer at the data site, and a printout of the recording along with the computer-assisted interpretation is mailed back to the office the same day. Patient information and baseline data (e.g., age, sex, height, weight, blood pressure, medications) also need to be relayed to assist in the interpretation. Depending upon the type of electrocardiograph, this information is either relayed verbally to the data site or entered on the electrocardiograph and transmitted automatically. The Burdick EK-7 is an example of an electrocardiograph with telephone transmission capabilities.

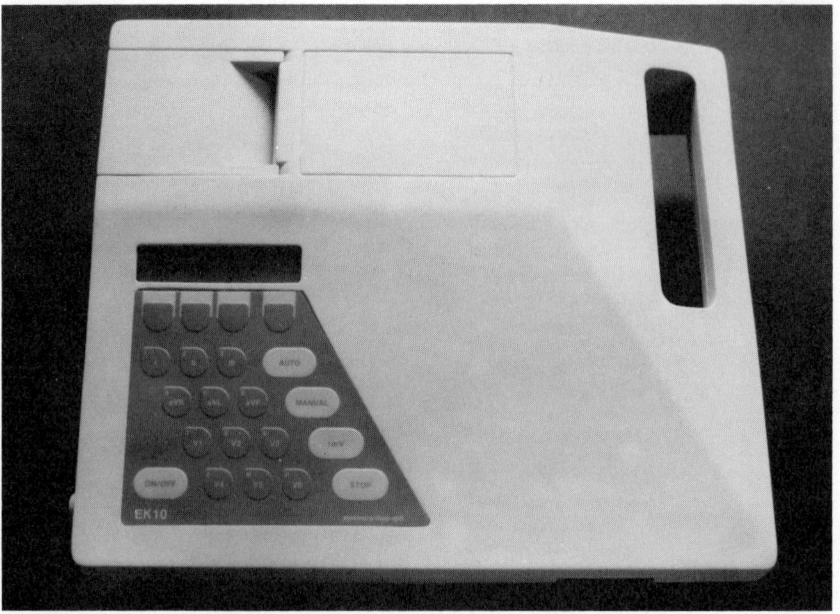

FIGURE 15–12. Example of a single-channel electrocardiograph with automatic capability: Burdick EK10. (Courtesy of the Burdick Corporation, Milton, Wisconsin.)

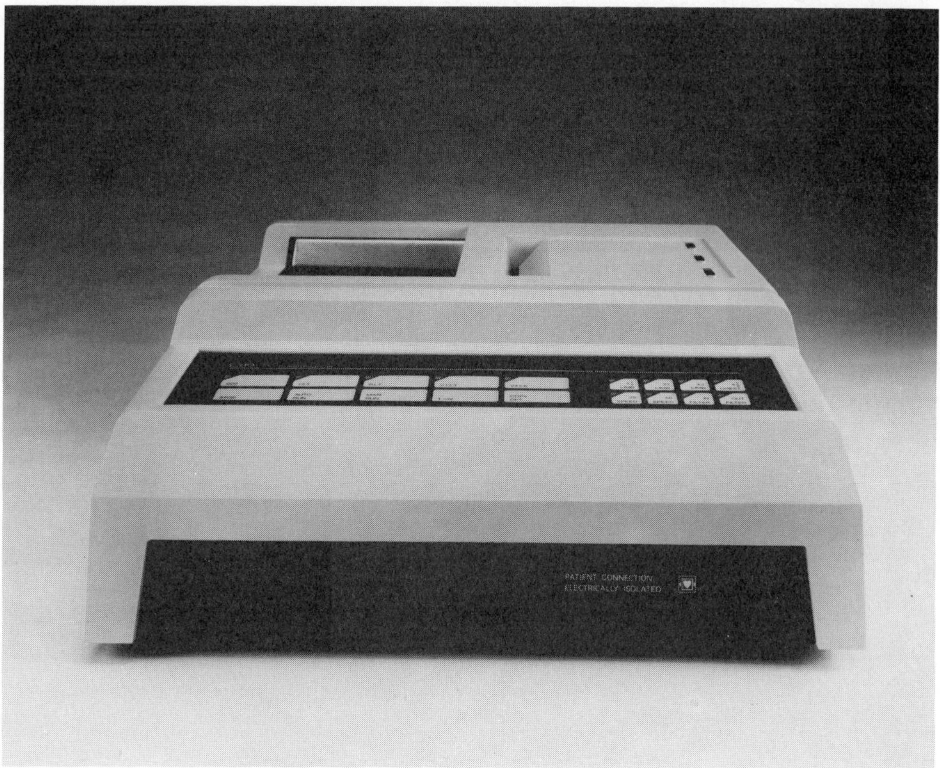

FIGURE 15–13. Example of a three-channel electrocardiograph: Burdick E310. (Courtesy of the Burdick Corporation, Milton, Wisconsin.)

Interpretive Electrocardiographs

An electrocardiograph with interpretive capabilities has a built-in computer program that analyzes the recording as it is being run. Interpretive electrocardiographs provide immediate information on the heart's activity leading to earlier diagnosis and treatment. Patient data are used in the interpretation of the ECG and must therefore be entered into the computer before running the recording. The data generally required include the patient's age, sex, race, height, weight, blood pressure, and medications. The computer analysis of the ECG is printed out at the top of the recording along with the reason for each interpretation (Fig. 15–14).

Artifacts

The medical assistant is responsible for producing a clear and concise ECG recording that can be easily read and interpreted by the physician. At times, structures appear in the recording that are not natural and that interfere with the normal appearance of the ECG cycles. They are known as *artifacts* and represent additional electrical activity that is picked up by the electrocardiograph. The medical assistant should be able to identify artifacts and correct them.

There are several types of artifacts; the most common ones are muscle, wandering baseline, and alternating current (AC) (Fig. 15–15).

Muscle

A muscle artifact (Fig. 15–15*A*) can be identified by its fuzzy irregular baseline. There are two types of muscle artifacts: those resulting from involuntary muscle movement (somatic tremor) and those resulting from voluntary muscle movement. Muscle artifacts may be caused by the following:

1. An apprehensive patient. Explaining the procedure and reassuring the patient that having an ECG recorded is a painless procedure can help reduce apprehension and relax muscles.

2. Patient discomfort. Make sure the table is wide enough to support the patient's arms and legs adequately. The patient can be made more comfortable by placing a pillow under his or her head. Check to make sure that the room temperature is comfortable for the patient. A temperature that is warm enough for the medical assistant may be too cold for the patient who has removed clothing. This could result in shivering, which would also produce a muscle artifact on the ECG.

3. Patient movement. The patient must be instructed to lie still and not talk during the recording.

Name JOHN DOE
ID 12345
36YR Male

SINUS BRADYCARDIA
POSSIBLE LEFT VENTRICULAR HYPERTROPHY [VOLTAGE CRITERIA PLUS LAE OR QRS WIDENING]
ABNORMAL ECG

14:04 11/22/88

Vent Rate	Durations PR	QRS	QT/QTC	Axes P	QRS	T
48	176	100	428/396	77	75	51

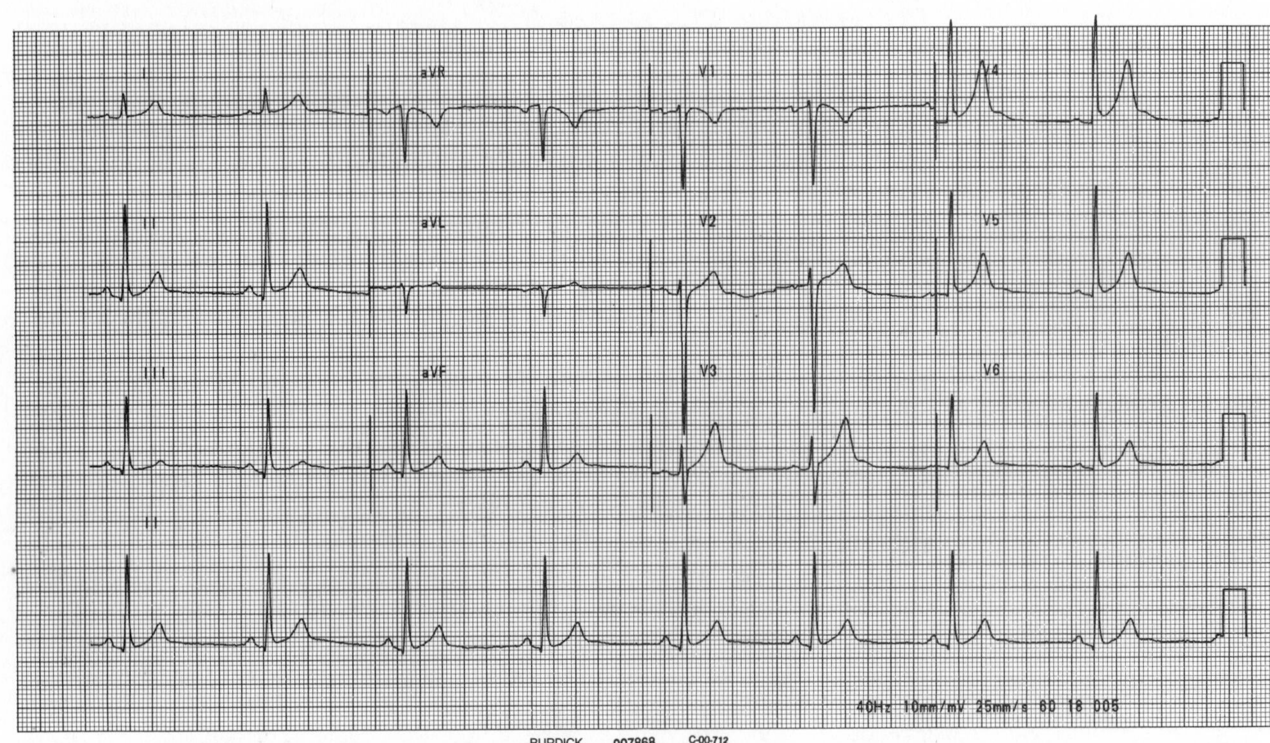

FIGURE 15–14. Example of an ECG recording that has been analyzed by an interpretive electrocardiograph. The computer analysis is printed out at the top of the recording, along with the reason for each interpretation. (Courtesy of the Burdick Corporation, Milton, Wisconsin.)

4. A physical condition. Several nervous system disorders, such as Parkinson's disease, prevent relaxation and the patient trembles continuously. The medical assistant must be understanding and try to record while the tremor is at a minimum.

Wandering Baseline

A wandering baseline (Fig. 15–15*B*) may be caused by the following:

1. Electrodes that are too tight or too loose. The medical assistant should follow proper procedure (see Procedure 15-1: Running a 12-Lead Electrocardiogram, Procedural Step 6) when applying limb electrodes to create equal tension in all four of them. The metal tips of the lead wires should also be firmly attached to the electrodes; the patient cable should be firmly supported and should not be allowed to dangle (this prevents pulling or twisting of the cable).
2. Dirty or corroded electrodes. Dirty or corroded electrodes are poor conductors of electrical current. The metal electrodes should be washed after use and cleansed periodically with kitchen cleanser until they are clean and bright. The metal tips of the lead wires may also become corroded and should be cleaned with kitchen cleanser.
3. An unequal amount of electrolyte on each electrode. The same amount of paste or gel should be applied to each electrode (see Procedure 15-1: Running a 12-Lead Electrocardiogram, Procedural Step 6). The electrolyte should be rubbed onto the patient's skin to ensure good contact between the skin and electrode.
4. Body creams, oils, or lotions present on the skin in the area where the electrode is applied. The medical assistant should remove these by rubbing with alcohol, using friction.

Alternating Current

Alternating current artifacts (Fig. 15–15*C*) are caused by electrical interference. Alternating current can "leak" or spread out from the power used by other electrical appliances in the medical office. This current may be picked up by the patient and carried into the electrocardiograph, where it would show up on the ECG recording as an AC artifact. An AC artifact appears as small straight spiked lines that are consistent in nature. Alternating current artifacts may be caused by the following:

1. Improper grounding of the electrocardiograph. The machine is automatically grounded when it is plugged in. Make sure the plug is firmly secure to the wall outlet. The right leg electrode is not used for recording the leads but picks up alternating current present on the patient and carries it into the electrocardiograph. The alternating current is then carried away by means of the machine's grounding system. To prevent AC artifacts, it is advisable to ground a metal patient table by connecting it to the electrocardiograph ground outlet using the auxiliary ground lead.
2. Electrical equipment present in the room. Lamps, sterilizers, x-ray equipment, electrical examining tables, or other electrical equipment that is plugged in may be leaking alternating current. Unplug all nearby electrical equipment in the room.
3. Wiring present in the walls, ceilings, or floors. Try moving the patient table to a new location away from the walls.
4. Dirty or corroded electrodes. Refer to Item 2 in the previous section to learn how to correct this problem.
5. Lead wires not following body contour. Dangling lead wires can pick up alternating current. Arrange the wires to follow body contour (see Procedure 15-1: Running a 12-Lead Electrocardiogram, Procedural Step 9).

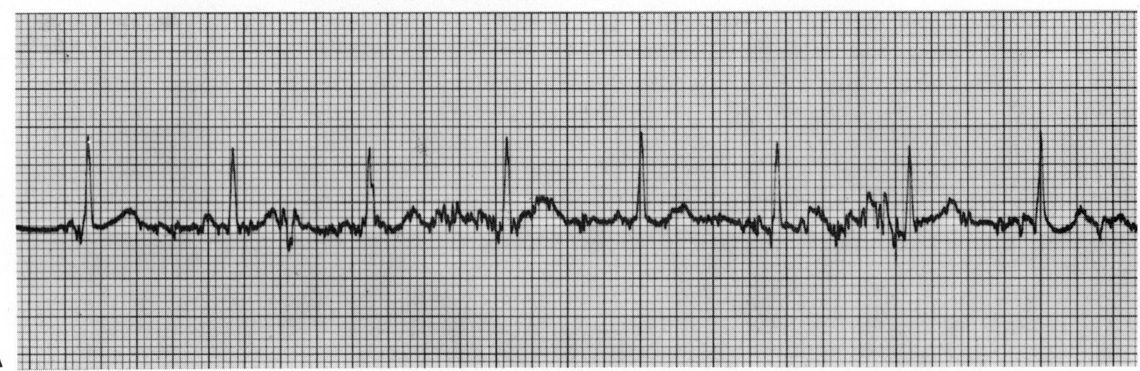

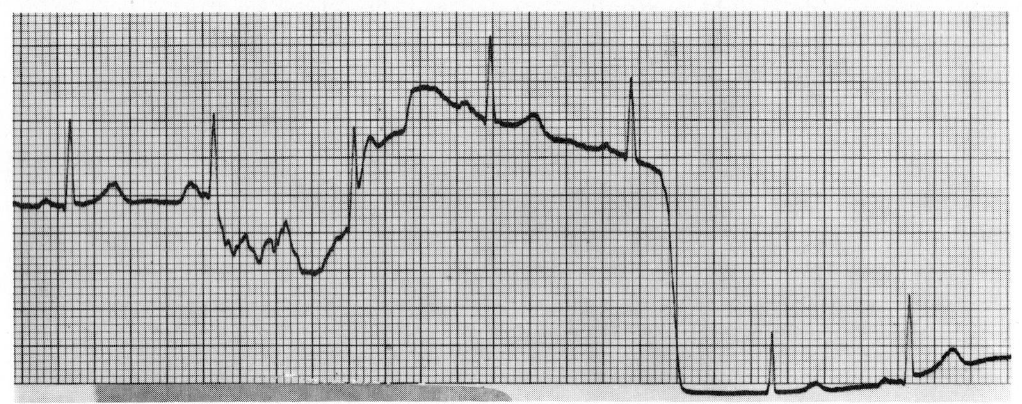

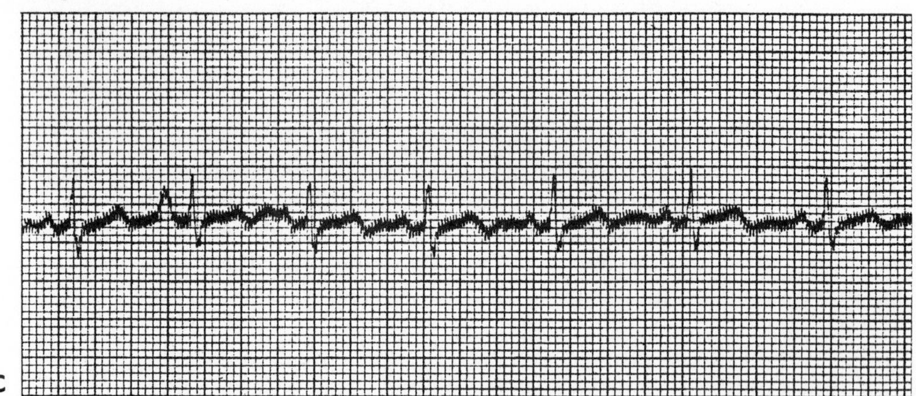

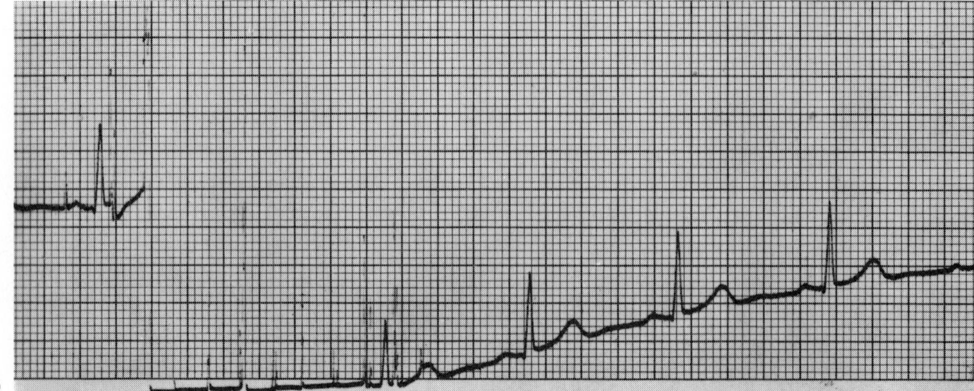

FIGURE 15–15. Examples of artifacts. (Courtesy of the Burdick Corporation, Milton, Wisconsin.)

Muscle, wandering baseline, and alternating current are the artifacts that the medical assistant observes most frequently on the ECG recording. Occasionally, an interrupted baseline (Fig. 15–15*D*) occurs that may be caused by the metal tip of a lead wire becoming detached from an electrode or by a broken patient cable. If the latter is the case, the manufacturer should be contacted for directions on replacing the patient cable.

In some circumstances, as when individuals have trouble holding still or in buildings with older electrical systems, normal methods to eliminate muscle and AC artifacts may not be successful. Electrocardiographs have an *artifact filter,* controlled by a frequency-response switch, which can be used to reduce artifacts when all else fails. However, because the artifact filter also affects the diagnostic accuracy of the ECG, it should be used as little as possible.

If the medical assistant is unable to correct an artifact, the physician should be consulted. It is possible that the machine itself is broken. If an electrocardiograph repairman has to be contacted, the medical assistant should have the following information available to aid the repairman in locating the problem:

1. What has already been done to locate and correct the problem.
2. Leads in which the artifacts occur.
3. A sample of the artifact as recorded by the machine.

Marking and Mounting the Electro-cardiogram

Each lead must be marked while it is being recorded so that it can be identified later and properly mounted. Most machines automatically mark the leads during recording in the upper margin of the paper, which relieves the medical assistant of having to manually mark each lead. Two examples of marking codes that may be used are diagrammed in Table 15–1.

The assistant should mount the completed recording following the medical office policy. There are commercially prepared mounting forms available, or the completed ECG may be mounted on sheets of plain paper. Each lead must be clearly and properly identified as leads I, II, III, aVR, aVL, and so forth. Also include the date, the patient's name, address, occupation, age, sex, height, weight, and blood pressure, and any other information requested by the physician. It is important that any drugs that the patient is taking also be recorded (particularly the cardiac drugs such as digitalis, propranolol hydrochloride [Inderal], and quinidine). If the medical office uses commercially available mounts, these categories are printed on the form with a space next to each category for entering the required data.

TABLE 15–1. Methods for Coding Leads*

LEAD	CODE I	CODE II
I	—	———
II	— —	——— ———
III	— — —	——— ——— ———
aVR	———	——— —
aVL	——— ———	——— — —
aVF	——— ——— ———	——— — — —
V_1	——— —	—
V_2	——— — —	— —
V_3	——— — — —	— — —
V_4	——— — — — —	— — — —
V_5	——— — — — — —	— — — — —
V_6	——— — — — — — —	— — — — — —

* Two examples for methods of coding ECG leads.

PROCEDURE 15-1
RUNNING A 12-LEAD ELECTROCARDIOGRAM

The procedure for running a 12-lead ECG is based upon the conventional single-channel electrocardiograph using one chest electrode. Regardless of the type of machine being used, however, most aspects of the procedure do not vary; these include patient preparation, placement of limb leads, placement of chest leads, attachment of lead wires, and guidelines for avoiding and eliminating artifacts. The procedure varies from one machine to another only in terms of the type and number of controls used to run the recording. Therefore, the medical assistant should be able to operate different types of electrocardiographs with a knowledge of the basic recording procedure.

1. **PROCEDURAL STEP.** Wash the hands; greet and identify the patient.

2. **PROCEDURAL STEP.** Work in a quiet, relaxing atmosphere away from nearby sources of electrical interference.

3. **PROCEDURAL STEP.** Prepare the patient. Ask him or her to remove clothing from the waist up. The lower legs must also be uncovered. Properly drape the patient over the uncovered body parts to prevent exposure and to provide warmth. The patient should be placed in a supine position on the table. The table should support the arms and legs adequately, so that they do not dangle. A pillow can be used to support the patient's head.
   PRINCIPLE. The chest, upper arms, and lower legs must be uncovered to allow for proper placement of the electrodes. The patient should be kept warm and the arms and legs should not be allowed to dangle; otherwise, muscle artifacts could result.

4. **PROCEDURAL STEP.** Help the patient to relax by explaining the procedure. Tell the individual that having an ECG recording is painless. Explain that he or she must lie still and not talk in order for an accurate recording to be obtained.
   PRINCIPLE. The patient should be mentally and physically relaxed for an accurate ECG recording, because an apprehensive or moving patient produces muscle artifacts.

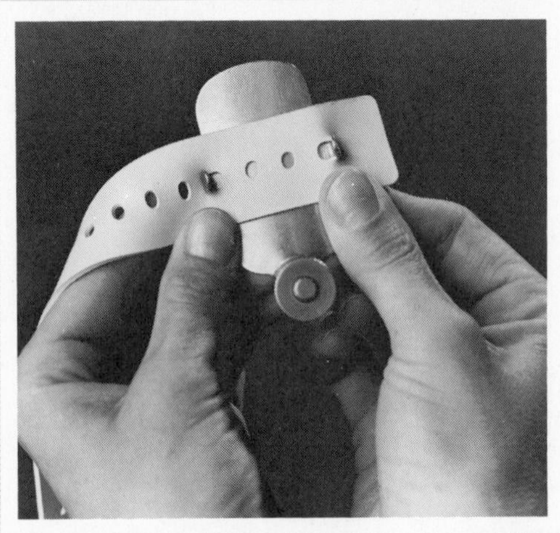

5. **PROCEDURAL STEP.** Position the electrocardiograph so that the power cord points away from the patient and does not pass under the table. It is usually easier for the medical assistant to work on the left side of the patient.
   PRINCIPLE. Proper positioning of the electrocardiograph reduces AC artifacts.

6. **PROCEDURAL STEP.** Apply the limb electrodes. Connect the rubber straps to the "ears" of the electrodes and apply the electrolyte to each one. If it appears that the patient has cream, oil, or lotion on the skin, remove it with alcohol, using friction.
   When using a paste or gel, apply the same amount to each electrode; a small amount of the paste or gel (about the size of a pea) should be applied.

Place the electrodes on the fleshy part of each of the four limbs (upper arms and lower legs) with the lead connectors pointing toward the patient's feet. Rub the electrolyte into the skin with the edge of the electrode. Tell the patient that the electrolyte will feel cold as it comes in contact with his or her skin. Pull the rubber strap around until the hole just meets the ear with no tension, then pull the strap one hole tighter and fasten.

PRINCIPLE. The lead connectors are pointed toward the patient's feet to provide a more stable connection when the lead wire is attached to the electrode. The electrolyte should be rubbed into the skin to ensure good contact between the skin and electrode. The limb electrodes should not be too tight or too loose and should be applied with the same amount of tension to reduce the possibility of artifacts.

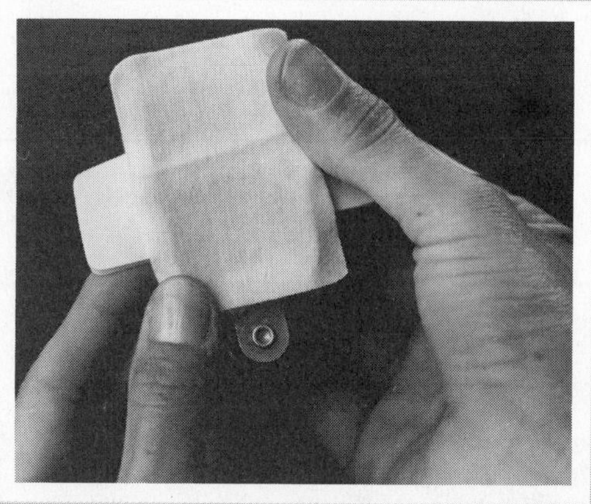

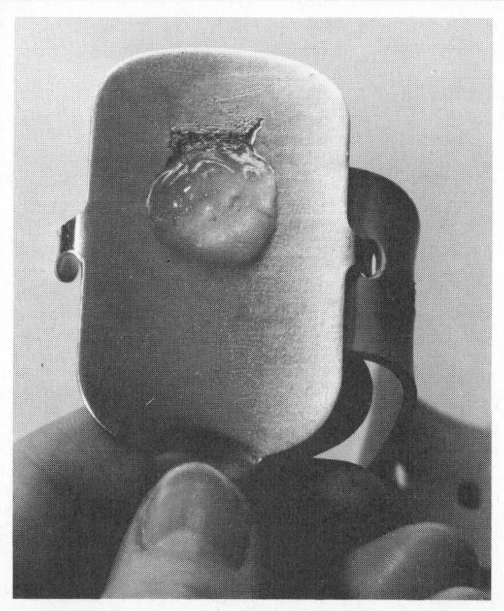

(Courtesy of the Burdick Corporation, Milton, Wisconsin.)

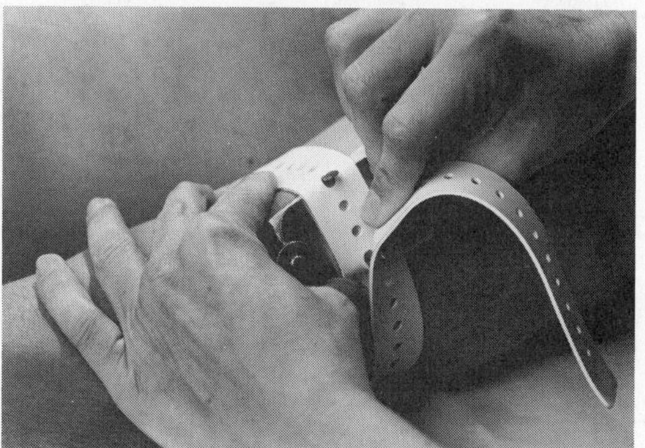

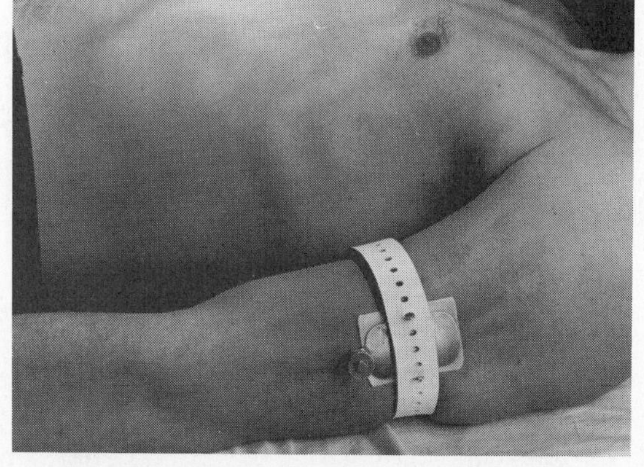

(Courtesy of the Burdick Corporation, Milton, Wisconsin.)

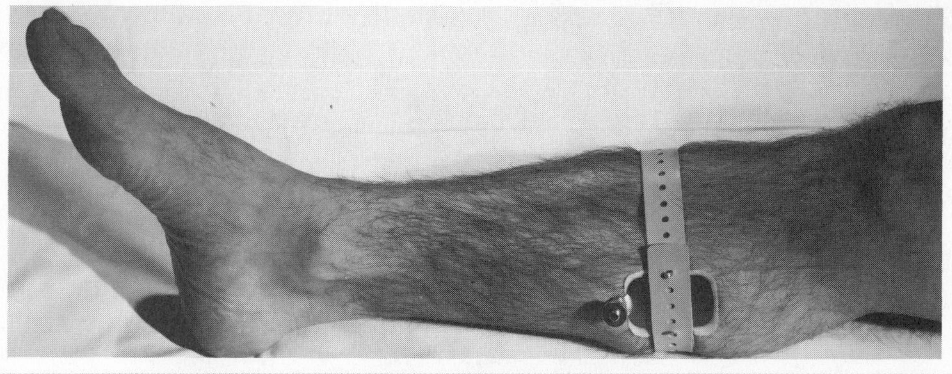

(Courtesy of the Burdick Corporation, Milton, Wisconsin.)

Continued

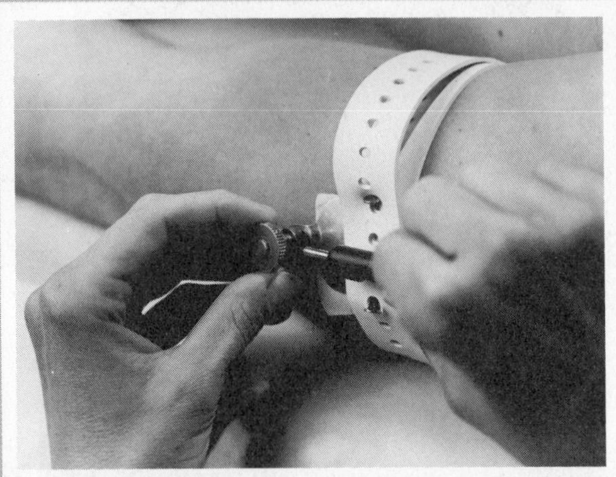

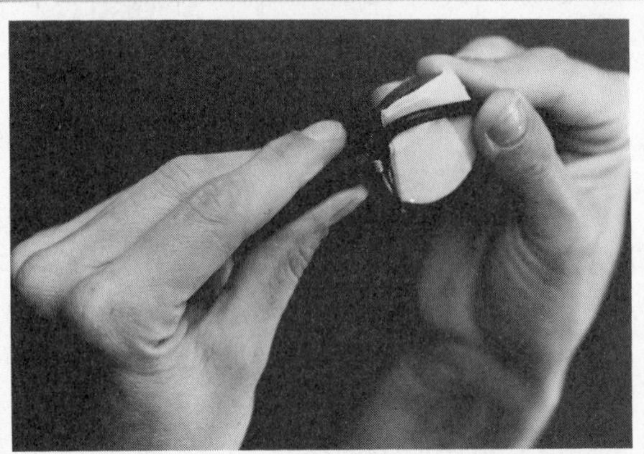

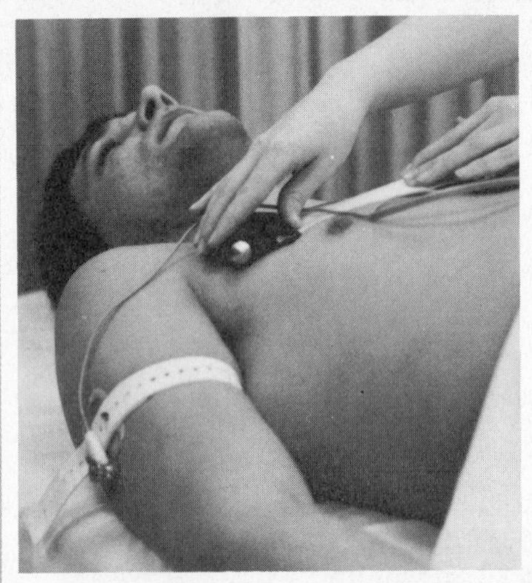

7. **Procedural step.** If using the metal disc chest electrode, position the chest strap under the patient's left side. The curved, concave surface of the weighted end of the strap should lie against the patient's chest.

8. **Procedural step.** Connect the lead wires to the lead connectors of the electrodes. The ends of these wires are usually color coded and are identified with abbreviations (RA, LA, LL, RL, and C or V) to help the medical assistant connect the proper one to each electrode. The connection between the lead wire and the lead connector of the electrode should be tight, and the lead wires should be arranged to follow body contour.
Principle. Arranging the lead wires to follow body contour reduces the possibility of AC artifacts.

9. **Procedural step.** Apply the electrolyte to the chest electrode and place it on the first chest lead position (V_1). Rub the electrolyte into the skin with the electrode. The Welsh vacuum cup electrode is held in place by depressing the rubber bulb, which creates a suction effect. Only a small dimple should remain in the bulb when it is released. The metal disc electrode is held in place with the chest strap.

10. **Procedural step.** Plug the patient cable into the machine. The cable should be supported on the table or on the patient's abdomen to prevent pulling or twisting.
Principle. Twisting or pulling of the cable would reduce chest electrode contact with the patient's skin, as well as cause patient discomfort.

11. **Procedural step.** Turn the machine ON. Some machines require a warm-up period of several minutes before the ECG can be recorded. Check the instruction manual to determine whether the machine requires this.

12. **Procedural step.** Position the Lead Selector Switch on STD and center the stylus. Place the Record Switch on RUN (25 mm/sec) and check the standardization of the machine by momentarily pressing the Standardization Button. The standardization mark should be 2 mm wide; if the width of the standardization mark is less or more than 2 mm, the Standardization Button should be depressed again for a longer or shorter period of time as required. Turn the machine to AMP OFF and determine the amplitude of the standardization mark by counting the small (1-mm) squares on the ECG graph paper. The standardization mark should be 10 mm (i.e., 10 small squares) high. If it is more or less than this, adjust the machine until the proper standardization is reached.
Principle. Standardizing the machine assures an accurate and reliable ECG.

13. **PROCEDURAL STEP.** Center the stylus and run 8 to 10 inches of leads I, II, and III by placing the Record Switch on RUN (25 mm/sec) and turning the Lead Selector Switch to the appropriate position. If the physician requests that a standardization mark be included with each lead, insert a standardization mark between the T wave of one ECG cycle and the P wave of the next cycle. (A standardization mark should always be inserted on the leads if the standard is changed to one-half or two times normal standard.) Mark the recording, unless the machine automatically marks it. When recording, do the following:

a. Make sure the recording stays near the center of the page. Use the Position Control knob if stylus adjustment is necessary. The entire ECG cycle must be recorded on the graph of the ECG paper. If any part of the cycle, such as the Q wave, is permitted to fall into the margin of the paper (which is not divided into a graph), it is difficult for the physician to interpret.
b. Observe the amplitude of the R wave to determine whether a change in standard or stylus position is needed.
c. Watch for artifacts appearing in the recording. If they occur, correct the problem.

14. **PROCEDURAL STEP.** Record 5 to 6 inches of leads aVR, aVL, and aVF by turning the Lead Selector Switch to the appropriate position. Insert a standardization mark with each lead if requested by the physician. Continue to mark the recording, unless the machine automatically marks it.

15. **PROCEDURAL STEP.** Record 5 to 6 inches of each chest lead (V_1 to V_6) by turning the Lead Selector Switch to the appropriate position. Most machines require that the machine be turned to AMP OFF when the chest leads are changed, to prevent the stylus from thrashing. Insert standardization marks and mark the recording as described previously.

Note: Since the first chest lead (V_1) is already positioned, most machines allow you to run the first 7 leads (I, II, III, aVR, aVL, aVF, and V_1) without having to turn the machine to AMP OFF.

16. **PROCEDURAL STEP.** Position the Lead Selector Switch on STD and run off the recording; it should be identified with the patient's name, the date, and your initials. Turn the machine OFF and unplug the power cord.

17. **PROCEDURAL STEP.** Disconnect the lead wires and remove the electrodes and rubber straps from the patient. If a paste or gel electrolyte was used, remove it from the patient's skin with a warm, damp cloth or paper towel. If flannel or cotton (saturated with an electrolyte) was used, discard it in a waste container.

18. **PROCEDURAL STEP.** Assist the patient in stepping down from the table.

19. **PROCEDURAL STEP.** Clean and return all equipment to its proper place.

Continued

20. **PROCEDURAL STEP.** Wash the hands.

21. **PROCEDURAL STEP.** Record the procedure in the patient's chart, making sure to initial the recording. Cut, mount, and identify the completed recording. Include the date and the patient's name, address, occupation, age, sex, height, weight, and blood pressure. Also record any drugs that the patient is taking and any other information requested by the physician. Handle the recording carefully to prevent pressure marks on it, which may interfere with accurate interpretation of it by the physician. Discard the excess ECG "scraps" in a waste container. Place the mounted recording in the appropriate place to be reviewed by the physician.

Record data below.

DATE	TIME	PATIENT'S NAME	RECORDING

Holter Monitor Electrocardiography

A Holter monitor is a portable ambulatory monitoring system for recording the cardiac activity of a patient over a 24-hour period. The system is designed so that the patient is able to maintain his or her usual daily activities with minimal inconvenience while being monitored. Holter monitor electrocardiography is an important noninvasive procedure used to diagnose cardiac rhythm and conduction abnormalities. It is most frequently used to evaluate patients with unexplained syncope, to discover cardiac arrhythmias that are intermittent in nature and not picked up on a routine 12-lead ECG, to assess the effectiveness of antiarrhythmic medications (e.g., digitalis and antianginal drugs), and to assess the effectiveness of the functioning of an artificial pacemaker.

The Holter monitor consists of electrodes that are placed on the patient's chest and a special portable magnetic tape recorder that continuously monitors the heart's activity (Fig. 15–16). The lightweight, battery-powered recorder is held in a protective case, which is worn either on a belt around the patient's waist or hung over the patient's shoulder by a strap. Throughout the 24-hour period, the system continuously records the patient's heart beat on the magnetic tape. An increasing number of physicians have Holter monitors in their offices. The medical assistant is responsible for preparing the patient, applying and removing the monitor, and instructing the patient in the guidelines for the procedure.

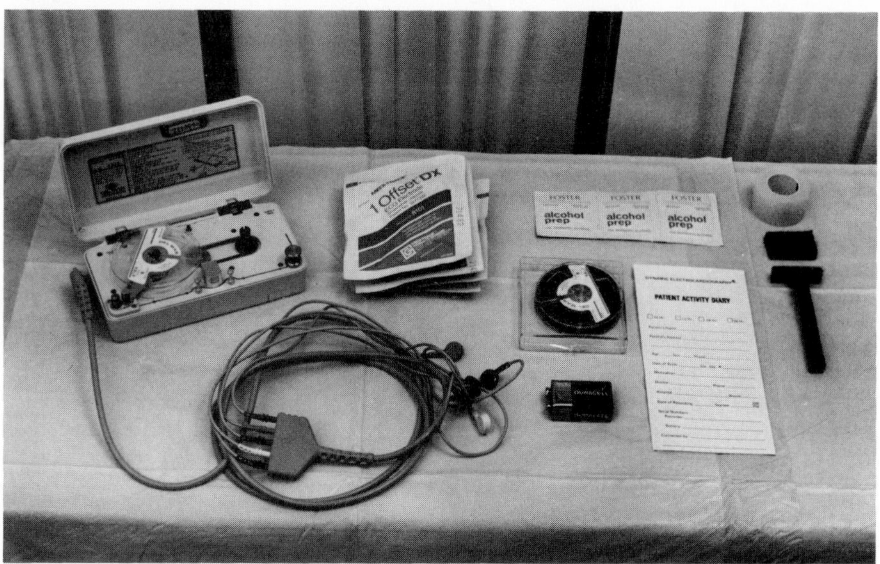

FIGURE 15–16. Holter monitor, including the supplies required for its application.

The effectiveness of the monitor should be checked after hooking up the patient to make sure a clear signal is being relayed from the electrodes to the recorder. This is performed by attaching one end of an accessory device known as a *test cable* to the recorder and the other end to an electrocardiograph machine. A short baseline strip is then recorded and observed for correct waveforms and the absence of artifacts. If the waveforms are incorrect and/or if artifacts are present, the patient may not be hooked up properly or a cable or lead malfunction may exist. The medical assistant should reconnect the leads and reposition the electrodes. If a problem still exists, the monitor may be malfunctioning and in need of repair.

An important aspect of the Holter monitor procedure is the completion of an activity diary by the patient (Fig. 15–17). All activities and emotional states (e.g., stress, anger) must be recorded during the monitoring period, along with the time of their occurrence. In addition, any symptoms experienced by the patient, such as vertigo, syncope, palpitations, chest pain, and dyspnea, must be recorded, along with the time of their occurrence. As a result, any arrhythmia recorded on the magnetic tape can be compared with the patient's diary to correlate patient symptoms with cardiac activity. Some monitors have an event marker mounted on one end of the recorder; the event marker is used along with the patient diary for patient evaluation. The patient should be told to momentarily depress the event marker when experiencing a symptom as described above. Depressing the marker places an electronic signal on the magnetic tape. This signal will later alert the technician to a significant event on the tape.

At the end of the 24-hour period, the Holter monitor system is removed from the patient and the tape is evaluated either by displaying it on a special Holter scanning screen or through computer analysis. Printouts of any portion of the electrocardiographic recording can be obtained for further study. The tape must be analyzed where a trained technician and Holter scanner or computer are available. This usually involves transferring the tape and diary to the cardiac department of a hospital for evaluation. The physician is provided with a written data report of the 24-hour period along with selected printouts of the patient's cardiac activity, including samples of any arrhythmias or abnormalities exhibited by the patient.

PATIENT ACTIVITY DIARY

TIME	ACTIVITY	SYMPTOM
AM PM	START RECORDING	
8:30 AM.	ATE BREAKFAST SMOKED CIGARETTE	
9:15	DRIVING FREEWAY	CHEST POUNDING
10:35	ARGUED WITH BOSS	CHEST POUNDING
10:45	TOOK MEDICATION	
12:30	ATE LUNCH	RELAXED
1:15	WALKED UP TWO FLIGHTS OF STAIRS	STOMACH BURNING- PAIN LEFT ARM

Page 1

TIME	ACTIVITY	SYMPTOM

Page 2

FIGURE 15–17. Holter monitor activity diary.

Holter Monitor Electrode Placement

A special type of electrode, known as a floating electrode, is used with the Holter monitor. It consists of a round plastic electrode plate with an adhesive backing and a central sponge pad containing an electrolyte gel (Fig. 15–18). This type of electrode is disposable and must be discarded after use.

Most Holter monitors are dual-channel systems, which means that two leads are recorded at the same time. A dual-channel monitor requires the use of five electrodes, one of which is the ground electrode. Some dual-channel monitors have the ground built into the monitor, in which case only four electrodes are required. The electrodes must be properly placed to ensure an accurate recording. Figure 15–19 shows the location of each of the electrode positions for the dual-channel Holter monitor. When one is learning to place these leads, it may help to mark their location on the patient's chest with a felt-tipped pen.

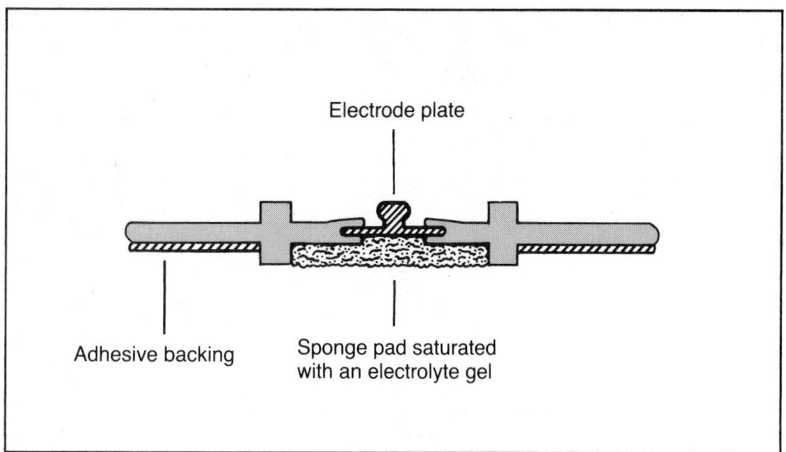

FIGURE 15–18. Floating electrode used with a Holter monitor.

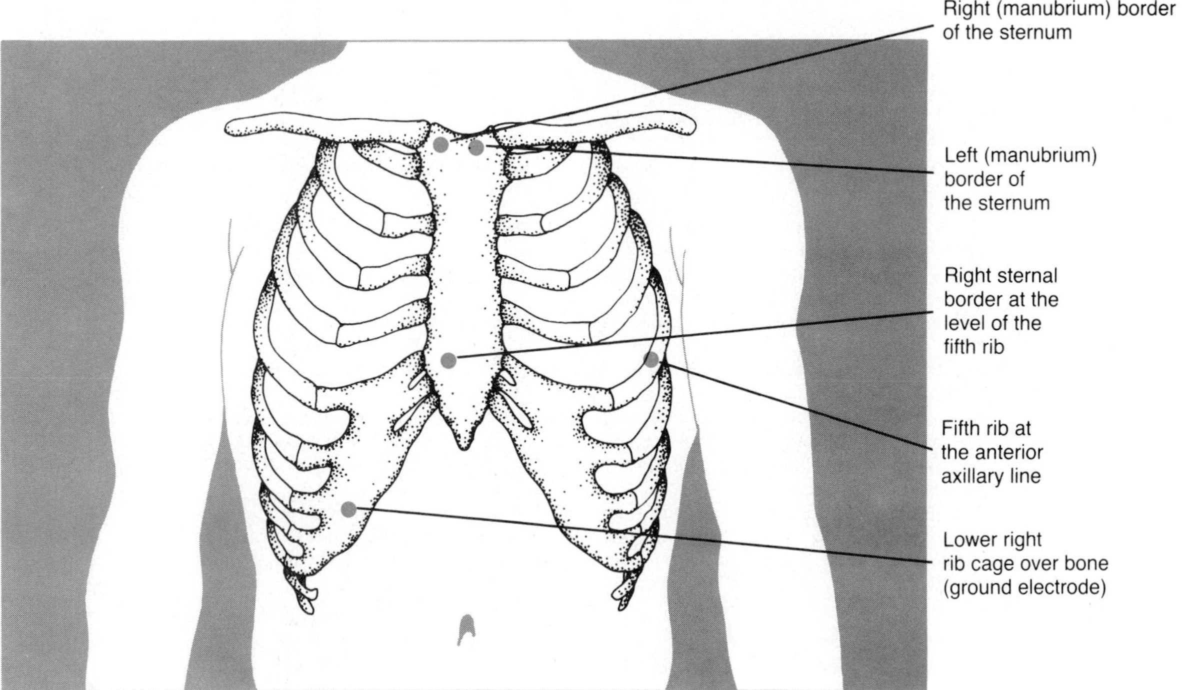

FIGURE 15–19. Holter monitor electrode positions (dual-channel).

PROCEDURE 15-2
APPLYING A HOLTER MONITOR

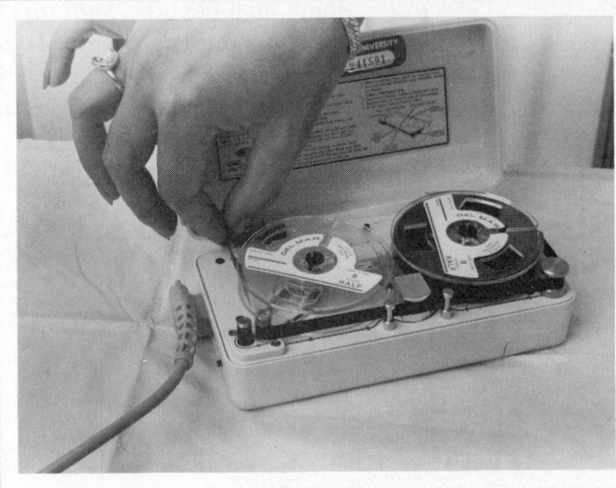

1. **PROCEDURAL STEP.** Assemble the equipment, which includes the **monitor**, a **blank magnetic tape**, a **battery**, the **carrying case**, a **belt or shoulder strap, skin electrodes, alcohol swabs, gauze, razor and blade, nonallergenic tape**, and the **patient diary.**

2. **PROCEDURAL STEP.** Prepare the equipment as follows: Remove the old battery from the recorder (if present), and install a new high-quality alkaline battery according to the markings on the battery holder. Insert a blank magnetic tape into the monitor according to the manufacturer's instructions.
PRINCIPLE. A new battery must be installed each time the monitor is used to ensure sufficient power throughout the 24-hour monitoring period.

3. **PROCEDURAL STEP.** Wash the hands and identify the patient.

4. **PROCEDURAL STEP.** Explain the procedure. Tell the patient that the Holter monitor will record the heart beat without interfering with his or her daily activities. Tell the patient that, because of its small size, the monitor will be fairly inconspicuous. Instruct the patient in the guidelines for wearing a Holter monitor (Table 15-2).
PRINCIPLE. The patient guidelines must carefully be followed to ensure an accurate recording.

5. **PROCEDURAL STEP.** Prepare the patient by asking him or her to remove clothing from the waist up.
PRINCIPLE. Clothing must be removed for placement of the chest electrodes.

TABLE 15-2. Holter Monitor Patient Guidelines

The following guidelines must be relayed to the patient to ensure an accurate and reliable electrocardiographic recording.

1. The electrodes and monitor must be kept dry. The patient is not permitted to shower, bathe, or swim while wearing the monitor.
2. The electrodes should not be touched or moved during the monitoring period to prevent artifacts from appearing in the recording.
3. The monitor should not be handled or taken out of its carrying case.
4. The event marker should be depressed only momentarily when a significant symptom or event is recorded. Overuse of the marker may cause masking of the ECG signals that are being relayed from the electrodes.
5. An electric blanket should not be used during the monitoring period.
6. The patient must keep a diary of activities, emotional states, and symptoms experienced during the monitoring period. The time of occurrence of each of the above must accompany each entry in the diary.
7. The patient should record the following activities in his or her diary: physical exercise, walking up or down stairs, emotional states, smoking, bowel movements, urination, meals (including alcohol and caffeine beverages), sexual intercourse, medications consumed, and sleep periods.

6. **PROCEDURAL STEP.** Place the patient in a sitting position.

7. **PROCEDURAL STEP.** Locate the electrode placement sites (Fig. 15–19), and at each site prepare an area of skin slightly larger than an electrode as follows:

a. If the patient's chest is hairy, dry shave it at each position site.
b. Swab the skin with an alcohol wipe and allow the area to dry completely.
c. Slightly abrade the skin with a 4 × 4-inch gauze square until it is visibly reddened.

PRINCIPLE. Shaving the chest improves the adherence of the electrodes and makes them easier to remove. The placement sites must be abraded with gauze to improve the adherence of the electrodes.

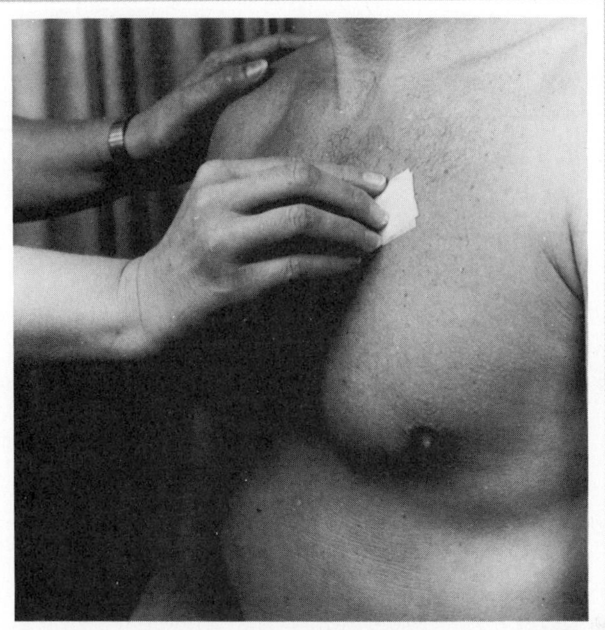

8. **PROCEDURAL STEP.** Remove the electrodes from their package. Peel the electrode backing from one of the electrodes. Avoid touching the adhesive as much as possible to prevent loss of stickiness from the adhesive. Check to make sure the electrolyte is moist. If it is dry, a new electrode must be obtained.
PRINCIPLE. The electrolyte should be moist to ensure good conduction of electrical impulses.

9. **PROCEDURAL STEP.** Apply the electrode to the first electrode position site with the adhesive side facing downward. Apply firm pressure beginning at the center of the electrode and moving outward. Ensure a firm seal by running your finger around the outer edge of the electrode until it is firmly attached to the skin.
PRINCIPLE. If pressure is applied by starting at one side and moving to the other, some of the electrolyte gel may be forced out from under the electrode, interfering with good conduction. The electrodes must be firmly attached to prevent distortion of the ECG recording.

10. **PROCEDURAL STEP.** Repeat Procedural Step 8 until all five electrodes have been applied.
PRINCIPLE. The electrodes pick up and conduct the electrical impulses given off by the heart.

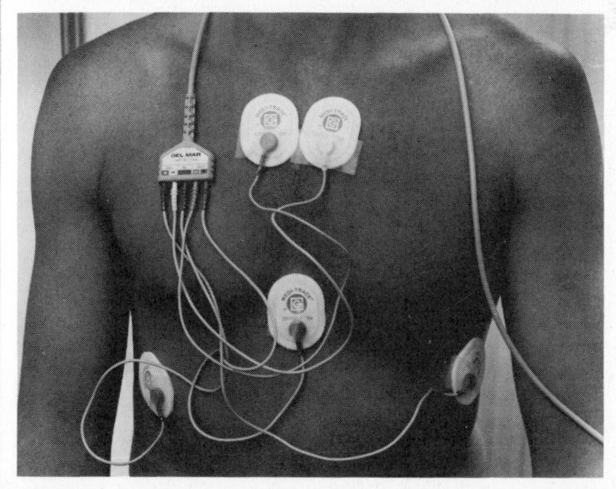

11. **PROCEDURAL STEP.** Attach the lead wires to the electrodes, and connect the lead wires to the patient cable.
PRINCIPLE. The lead wires transmit the electrical impulses to the cardiac monitor.

12. **PROCEDURAL STEP.** Place a strip of nonallergenic tape over each electrode.
PRINCIPLE. Applying tape facilitates secure attachment of the electrodes by reducing strain and pulling on them.

13. **PROCEDURAL STEP.** Check the recorder's effectiveness by connecting it to an electrocardiograph machine by way of the test cable and running a short baseline recording.
PRINCIPLE. Checking the recorder verifies that the patient is properly hooked up and that no cable or lead malfunction exists.

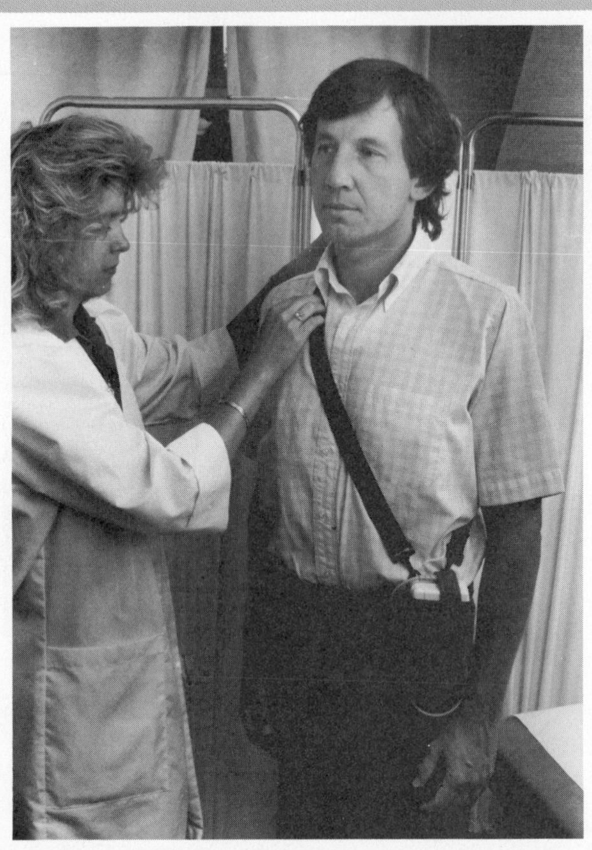

14. **PROCEDURAL STEP.** Tell the patient to redress while being careful not to pull on the lead wires. The electrode cable should extend from under the patient's garment or between buttons of the patient's garment.

15. **PROCEDURAL STEP.** Insert the recorder into its carrying case and strap it over the patient's clothing, using either a waist belt or shoulder strap. Make sure the strap is properly adjusted so the weight of the recorder does not cause straining or pulling on the lead wires.
PRINCIPLE. Straining or pulling on the lead wires may cause detachment of the electrodes.

16. **PROCEDURAL STEP.** Plug the electrode cable into the recorder. Check the time and turn on the recorder according to the manufacturer's instructions. Record the starting time in the patient diary.
PRINCIPLE. The beginning time must be recorded for later correlation of the patient diary with cardiac activity.

17. **PROCEDURAL STEP.** Complete the patient information section of the diary notebook. Give the diary to the patient and provide him or her with instructions on completing it.
PRINCIPLE. The patient diary is used to correlate patient symptoms with cardiac activity.

18. **PROCEDURAL STEP.** Instruct the patient when to return for removal of the monitor. Be sure to remind the patient not to forget the diary.

19. **PROCEDURAL STEP.** Wash the hands and record the procedure in the patient's chart. Include the patient's name, the date and time, the name of the procedure (application of a Holter monitor), the beginning time, and your initials.

Record data below.

DATE	TIME	PATIENT'S NAME	RECORDING

Cardiac Arrhythmias

The normal ECG graph cycle consists of a P wave, QRS complex, and a T wave, which repeats itself in a regular pattern (see Fig. 15–3). The term ***normal sinus rhythm*** refers to an ECG that is within normal limits. This means that the waves, intervals, segments, and cardiac rate fall within normal range. The normal heart rate ranges from 60 to 100 beats per minute. A rate falling below 60 beats per minute is termed ***sinus bradycardia,*** whereas a rate above 100 beats per minute is termed ***sinus tachycardia.***

Each ECG graph cycle is separated from the next one by a flat length of baseline termed the T–P segment. Any change in the baseline distance between graph cycles indicates the presence of a cardiac abnormality falling into one of the following categories: (1) the presence of extra beats, (2) an abnormal rhythm, or (3) an abnormal heart rate. The medical assistant should be able to recognize basic cardiac arrhythmias on an electrocardiographic recording for the purpose of alerting the physician to their presence. If the recording is to be mounted, the arrhythmia(s) must be included in the report. The arrhythmias the medical assistant should be able to identify are presented below, and a brief description of each and significant clinical aspects are included (see Fig. 15–20 for an illustration of each arrhythmia described).

Atrial Premature Contraction

Description. An atrial premature contraction (APC) is characterized by a beat that comes before the next normal beat is due. The most distinguishing feature is that the P wave of the premature beat has a different shape than the P wave of the normal beat. The APC has a normal QRS complex and a normal T wave, similar to the other ECG graph cycles.

Clinical Aspects. Atrial premature contractions are common in healthy individuals and are often associated with the intake of stimulants such as caffeine or tobacco. They may also be associated with more serious atrial arrhythmias and structural heart disease.

Paroxysmal Atrial Tachycardia

Description. Paroxysmal atrial tachycardia (PAT) is an abrupt episode of tachycardia with a constant heart rate that usually falls between 150 and 250 beats per minute. PAT is characterized by a rhythm that has a sudden onset and termination. The sudden increase in rate occurs in short bursts and lasts a few seconds only, after which the rate returns to what it was before the PAT occurred. Because of the increase in heart rate, the ECG graph cycles are very close together. With PAT, the patient experiences a sudden pounding or fluttering of the chest associated with weakness or breathlessness and acute apprehension. Occasionally, the patient experiences syncope.

Clinical Aspects. Paroxysmal atrial tachycardia is one of the most common rhythm disorders, often occurring in healthy patients with no underlying heart disease and young adults with normal hearts. It may also occur in individuals with organic heart disease.

Atrial Flutter

Description. Atrial flutter is a rapid, regular fluttering of the atrium in which the heart rate falls between 250 to 350 beats per minute. More than one P wave precedes each QRS complex, and the P waves appear as saw-toothed spikes be-

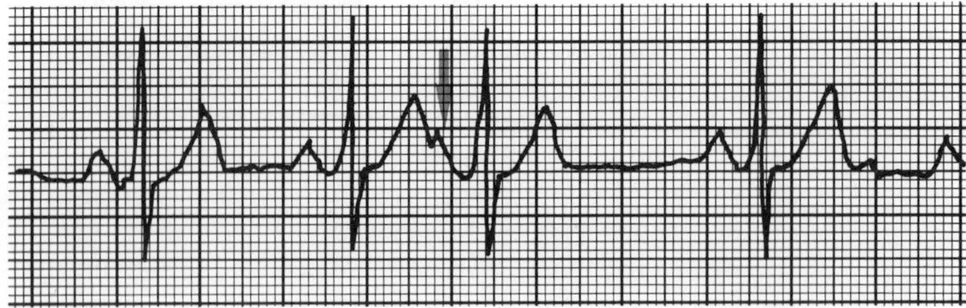

A Atrial premature contraction (APC)

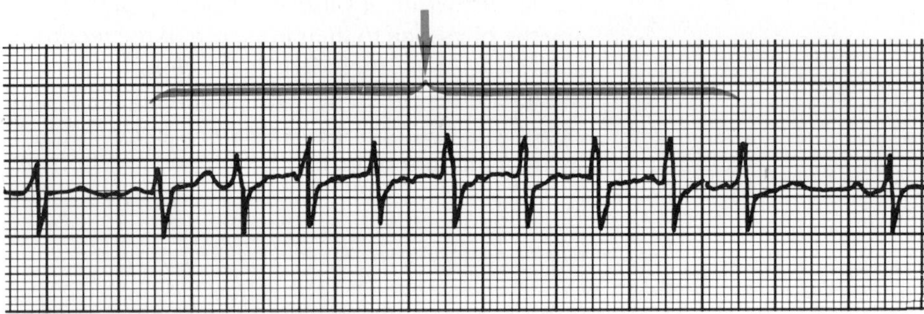

B Paroxysmal atrial tachycardia (PAT)

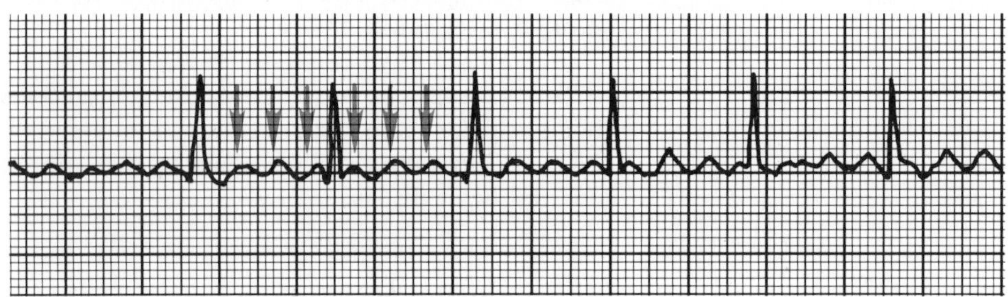

C Atrial flutter

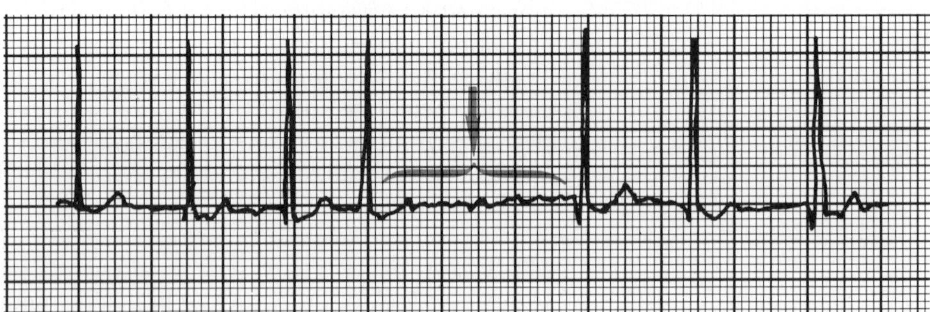

D Atrial fibrillation

FIGURE 15–20. Cardiac arrhythmias. (*A, B, D* to *G* from *Coronary Care Nursing. C, H* from *A Simplified Approach to Electrocardiography.*)

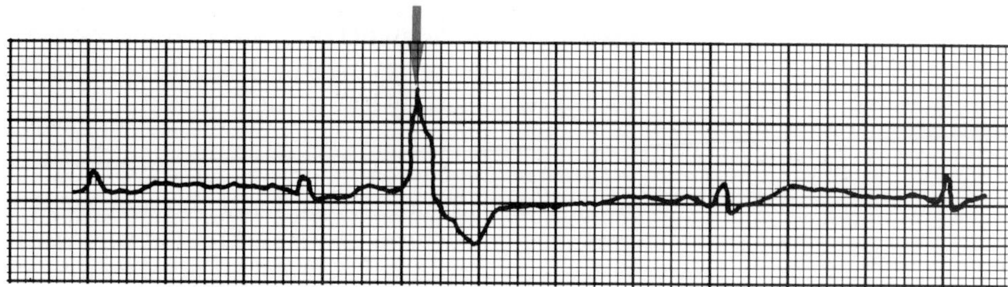

E Premature ventricular contraction (PVC)

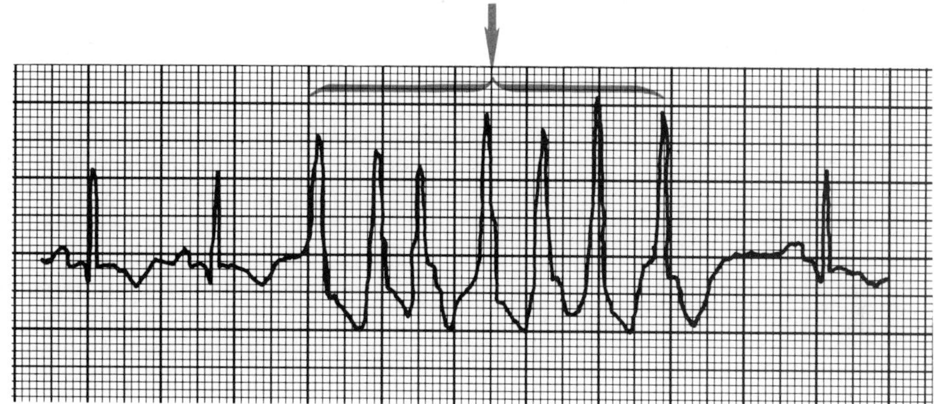

F Ventricular tachycardia

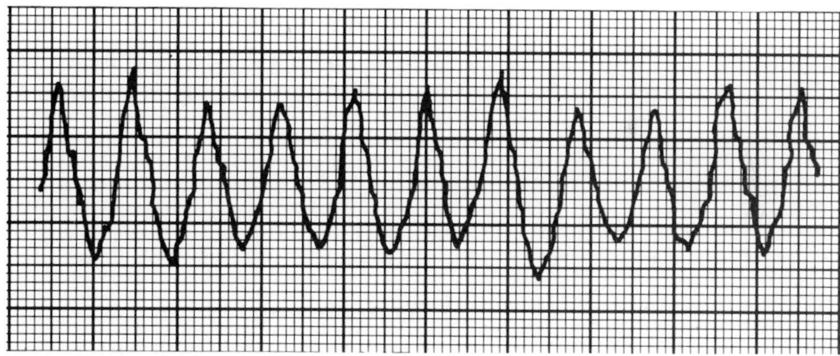

G Ventricular flutter

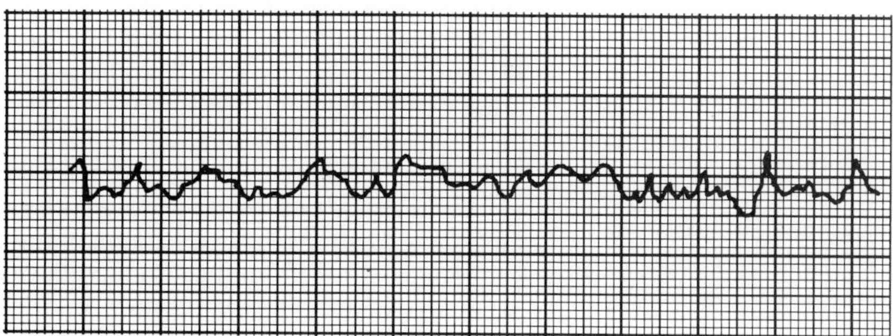

H Ventricular fibrillation

FIGURE 15–20 *Continued*

tween the QRS complexes. The number of waves can range from just one extra P wave to as many as eight falling in rapid succession, but all have the same size and shape. The QRS complexes of an atrial flutter configuration are normal; however, the T wave is usually lost in the P waves.

Clinical Aspects. Atrial flutter is rarely seen in healthy individuals. It is found in patients with underlying heart disease. Atrial flutter is not specific for any particular type of heart disease and can occur in patients with mitral valve disease, coronary artery disease, acute myocardial infarction, chronic lung disease, hypertensive heart disease, and pulmonary emboli, and in those who have undergone cardiac surgery.

Atrial Fibrillation

Description. Atrial fibrillation is characterized by an ECG tracing in which the P waves have no definite pattern or shape. The P waves appear as irregular wavy undulations between the QRS complexes. The QRS complexes in atrial fibrillation are normal but do not have a definite pattern. It is difficult to accurately measure the atrial rate because the P waves are not discernible; however, the atria are contracting between 400 and 500 times per minute.

Clinical Aspects. Atrial fibrillation is a commonly seen arrhythmia and may occur both in healthy individuals and in patients with a variety of cardiac diseases. In healthy individuals, it can be initiated by emotional stress, excessive alcohol consumption, and vomiting. In individuals under 50 years of age, the common causes of atrial fibrillation are congenital heart disease and rheumatic heart disease with mitral valve involvement. In individuals over 50 years of age, atrial fibrillation is caused by diseases capable of producing ischemia or hypertrophy of the atria, such as coronary artery disease, mitral valve disease, and hypertensive heart disease.

Premature Ventricular Contraction

Description. Premature ventricular contractions (PVCs) are among the most common rhythm disturbances seen on an ECG. The PVC is characterized by a beat that comes early in the cycle, is not preceded by a P wave, has a wide and distorted QRS complex, and has a T wave opposite in direction to the R wave of the QRS complex. Because of the unusual configuration of the QRS complex, the PVC easily stands out from the normal ECG graph cycles. The baseline distance after the PVC is normally longer than the usual distance between the other cycles. In other words, the PVC is followed by a pause before the next normal beat occurs.

Clinical Aspects. Premature ventricular contractions are seen in normal individuals in all age groups and are caused by anxiety, smoking, caffeine, alcohol, and certain medications (epinephrine, isoproterenol, and aminophylline). Premature ventricular contractions may occur with virtually any type of heart disease but are seen most often in patients with hypertensive heart disease, ischemic heart disease, lung disease with hypoxia, and digitalis toxicity. PVCs are also common in individuals with mitral valve prolapse.

Ventricular Tachycardia

Description. Ventricular tachycardia consists of a series of three or more consecutive premature ventricular contractions occurring at a rate of between 150 and

250 per minute. The tachycardia may occur paroxysmally and last only a short period of time or it may persist for a long time. The QRS complexes are bizarre and widened and no P waves are present. Sustained ventricular tachycardia is a life-threatening arrhythmia because the rapid ventricular rate prevents adequate filling time for the heart, leading to reduced cardiac output that often degenerates into ventricular fibrillation and cardiac arrest.

Clinical Aspects. Ventricular tachycardia is usually seen in patients with acute or chronic heart disease. Runs of ventricular tachycardia are indicative of coronary artery disease. Ventricular tachycardia also occurs as a complication of a myocardial infarction.

Ventricular Flutter

Description. In ventricular flutter, the QRS complex loses its sharp-peaked wave and becomes widened, resembling a stretched spring. No other waves are present with ventricular flutter other than the widened QRS complexes. Ventricular flutter is caused by a rapid, feeble contraction of the ventricles and a rate of 150 to 300 beats per minute. It is a dangerous rhythm and should be reported immediately. Ventricular flutter is almost always followed by ventricular fibrillation.

Clinical Aspects. Ventricular flutter is seen in patients with existing heart disease and cardiac arrhythmias.

Ventricular Fibrillation

Description. Ventricular fibrillation is the most serious arrhythmia. With this type of arrhythmia, the ventricles do not beat in any coordinated manner but instead they twitch or fibrillate. Because of this, virtually no blood is ejected into the systemic circulation. On an ECG recording, ventricular fibrillation is characterized by irregular, chaotic undulations of the baseline. There are no recognizable P waves, QRS complexes, or T waves in the irregular line of jagged spikes. Because the ventricles are twitching irregularly, there is no effective ventricular pumping action, resulting in no circulation. Ventricular fibrillation is a serious arrhythmia that must immediately be cared for because it can lead to sudden death.

Clinical Aspects. The most common cause of ventricular fibrillation is an acute myocardial infarction. It can also occur in patients with existing organic heart disease and cardiac arrhythmias. It may be preceded by an arrhythmia such as premature ventricular contractions or ventricular tachycardia, or it may occur spontaneously.

Study Questions

1. What is the purpose of electrocardiography?
2. What do each of the following ECG components represent: P wave, QRS complex, T wave, P–R interval, Q–T interval, P–R segment, S–T segment, and the baseline following the T wave?
3. What are the 12 leads recorded during an ECG?
4. What causes each of the following artifacts: muscle, wandering baseline, alternating current, and interrupted baseline?
5. What is the purpose of applying a Holter monitor?

16 X-RAY EXAMINATIONS

CHAPTER OUTLINE

X-rays
The X-ray Machine
Contrast Media
Fluoroscopy
Positioning the Patient
X-ray Precautions
The Darkroom
Specific Radiographic Examinations

COMPETENCIES

After completing this chapter, you should be able to demonstrate the proper procedure to perform the following:

1. Instruct a patient in the proper preparation required for each of the following types of x-ray examinations: barium meal, barium enema, cholecystography, and intravenous pyelography.
2. Position a patient for an x-ray examination.
3. Take and develop a radiograph.

LEARNING OBJECTIVES

After completing this chapter, you should be able to do the following:

1. Define the words listed in the vocabulary.
2. State the function of x-rays in medicine.
3. Explain why it is important for a patient to prepare properly for an x-ray examination.
4. Describe how x-rays are produced.
5. State the purpose of the grid and intensifying screen.
6. Describe the following positions used for x-ray examinations: anteroposterior, posteroanterior, right and left lateral, supine, and prone.
7. Explain the function of the processing cycle, and list the series of steps included in the cycle.
8. Explain the function of a contrast medium.
9. Describe the purpose of a fluoroscope.
10. Explain why precautions must be taken when one is working with x-rays, and list three types of precautionary measures.
11. Explain the purpose of each of the following types of x-ray examinations: barium meal, barium enema, cholecystography, and intravenous pyelography.

• VOCABULARY •

contrast medium (kon' trast me' de-um)—A substance that is used to make a particular structure visible on a radiograph.

enema (en' ĕ-mah)—An injection of fluid into the rectum to aid in the elimination of feces from the colon.

fluoroscope (floo' or-o-skōp")—An instrument used to view internal organs and structures directly.

fluoroscopy (floo" or-os' ko-pe)—Examination of a patient using the fluoroscope.

radiograph (ra' de-o-graf")—A permanent record of a picture of an internal body organ or structure produced on radiographic film. Also known as a roentgenogram.

radiography (ra" de-og' rah-fe)—The taking of permanent records (radiographs) of internal body organs and structures by passing x-rays through the body to act upon a specially sensitized film.

radiologist (ra" de-ol' o-jist)—A medical doctor who specializes in the diagnosis and treatment of disease using radiant energy such as x-rays, radium, and radioactive material.

radiology (ra" de-ol' o-je)—The branch of medicine that deals with the use of radiant energy in the diagnosis and treatment of disease.

radiolucent (ra" de-o-lu' sent)—Describing a structure that permits the passage of x-rays.

radiopaque (ra" de-o-pāk')—Describing a structure that obstructs the passage of x-rays.

roentgenologist (rent" gĕ-nol' o-jist)—A medical specialist who is qualified in the use of x-rays (but not other kinds of radiant energy) for the diagnosis and treatment of disease.

Introduction

Wilhelm Konrad Roentgen, a German physicist, discovered x-rays on November 8, 1895, while working with a cathode ray tube. He noticed that these rays could pass through solid materials such as paper, wood, and human skin. He did not know what they were, so he named them x-rays. They have since been renamed *roentgen rays* after their discoverer; however, they are better known as x-rays. X-rays are used to visualize internal organs and structures and serve as a diagnostic aid to determine the presence of disease. They are also used therapeutically to treat disease conditions such as malignant neoplasms.

The medical office may have its own x-ray machine, but more often the radiographs are taken at a hospital or medical laboratory. Some radiographs, such as a bone study, require no advance preparation, whereas others such as the barium enema require a great deal of special preparation. The medical assistant is usually responsible for instructing the patient in the type of preparation required for a particular x-ray examination and for making sure he or she understands the importance of the preparation. If the patient fails to prepare properly, a radiograph of poor quality may result. This may even necessitate rescheduling the procedure. This chapter provides an introduction to the study of x-rays, focusing on the patient preparation required for common radiographs.

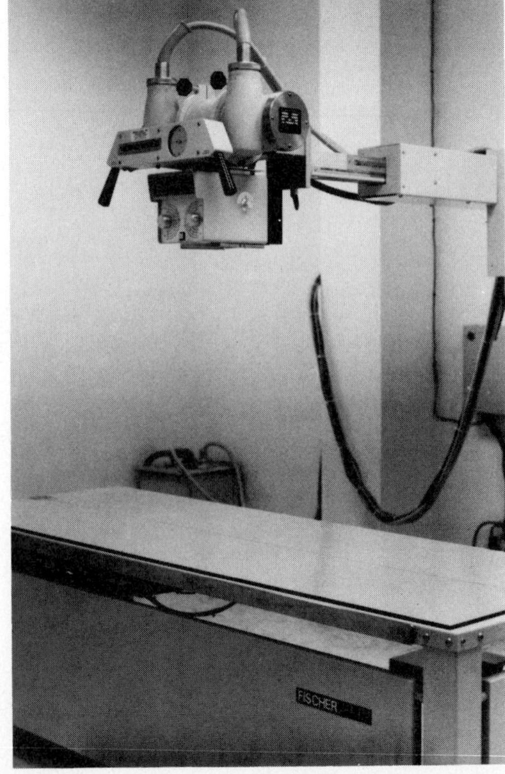

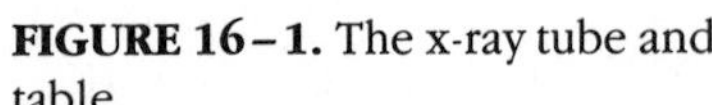
FIGURE 16–1. The x-ray tube and table.

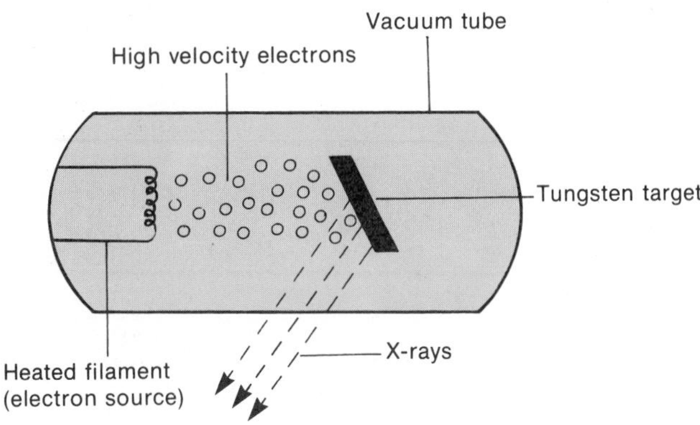

FIGURE 16–2. The production of x-rays. Fast-moving electrons strike a tungsten target, producing x-rays.

X-rays

X-rays are high-energy electromagnetic waves that are invisible and have a very short wavelength that enables them to penetrate solid materials. A special radiographic film is placed behind the part being examined, and a shadow or image of the internal body structure being photographed is produced on the film. *Radiograph* or *roentgenogram* is the term given to the permanent record of the picture produced on the radiographic film. *Radiology* is the branch of medicine that deals with the use of radiant energy in the diagnosis and treatment of disease. A *radiologist* is a medical doctor who specializes in the diagnosis and treatment of disease using any of various forms of radiant energy, such as x-rays, radium, and radioactive material. A medical doctor who is qualified only in the use of x-rays for the diagnosis and treatment of disease is known as a *roentgenologist.*

The X-ray Machine

The x-ray machine consists of three main parts: the x-ray table, the x-ray tube, and the control panel. Radiographs are taken with the table in a horizontal position, but some tables are moveable and may be placed in an upright or angled position for use in a particular type of x-ray examination. Situated above the table is a moveable x-ray tube that functions to produce the x-radiation (Fig. 16–1). X-rays are produced in a vacuum tube by high-velocity electrons that strike a solid target that is usually made of a tungsten alloy. When these fast-moving electrons strike the target, x-radiation is produced (Fig. 16–2). The control panel (Fig. 16–3) contains knobs for regulating the x-ray machine and is positioned behind a specially

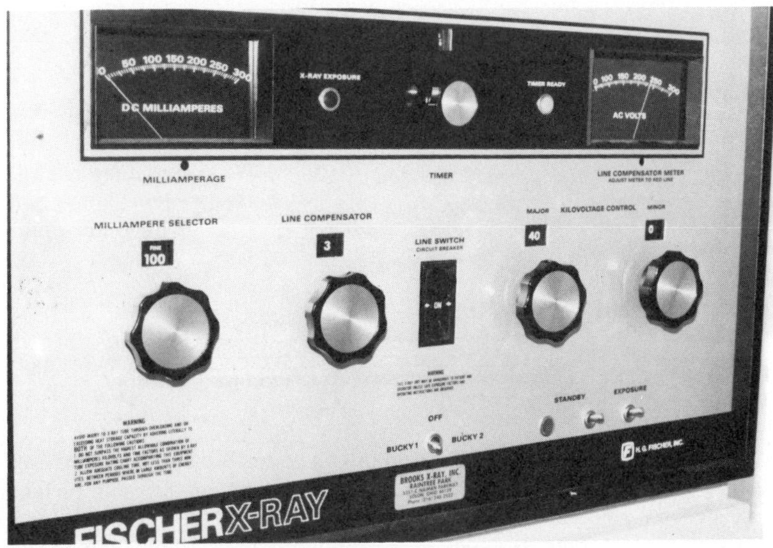

FIGURE 16–3. The x-ray control panel.

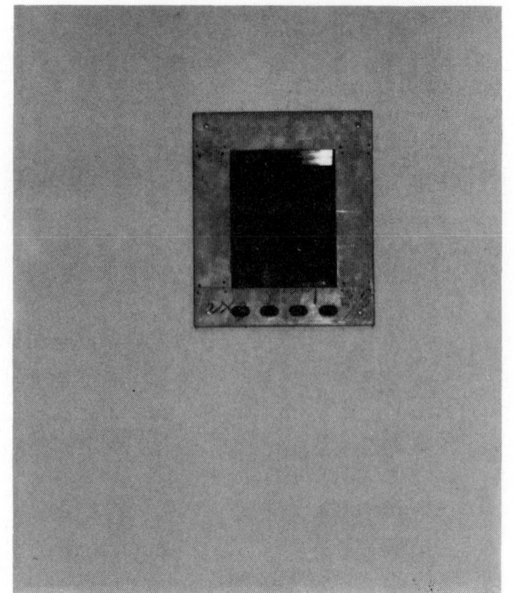

FIGURE 16–4. The control panel is situated behind a lead-lined wall with a lead-treated window to protect the radiation worker.

constructed lead-lined wall to protect the radiation worker. The wall contains a lead-treated window to permit observation of the patient during the x-ray exposure (Fig. 16–4).

X-rays travel in a straight line, but when they pass through a radiopaque object such as bone, the rays are scattered. To absorb this scattered or secondary radiation and prevent it from blurring the x-ray film and hindering good visibility of the image, a *grid* may be used. A grid is composed of numerous lead strips alternating with radiolucent strips. The lead strips are arranged parallel to the x-ray beams. The grid is placed between the patient and the film and functions to absorb the secondary radiation before it can strike the film. Stationary grids may be used; however, the image of the lead strips is superimposed on the radiograph. If the grid is set in motion, these lines are blurred out of the image. The *Potter-Bucky diaphragm,* or simply *Bucky,* is the name given to this type of grid and its moving mechanism (Fig. 16–5). Grids are generally used when a radiograph of a thicker part of the body is being taken.

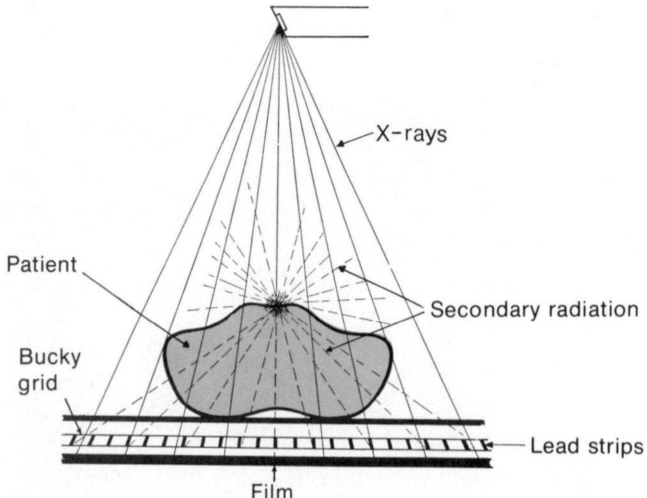

FIGURE 16–5. Diagram of a Potter-Bucky diaphragm used to absorb secondary radiation and prevent it from blurring the x-ray film. (Modified from Meschan, I.: *Synopsis of Radiologic Anatomy with Computed Tomography.* Philadelphia, W. B. Saunders Company, 1980.)

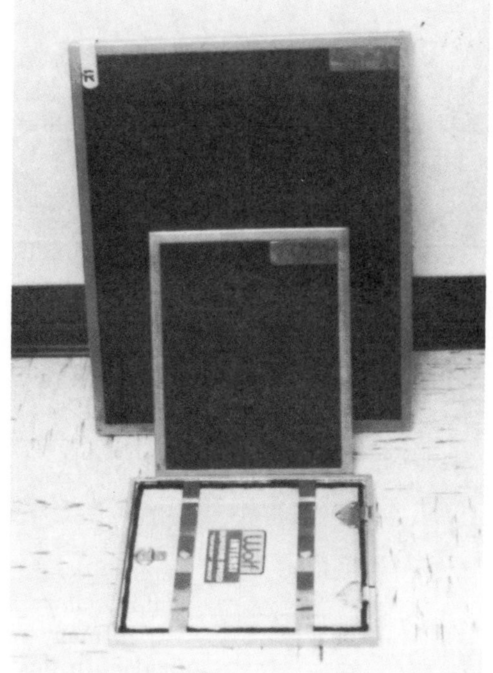

FIGURE 16–6. Examples of cassettes of various sizes. The locking mechanism is exhibited on the bottom cassette.

Intensifying screens may also be used to help obtain an image on the radiographic film in a shorter period of time, thus reducing the amount of radiation exposure to the patient. They may be housed in a permanent or disposable cardboard holder or in a cassette. A *cassette* is a framelike container that acts as a holder for the screens and film and protects the film from light. It contains a locking mechanism to close it securely (Figs. 16–6 and 16–7).

Contrast Media

Radiography relies upon differences in density between various body structures to produce shadows of varying intensities on the radiographic film. For example, there is a difference in density between bone and flesh (bone is more dense than flesh). The bone absorbs more x-rays and does not allow them to reach the radiographic film. This leaves that part of the film unexposed and causes white areas to appear on the processed film. If the x-rays penetrate an organ or structure, it will appear black on the film. For example, the lungs contain air and therefore

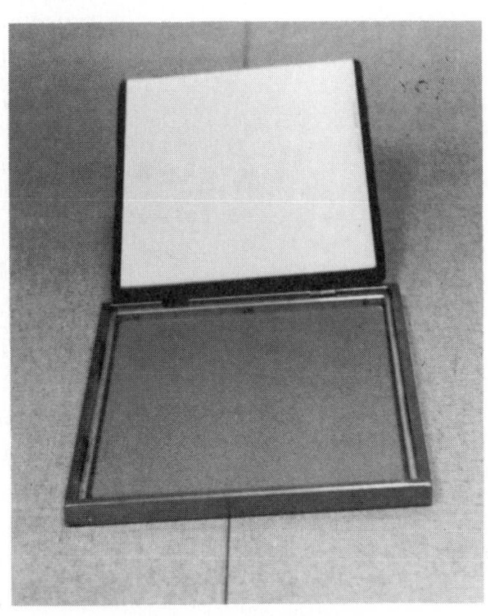

FIGURE 16–7. The cassette acts as a holder for the intensifying screens (upper white portion) and film (lower shaded portion).

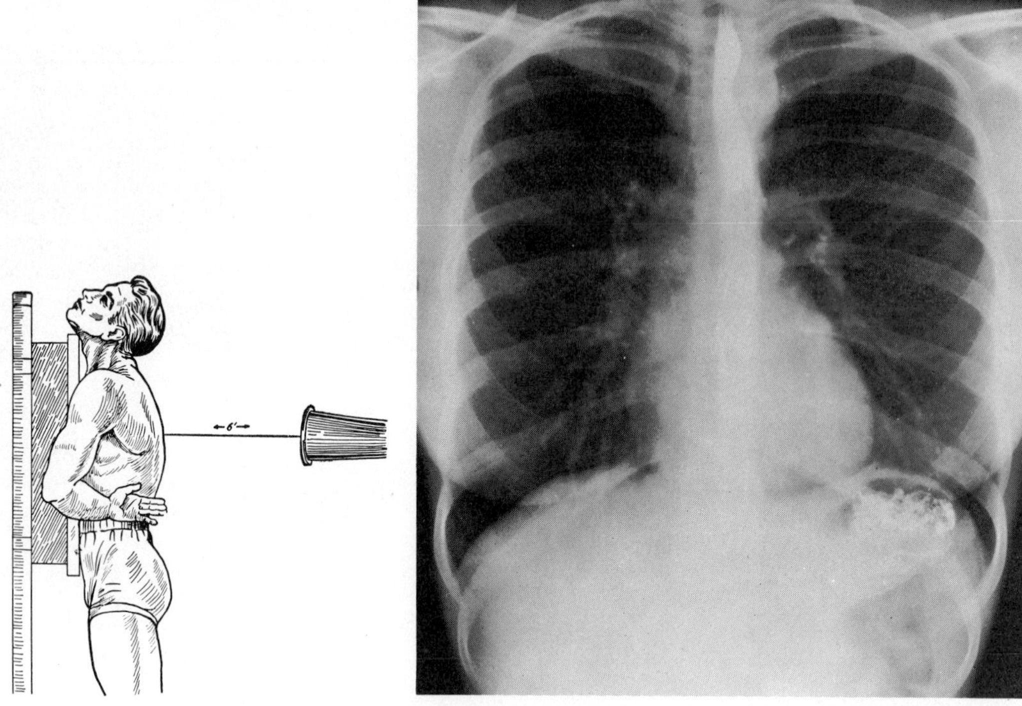

FIGURE 16–8. Posteroanterior projection of the chest: position of patient and radiograph. (From Meschan, I.: *Synopsis of Radiologic Anatomy with Computed Tomography.* Philadelphia, W. B. Saunders Company, 1980.)

x-rays are able to penetrate them easily; as a result, the lungs appear black on the processed film. The ribs, on the other hand, absorb many of the x-rays and appear as white shadows on the film (Fig. 16–8). A structure that permits the passage of x-rays, such as lung tissue, is *radiolucent.* A structure, such as bone, that obstructs the passage of x-rays and causes an image to be cast on the film is *radiopaque.*

In many cases, the natural densities of two adjacent organs or structures are similar. In this instance, in order to make a particular structure become visible on the radiograph, a *contrast medium* must be used. Substances used as contrast media are usually radiopaque chemical compounds that cause the body tissue or organ to absorb more radiation. This provides a contrast in density between the tissue or organ being filmed and the surrounding area. The tissue or organ becomes visible and appears white on the processed radiograph. Substances used as contrast media must be able to be ingested or injected into the body tissues or organs without causing harm to the patient. Barium sulfate and organic iodine compounds are commonly used radiopaque contrast media. Barium sulfate is a chalky compound that is water-insoluble and does not allow x-rays to penetrate it. It is frequently used for examination of the gastrointestinal tract, because barium is not absorbed into the body through the GI tract and does not alter its normal function. Iodine salts are radiopaque and are combined with other compounds for x-ray examination of structures such as the gallbladder and kidneys. Iodine may sometimes produce an allergic reaction, and before it is administered, the patient should be asked whether he or she is allergic to iodine or foods containing iodine. Those patients who have known allergies may be given an iodine-sensitivity test as a precautionary measure.

Another type of contrast medium causes the structure to become less dense than the surrounding area. The x-rays are able to easily penetrate the structure, which appears as darker areas on the radiograph. This type of contrast medium includes such substances as air and carbon dioxide.

Fluoroscopy

A *fluoroscope* is an instrument used in a darkened room to view internal organs and structures of the body directly. Examination of a patient using the fluoroscope is known as *fluoroscopy.* A radiopaque medium is often used with fluoroscopy to outline various parts of the body. The patient is positioned between the x-ray tube and a fluorescent screen composed of zinc cadmium sulfide crystals. When the x-rays pass through the body and strike the crystals, they cause visible light to be given off so that the radiologist can view the action of body organs or structures such as the heart, stomach, and intestines on a television screen. During fluoroscopy, the radiologist can take radiographs that permit him or her to study the structure in detail and that also serve as a permanent record.

Positioning the Patient

The position of the patient is determined by the purpose of the examination and the part being examined. The patient is generally positioned so that several different views can be taken to provide a complete three-dimensional picture of the part being examined. Articles such as jewelry and hairpins must be removed so that they do not obscure the image on the radiograph. To prevent blurring of the image on the film, the patient must be instructed to maintain the position in which he or she is placed and not to move during the x-ray examination. Blurring prevents good visualization of the part and may warrant retaking of the film. Types of x-ray views and the method used to position the patient for each is described below.

Anteroposterior view (AP): The x-rays are directed from the front toward the back of the body. The patient is positioned with the anterior aspect of the body facing the x-ray tube and the posterior aspect facing the radiographic film (see Fig. 16–10).

Posteroanterior view (PA): The x-rays are directed from the back toward the front of the body. The patient is positioned with the posterior aspect of the body facing the x-ray tube and the anterior aspect facing the radiographic film (see Fig. 16–8).

Lateral view: The x-ray beam passes from one side of the body to the opposite side (Fig. 16–9).

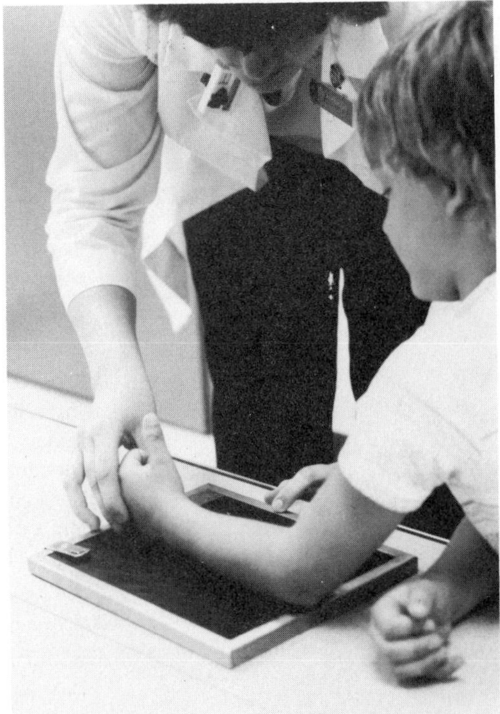

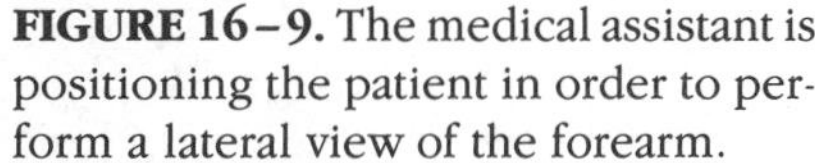

FIGURE 16–9. The medical assistant is positioning the patient in order to perform a lateral view of the forearm.

Right lateral view (RL): The right side of the body is positioned next to the radiographic film, and the x-rays are directed through the body from the left to the right side.

Left lateral view (LL): The left side of the body is positioned next to the radiographic film, and the x-rays are directed through the body from the right to the left side.

Oblique view: The body is positioned at an angle or semilateral position.

Supine position: The patient is positioned on his or her back with the face upward.

Prone position: The patient is positioned face down with the head turned to one side.

X-ray Precautions

Precautions must be taken when one is working with x-rays because excessive radiation exposure can cause tissue damage, producing somatic and genetic effects. Somatic effects involve an injury to the body tissues. Damage to the reproductive organs possibly induces genetic mutation that may produce a hereditary defect in future generations. A radiation worker who holds or positions the patient as the radiograph is being taken must wear a lead apron and gloves. Lead absorbs radiation and provides protection (Fig. 16–10).

The patient's gonads should be protected from x-rays by a gonad shield containing lead (Fig. 16–11). This is especially important for women in the first 3 months of pregnancy because the x-rays can produce harmful effects on the developing embryo or fetus.

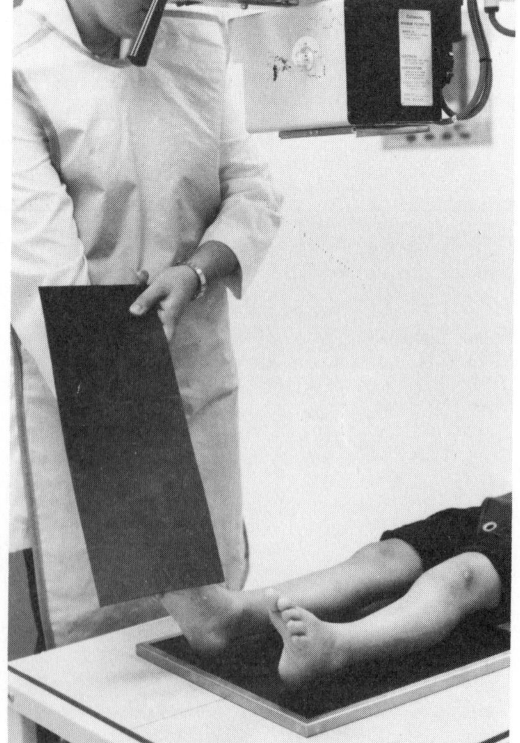

FIGURE 16–10. The medical assistant is wearing a lead apron and holding a lead shield to protect herself from radiation exposure while the radiograph is being taken. She is helping to maintain the patient's position for an anteroposterior view of the lower leg.

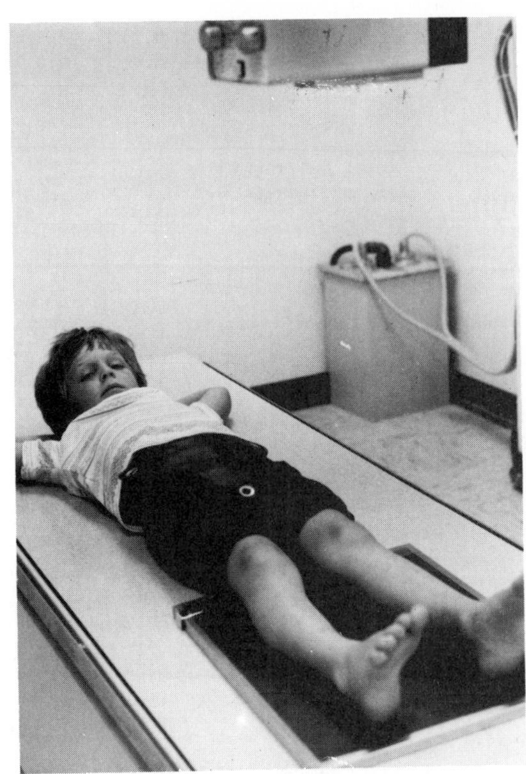

FIGURE 16–11. The patient's gonads should be protected from x-rays by a shield containing lead.

Radiation workers must wear film badges, which detect and record the amount of radiation received (Fig. 16–12). Periodically, the film in the badge is sent away for evaluation to determine the amount of radiation an individual is receiving. The film detects an overexposure to x-rays before the individual has been exposed to dangerous amounts of radiation. A radiation worker whose film badge shows that too many x-rays are being received must exercise greater caution.

The room containing the x-ray machine is constructed with specially made lead-lined walls, floors, and doors to protect individuals outside the room when the machine is in operation. The radiation worker should be sure to close the door while operating the machine.

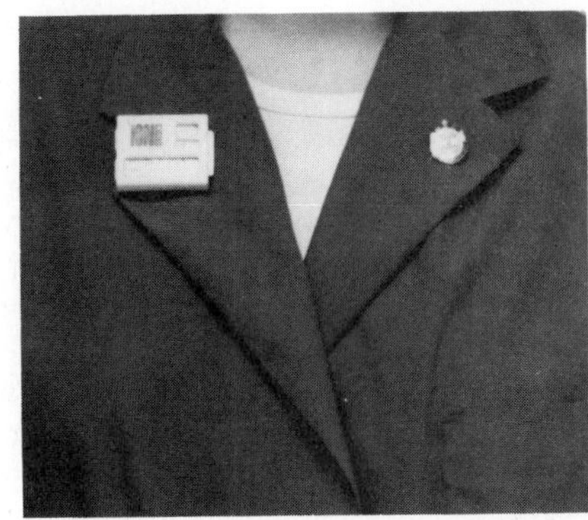

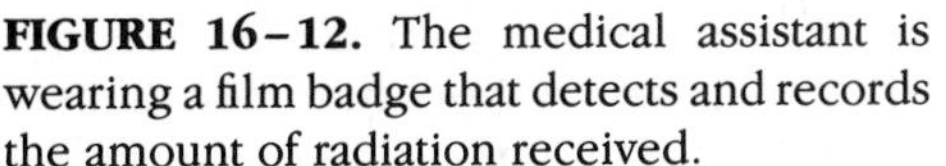

FIGURE 16–12. The medical assistant is wearing a film badge that detects and records the amount of radiation received.

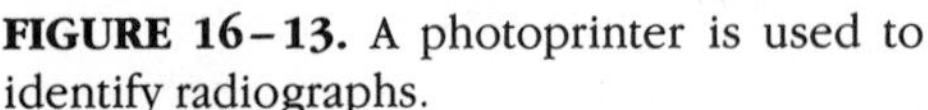

FIGURE 16–13. A photoprinter is used to identify radiographs.

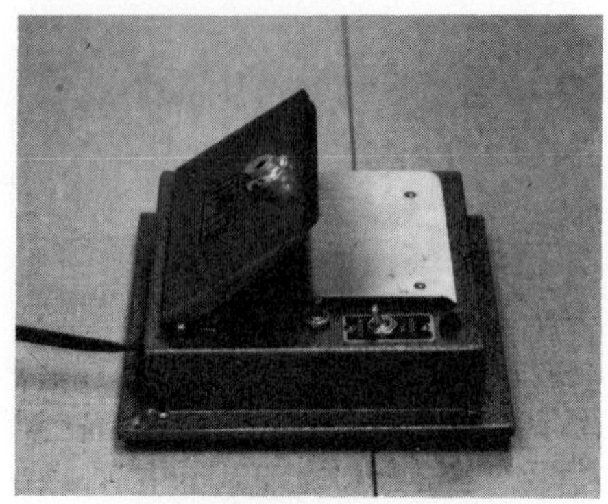

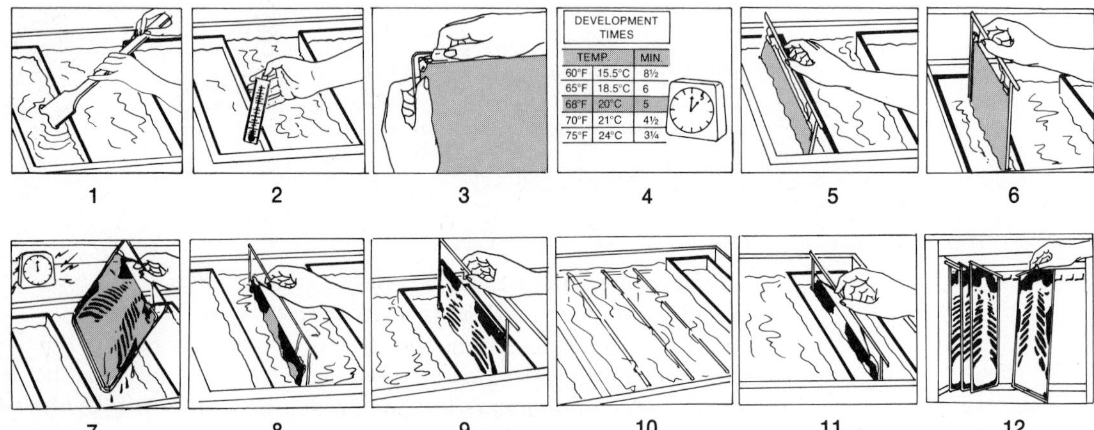

FIGURE 16–14. The steps involved in x-ray film processing. *1,* Stir developer and fixer solutions to equalize their temperature. (Use a separate paddle for each to avoid possible contamination.) *2,* Check temperature of solutions with accurate thermometer. (Rinse off each solution before checking next one.) Adjust to 68°F (20°C), if possible. *3,* Attach film carefully to hanger of proper size. (Attach at lower corners first.) Avoid finger marks, scratches, or bending. *4,* Set timer for desired period of development based on temperature of developer. See chart on reverse side for temperature and time. *5,* Completely immerse film. Do it smoothly and without pause to avoid streaking. Start timer. *6,* Raise and lower hanger several times to bathe film surfaces thoroughly. Repeat once each time. For asterisked films, tap hanger at start only (see chart). *7,* When alarm rings, lift hanger out quickly. Then drain film for a moment *into space between tanks.* For fast drainage, tilt hanger. *8,* Place film in acid rinse bath or running water. Agitate hanger vigorously. Rinse for 30 seconds. If water rinse is used, lift film and drain well; if an acid stop bath, plunge film immediately into the fixer. *9,* Immerse film. Agitate hanger vigorously. Fix most films at 60 to 75°F (15.5 to 24°C), 5 to 10 minutes in Kodak X-ray Fixer; 2 to 4 minutes in Kodak Rapid Fixer. No-Screen Film, 10 to 15 minutes or 8 to 10 minutes respectively. *10,* Place films in tank of running water, with ample space between hangers. Times: X-Omat Films (except duplicating), PF, and PFC—5 minutes; Blue Brand—20 minutes; SB, X-Omat Duplicating, Industrex, and No-Screen—30 minutes. *11,* If facilities permit, use a final rinse of Kodak Photo-Flo Solution to speed drying time and prevent water marks. Immerse film for about 30 seconds, and drain for several seconds. *12,* Place in dryer, or rack in current of air. Keep films well separated. When dry, remove films from hangers and trim corners to remove clip marks. Insert in identified envelopes. (Courtesy of Radiography Market Division, Eastman Kodak Company.)

The Darkroom

Radiographic film must always be stored and handled in a way that prevents it from being exposed to light or excessive heat and dampness, which would ruin it. A darkroom is especially designed for this function. It is a room that is free from light, except for a safelight that utilizes a low-wattage bulb. The safelight provides a small amount of illumination for the radiation worker to perform procedures accurately but at the same time does not harm the radiographic film. The film must be loaded into its holder or cassette, unloaded, and processed in the darkroom.

Once the radiograph of a particular organ or structure has been taken, it must be properly identified using a photoprinter (Fig. 16–13) or other suitable labeling device. The radiographic film then goes through a processing cycle that makes the exposed image visible and permanent. The cycle consists of a series of steps including developing, rinsing, fixing, washing, and drying. The film may be manually moved from one step to the next (Fig. 16–14) or it may be automatically moved by a roller system using an automatic processor (Fig. 16–15). Automatic processing is generally used because of its convenience and uniform processing results.

The processed radiograph is placed on an illuminated viewbox for interpretation by the physician and is then stored in a specially designed file envelope labeled with the patient's name, the date, and any other necessary information.

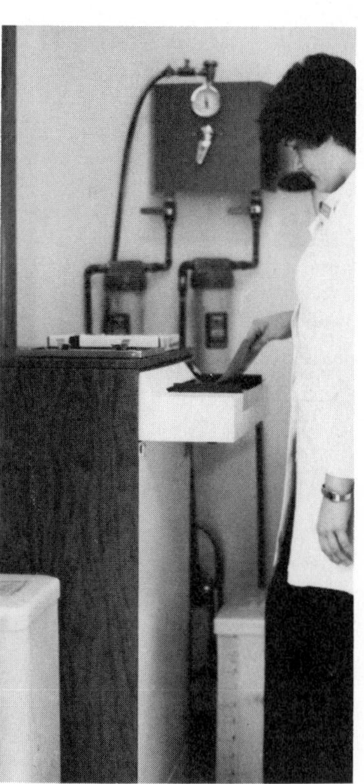

FIGURE 16–15. The medical assistant is developing a radiograph using an automatic processor. (*Note:* The film is processed in the dark using a safelight.)

PROCEDURE 16-1

PRODUCING A RADIOGRAPH (GENERAL PROCEDURE)

The steps involved in the production of a radiograph vary, depending on the type of equipment utilized and the medical office policy. A general procedure is outlined here to serve as a basic guideline.

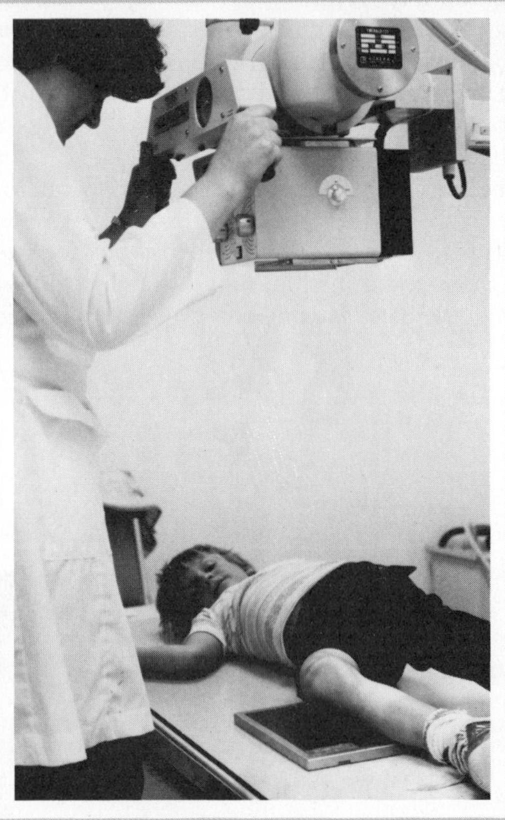

1. Load the holder or cassette with radiographic film in the darkroom.

2. Identify the patient and explain the procedure.

3. Position the patient and center the x-ray tube. Instruct the patient to maintain the position and not to move. Protect the patient's gonads with a gonad shield.

4. Set and operate the x-ray machine from the control panel situated behind the lead-lined wall according to the manufacturer's and physician's instructions. Observe the patient through the lead-treated window.

5. Take the exposed film into the darkroom and unload it from the holder or cassette.

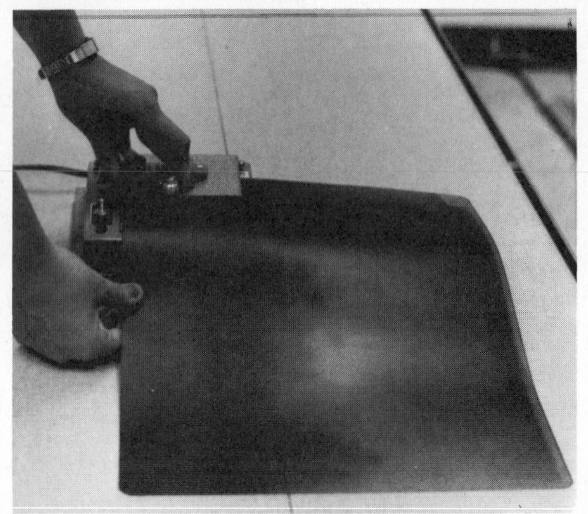

6. Identify the film using a photoprinter or other suitable labeling device.

7. Process the film in the darkroom.

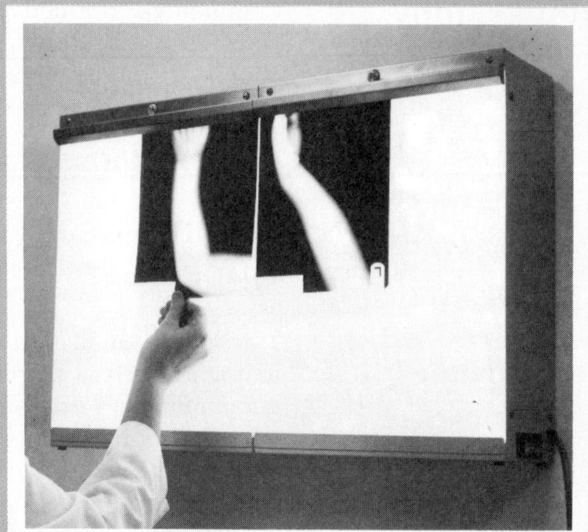

8. Place the processed radiograph on an illuminated viewbox for interpretation by the physician.

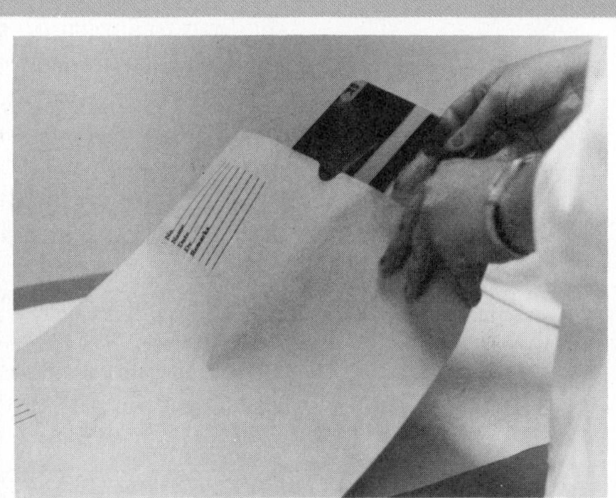

9. Place the film in a labeled film envelope and file it according to the policy of the medical office.

Specific Radiographic Examinations

The medical assistant should understand the purpose of preparing for an x-ray examination and should be able to instruct a patient in the proper preparation. Commonly performed radiographic examinations and the special advance preparation required for each are described here. The preparation may vary somewhat, depending on the medical office.

Gastrointestinal Series

Barium Meal (Also Termed Upper GI)

This is an examination of the upper digestive tract using both fluoroscopy and radiography. It is helpful in diagnosing disorders of the esophagus, stomach, duodenum, and small intestine, such as peptic ulcers or benign and malignant tumors. Proper patient preparation is very important for this procedure. The patient's stomach must be empty at the beginning of the study so that food does not obscure the radiographic image. To prepare for the examination, the patient must be instructed to eat a light evening meal only and then not to eat or drink anything, including water and medications, after midnight on the day before the examination. Food or fluid in the GI tract has a degree of density and could cause confusing shadows to appear on the radiograph.

The stomach varies little in density from the structures around it, and in order to make it show up on a radiograph, a contrast medium must be used. A suspension of barium mixed with water and a flavoring is given to the patient to drink. The mixture is known as the "barium meal" and has a chalky taste. As the patient swallows the barium, the radiologist observes its passage down the esophagus and into the stomach and duodenum by fluoroscopy. Radiographs are taken periodically during the examination to allow a detailed study of the upper GI tract and to provide a permanent record. The patient's position is changed at various times so that the upper digestive tract can be visualized from different profiles. If the radiologist wants to observe the passage of the barium through the small and large intestines, the patient will have to return several times for additional radiographs.

The medical assistant should explain to the patient that the barium suspension will appear in his or her stool the following day, causing it to have a lighter color. The barium mixture may cause the patient to become constipated and require a laxative.

Barium Enema (Also Termed Lower GI)

A barium enema involves filling the colon with a barium sulfate mixture by means of a tube inserted into the colon. The examination utilizes both fluoroscopy and radiography to observe and obtain permanent pictures of the colon (Fig. 16–16). A barium enema assists in diagnosing disorders of the lower intestines such as polyps, tumors, lesions, and diverticulosis. The colon must be thoroughly cleansed in advance to remove gas and fecal material. Gas has a certain degree of density and shows up as confusing shadows on the radiograph. If fecal material appears on the film, it obscures the image of the colon. The instructions a patient is given for cleansing the colon may vary somewhat from one medical office to another, but in general the patient is instructed to eat a light evening meal. A cathartic such as bisacodyl (Dulcolax) is taken on the day before the scheduled examination, and a cleansing enema may also be required. The patient must not eat anything after midnight on the day before the examination. Water may be taken when desired.

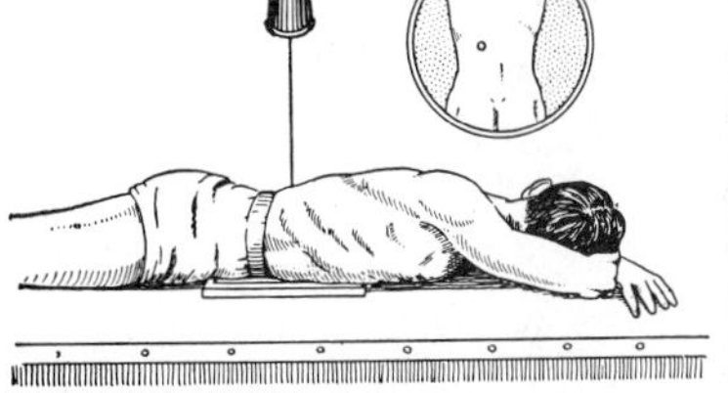

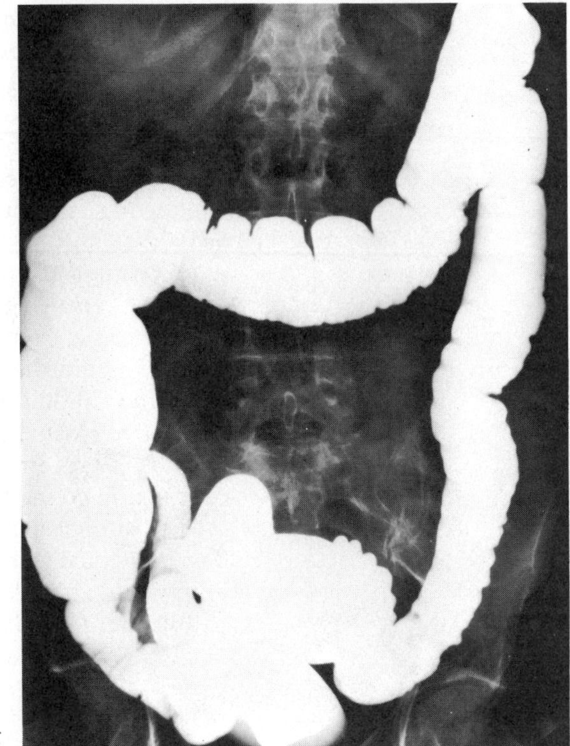

FIGURE 16–16. Colon distended with barium: positioning of patient and radiograph. (From Meschan, I.: *Synopsis of Radiologic Anatomy with Computed Tomography.* Philadelphia, W. B. Saunders Company, 1980.)

On the morning of the examination, the patient takes warm water cleansing enemas. He or she should be instructed to use 500 to 1000 ml of tap water at a temperature of approximately 105°F (40.5°C). The enema solution container should be held approximately 12 to 18 inches above the anus. With the patient lying on the left side, one-third of the enema solution is allowed to run slowly into the colon. The patient then turns on the right side for another third and finally turns on the back for the remainder of the solution. The patient retains the solution until the urge to defecate occurs, usually in 5 to 10 minutes. This procedure should be repeated until the returns are clear.

The patient reports at the scheduled time and is instructed to relax on one side while the rectal tube is inserted. As the barium enters the colon, the radiologist watches it on the fluoroscopic screen and periodically takes radiographs. The patient feels a sensation of fullness and the urge to defecate as the barium enters the colon. The patient is moved into various positions to allow the barium to fill the colon completely and to obtain better visualization of the colon. He or she is then allowed to evacuate, and another radiograph is taken to finish the x-ray study.

Cholecystography

Cholecystography is an x-ray examination of the gallbladder used to determine the presence of pathologic conditions such as gallstones.

The gallbladder is a pear-shaped sac located on the undersurface of the liver. It stores bile until it is needed by the body. Bile is produced by the liver and functions to break down fat. When fat enters the small intestine, the gallbladder contracts, releasing bile, which enters the small intestine by way of the common bile duct.

Because the gallbladder does not normally show up on a radiograph, a contrast medium must be used to make it radiopaque. The patient is instructed to eat an evening meal consisting of nonfatty food such as lean meat, fresh fruit and vegetables, toast or bread, jelly, and tea or coffee. The patient should not consume foods containing fat, such as milk, butter, cheese, cream, eggs, or chocolate, or fried or greasy foods. The reason for this is to prevent the gallbladder from functioning and contracting and thus emptying the contrast medium before the radiograph is taken.

The patient is given some tablets containing the contrast medium to take at regular intervals (generally 5 to 10 minutes) during or after the meal. Specific instructions are given with the tablets regarding how they should be taken. The contrast medium is absorbed by the gallbladder. Once the tablets have been taken, the patient should have nothing to eat or drink. The individual may also be instructed to cleanse the intestinal tract by means of a mild cathartic and cleansing enemas to prevent gas and fecal material from appearing on the radiograph and obstructing good visualization of the gallbladder.

The patient reports at the scheduled time, and a series of radiographs is taken. The individual is then given a meal containing fat to stimulate the gallbladder to empty, and another radiograph is taken to evaluate the functioning ability of the gallbladder (Fig. 16–17).

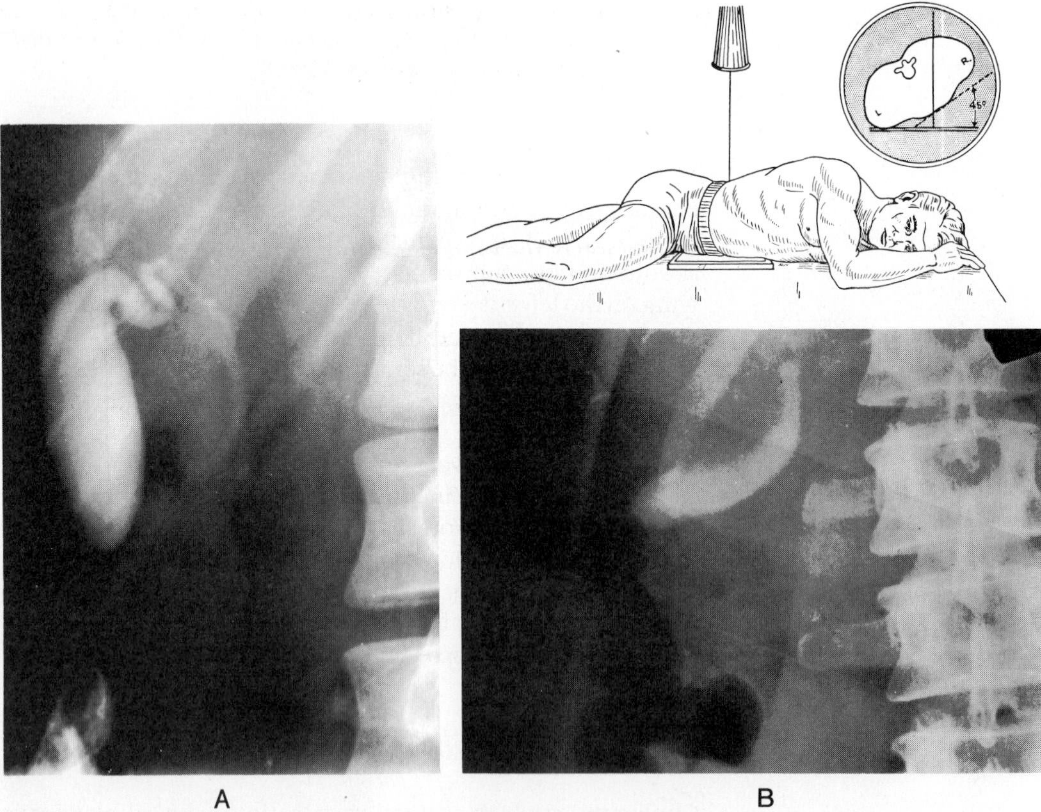

FIGURE 16–17. Radiographic study of the gallbladder: positioning of patient and radiographs obtained before *(A)* and after *(B)* fatty stimulation. (From Meschan, I.: *Synopsis of Radiologic Anatomy with Computed Tomography.* Philadelphia, W. B. Saunders Company, 1980.)

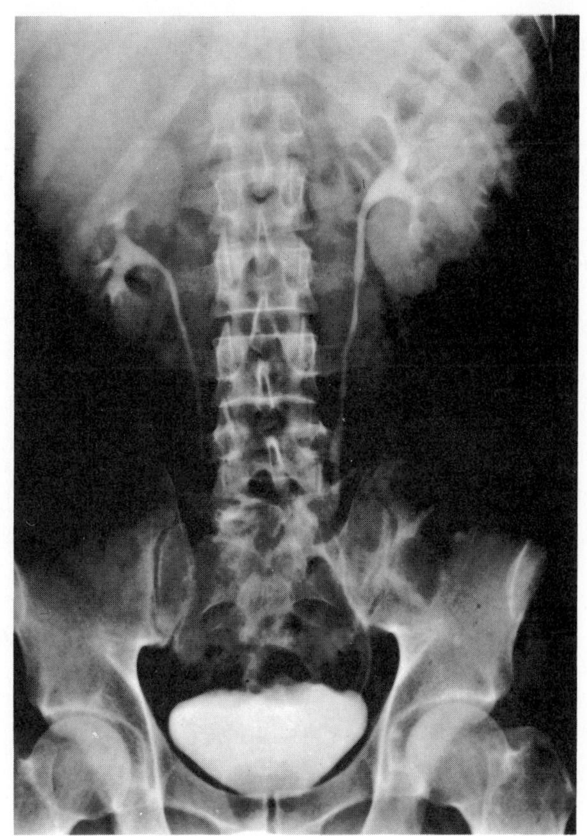

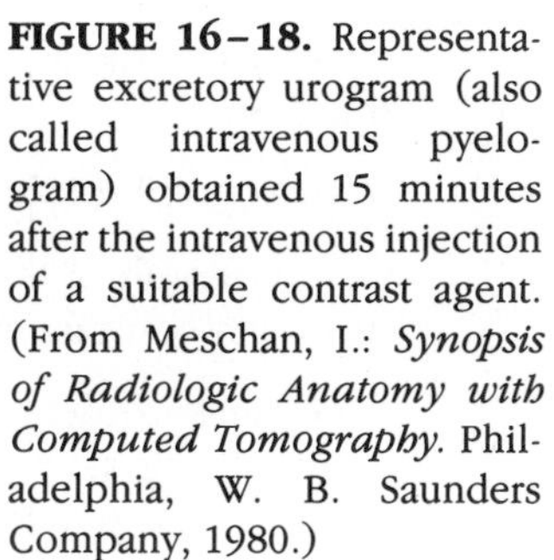

FIGURE 16–18. Representative excretory urogram (also called intravenous pyelogram) obtained 15 minutes after the intravenous injection of a suitable contrast agent. (From Meschan, I.: *Synopsis of Radiologic Anatomy with Computed Tomography.* Philadelphia, W. B. Saunders Company, 1980.)

Intravenous Pyelography

An intravenous pyelogram, more commonly known by its abbreviation, IVP, is a radiograph of the kidneys and urinary tract (Fig. 16–18). The patient is instructed to eat a light evening meal and not to eat or drink anything after 9:00 PM. He or she must remove gas and fecal material from the intestines with a cathartic (e.g., Dulcolax) and cleansing enemas. This permits proper visualization of the urinary tract. A contrast medium consisting of iodine must be used and is intravenously administered to the patient. Some patients are allergic to iodine. Therefore, the medical assistant should ask the patient if he or she is allergic to iodine or foods containing iodine, such as seafood.

Other Types of Radiographs

The following is a list of other types of radiographs that the medical assistant may encounter.

Angiocardiogram — A radiograph of the heart and great vessels taken after introduction of a radiopaque contrast medium.

Aortogram — A radiograph of the aorta taken after injection of a radiopaque contrast medium.

Bronchogram — A radiograph of the bronchial tree taken after introduction of a radiopaque contrast medium.

Cerebral angiogram	A radiograph of the arteries of the brain taken after injection of a radiopaque contrast medium.
Cholangiogram	A radiograph of the bile ducts taken after administration of a radiopaque contrast medium.
Cystogram	A radiograph of the urinary bladder taken after injection of a radiopaque contrast medium.
Hysterosalpingogram	A radiograph of the uterus and fallopian tubes taken after injection of an oily radiopaque contrast medium.
Mammogram	A radiograph of the breast.
Myelogram	A radiograph of the spinal canal taken after injection of a contrast medium.
Pelvimetry	The measurement of the pelvic dimensions, either manually or with the use of x-rays, to determine whether the pelvis is large enough for the fetus to pass through normally during delivery.
Pneumoencephalogram	A radiograph of the brain taken after introduction of air as a radiolucent contrast medium.
Retrograde pyelogram (RP)	A radiograph of the kidneys and urinary tract taken after injection of radiopaque contrast medium directly into the ureter through a ureteral catheter. The dye flows to the kidneys through the ureters.
Sialogram	A radiograph of the salivary ducts taken after injection of a radiopaque contrast medium.

Study Questions

1. Why is it important for the patient to prepare properly for an x-ray examination?
2. How must the patient be positioned for each of the following views: anteroposterior, posteroanterior, right and left lateral, supine, and prone?
3. What is the function of a contrast medium?
4. What is the purpose of each of the following types of x-ray examinations: barium meal, barium enema, cholecystography, and intravenous pyelography?

17

SPECIALTY EXAMINATIONS AND PROCEDURES

CHAPTER OUTLINE

THE PEDIATRIC EXAMINATION
- Pediatric Office Visits
- Understanding the Child
- Carrying the Infant
- Growth Patterns
- Pediatric Intramuscular Injections
- Immunizations
- The PKU Screening Test

THE GYNECOLOGIC EXAMINATION
- Gynecology
- The Breast Examination
- The Pelvic Examination
- The Papanicolaou Test
- Vaginal Infections
- Bimanual Pelvic Examination

PRENATAL CARE
- Obstetrics
- The First Prenatal Visit
- The Prenatal Record
- Initial Prenatal Examination
- Return Prenatal Visits
- Six-Weeks Postpartum Visit

COLON PROCEDURES
- Fecal Occult Blood Testing
- Quality Control for the Guaiac Slide Test
- Proctoscopy and Sigmoidoscopy

INTRODUCTION

Specialty examinations and procedures are often performed in the medical office, the most common being the pediatric examination, the gynecologic examination, the prenatal examination, the proctoscopic and sigmoidoscopic examinations, and the fecal occult blood determination, all of which are presented in this chapter. The medical assistant helps the physician during each of these in varying capacities. He or she should have a thorough knowledge of the responsibilities regarding each and perform them with skill and competence.

Obtaining the patient's cooperation helps to make the examination proceed more smoothly and, as a result, makes the patient feel more comfortable. The medical assistant can help by explaining the purpose of the procedure to the patient. If the individual understands the beneficial results to be derived from the examination, he or she is more likely to participate as required.

Safety precautions are of primary importance before, during, and after the examinations to prevent accidents that could result in harm to the patient. Additional precautionary measures should be taken with children and elderly patients. For instance, instruments and supplies should be kept out of the reach of young children. Elderly patients should be helped into the examination room and assisted in getting on and off the examining table. The medical assistant should always be alert to any potential hazards that may exist in the medical office.

This chapter is divided into four units covering four specialty areas: the pediatric examination, the gynecologic examination, the prenatal examination, and colon procedures. Each unit has separate objectives, vocabulary lists, procedures, and study questions.

• VOCABULARY •

immunity (i-mu' ni-te)—The resistance of the body to the effects of a harmful agent such as a pathogenic microorganism or its toxins.

immunization (active, artificial) (im" u-ni-za' shun)—The process of becoming immune or of rendering an individual immune through the use of a vaccine or toxoid.

infant (in' fant)—A child from birth to 1 year of age.

length (recumbent) (lĕngkth)—The measurement from the vertex of the head to the heel of the foot in a supine position.

pediatrician (pe" de-ah-trish' an)—A medical doctor who specializes in the care and development of children and the diagnosis and treatment of diseases of children.

pediatrics (pe" de-at' riks)—The branch of medicine dealing with the care and development of children and the diagnosis and treatment of diseases of children.

stature (stat' ūr)—The height of the body in a standing position.

toxoid (tok' soid)—A toxin (poisonous substance produced by a bacterium) that has been treated by heat or chemicals to destroy its harmful properties. It is administered to an individual to prevent an infectious disease by stimulating the production of antibodies in that individual.

vaccine (vak' sēn)—A suspension of attenuated (weakened) or killed microorganisms administered to an individual to prevent an infectious disease by stimulating the production of antibodies in that individual.

vertex (ver' teks)—The summit, or top, especially the top of the head.

COMPETENCIES

After completing this unit, you should be able to demonstrate the proper procedure to perform the following:

1. Carry an infant, using the following positions: cradle, upright, and football.
2. Measure the weight and length of an infant, and record the results.
3. Plot pediatric growth values on a growth chart, and record the results.
4. Collect a urine specimen from an infant, using a pediatric urine collector bag, and record the procedure.
5. Administer an intramuscular injection to an infant, and record the procedure.
6. Collect a specimen for a phenylketonuria (PKU) screening test and record the procedure.

LEARNING OBJECTIVES

After completing this unit, you should be able to do the following:

1. Define the terms listed in the vocabulary.
2. List the two categories of pediatric patient office visits and what functions are performed during each.
3. Explain why it is important to develop a rapport with the pediatric patient.
4. State the importance of measuring the child's weight and height (or length) during each office visit.
5. Locate the following pediatric intramuscular injection sites and explain the use of each in regard to the age of the pediatric patient: gluteus medius, vastus lateralis, and deltoid.
6. Describe the schedule for immunization of infants and children recommended by the American Academy of Pediatrics.
7. Explain the purpose for performing a PKU screening test.

The Pediatric Examination

Pediatric Office Visits

Pediatrics is the branch of medicine dealing with the care and development of children and the diagnosis and treatment of diseases in children. A *pediatrician* is a medical doctor who specializes in pediatrics. Many physicians involved in general practice also handle pediatric patients. It is essential that the medical assistant develop the skills needed to assist the physician in the care and treatment of children.

There are two broad categories of pediatric patient office visits. The first is the *well-child visit,* in which the physician progressively evaluates the growth and development of the child. A physical examination is performed during each well-child visit and is directed toward discovering any abnormal conditions commonly associated with the stage of development reached by the child. He or she will also receive any necessary immunizations during these visits. The interval between well-child visits depends on the medical office, but it frequently follows this schedule after birth: 1 month, 2 months, 4 months, 6 months, 9 months, 12 months, 15 months, 18 months, 24 months, and yearly thereafter.

The other category is the *sick-child visit.* The child is exhibiting the signs and symptoms of disease, and the physician evaluates the patient's condition to arrive at a diagnosis and to prescribe treatment.

During both the well- and sick-child visits, the medical assistant utilizes many of the same techniques that have been presented in previous chapters (e.g., temperature and pulse readings, measurement of respiration and blood pressure, measurement of visual acuity, assisting with the patient examination, and others). Techniques relating specifically to the pediatric patient and variations in techniques already presented are discussed in this unit.

Understanding the Child

The medical assistant must establish a rapport with the pediatric patient. If he or she gains the child's trust and confidence, the child is more likely to cooperate during an examination or procedure. Interacting with children requires special techniques, depending on the age of the child. For example, children in the age group of 2 to 4 years often respond well to making a game of the procedure. Explaining the purpose of an instrument (e.g., the stethoscope) and allowing the child to hold the instrument or even to help during the procedure may also aid in overcoming fears (Fig. 17–1).

The medical assistant should always explain the procedure to children who are able to understand. Each child must be approached at his or her level of understanding. In order to do this, the medical assistant should have a knowledge of what to expect from a child at a particular age, in terms of both motor and social development. It should be kept in mind, however, that each child has his or her own rate of development. The descriptions of normal development based on age are meant to serve as a guide only and may have to be modified to meet individual needs. It is also important to realize that it is normal for an ill child to regress to an earlier level of behavior.

Carrying the Infant

The medical assistant needs to lift and carry the infant in order to perform various procedures, such as measurement of length and weight. The infant should be lifted and carried in a manner that is both safe and comfortable. The three basic positions are described here.

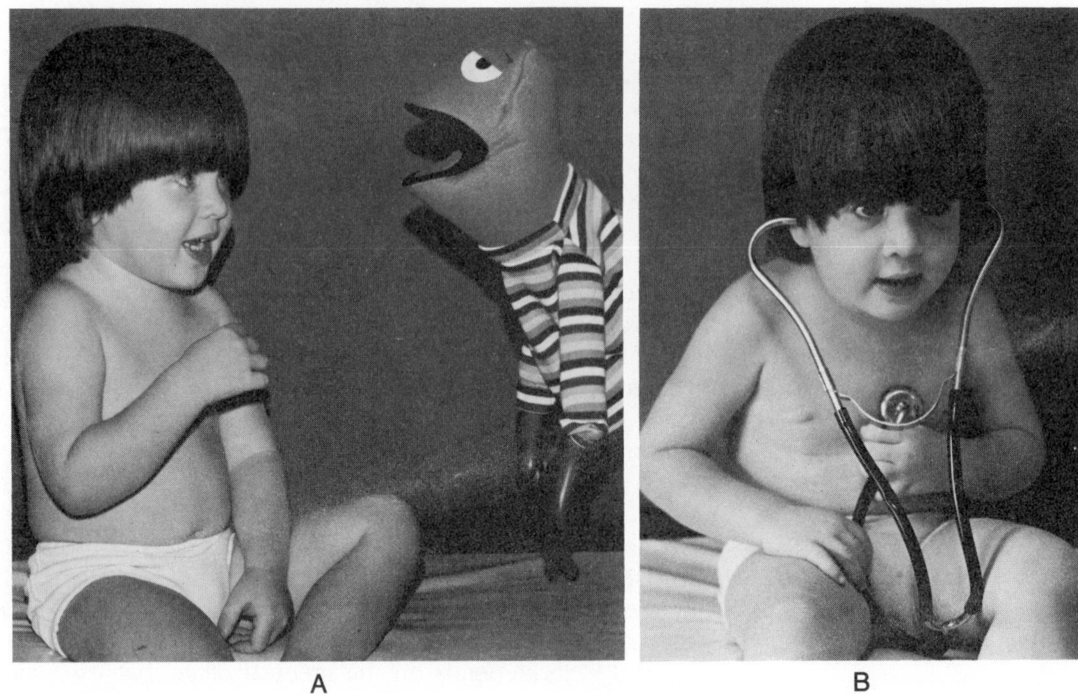

FIGURE 17–1. The medical assistant should develop a rapport with young children in order to gain their trust and cooperation. Making a game of the procedure *(A)* and explaining the purpose of the stethoscope and allowing the child to hold it *(B)* help the child to overcome fears.

Cradle Position. The medical assistant slides his or her left hand and arm under the infant's back and grasps the baby's upper arm from behind. The thumb and fingers should encircle the infant's upper arm. The infant's head, shoulders, and back are supported by the medical assistant's arm. Next the medical assistant slips his or her right arm up and under the baby's buttocks. The infant is cradled in the arm with the child's body resting against the medical assistant's chest (Fig. 17–2).

Upright Position. The medical assistant slips his or her right hand under the infant's head and shoulders. The fingers should be spread apart to support the infant's head and neck. The left forearm is then slipped under the infant's buttocks

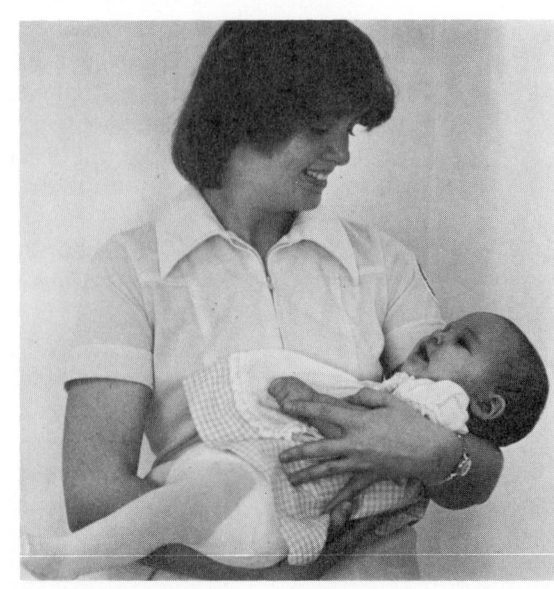

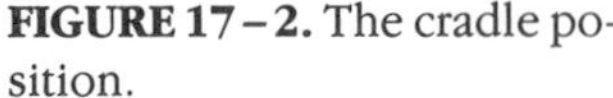

FIGURE 17–2. The cradle position.

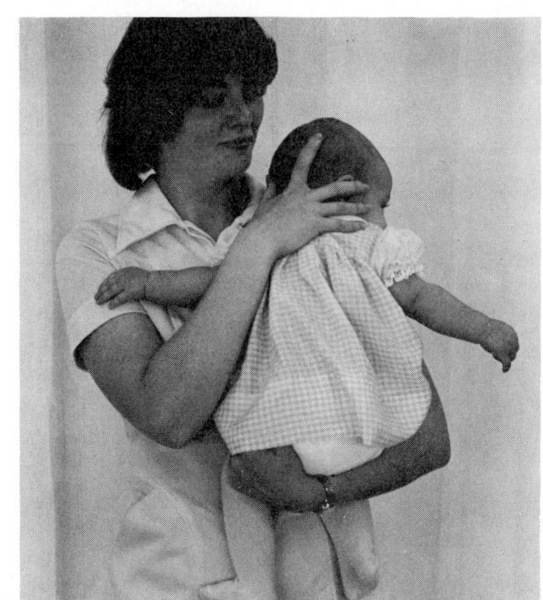

FIGURE 17–3. The upright position.

to help support the baby's weight. The infant should be allowed to rest against the medical assistant's chest with the cheek resting on the medical assistant's shoulder (Fig. 17–3).

Football Position. The medical assistant slips his or her left hand under the baby's head and shoulders. The fingers should be spread apart to support the infant's head and neck. The hips of the infant are supported against the medical assistant's hip and the bend of the elbow. The football position is utilized more in the home than in the medical office and is useful for washing and rinsing the baby's head during bathing (Fig. 17–4).

Each infant prefers a particular position in which to be held and may feel insecure when held any other way. The way in which the mother holds the baby can serve as a guide. In general, most babies seem to prefer the upright position rather than the cradle or football position.

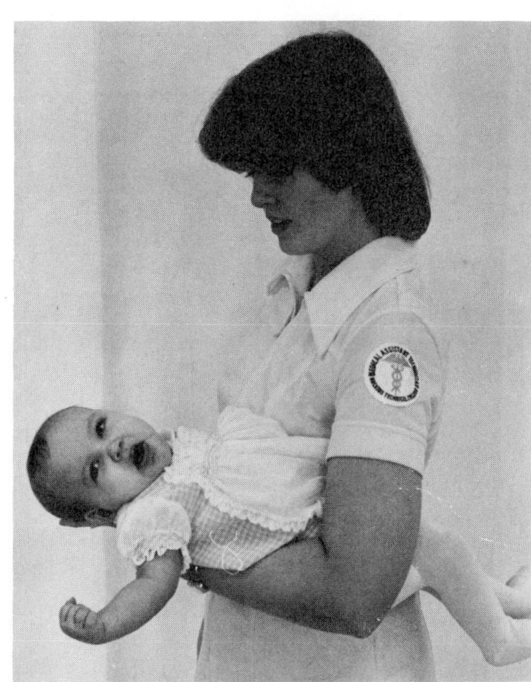

FIGURE 17–4. The football position.

Growth Patterns

One of the best methods used to evaluate the progress of a child is to measure his or her growth. The weight and height (or length) of a child should be measured during each office visit and plotted on a growth chart (Fig. 17–5). Growth charts should be included in every child's permanent record. They provide a means for assessing the child's rate of growth and for comparing it with that of other children of the same age. The physician will want to investigate any significant change or rapid rise or drop in the child's growth pattern. The charts can be used to identify children with growth or nutritional abnormalities. Head circumference should routinely be measured on all children under 3 years of age. It is an important screening measurement for microcephaly and macrocephaly.

The medical assistant may be responsible for plotting the child's growth measurements on the chart. The procedure for using the National Center for Health Statistics (NCHS) growth charts is as follows: Locate the growth value in the vertical column under the appropriate category (stature, length, or weight). Next, locate the child's age in the horizontal column. Find the site at which the two lines (extending from these values) intersect on the graph. Place an **X** on this site. To determine the percentile in which the child falls in relation to other children of the same age, follow the percentile line upward to read the value located on the side of the chart. (Interpolation is needed if the value does not fall exactly on a percentile line.) Record results as instructed by the physician.

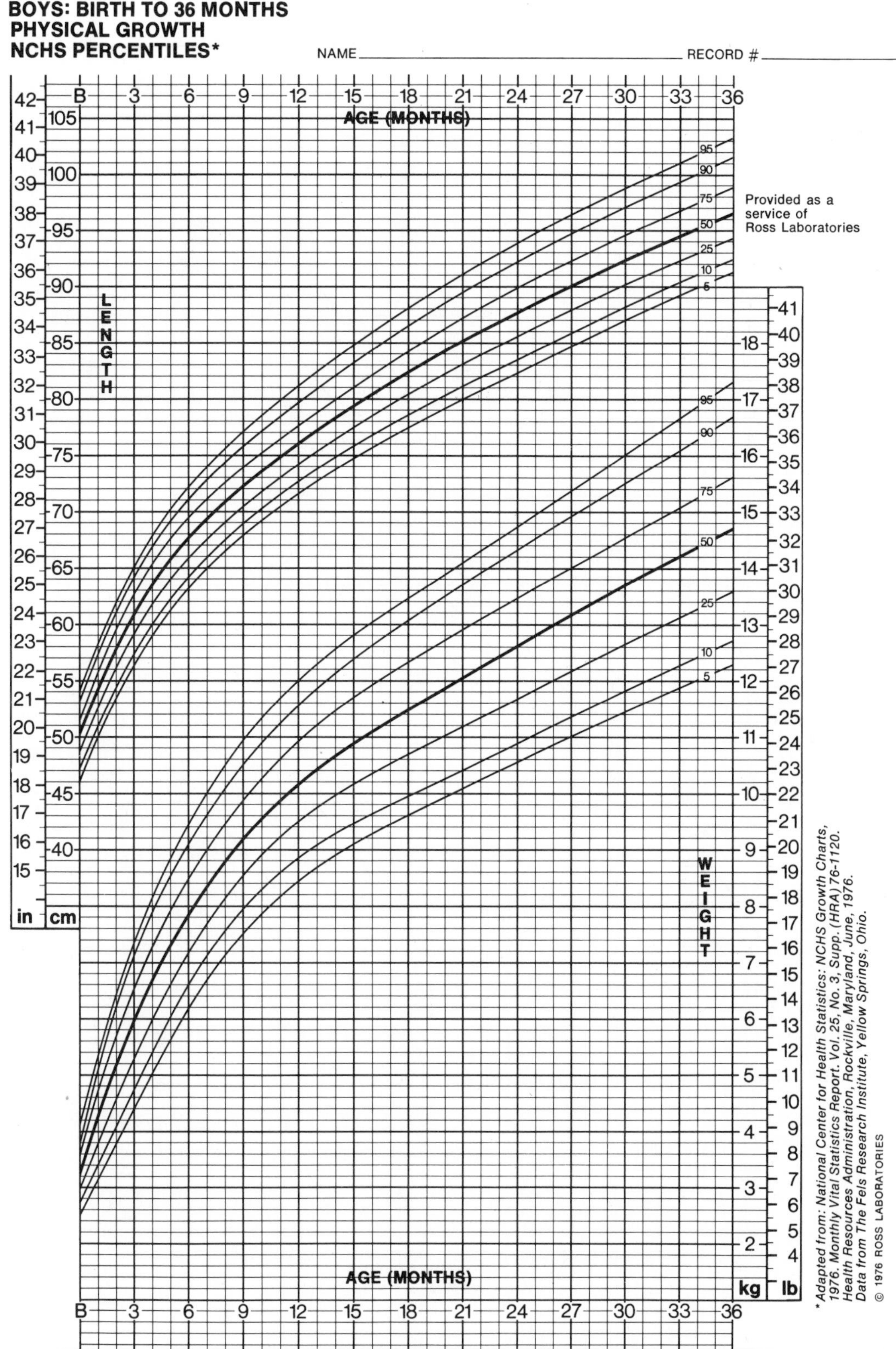

FIGURE 17–5. Growth charts. (Courtesy of Ross Laboratories, © 1976.)

Illustration continued on following page

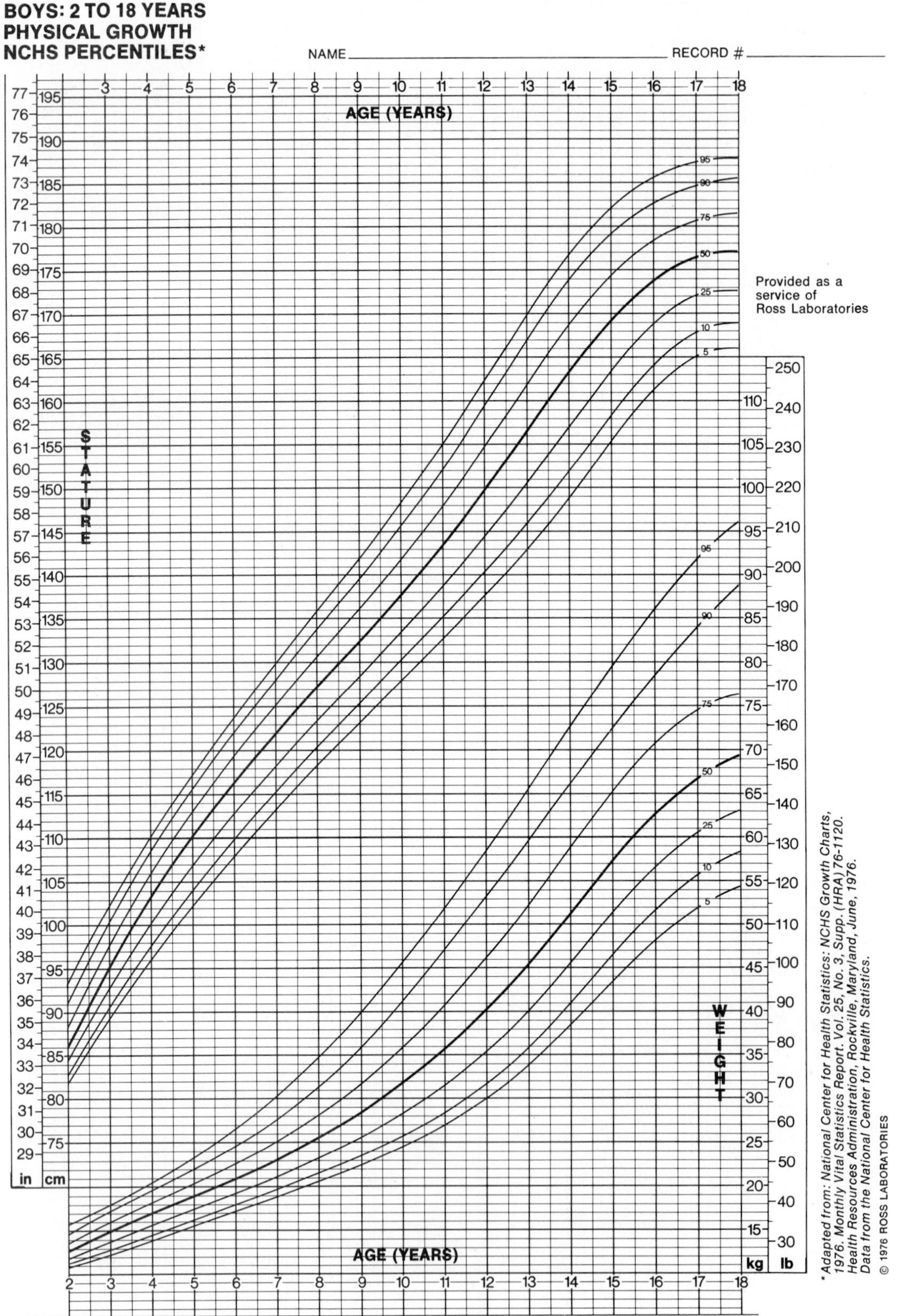

FIGURE 17–5 *Continued*

Illustration continued on opposite page

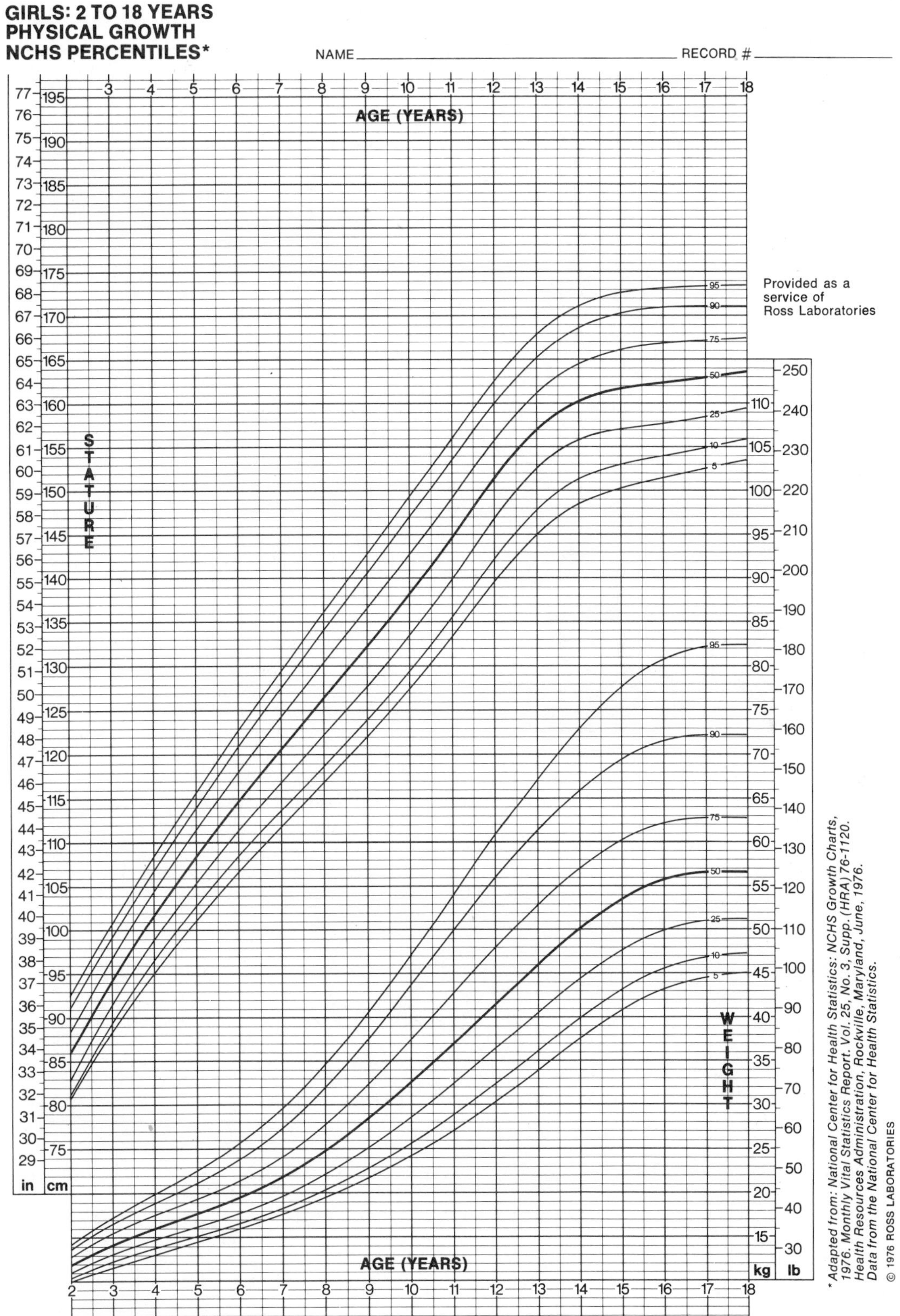
GIRLS: 2 TO 18 YEARS
PHYSICAL GROWTH
NCHS PERCENTILES*
NAME
RECORD #
AGE (YEARS)
STATURE
WEIGHT
in
cm
kg
lb
Provided as a service of Ross Laboratories
*Adapted from: National Center for Health Statistics: NCHS Growth Charts, 1976. Monthly Vital Statistics Report. Vol. 25, No. 3, Supp. (HRA) 76-1120. Health Resources Administration, Rockville, Maryland, June, 1976. Data from the National Center for Health Statistics.
© 1976 ROSS LABORATORIES

FIGURE 17–5 *Continued*

PROCEDURE 17-1
MEASURING THE WEIGHT OF AN INFANT

The medical assistant should exercise care in measuring the weight of an infant. The weight is often utilized to determine the infant's nutritional needs and the proper dosage of medication to administer to the child. The infant is weighed in a recumbent position as described here. Older children are weighed in a standing position (see Chapter 3).

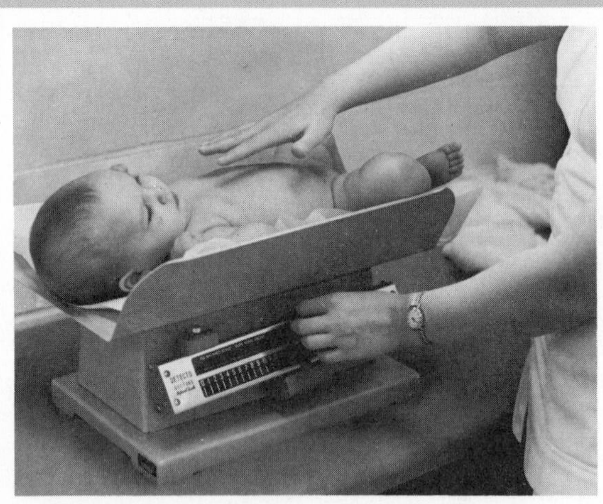

1. **PROCEDURAL STEP.** Wash the hands.

2. **PROCEDURAL STEP.** Remove the infant's clothing, including the diaper.
   PRINCIPLE. Bulky diapers tend to increase the child's weight considerably. In addition, growth charts for infants and young children generally base their percentiles on the weight of the child without clothing.

3. **PROCEDURAL STEP.** Unlock the pediatric scale (if necessary) and place a clean paper protector on it. Check the balance scale for accuracy, making sure to compensate for the weight of the paper.
   PRINCIPLE. The paper protector prevents cross-contamination and reduces the spread of disease from one patient to another. If the scale is metal, the paper provides warmth and protection from the cold metal.

4. **PROCEDURAL STEP.** Gently place the infant on his or her back on the scale. Place one hand slightly above the infant to make sure that he or she does not fall.

5. **PROCEDURAL STEP.** Balance the scale and read the results in pounds and ounces while the infant is lying still.

6. **PROCEDURAL STEP.** Return the balance to its resting position and lock the scale (if necessary).

7. **PROCEDURAL STEP.** Gently remove the infant from the scale and record results.

Record data below.

DATE	TIME	PATIENT'S NAME	RESULTS

PROCEDURE 17-2
MEASURING THE LENGTH OF AN INFANT

The recumbent length is a measurement from the vertex of the head to the heel of the infant in a supine position. Older children have their height measured in a standing position, as described in Chapter 3. Two people are needed to accurately determine the length of an infant. The parent's help can be solicited if the medical assistant gives explicit instructions on what is to be done.

1. **PROCEDURAL STEP.** Place the infant on his or her back on a flat table. Be careful not to let him or her roll off the table.

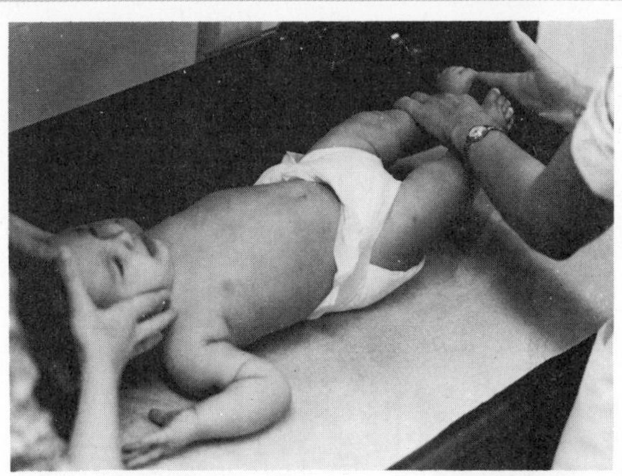

2. **PROCEDURAL STEP.** Place the vertex of the infant's head at the beginning of the measure (measuring tape, rod, or table). Ask the helper to hold the infant's head in this position.

3. **PROCEDURAL STEP.** Straighten the infant's knees and place the soles of his or her feet firmly against an upright foot board (to create a right angle).

4. **PROCEDURAL STEP.** Read the infant's length in inches from the measure and return the footboard to its resting position.

5. **PROCEDURAL STEP.** Properly record the results in the patient's chart. Place your initials next to the recording.

6. **PROCEDURAL STEP.** If directed by the physician, plot the growth values on the infant's growth chart.

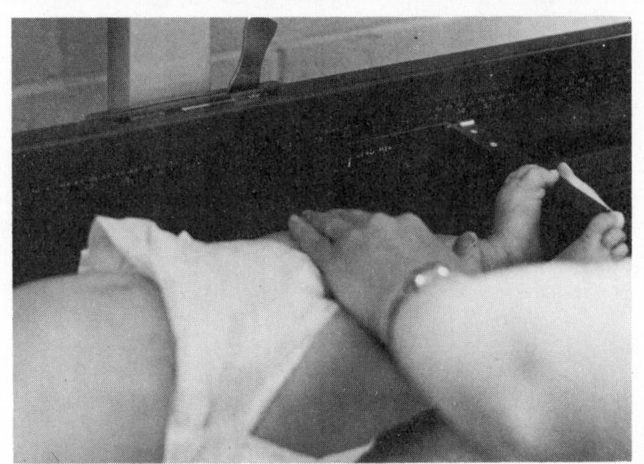

Record data below.

DATE	TIME	PATIENT'S NAME	RESULTS

PROCEDURE 17-3
APPLYING A PEDIATRIC URINE COLLECTOR

A urine specimen may be required from a pediatric patient as part of a general physical examination, to assist in the diagnosis of a pathologic condition, or to evaluate the effectiveness of therapy.

The collection of a urine specimen in a child exhibiting bladder control is performed using the technique outlined in Chapter 10. Collecting a urine specimen from an infant or young child who cannot urinate voluntarily involves the use of a pediatric urine collector. The urine collector consists of a clear plastic bag containing a soft sponge ring coated with a pressure-sensitive adhesive around the opening. The adhesive firmly attaches the urine collector to the genitalia. Most pediatric urine collectors are designed to be used with both sexes.

1. **PROCEDURAL STEP.** Wash the hands.

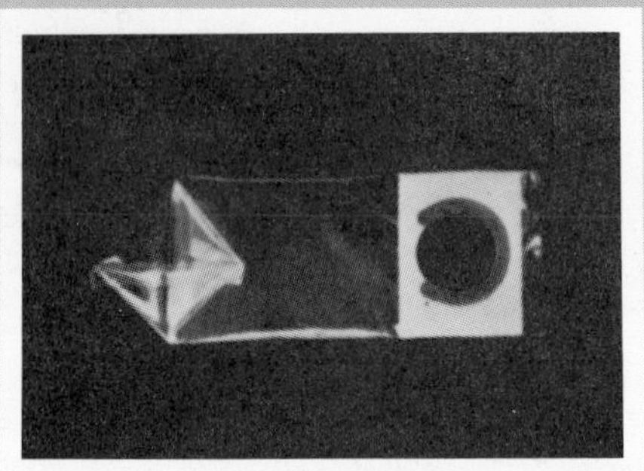

2. **PROCEDURAL STEP.** Assemble equipment. The equipment needed includes a **cleansing agent, cotton balls (or 4 × 4-inch gauze)**, a **pediatric urine collector bag**, and a **urine specimen container.**

3. **PROCEDURAL STEP.** Position the child. The child should be placed on his or her back with the legs spread apart. The medical assistant may need another individual to hold the child's legs apart.

   PRINCIPLE. This position facilitates cleansing of the genitalia and permits proper application of the urine collector bag.

4. **PROCEDURAL STEP.** Cleanse the child's genitalia.

   Female: Using a front-to-back motion (pubis to anus), cleanse each side of the meatus with a separate cotton ball and then, with a third cotton ball, cleanse directly down the middle (directly over the urinary meatus). Thoroughly rinse the area and wipe it dry.

   Male: If the child is not circumcised, retract the foreskin of the penis. Cleanse the area around the meatus and the urethral opening (meatal orifice) in a manner similar to that used in the female patient. Be sure to use a separate cotton ball for each swipe. Cleanse the scrotum last, using a fresh cotton ball. Rinse the area and thoroughly wipe it dry.

   PRINCIPLE. The urinary meatus and surrounding area must be cleansed to prevent contaminants such as baby powder, fecal material, and microorganisms from entering the urine specimen, which could affect the test results. A front-to-back motion must be used to prevent drawing microorganisms from the anal area into the area being cleansed. The cleansing agent must be rinsed off to prevent it from entering the urine specimen, which could affect the accuracy of the test results. The area must be wiped dry to assure an airtight adhesion of the collection bag to prevent leakage of urine.

5. **PROCEDURAL STEP.** Remove the paper backing from the urine collector bag, thereby exposing the adhesive surface. Firmly attach the bag in the following manner:

Female: The round opening of the bag should be placed so as to cover the upper half of the external genitalia. The opening of the bag should be directly over the urinary meatus.

Male: The bag should be positioned so the child's penis and scrotum are projected through the opening of the bag.

PRINCIPLE. The urine collector bag must be attached securely to prevent leakage.

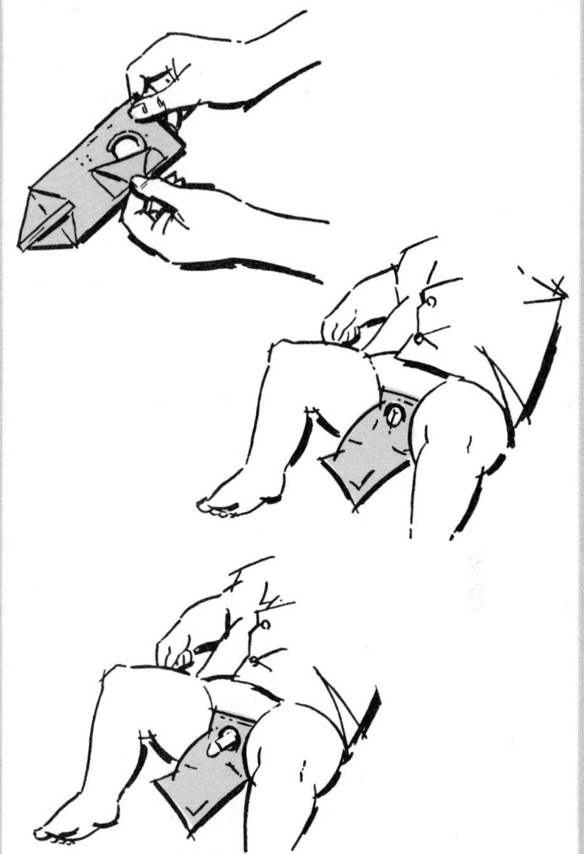

6. **PROCEDURAL STEP.** Loosely diaper the child. Check the urine collector bag every 15 minutes until a urine specimen is obtained.

PRINCIPLE. The diaper helps to hold the urine collector bag in place.

7. **PROCEDURAL STEP.** Once the child has voided, gently remove the urine collector bag.

PRINCIPLE. The bag must be removed gently because pulling the adhesive away too quickly may cause discomfort and irritation of the child's skin.

8. **PROCEDURAL STEP.** Clean the genital area and rediaper the child.

9. **PROCEDURAL STEP.** Transfer the urine specimen into a urine specimen container and tightly apply the lid. Label the container with the child's name, the date, the time of collection, and the type of specimen (i.e., urine). Dispose of the collector bag. Based on the medical office routine, test the urine specimen or prepare it for transfer to an outside laboratory, making sure to include a completed laboratory request. If the specimen cannot be tested or transferred immediately, preserve it by placing it in the refrigerator.

PRINCIPLE. Changes take place in a urine specimen that is left sitting out.

10. **PROCEDURAL STEP.** Wash the hands.

11. **PROCEDURAL STEP.** Record the procedure in the patient's chart, including the patient's name, the date, the time of collection, and the type of specimen (i.e., urine). If the specimen is to be transported to an outside laboratory, indicate this information, including the laboratory tests ordered. Place your initials next to the recording.

Record data below.

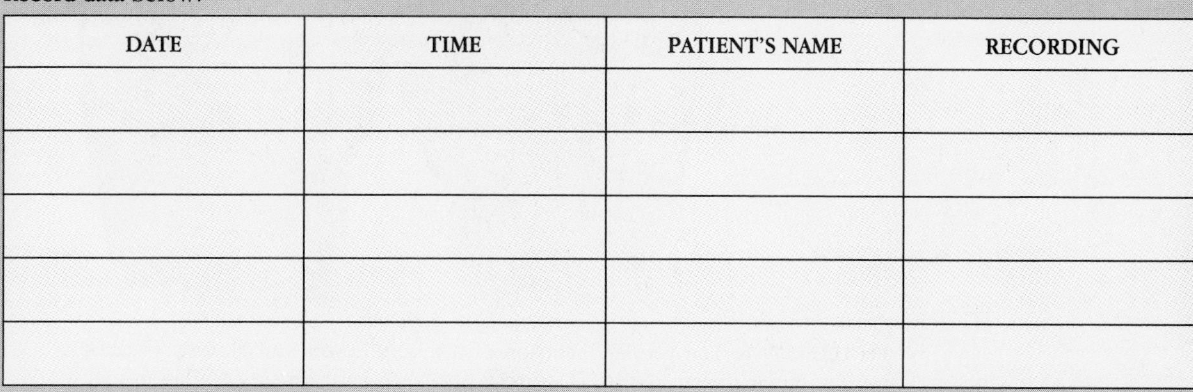

DATE	TIME	PATIENT'S NAME	RECORDING

Pediatric Intramuscular Injections

Administering an intramuscular (IM) injection to a child is an important responsibility. The experience a child has with early injections influences his or her attitude toward later ones. If the child is old enough to understand, the procedure should be explained. The medical assistant should be honest and attempt to gain the child's trust and cooperation. The child should be told the truth about the injection—that it will hurt but only for a short time. It is also advisable to explain that the medicine will help him or her get better. Another person should be present to assist. The assistant can help to position the child and can divert or restrain him or her if necessary. If the child struggles and fights excessively, however, the medical assistant should delay the injection and consult the physician.

The administration of IM injections has already been described in Chapter 8. Before undertaking the study of pediatric IM injections, the medical assistant should thoroughly review that chapter, concentrating on the location of injection sites and the procedure for the administration of an injection. The same basic technique used to administer an IM injection to an adult is used for a child. Variations in procedure are explained in the following section.

The gauge and length of the needle used for the IM injection varies, depending on the consistency of the medication to be administered and the size of the child. Thick or oily preparations require a larger needle lumen, and the needle must be of sufficient length to reach muscle tissue.

There are variations in pediatric injection sites based on the age of the child. The specific site to be utilized is stated in the package insert accompanying the medication. Until the child is walking, the gluteus muscle is small, not well developed, and primarily made up of fat. Moreover, an injection in this area may come dangerously close to the sciatic nerve. The danger is increased if the child is squirming or fighting. Because serious trauma can result from incorrect administration of an

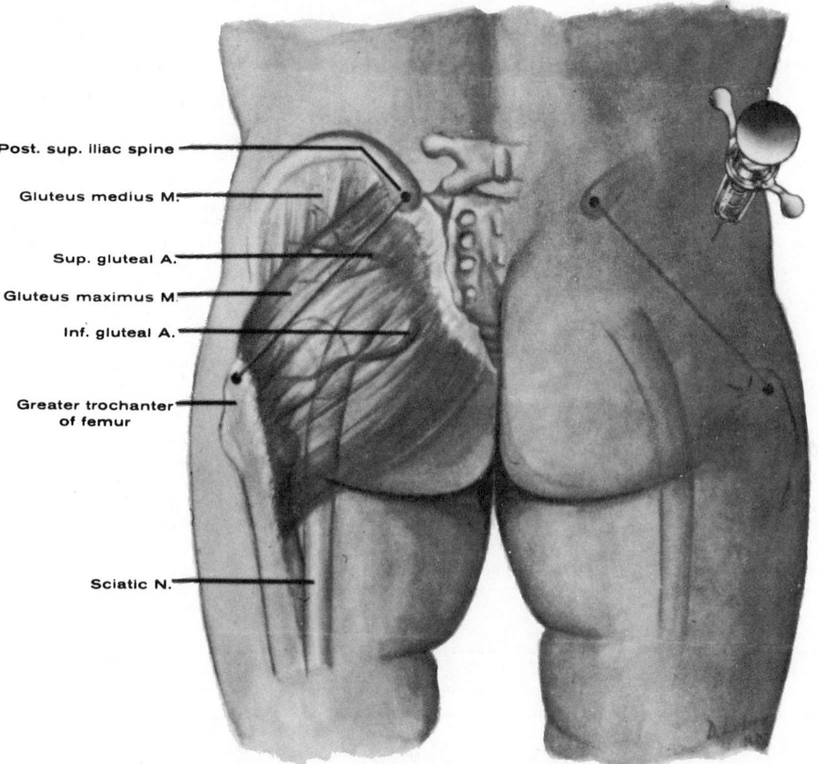

FIGURE 17-6. The proper insertion of the needle into the gluteus medius intramuscular injection site. (Courtesy of Wyeth Laboratories, Philadelphia, Pennsylvania.)

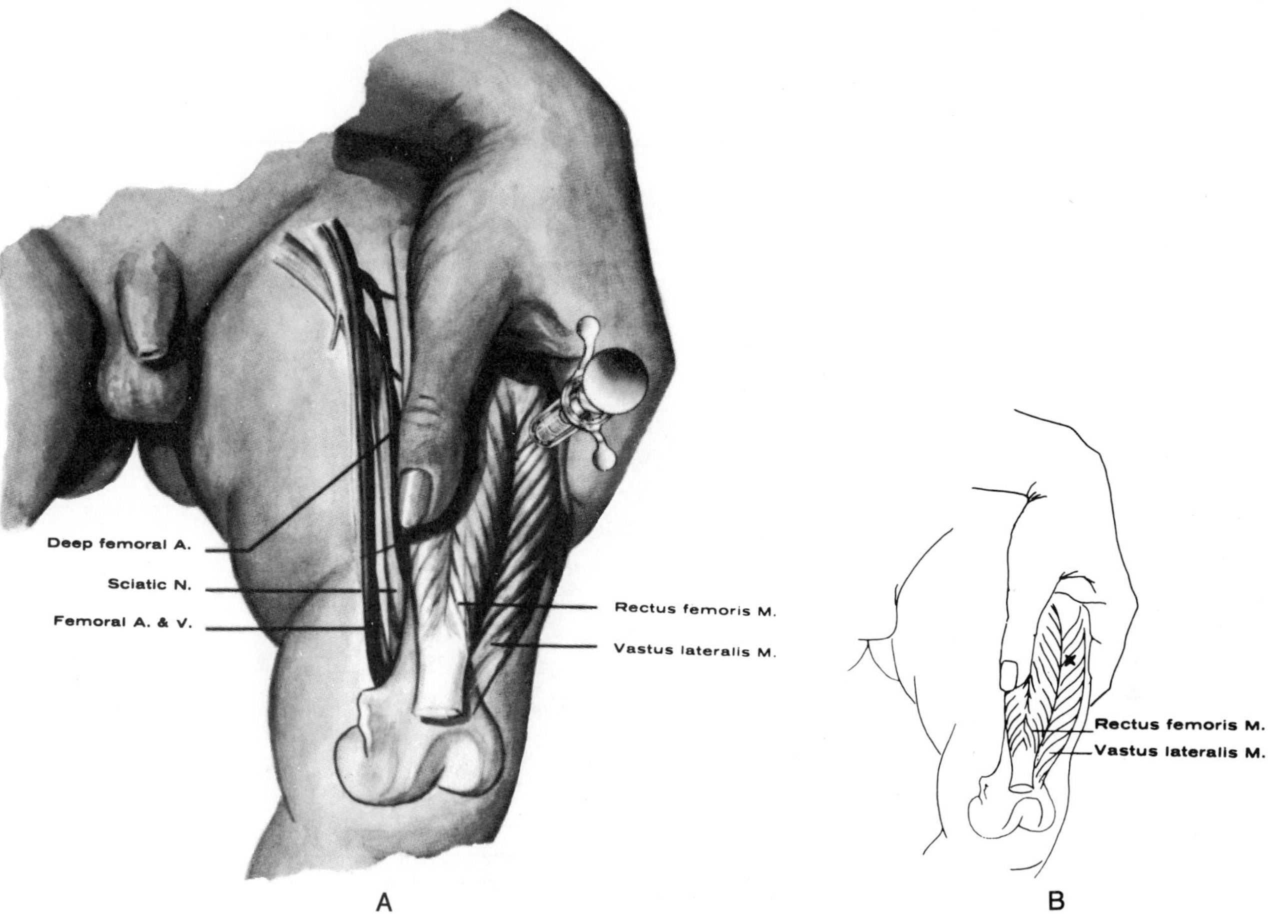

FIGURE 17–7. *A,* The proper insertion of the needle into the vastus lateralis intramuscular injection site. *B,* To compress the muscle tissue, grasp the thigh of an infant or young child when administering an injection into the vastus lateralis site. (Both figures courtesy of Wyeth Laboratories, Philadelphia, Pennsylvania.)

injection in this area, it is recommended that this site not be used until the child has been walking for at least a year (Fig. 17–6).

The vastus lateralis muscle site is recommended instead in infants and young children. It is located on the anterior surface of the midlateral thigh, away from major nerves and blood vessels, and it is large enough to accommodate the injected medication (Fig. 17–7). The length of the needle used depends on the overall size of the thigh. It should be long enough to penetrate the muscle belly for proper absorption to take place. A 1-inch needle is often utilized. To administer the injection, the infant is placed on his or her back. The thigh is grasped in order to compress the muscle tissue and to stabilize the extremity. The injection is administered following the procedure outlined in Chapter 8 (Procedure 8-6: Administering an Intramuscular Injection).

The deltoid muscle, another injection site in infants and young children, is shallow and can accommodate only a very small amount of medication. In addition, repeated injections to this site are painful. As during an injection into the vastus lateralis, the muscle mass should be grasped at the injection site and compressed between the thumb and fingers. The needle should be inserted pointing slightly upward toward the shoulder (Fig. 17–8).

After giving the injection, the medical assistant or the child's parent should hold the infant and show approval so that the child associates something other than pain with this procedure.

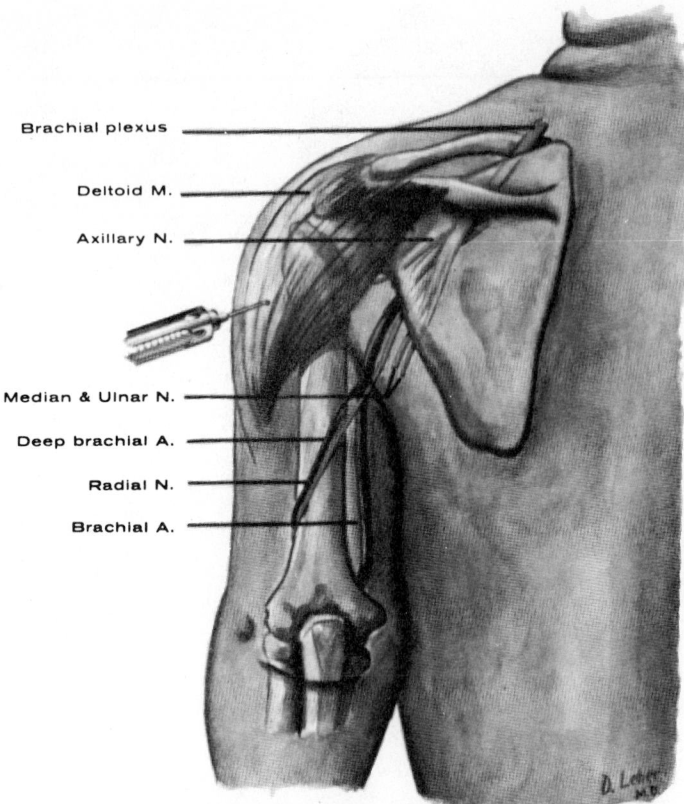

FIGURE 17–8. The proper insertion of the needle into the deltoid intramuscular injection site. (Courtesy of Wyeth Laboratories, Philadelphia, Pennsylvania.)

Immunizations

Immunity is the resistance of the body to the effects of harmful agents such as pathogenic microorganisms or their toxins. The process of becoming immune or rendering an individual immune through the use of a vaccine or toxoid is known as active, artificial *immunization.* Immunizations build up the body's defenses and protect an individual from attack by certain infectious diseases. Common immunizations administered to infants and children include the following: diphtheria and tetanus toxoids combined with pertussis vaccine; trivalent oral polio vaccine; and measles (rubeola), mumps, and rubella combined vaccines. Prevention of disease is one of the most important goals in the care of children.

Immunizations should be administered to infants and young children during well-child visits according to an immunization schedule. The American Academy of Pediatrics recommends following the schedule outlined in Table 17–1. This schedule is intended as a guide to be used with any modifications needed to meet the requirements of an individual or group.

Medical assistants should be completely familiar with each type of immunization that is given. They should have a knowledge of its use, precautions to be taken, common side effects and adverse reactions, the route of administration, the dosage, and the method of storage. The drug manufacturer includes a package insert with each vaccine or toxoid that contains valuable information about the drug. Drug references, such as the *Physician's Desk Reference,* can also be utilized to locate information on immunizations.

Once the immunization has been given, the medical assistant should make sure to record the information on the patient's chart. Included should be the date and time, the name of the medication, the dosage given, the route of administration, the injection site used (if applicable), and any significant observations or patient reactions. The medical assistant should place his or her initials next to the entry.

TABLE 17-1. Recommended Schedule for Active Immunization of Normal Infants and Children

2 mo	DTP[1]	TOPV[2a]
4 mo	DTP	TOPV
6 mo	DTP	
1 yr		Tuberculin test[3]
15 mo	Measles,[4] rubella[4]	Mumps[4]
1½ yr	DTP	TOPV
4–6 yr	DTP	TOPV
14–16 yr	Td[5]—repeat every 10 years	

[1] DTP—diphtheria and tetanus toxoids combined with pertussis vaccine.

[2a] TOPV—trivalent oral poliovirus vaccine. This recommendation is suitable for breast-fed as well as bottle-fed infants.

[3] Frequency of repeated tuberculin tests depends on risk of exposure of the child and on the prevalence of tuberculosis in the population group. For the pediatrician's office or outpatient clinic, an annual or biennial tuberculin test, unless local circumstances clearly indicate otherwise, is appropriate. The initial test should be done at the time of, or preceding, the measles immunization.

[4] May be given at 15 months as measles-rubella or measles-mumps-rubella combined vaccines.

[5] Td—combined tetanus and diphtheria toxoids (adult type) for those over 6 years of age, in contrast to diphtheria and tetanus (DT) toxoids, which contain a larger amount of diphtheria antigen. *Tetanus toxoid at time of injury:* For clean, minor wounds, no booster dose is needed by a fully immunized child, unless more than 10 years have elapsed since the last dose. For contaminated wounds, a booster dose should be given if more than 5 years have elapsed since the last dose.

Concentration and Storage of Vaccines: Because the concentration of antigen varies in different products, the manufacturer's package insert should be consulted regarding the volume of individual doses of immunizing agents. Because biologics are of varying stability, the manufacturer's recommendations for optimal storage conditions (e.g., temperature, light) should be carefully followed. Failure to observe these precautions may significantly reduce the potency and effectiveness of the vaccines.

From American Academy of Pediatrics: *Active Immunization Procedures. Report of the Committee on Infectious Diseases.* 18th edition, 1977.

It is helpful for parents to have an immunization record card (Fig. 17–9). They should be encouraged to bring this card on each visit so that their child's immunizations can be recorded. It is important for parents to understand the benefits of having their children protected against infectious diseases. They should also be informed of the possible side effects from the immunization and given instructions for responding to them if they occur.

The PKU Screening Test

Phenylketonuria (PKU) is a congenital hereditary disease caused by a lack of the enzyme *phenylalanine hydroxylase.* This enzyme is needed to convert phenylalanine, an amino acid, into tryosine which is necessary for normal metabolic functioning. Without this enzyme, phenylalanine accumulates in the blood and, if left untreated, results in mental retardation and other abnormalities such as tremors and poor muscular coordination. In most cases, upon early detection, a special low-phenylalanine diet and close periodic monitoring can prevent adverse effects. Normal development usually occurs if treatment is started before the child reaches 3 to 4 weeks of age.

Phenylalanine can be detected in the blood of an abnormal child once the child has been on a breast or formula milk intake for several days. Most states require, by law, that infants undergo PKU screening. Although PKU is not a common condition (affecting 1 in every 10,000 births), early diagnosis and treatment lead to a better patient prognosis. Infants on formula can be tested earlier than breast-fed babies because formula contains phenylalanine whereas the "first breast-milk" or colostrum does not. Therefore the test results of breast-fed babies are usually invalid until the mother begins producing milk.

FAMILY IMMUNIZATION RECORD Metropolitan

- Ask your doctor when shots are due.
- When shots are given, have your doctor enter dates under child's name.

SHOTS FOR ▼	CHILD'S NAME ▶				
• DIPHTHERIA • TETANUS • WHOOPING COUGH One immunization (one shot each date) can immunize for all three if doctor recommends.	AT AGE 2 MOS.*				
	2 MOS. LATER				
	2 MOS. LATER				
	12 MOS. LATER				
	BOOSTER 4-6 YRS. OLD				
• POLIO One oral immunization each date.	AT AGE 2 MOS.*				
	2 MOS. LATER				
	2 MOS. LATER				
	12 MOS. LATER				
	BOOSTER 4-6 YRS. OLD				
•MEASLES •MUMPS •RUBELLA (German measles) Triple immunization (one shot for all three). Measles booster at 15 mos. if first immunized before 1 year.	AFTER 1 YEAR OLD				
	AFTER 1 YEAR OLD				
	AFTER 1 YEAR OLD				
	*For children already beyond infancy, don't delay. See your physician and start series now.				

FIGURE 17–9. Parents should maintain an up-to-date immunization record for each child in their family. (Courtesy of the Metropolitan Life Insurance Company.)

PKU testing is performed on either the urine or blood of an infant within 2 to 7 days after birth. The testing procedure considered most accurate and used most often is the blood phenylalanine test performed on capillary blood obtained from the plantar surface of the infant's heel. The blood specimen is placed on a special filter paper attached to the PKU test card (Fig. 17–10) and mailed to an outside laboratory for analysis.

DO NOT WRITE IN BLUE SHADED AREAS - DO NOT WRITE ON BARCODE

CC040H1088462C

ALL INFORMATION MUST BE PRINTED

BIRTHDATE: / / MM/DD/YY TIME: : (USE 24 HOUR TIME ONLY)
BABY'S NAME: (last, first)
HOSPITAL PROVIDER NUMBER: (MANDATORY)
HOSPITAL NAME:
MOTHER'S NAME: (last, first, initial)
MOTHER'S ID: BABY'S ID:
MOTHER'S ADDRESS:
MOTHER'S PHONE: ( ) -
SPECIMEN DATE: / / MM/DD/YY TIME: : (USE 24 HOUR TIME ONLY)
PHYSICIAN NAME:
PHYSICIAN ADDRESS:
CITY: OHIO ZIP: -
PHYSICIAN PHONE NUMBER: ( ) -
PHYSICIAN PROVIDER NUMBER: (MANDATORY)
ODH ONLY: ☐ SPECIAL:

ODH COPY

TEST RESULTS:
☐ SCREENING TEST NORMAL FOR: PKU, HOM, GAL, HYPOTHYROIDISM
☐ SCREENING TEST NORMAL FOR: PKU, AND HOM ONLY
☐ SCREENING TEST NORMAL: ☐ PKU ☐ HOM ☐ GAL ☐ HYPOTHYROIDISM
☐ SCREENING TESTS ABNORMAL:
SEE FOOTNOTE ________ ON BACK
☐ SPECIMEN REJECTED FOR REASON:

BABY SEX: ☐ MALE ☐ FEMALE
BIRTH WEIGHT: GRAMS
PREMATURE: ☐ YES ☐ NO
ANTIBIOTICS: ☐ YES ☐ NO
TRANSFUSION: ☐ YES ☐ NO
SPECIMEN: ☐ FIRST ☐ SECOND
SUBMITTOR: ☐ HOSPITAL ☐ PHYSICIAN ☐ HEALTH DEPARTMENT ☐ OTHER: (name below)

HEA 2518

FILL ALL CIRCLES WITH BLOOD
BLOOD MUST SOAK COMPLETELY THROUGH
DO NOT APPLY BLOOD TO THIS SIDE

FIGURE 17–10. PKU test card.

PROCEDURE 17-4
PKU SCREENING TEST

1. **PROCEDURAL STEP.** Wash the hands.

2. **PROCEDURAL STEP.** Assemble the equipment. The equipment includes an **alcohol pledget, cotton balls,** a **sterile lancet, clean gloves,** and the **PKU test card** and **mailing envelope.** Complete the information section of the PKU card.

3. **PROCEDURAL STEP.** Select an appropriate puncture site. The lateral and medial curves of the plantar surface of the heel can be used.
PRINCIPLE. The lateral and medial curves are used to avoid calcaneal complications.

4. **PROCEDURAL STEP.** Cleanse the puncture site with an alcohol pledget and allow it to dry.

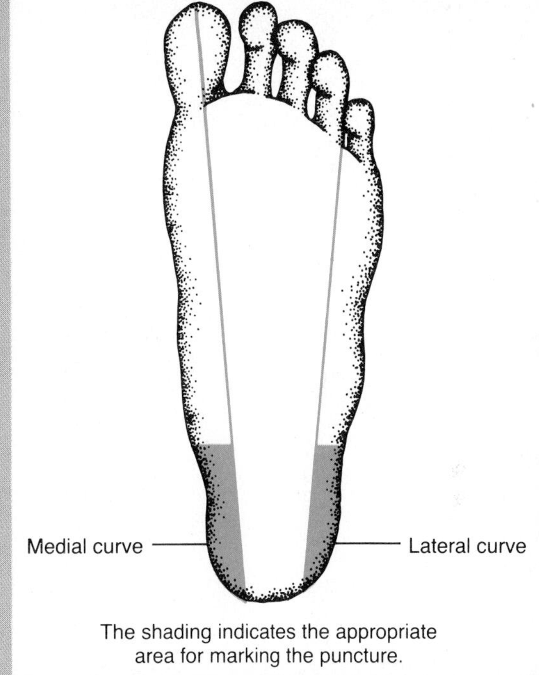

The shading indicates the appropriate area for marking the puncture.

5. **PROCEDURAL STEP.** Apply gloves. Grasp the infant's foot around the heel and, without touching the cleansed site, make a puncture with the sterile lancet. The puncture should be made at a right angle to the lines of the skin and be approximately 2 to 3 mm deep.
PRINCIPLE. Touching the site after cleansing will contaminate it and the cleansing process will have to be repeated.

6. **PROCEDURAL STEP.** Wipe away the first drop of blood with a cotton ball.
PRINCIPLE. The first drop of blood is diluted with alcohol and tissue fluid and is not a suitable specimen.

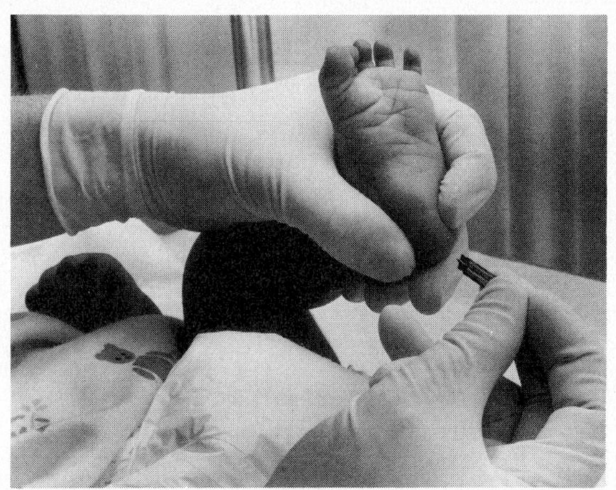

Continued

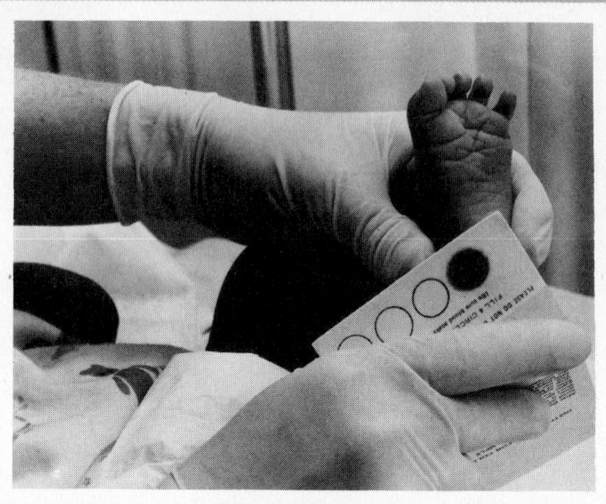

7. **PROCEDURAL STEP.** Use the second drop of blood for the test by placing the backside of the filter paper (side opposite the circles) against the baby's heel and exerting gentle pressure without excessively squeezing the heel.

PRINCIPLE. Excessive squeezing will cause dilution of the blood sample with tissue fluid leading to inaccurate test results.

8. **PROCEDURAL STEP.** Completely fill each of the circles on the PKU test card with a large drop of blood. The proper amount of specimen is obtained when the blood can be observed soaking completely through the filter paper from one side to the other.

PRINCIPLE. The circles must be completely filled to ensure enough of a blood sample to perform the test. Most repeat tests are required because of an inadequate blood specimen.

9. **PROCEDURAL STEP.** Hold a piece of gauze or cotton over the puncture site and apply pressure to control the bleeding. Remain with the infant until the bleeding stops.

10. **PROCEDURAL STEP.** Remove the gloves and wash hands.

11. **PROCEDURAL STEP.** Allow the test card to dry for 2 hours at room temperature on a nonabsorbent surface. Cards should not be stacked together while drying.

12. **PROCEDURAL STEP.** After the blood is completely dry, place the test card in its protective envelope and mail it to an outside laboratory for testing within 48 hours.

PRINCIPLE. The test card should be mailed within 48 hours to ensure accurate test results.

13. **PROCEDURAL STEP.** Record the procedure in the patient's chart. Include the patient's name, the date and time, the type of procedure (collection of a capillary blood specimen for PKU screening), the puncture site location, and any unusual patient reactions. Place your initials next to the recording.

Record data below.

DATE	TIME	PATIENT'S NAME	RECORDING

Study Questions

1. What are the two categories of pediatric patient office visits? What functions are performed during each?
2. Why is it important to measure the child's weight and height during each office visit?
3. What is the purpose of performing the PKU screening test?

• VOCABULARY •

atypical (a-tip' i-kal)—Deviation from the normal.

adnexal (ad-nek' sal)—Adjacent.

cytology (si-tol' o-je)—The science that deals with the study of cells, including their origin, structure, function, and pathology.

dilation and curettage (di-la' shun and ku" rē-tahzh')—The process of expanding the opening of the uterus to permit scraping of its walls; also called D and C.

endocervix (en" do-ser' viks)—The mucous membrane lining the cervical canal.

exfoliated cells (eks-fo" le-a' ted selz)—Cells that have been sloughed off from the surface of tissues into the secretions bathing those tissues.

external os (eks-ter' nal os)—The opening of the cervical canal of the uterus into the vagina.

gynecology (gi" nĕ-kol' o-je)—The branch of medicine that deals with the diseases of the reproductive organs of women.

internal os (in-ter' nal os)—The internal opening of the cervical canal into the uterus.

perineum (per" i-ne' um)—The external region between the vaginal orifice and the anus in a female and between the scrotum and the anus in a male.

vulva (vul' vah)—The region of the external genital organs in the female.

COMPETENCIES

After completing this unit, you should be able to demonstrate the proper procedure to perform the following:

1. Instruct an individual in the procedure for a breast self-examination.
2. Prepare a patient for a gynecologic examination.
3. Assist the physician with a gynecologic examination.
4. Complete a cytology laboratory requisition for a Papanicolaou test.

LEARNING OBJECTIVES

After completing this unit, you should be able to do the following:

1. Define the terms listed in the vocabulary.
2. List the parts of the pelvic examination.
3. Explain the purpose of performing each of the following: breast examination; inspection of the external genitalia, vagina, and cervix; Papanicolaou test; bimanual pelvic examination; and rectal-vaginal examination.
4. List and explain the five classifications for the results of the Pap smear test.
5. Explain the methods used to identify each of the following vaginal infections and the supplies required for the collection and evaluation of each: trichomoniasis, candidiasis, gonorrhea, and chlamydia.

The Gynecologic Examination

Gynecology

Gynecology is the branch of medicine that deals with disease of the reproductive organs of women. Gynecologic examinations are frequently and routinely performed in the medical office and generally include a breast and a pelvic examination. The gynecologic examination may be included as part of the physical examination or may be performed by itself. The purpose of the gynecologic examination is to assess the health status of the female reproductive organs in order to detect the early signs of disease, leading to early diagnosis and treatment. Although assisting with the gynecologic examination is a routine procedure for the medical assistant, the patient may not consider it a routine examination. The medical assistant should fully explain the procedure and offer to answer any questions to reduce the patient's possible, apprehension or embarrassment.

The Breast Examination

The physician generally begins with the breast examination. The medical assistant helps the patient into the horizontal recumbent (or supine) position. The physician inspects the breasts for any localized redness or inflammation. The nipples are checked for abnormalities such as bleeding or discharge, and the breasts and axillary lymph nodes are palpated for lumps.

The patient should know how to examine her breasts at home for the presence of lumps. Most breast cancers are first discovered by women themselves. The medical assistant may be responsible for instructing the patient in this procedure. The American Cancer Society recommends that a woman examine her breasts monthly, approximately 1 week after the menstrual period, when the breasts are usually not tender or swollen. Figure 17–11 demonstrates the procedure for performing a breast self-examination. If a lump or discharge is discovered, the woman should schedule an appointment with her physician as soon as possible. Most breast lumps are not cancerous, but the physician is the one to make that diagnosis.

The Pelvic Examination

The most common position for the pelvic examination is the dorsal lithotomy position. The patient should lie on the table on her back, with her feet in the stirrups and her buttocks at the bottom edge of the table. The stirrups should be level with the examining table and pulled out approximately 1 foot from the edge of the table. The patient's knees should be bent and relaxed, and her thighs should be rotated outward as far as is comfortable. This position helps to relax the vulva and perineum and facilitates insertion of the vaginal speculum. The patient should be properly draped to reduce exposure and to provide warmth. The dorsal lithotomy position is difficult to maintain, and the patient should not be placed in this position until the physician is ready to begin the examination. The medical assistant can help the patient relax her abdominal muscles by telling her to breathe deeply, slowly, and evenly through the mouth during the examination. If the patient is relaxed, it is easier for the physician to insert the vaginal speculum and to perform the bimanual pelvic examination; it is also more comfortable for the patient. It is recommended that the medical assistant remain in the room during the pelvic examination to provide legal protection for the physician, to reassure the patient, and to assist the physician.

The pelvic examination consists of several parts. The physician begins the examination with inspection of the external genitalia. The vulva is inspected for swelling, ulceration, or redness.

How to examine your breasts

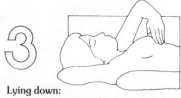

In the shower:

Examine your breasts during bath or shower; hands glide easier over wet skin. Fingers flat, move gently over every part of each breast. Use right hand to examine left breast, left hand for right breast. Check for any lump, hard knot or thickening.

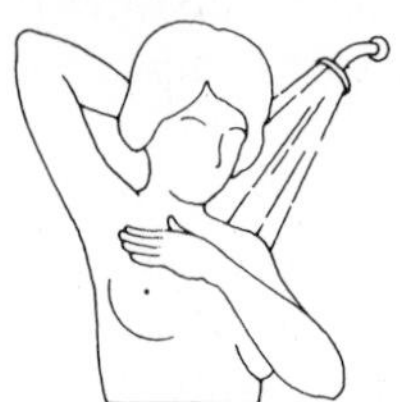

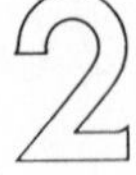

Before a mirror:

Inspect your breasts with arms at your sides. Next, raise your arms high overhead. Look for any changes in contour of each breast, a swelling, dimpling of skin or changes in the nipple.

Then, rest palms on hips and press down firmly to flex your chest muscles. Left and right breast will not exactly match—few women's breasts do.

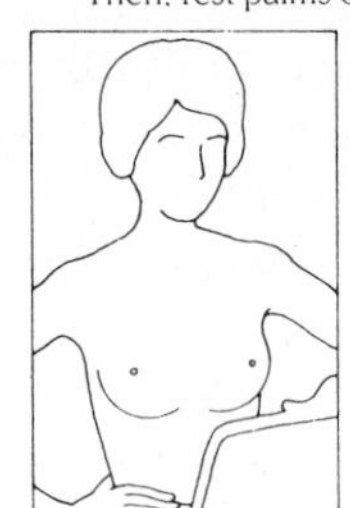

Regular inspection shows what is normal for you and will give you confidence in your examination.

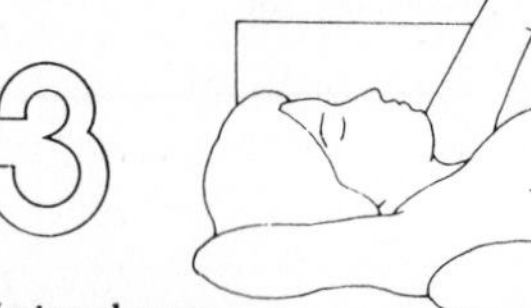

Lying down:

To examine your right breast, put a pillow or folded towel under your right shoulder. Place right hand behind your head—this distributes breast tissue more evenly on the chest. With left hand, fingers flat, press gently in small circular motions around an imaginary clock face. Begin at outermost top of your right breast for 12 o'clock, then move to 1 o'clock, and so on around the circle back to 12. A ridge of firm tissue in the lower curve of each breast is normal. Then move in an inch, toward the nipple, keep circling to examine *every part of your breast*, including nipple. This requires at least three more circles. Now slowly repeat procedure on your left breast with a pillow under your left shoulder and left hand behind head. Notice how your breast structure feels.

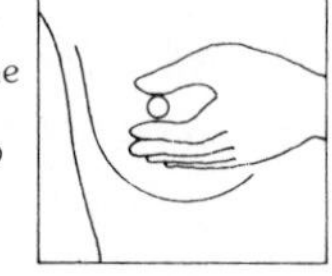

Finally, squeeze the nipple of each breast gently between thumb and index finger. Any discharge, clear or bloody, should be reported to your doctor immediately.

FIGURE 17–11. Breast self-examination. (Courtesy of American Cancer Society, Inc., © 1975.)

Next, the physician inserts a vaginal speculum into the vagina. Specula are available in two forms—metal and plastic. Metal specula are reusable and therefore must be sanitized and sterilized after each use. Plastic specula are disposable and are designed for one use only. Vaginal specula come in three sizes: small, medium, and large. The physician determines the size required based on the physical and sexual maturity of the patient. The function of the speculum is to hold the walls of the vagina apart to allow visual inspection of the vagina and cervix (Fig. 17–12). If a Papanicolaou (Pap) smear or a specimen for microbiologic examination is to be obtained, the speculum should not be lubricated because this would interfere with the test results. It should be warmed before use by moistening it with warm water, by placing it on a heating pad, or by storing it in an examining table that has a warming drawer. Moistening the speculum helps to lubricate it, which allows easier insertion when a lubricant cannot be used. The physician inspects the vagina and cervix for color, lacerations, ulcerations, tenderness, nodules, or discharge. If an abnormal discharge is present, the physician obtains a specimen for microbiologic examination. Examples of pathologic conditions producing a discharge include vaginal infections such as *trichomoniasis, candidiasis, gonorrhea,* and *chlamydia.* The Pap test and the collection of a specimen for detection of the presence of a vaginal infection are described in more detail below.

The Papanicolaou Test

A Pap test is usually included as part of the pelvic examination. It is a simple and painless cytologic screening test named after its discoverer, Dr. George Papanicolaou. It is used for early detection of precancerous or cancerous conditions of the cervix and endometrium and makes early treatment possible, which may lead to a cure. The American Cancer Society recommends that women age 20 and older (or

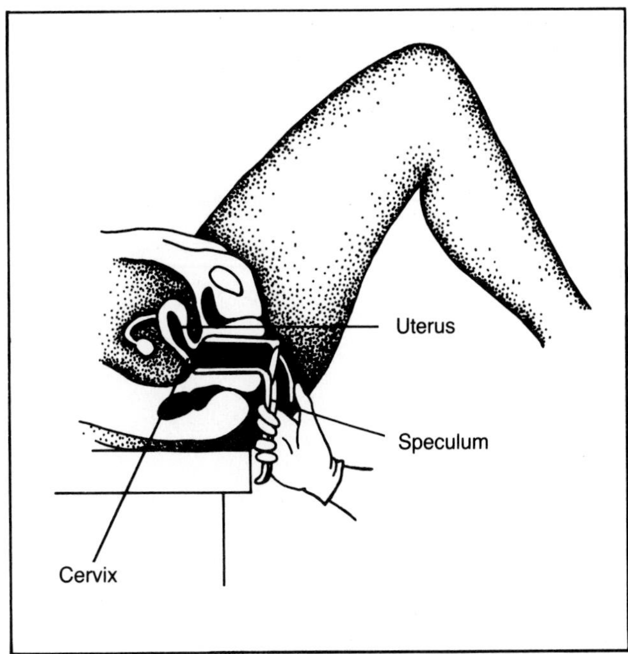

FIGURE 17–12. Insertion of the vaginal speculum for visualization of the vagina and cervix.

at the onset of sexual activity) have a Pap test performed every 3 years, except for those at high risk of cervical cancer; these women should undergo a Pap test more frequently.

The Pap test is based on the fact that tissues, including malignant uterine tumors, slough off cells into the surrounding cervical and vaginal mucus; these are known as *exfoliated* cells. A scraping of mucus containing these exfoliated cells is taken from the cervix and vagina, using a specially designed plastic or wooden spatula known as an Ayre spatula. The mucus is thinly spread on a glass slide having a frosted edge; smears should always be made on the slide surface that carries the frosted edge. This frosted edge permits the recording of data with a lead pencil. The medical assistant must label each slide according to the source of the specimen as follows: C (cervical), V (vaginal), and E (endocervical).

The physician obtains the cervical specimen by placing the **S**-shaped end of the Ayre spatula just inside the cervical canal at the cervical os and then rotating the blade 360 degrees over the surface of the cervix at the squamocolumnar junction, where cervical cancer is most often found (Fig. 17–13*A*). The physician then thinly spreads the mucus specimen on the appropriate slide. The physician obtains the vaginal specimen from the vaginal pool in the posterior fornix of the vagina (just below the cervix), using the rounded end of the wooden spatula and thinly spreading the mucus on another slide. The physician may want to collect a specimen from the cervical os; this is accomplished by taking a sterile cotton-tipped applicator and moistening it with normal saline, inserting it into the cervical os, and then rotating the applicator. The specimen obtained is known as an endocervical specimen (Fig. 17–13*B*). The physician may obtain an endocervical specimen in place of the vaginal specimen. This means that the physician collects an endocervical and cervical specimen for the Pap test. In collecting these specimens, the endocervical specimen is always obtained first because the collection of the cervical specimen may result in bleeding; these red blood cells would obscure the endocervical smear if it were to be collected second.

The smears must immediately be fixed by lightly spraying the slides with a commercial cytology spray fixative (brand names include Cytospray and Spray-

A. **Cervical Specimen**

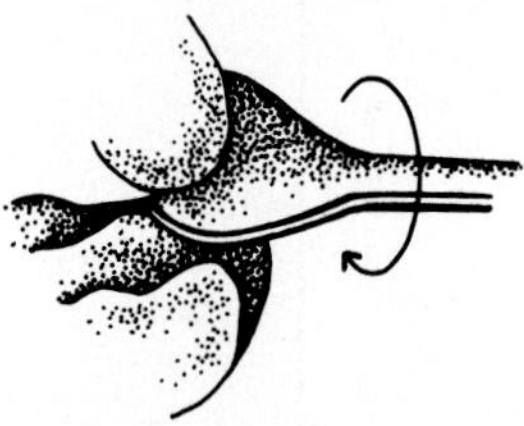

The S-shaped end of the spatula is placed inside the cervical canal and rotated 360 degrees over the surface of the cervix.

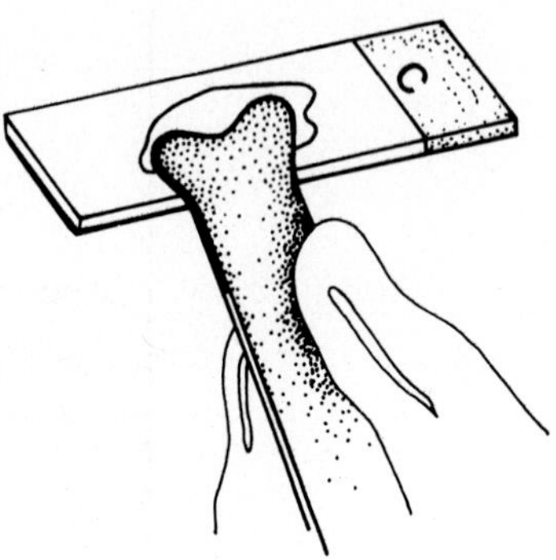

The sample is thinly smeared onto a glass slide.

B. **Endocervical Specimen**

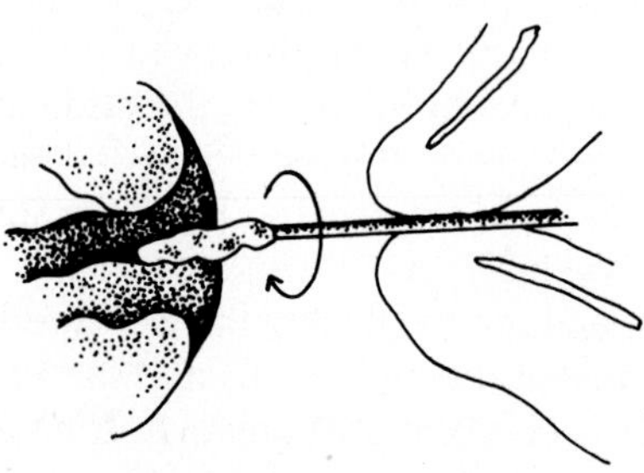

A cotton applicator is twirled inside the cervix to pick up some cells.

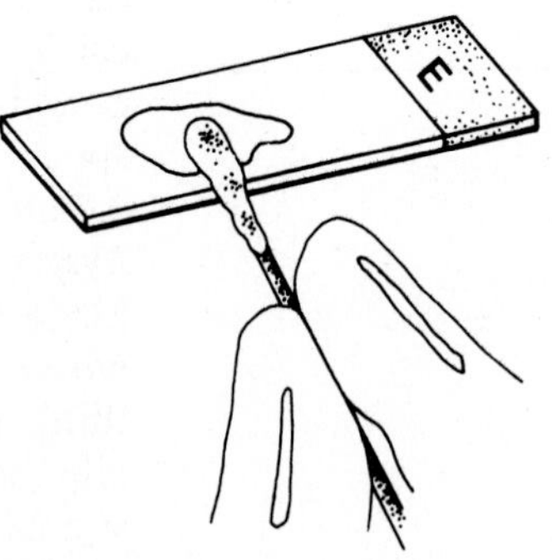

The sample is thinly smeared onto a glass slide.

FIGURE 17–13. Obtaining the Pap smear.

CYTOLOGY - PAP TECHNIQUE

PLEASE DO NOT WRITE IN THIS SPACE

PLEASE PRINT

Patient's Name ______ Date ______

☐ PAP ONLY
☐ PAP & M.I.
☐ ______

THIS SPACE FOR INFORMATION DESIRED ON REPORT.

Address Line Should Only Be Filled In When Address Is Desired On Report.

Separate Address Forms Required For Bill Patients.

PLEASE PENCIL PATIENT'S NAME ON FROSTED END OF SLIDE.

Physician's Name ______ 24716

Address ______

City ______ State ______ Zip ______

DIAGNOSTIC INFORMATION
(Please complete this section)

Patient's Age ______ Sex ______
Source of Material ______
Last Menstrual Period (First Day) ______
Vag. Bleeding ☐ Vag. Discharge ☐
No. of Pregnancies ______
Menopause ______
Hormone Therapy ______
Irradiation ______
Chief Complaint ______
Clinical Diagnosis ______
☐ Additional information or instructions to Laboratory on reverse side of form.

FIGURE 17–14. Cytology request form.

Cyte). The purpose of the fixative is to maintain the normal appearance of the cells, to protect the slides from contaminants in the air such as dust and bacteria, and to firmly attach the smear to the slide. The cytology fixative must be allowed to dry thoroughly; the slides are then ready for transport to an outside medical laboratory for evaluation.

A cytology request must accompany all Pap smears. It should include the physician's name and address; the date; the source of the specimen; the patient's name, address, age, and date of last menstrual period (abbreviated LMP); and other essential data as indicated in Figure 17–14, which is an example of a cytology request form. If the results of the Pap smear are abnormal, the physician may want to repeat the test. On repeat smears, the previous laboratory number and date must also be included on the request form.

The maturation index (MI) provides the physician with an endocrine evaluation of the patient, which can assist in evaluating the cause of infertility, menopausal or postmenopausal bleeding, or amenorrhea and can help assess the results of treatment with hormones. The maturation index refers to the percentage of parabasal, intermediate, and superficial cells present in the smear. If the physician orders a maturation index along with the Pap test, the medical assistant must be sure to indicate this on the cytology request by checking the appropriate square labeled Pap and MI (see Fig. 17–14). Numerous factors may affect the results of the maturation index; therefore, it is important to indicate on the cytology request the presence of abnormal bleeding, hormone treatment, or treatment with digitalis, corticosteroids, and thyroid medication.

To protect the slides during transport to an outside laboratory, they must be carefully placed in a slide container designed especially for this purpose and bearing a label indicating that the contents include a medical specimen. The smears are then mailed to a laboratory where they are stained and studied under a microscope by a pathologist for evidence of abnormal or cancerous cells.

Women should be instructed not to douche for 24 hours before having a Pap smear taken, because douching causes the cells that have been sloughed off to wash away, making the specimen nonrepresentative or invalid. A Pap smear must not be taken from a woman during her menstrual period, because the red blood cells obscure the smear and interfere with an accurate reading.

The pathologist examines the Pap smear and determines the results, which are recorded on a cytologic report form (Fig. 17–15) and returned to the medical office.

Report of Cytological Examination
Papanicolaou Technique

Laboratory I.D. | Patient Age | Date Received
Source of Material
Other Information
Patient Name | Physician Name

MATURATION INDEX

Estrogen (0-3+)	*Trichomonas*	% Superficial
Inflammation (0-3+)	*Candida*	% Intermediate
Blood (0-3+)	Erosion Cells	% Parabasal

Class I Negative...................... Absence of abnormal or atypical cytology.

Class II Doubtful...................... Atypical cytology not suggestive of malignancy.

Class III Suspicious.................... Cytology compatible with malignancy or other etiology.

Class IV Highly Susp. .... Cytology strongly suggestive of malignancy.

Class V Positive....................... Cytology practically conclusive of malignancy.

Class C .... Insufficient for examination.

REMARKS & RECOMMENDATIONS

screened by

FIGURE 17–15. Cytology report form.

Results of the Pap Test

The results of the Pap test will fall under one of the five cytologic classifications listed here.

Class I: Negative, absence of abnormal cells.

Class II: Atypical cytology, but no evidence of malignancy. The atypical cells may be due to inflammation, which causes them to change in character.

Class III: Atypical cytology, suggestive of but not conclusive for malignancy.

Class IV: Abnormal cytology, strongly suggestive of malignancy.

Class V: Abnormal cytology, positive for malignancy.

If the patient has an abnormal Pap smear, it doesn't necessarily mean that cancer is present, except in the case of Class V. The Class II category usually indicates the presence of a vaginal infection. Abnormal cytologic findings indicate that further tests should be done to determine whether a malignancy is present. Examples of additional procedures that may be performed include colposcopy and cervical biopsy.

Vaginal Infections

The vagina provides a warm, moist environment, which tends to encourage the growth of various organisms, resulting in a vaginal infection or ***vaginitis.*** If an unusual vaginal discharge is present, suggesting a vaginal infection, a specimen is obtained for culture or microscopic examination to identify the invading organism. A specimen of the discharge is collected at the medical office and is either evaluated there or placed on a culture or transport medium that is picked up or sent to an outside medical laboratory for evaluation. The patient should be instructed not to douche before coming to the medical office, because the physician will be unable to observe the discharge or to obtain a specimen for microbiologic analysis.

The medical assistant is responsible for assembling the appropriate supplies for the collection and evaluation of the suspected invading organism. She or he must be sure to label all specimens with the patient's name, the date, and the source of the specimen. If it will be transported to an outside medical laboratory for evaluation, a request form must be completed, including the source of the specimen, the physician's clinical diagnosis, the microbiologic examination requested, and any other pertinent information such as medications the patient is taking. The physician's clinical assessment of the patient's signs and symptoms along with the results of the laboratory evaluation of the specimen are used to diagnose the presence of a vaginal infection. Medical assistants should take precautions to protect themselves from being infected with a pathogen while assisting with the collection and evaluation of the specimen by practicing good techniques of medical asepsis. Methods used to identify the invading organism and the supplies required for the collection and evaluation of organisms causing common vaginal infections are presented in the following paragraphs.

Trichomoniasis

Trichomonas vaginalis, the causative agent of trichomoniasis (trich), is a pear-shaped protozoan possessing flagella, which allows for the motility of the organism (see Fig. 10–7). Trichomoniasis is most commonly spread through sexual intercourse. Symptoms of this infection include a profuse frothy vaginal discharge that is usually yellowish green in color, itching and irritation of the vulva and vagina, and dysuria. The cervix may exhibit red spots, a condition known as "strawberry cervix." *Trichomonas* may be identified at the medical office by the preparation of a wet mount, which involves placing a small amount of the discharge on a microscope slide using a sterile swab, adding a drop of isotonic saline to it, and then placing a coverslip over the mixture to protect it. The slide is then examined under the microscope and observed for the presence of the lashing movements of the flagella and the motility of the organism. If the physician prefers to have an outside laboratory evaluate the specimen, it must be placed in a sterile culture tube containing isotonic saline; a brand name of a commercially available form is the Culturette. It is important that the specimen be transported as soon as possible to prevent it from dying, which would impede visualization of the motility of the organism.

The treatment of trichomoniasis involves the oral administration of metronidazole (Flagyl). Both the woman and her sexual partner must be treated at the same time to prevent reinfection, because the partner may harbor the organism without displaying noticeable symptoms. Trichomoniasis is often responsible for a Class II Pap smear.

Candidiasis

Candida albicans is a yeastlike fungus normally found in the intestinal tract and is therefore a frequent contaminant of the vagina; however, it usually does not produce symptoms indicating a vaginal infection. Conditions such as pregnancy, diabetes mellitus, and prolonged antibiotic therapy produce changes within the vagina that may precipitate a candidal infection of the vagina, commonly referred to as a yeast infection. Symptoms of candidiasis include white patches on the mucous membrane of the vagina along with a thick, odorless cottage cheese-like discharge. The discharge is extremely irritating and usually results in burning and pruritus. The patient generally experiences severe vulval irritation and dysuria.

Candida may be identified in the medical office by placing a specimen of the vaginal discharge on a slide using a sterile swab and adding a drop of a 10 to 20 per cent solution of potassium hydroxide (KOH). The KOH dissolves cellular debris present in the smear and allows for better visualization of yeast buds, spores, or hyphae (fungus filaments), indicating the presence of *Candida albicans.*

If the specimen is to be transported to a medical laboratory for identification, it must be placed on a transport medium to prevent drying and death; a commonly used medium is the Culturette.

The treatment of candidiasis generally involves mild acid (vinegar) douches and drug therapy with nystatin (Mycostatin) vaginal cream or suppositories. Candidiasis has a tendency to recur; therefore, the woman should be instructed to contact the medical office if the symptoms of the yeast infection reappear.

Gonorrhea

Neisseria gonorrhoeae, a gram-negative diplococcus, is the causative agent of gonorrhea, the most common venereal disease. Gonorrhea is an infection of the genitourinary tract that is transmitted through sexual intercourse.

Women who have contracted gonorrhea may be asymptomatic or may exhibit a purulent vaginal discharge. As the disease progresses, it may spread to the lining of the uterus, resulting in pelvic inflammatory disease (PID) with the symptoms of lower abdominal pain, fever, nausea, and vomiting. If gonorrhea is left undiagnosed or untreated, it could result in sterility.

Neisseria gonorrhoeae is a fastidious organism, meaning it is difficult to grow and requires specialized growth conditions; therefore, special precautions must be followed when culturing the organism to prevent it from dying. It does not survive for long on a swab placed in a transfer medium; therefore, a culture is the diagnostic procedure of choice for women. The physician collects the specimen from the endocervical canal using a sterile swab. Specimens from the vagina and rectum may also be collected. Because gonococcus is a fastidious organism, the specimen must be inoculated on the culture medium immediately after collection to prevent death of the organism. The medical assistant is responsible for removing the lid and holding the plate while the physician inoculates it. The lid must be removed during inoculation only; unnecessary removal results in contamination of the specimen with extraneous microorganisms.

The growing conditions for *Neisseria gonorrhoeae* must include an atmosphere of carbon dioxide (devoid of oxygen) as well as a specially enriched blood medium known as chocolate agar. Thayer-Martin medium contains chocolate agar, which should be kept refrigerated and then warmed to room temperature just before using to provide the proper temperature growth requirement. Using a cold medium results in the death of any gonococci present in the specimen. The physician inoculates the Thayer-Martin medium and then places it in an atmosphere of carbon dioxide. This may be accomplished by several different methods. In one, a Thayer-Martin plate containing a well is used. A carbon dioxide–

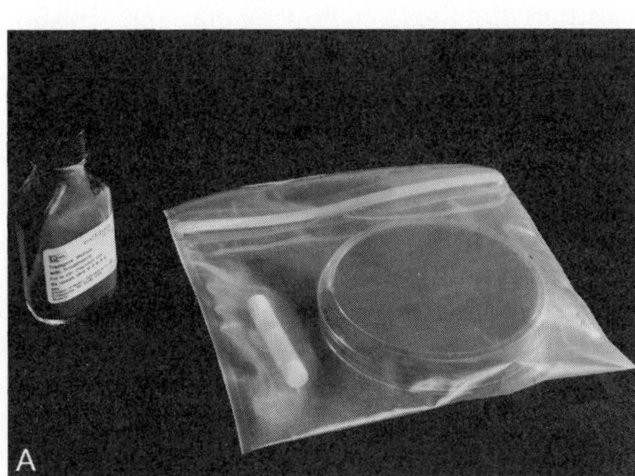

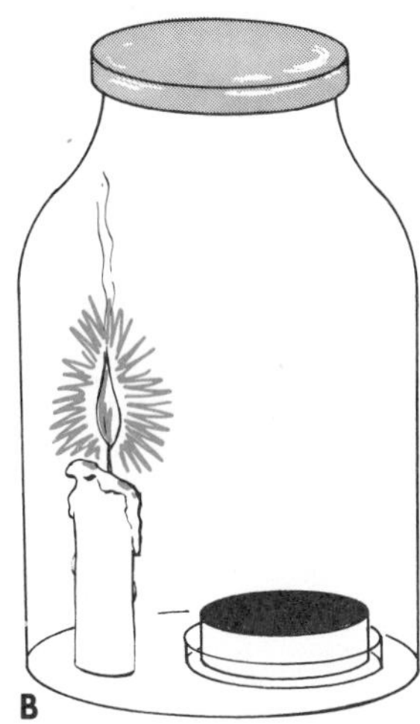

FIGURE 17–16. Growth requirements for *Neisseria gonorrhoeae. A,* The inoculated Thayer-Martin plate (right) is placed upside-down in a plastic bag along with a carbon dioxide–generating ampule. The bag is tightly sealed, and the ampule is crushed by pressing it between the sides of the bag with the fingers to provide a carbon dioxide atmosphere within the bag. Transgrow medium is contained in a bottle with flat sides (left). The bottle contains carbon dioxide and must not be turned upside-down when the cap is removed to prevent the carbon dioxide from flowing out. *B,* Candle jar with the inoculated Thayer-Martin plate placed upside-down in the jar. The lighted candle removes oxygen from the jar to provide the proper growth conditions for *Neisseria gonorrhoeae.*

generating tablet or ampule packed in a foil pouch is unwrapped and placed in this well, and the lid is placed back on the plate. The Thayer-Martin plate is then turned upside-down and placed in a gas-impermeable plastic bag, which is sealed tightly to maintain the carbon dioxide atmosphere, which allows for proper growth of the gonococci, and to prevent air from entering and killing the gonococci. If a plate is used that does not contain a well, the carbon dioxide tablet or ampule should be placed in the plastic bag (Fig. 17–16*A*).

Another way to provide a carbon dioxide atmosphere is by using a candle jar (Fig. 17–16*B*). The inoculated Thayer-Martin plate is placed upside down in the jar and a candle contained in the jar is lit; the lid is then screwed on tightly. Each time a new plate is introduced into the jar, the candle must be relit as described. The burning candle removes oxygen from the jar, thus providing an atmosphere of carbon dioxide; when the candle goes out, all of the oxygen has been removed. The reason for turning the plate upside down (with the agar facing up) is that otherwise water droplets may form on the top of the lid, owing to water condensation, and may drip down into the inoculated specimen, interfering with its growth and multiplication. If the Thayer-Martin medium is used, it is preferable that the specimen be transported as soon as possible to a medical laboratory; therefore, this method is best used when a local laboratory performs the evaluation. The inoculated Thayer-Martin plate is either stored at room temperature or placed in an incubator in its carbon dioxide environment (i.e., candle jar, plastic bag) until transport to the laboratory.

If the specimen is to be mailed to an outside reference laboratory, Transgrow medium is generally recommended for use in culturing it. Transgrow medium is a modified Thayer-Martin medium (MTM) contained in a bottle with flat sides (Fig. 17–16*A*). The medium must be stored in the refrigerator, then removed and allowed to warm to room temperature just before inoculation. The bottle already contains carbon dioxide to provide the proper atmospheric conditions for supporting the growth of the gonococci. Carbon dioxide is heavier than air, and therefore whenever the cap must be removed for inoculation of the specimen, the bottle must *not* be turned upside-down but held in an upright position to keep the carbon dioxide from flowing out. The cap should be removed only when the physician is ready to inoculate the specimen. It is important to recap the bottle as soon as possible to retain the carbon dioxide.

In males, gonorrhea can usually be identified with a gram-stained smear. The physician collects a specimen of the purulent urethral exudate and spreads the material on a slide. The slide should be allowed to air dry; a fixative should not be used. The laboratory stains the smear and then examines it for the presence of gram-negative intracellular diplococci, which indicates the presence of the gonococcus. A smear is not considered an accurate method of identification of *Neisseria gonorrhoeae* for women because other strains of gram-negative diplococci reside in the vagina that are not indicative of *Neisseria gonorrhoeae,* thereby confusing the diagnosis. Males who have contracted gonorrhea exhibit more symptoms than females, including urethritis, dysuria, and a profuse yellow purulent discharge.

Gonorrhea is usually treated with procaine penicillin G administered intramuscularly. Probenecid is administered by mouth ½ hour before the injection of penicillin. Probenecid delays the urinary excretion of penicillin, thereby maintaining higher and more prolonged blood levels of penicillin. Gonorrhea is one of the infectious diseases that must be reported to the local Department of Health, so that all contacts can be followed up and treated.

Chlamydia

Chlamydia is a gram-negative intracellular bacteria, meaning it grows and multiplies in the cytoplasm of the host cell. The name of the species affecting humans is *Chlamydia trachomatis.* Chlamydia is transmitted through sexual intercourse and in the past decade has become one of the most prevalent sexually transmitted diseases in the United States. Chlamydia often occurs in association with gonorrhea; approximately 25 to 50 per cent of patients with gonorrhea also have chlamydia.

Individuals with chlamydia may be asymptomatic, and therefore the patient may not be aware of having the condition. Because of this, the patient may not seek medical care until serious complications have occurred. Females with symptoms have itching and burning in the genital area, an odorless, thick, yellow-white vaginal discharge, dull abdominal pain, and bleeding between menstrual periods. The genital site most commonly affected in women is the cervix; chlamydial cervicitis can extend into the fallopian tubes resulting in salpingitis. Chlamydia is also thought to be a cause of PID, an inflammation of the cervix, uterus, fallopian tubes, and ovaries. If left untreated, a chlamydial infection in the female can lead to scarring in the fallopian tubes, infertility, and tubal pregnancy. In the male, symptoms of a chlamydial infection include dysuria and a watery discharge from the penis. A chlamydial infection in the male is often described as *nongonococcal urethritis* and, if left untreated, can lead to epididymitis and sterility.

Chlamydia can be diagnosed through cell culture isolation and examination of a stained smear, serum-antibody detection, and direct-antigen detection. The equipment and supplies needed for the tray set-up depend upon the method used to diagnose chlamydia. The cell culture isolation and direct antigen detection involve the collection of a specimen from the endocervix in the female, and the urethra in the male, using a sterile swab. The specimen must be placed in a tube containing a transport medium to preserve the specimen until it reaches the laboratory. The patient should be instructed not to void for 1 hour before the collection of the specimen to prevent any chlamydia organisms from being washed away. The serum antibody detection of chlamydia requires the collection of a blood specimen from the patient. Treatment of chlamydia consists of antibiotic drug therapy with tetracycline, doxycycline, erythromycin, or sulfonamides.

Bimanual Pelvic Examination

After obtaining the smear for the Pap test and any specimen required for the detection of a vaginal infection, the physician withdraws the speculum and performs a bimanual pelvic examination. The physician inserts the index and middle fingers of a lubricated gloved hand into the vagina. The fingers of the other hand are placed on the patient's lower abdomen. Between the two hands, the physician can palpate the size, shape, and position of the uterus and ovaries and detect tenderness or lumps (Fig. 17–17).

The last part of the pelvic examination is a rectal-vaginal examination. The physician inserts one gloved finger into the vagina and another gloved finger into the rectum to gain information about the tone and alignment of the pelvic organs and the adnexal region (the ovaries, fallopian tubes, and ligaments of the uterus). The presence of hemorrhoids, fistulas, and fissures can also be noted during the examination.

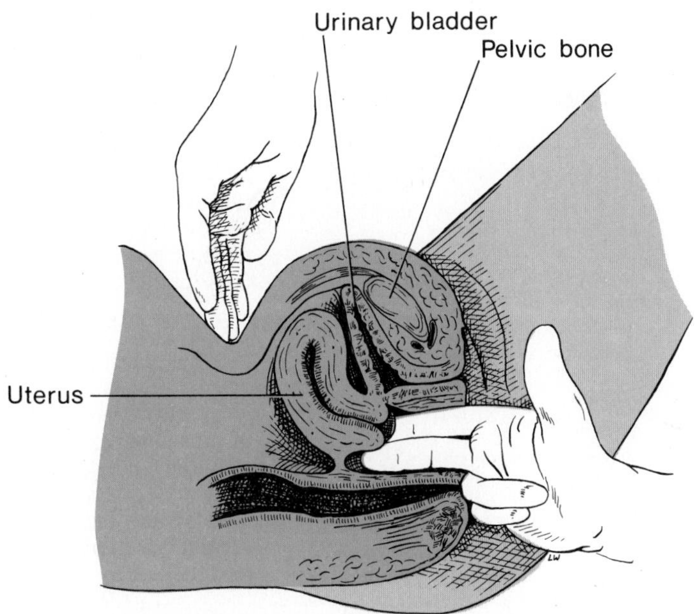

FIGURE 17–17. The bimanual pelvic examination.

PROCEDURE 17-5
ASSISTING WITH A GYNECOLOGIC EXAMINATION

The following procedure describes the medical assistant's role in assisting with a gynecologic examination consisting of a breast and pelvic examination, including a Pap smear, and the collection of a microbiologic specimen to detect the presence of a vaginal infection.

1. **PROCEDURAL STEP.** Wash the hands.

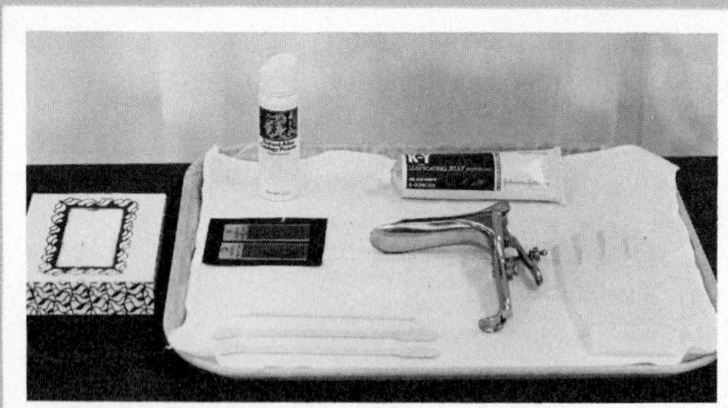

2. **PROCEDURAL STEP.** Assemble the equipment, which includes a **vaginal speculum of the appropriate size** (as designated by the physician), **Ayre spatula, clean glass slides with a frosted edge, spray fixative, nonsterile aseptic glove(s)**, a **lubricant**, and **tissues.** Using a lead pencil, identify the slides on the frosted edge with the patient's name, the date, and the source of the specimen. Use a C to identify the slide of the smear taken from the cervix and a V to identify the slide of the smear taken from the vagina. If an endocervical specimen is to be taken, a sterile cotton-tipped applicator and a slide labeled with an E (endocervical) must be included in the tray set-up. If a specimen is to be obtained to detect the presence of a vaginal infection, sterile swabs and the appropriate culture medium (at room temperature), transport medium, and slides must be assembled and properly labeled with the patient's name, the date, and the source of the specimen. Check the expiration date on the culture and transport media. Place the equipment and supplies within easy reaching distance of the physician.

3. **PROCEDURAL STEP.** Complete the cytology request form, making sure to include all essential information required by the outside medical laboratory. If the physician will be obtaining a vaginal specimen to be examined by an outside laboratory for the detection of a vaginal infection, an appropriate microbiologic laboratory request form must also be completed.

4. **PROCEDURAL STEP.** Identify the patient and explain the procedure. Ask the patient if she needs to empty her bladder before the examination. If a urine specimen is needed, she is requested to void into a specimen container.

   PRINCIPLE. An empty bladder makes the pelvic examination easier and is more comfortable for the patient.

5. **PROCEDURAL STEP.** Instruct and prepare the patient for the examination. The patient must completely undress and wear the examining gown with the opening positioned in front. Be sure to give complete and thorough instructions so the patient knows exactly what is expected of her. If the medical assistant senses that she may have trouble undressing, assistance should be offered.

   PRINCIPLE. Complete instructions reduce patient confusion.

6. **PROCEDURAL STEP.** Assist the patient onto the examining table, using the footstool. Position and drape her in a horizontal recumbent position for the breast examination.

7. **PROCEDURAL STEP.** Assist the patient into the dorsal lithotomy position for the pelvic examination. Properly drape the patient. Once the patient is positioned and draped, lower or push in the footboard (depending on the type of examining table). Adjust and focus the light for the physician. Reassure the patient and help her to relax the abdominal muscles during the examination by telling her to breathe deeply, slowly, and evenly through the mouth.
PRINCIPLE. Visualization of the vagina and cervix requires direct light. If the patient is relaxed, the examination proceeds more smoothly and is more comfortable for the patient.

8. **PROCEDURAL STEP.** Assist the physician as required for the pelvic examination. The medical assistant may be responsible for the following:

a. Warming the vaginal speculum before insertion by moistening it with warm water, by placing it on a heating pad, or by storing it in a warming drawer. Inserting a cold speculum into the vagina causes the patient discomfort and results in contraction of the vaginal muscles, making it difficult to insert the speculum.
b. Assisting the physician with the application of the gloves.
c. Immediately spraying the slides with a cytology spray fixative, following the directions on the spray container. The smears must be fixed immediately (within 10 seconds after collection) to maintain the normal appearance of the cells and to prevent the smears from being exposed to contaminants in the air. The medical assistant must be sure to hold the nozzle of the spray fixative the recommended distance from the slides (usually 5 to 6 inches). Holding the spray nozzle too close may result in blowing the cells off the slides. The slides should be sprayed lightly with a continuous motion from left to right, then right to left, and allowed to dry thoroughly, usually for 5 to 10 minutes.

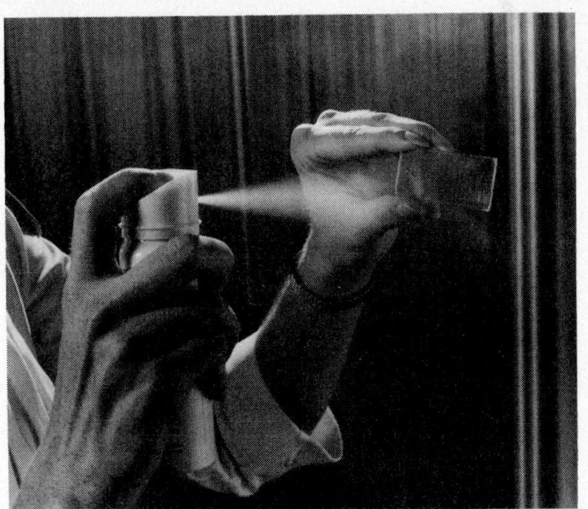

d. Assisting the physician with the collection of a vaginal specimen to detect the presence of a vaginal infection. The medical assistant will need to hold the appropriate medium and/or slide so that the physician can place the specimen on it. The medical assistant must be sure to follow the principles of medical asepsis during specimen collection to prevent infection with a pathogen.
e. Applying lubricant to the physician's glove for the bimanual and rectal examinations. Be careful not to allow the tube of lubricant to touch the physician's fingers to prevent contamination of the contents of the tube.
f. Preparing a wet mount of the vaginal specimen for viewing under the microscope by the physician to detect the presence of a vaginal infection.

Continued

9. **PROCEDURAL STEP.** After the examination, have the patient move back on the table (assist the patient if needed). Raise or pull out the footboard and remove both legs from the stirrups simultaneously. Allow the patient to rest for a minute in the recumbent position. Offer the patient tissues to remove excess lubricating jelly from the perineum. Help the patient into a sitting position, lower or push in the footboard, and assist the patient off the examining table so no falls will occur. Instruct the patient to get dressed, offering assistance if needed. Inform the patient of the method used by the medical office to relay test results.

PRINCIPLE. Patients (especially elderly ones) frequently become dizzy after being on the examining table and should be allowed to rest before sitting up.

10. **PROCEDURAL STEP.** Record information in the patient's chart as instructed by the physician. Be sure to include your initials next to the recording.

11. **PROCEDURAL STEP.** Prepare the Pap slides for transportation to the laboratory by placing them in a protective slide container. Be sure to include the completed cytology request form. If necessary, prepare any vaginal specimens collected (for the detection of a vaginal infection) for transport to an outside laboratory. Be sure to include the completed microbiologic laboratory request.

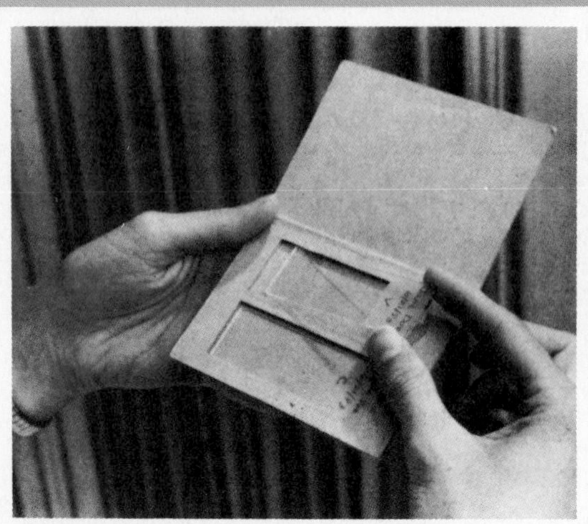

12. **PROCEDURAL STEP.** Clean the examining room in preparation for the next patient. Rinse the vaginal speculum in cold water to remove secretions or they will dry and be more difficult to remove later on. Then sanitize and sterilize the speculum when it is convenient to do so, according to the medical office policy.

Record data below.

DATE	TIME	PATIENT'S NAME	RECORDING

Study Questions

1. What are the parts of a pelvic examination?
2. What is the purpose of a Pap test?
3. What is the purpose of the bimanual pelvic examination?
4. What are the symptoms of each of the following vaginal infections: trichomoniasis, candidiasis, gonorrhea, and chlamydia?

COMPETENCIES

After completing this unit, you should be able to demonstrate the proper procedure to perform the following:

1. Complete a prenatal health history on a patient.
2. Prepare the patient and assist the physician with an initial prenatal examination.
3. Prepare the patient and assist the physician with a return prenatal examination.
4. Prepare the patient and assist the physician with a 6-weeks postpartum examination.

LEARNING OBJECTIVES

After completing this unit, you should be able to do the following:

1. Define the terms listed in the vocabulary.
2. Explain the purpose of prenatal care.
3. List the three different categories of medical office visits that provide prenatal and postpartum care to the pregnant woman.
4. Explain the purpose of each of the four components included in the first prenatal visit: prenatal record, initial prenatal examination, patient education, and laboratory tests.
5. Record the patient's pregnancy in terms of gravidity and parity.
6. Calculate the estimated date of confinement (EDC) using Nägele's rule and a gestation calculator.
7. List and explain the purpose of each procedure included in the initial prenatal examination.
8. List and explain the purpose of each laboratory test included in the prenatal laboratory work-up.
9. Explain the purpose of return prenatal visits.
10. List and explain the purpose of each of the procedures commonly included in the return prenatal examination.
11. Explain the purpose of the 6-weeks postpartum visit.
12. List and explain the purpose of each of the procedures commonly included in the 6-weeks postpartum examination.

• VOCABULARY •

abortion (ah-bor' shun)—The loss of a pregnancy before the stage of viability.

Braxton Hicks contractions (braks' ton hiks kon-trak' shuns)—Intermittent and irregular painless uterine contractions that occur throughout pregnancy. They occur more frequently toward the end of the pregnancy and are sometimes mistaken for true labor pains.

dilation (of the cervix) (di-la' shun)—The stretching of the external os from an opening a few millimeters in size to an opening large enough to allow the passage of an infant (approximately 10 cm).

EDC—Estimated date of confinement, or due date; so named because a long period of bed rest following childbirth used to be the norm.

effacement (i-fās' ment)—The thinning and shortening of the cervical canal from its normal length of 1 to 2 cm to a structure with paper-thin edges in which there is no canal at all. Effacement occurs late in pregnancy or during labor, or both. The purpose of effacement along with dilation is to permit the passage of the infant into the birth canal.

engagement (en-gāj' ment)—The entrance of the fetal head or the presenting part into the pelvic inlet.

fetal heart rate (fe' tal hart rāt)—The number of times the fetal heart beats per minute.

fetal heart tones (fe' tal hart tōnz)—The heart beat of the fetus as heard through the mother's abdominal wall.

fetoscope (fe' to-skōp)—An instrument for auscultation of the heart of the fetus.

fetus (fe' tus)—The child in utero, from the third month after conception to birth; during the first 2 months of development, it is called an embryo.

fundus (fun' dus)—The dome-shaped upper portion of the uterus between the fallopian tubes.

gestation (jes-ta' shun)—The period of intrauterine development from conception to birth; the period of pregnancy. The average pregnancy lasts about 280 days or 40 weeks from the date of conception to childbirth.

gravid (grav' id)—Pregnant.

gravida (grav' ĭ-dah)—A woman who is or has been pregnant.

gravidity (grah-vid' ĭ-te)—The total number of pregnancies a woman has had regardless of duration, including a current pregnancy.

high-risk (hī-risk)—Having an increased possibility of suffering harm, damage, or death.

infant (in' fant)—A child from birth to 1 year of age.

lochia (lo' ke-ah)—A discharge from the uterus after delivery consisting of blood, tissue, white blood cells, and some bacteria.

multipara (mul-tip' ah-rah)—A woman who has completed two or more pregnancies to the age of viability regardless of whether they ended in live infants or stillbirths.

multigravida (mul" tĭ-grav' ĭ-dah)—A woman who has been pregnant more than once.

nullipara (nuh-lip' ah-rah)—A woman who has not carried a pregnancy to the point of viability.

obstetrics (ob-stet' riks)—That branch of medicine concerned with the care of the woman during pregnancy, childbirth, and the postpartal period.

para (par' ah)—A term used to refer to past pregnancies that reached viability regardless of whether the infant was dead or alive at birth.

parity (par' ĭ-te)—The condition of having borne offspring who had attained the age of viability regardless of whether they were live infants or stillbirths.

pelvimetry (pel-vim' ĭ-tre)—Measurement of the capacity and diameter of the maternal pelvis, which helps to determine if it will be possible to deliver the infant through the vaginal route.

position (po-zish' un)—The relation of the presenting part of the fetus to the maternal pelvis.

postpartum (pōst-par' tum)—Occurring after childbirth.

Continued

pre-eclampsia (pre" e-klamp' se-ah)—A major complication of pregnancy of unknown cause characterized by increasing hypertension, albuminuria, and edema. If this condition is neglected or not treated properly, it may develop into eclampsia, which could cause maternal convulsions and coma. Eclampsia generally occurs between the twentieth week of pregnancy and the end of the first week postpartum.

prenatal (pre-na' tal)—Before birth.

presentation (prez" en-ta' shun)—The part of the fetus that is closest to the cervix and will be delivered first. A cephalic presentation is a delivery in which the fetal head is presenting against the cervix. A breech presentation is a delivery in which the buttocks or feet are presented instead of the head.

primigravida (pri" mi-grav' i-dah)—A woman who is pregnant for the first time (gravida I).

primipara (pri-mip' ah-rah)—A woman who has carried a pregnancy to viability regardless of whether the infant was dead or alive at birth (para I).

puerperium (pu" er-pe' re-um)—The period of time (usually 4 to 6 weeks) in which the uterus and the body systems are returning to normal following delivery.

quickening (kwik' en-ing)—The first movements of the fetus in utero as felt by the mother, which usually occurs between the sixteenth and twentieth weeks of gestation and are consistently felt thereafter.

sonography (so-nog' rah-fe)—A diagnostic aid in which high-frequency sound waves are directed toward a woman's abdomen. Sonography is used to detect the presence of pregnancy and to assess fetal maturity.

toxemia (tok-se' me-ah)—A pathologic condition occurring in pregnant women that includes pre-eclampsia and eclampsia. If pre-eclampsia goes undiagnosed or is not satisfactorily controlled, it could develop into eclampsia, characterized by convulsions and coma.

trimester (tri-mes' ter)—Three months, or one-third, of the gestational period of pregnancy.

Prenatal Care

Obstetrics

Obstetrics is the branch of medicine dealing with the supervision of women during pregnancy, childbirth, and the puerperium. *Prenatal* or *antepartal care* refers to the care of the pregnant woman before delivery of the infant. Prenatal care consists of a series of scheduled medical office visits for the promotion of the health of the mother and fetus through the prevention of disease and the provision of early detection, diagnosis, and treatment of problems common to pregnancy (e.g., anemia, urinary tract infection, and pre-eclampsia). Early detection of medical problems helps to prevent serious complications in the mother and/or fetus.

The medical office visits for providing prenatal and postpartal care to the pregnant woman can be grouped into three major categories as follows:

1. First prenatal visit.
2. Return prenatal visits.
3. Six-weeks postpartum visit.

Each of these categories and the responsibilities of the medical assistant during each is presented in this unit.

The First Prenatal Visit

The first prenatal visit generally occurs after the woman has missed her second menstrual period; if problems exist, the woman is seen after missing her first menstrual period. The first visit is often a stressful experience, and the medical assistant plays an important role in helping to relax the patient and relieve her anxiety.

The first prenatal visit requires more time than the subsequent or return prenatal visits; therefore, sufficient time should be scheduled to allow for a complete and accurate initial assessment of the pregnant woman. The components of the first prenatal visit vary, depending on the medical office, but generally include the following.

1. Completion of a prenatal record form.
2. Initial prenatal examination consisting of a complete physical examination: of particular importance are the breast, abdominal, and pelvic examinations. Pelvic measurements may also be taken at this time or during a return prenatal visit.
3. Prenatal patient education.
4. Laboratory tests.

Each component of the first prenatal visit is described in more detail on the following pages.

The Prenatal Record

The prenatal record provides information regarding the past and present health status of the patient and also serves as a data base and flow sheet for subsequent prenatal visits. The prenatal record is essential in helping to identify high-risk patients. The medical assistant is usually responsible for collecting a portion of the information required for the prenatal record. Many different types of printed prenatal record forms are available (see Fig. 17 – 18 for one example). The form utilized in your medical office will be based on physician preference and the method used for conducting the prenatal examination.

Obtaining and recording information in the prenatal record provides an excellent opportunity for the medical assistant to develop rapport with the patient. It is also an excellent time to relay information to her regarding various aspects of the prenatal and postnatal period such as an explanation of the changes taking place within her body, information relating to the Lamaze method of childbirth, the signs and symptoms of oncoming labor, nutrition of the infant (breast-feeding and bottle feeding), and care of the newborn. Providing a quiet setting free from

Prenatal Health History Summary

Date:

Patient's name ______

Age ____ Race ____ Religion ____ Marital status ____ Years married ____ Education ____ Occupation ____

Home address ____ Home tel. ____ Work tel. ____

Nearest relative ____ Relative's employer ____ Work tel. ____

Referring physician ____ Attending physician ____

PAST MEDICAL HISTORY	Patient	Family	Check and detail positive findings including date and place of treatment. Precede findings by reference number.
1. Congenital anomalies			
2. Genetic diseases			
3. Multiple births			
4. Diabetes mellitus			
5. Malignancies			
6. Hypertension			
7. Heart disease			
8. Rheumatic fever			
9. Pulmonary disease			
10. GI problems			
11. Renal disease			
12. Other urinary tract problems			
13. Genitourinary anomalies			
14. Abnormal uterine bleeding			
15. Infertility			
16. Venereal disease			
17. Phlebitis, varicosities			
18. Nervous/mental disorders			
19. Convulsive disorders			
20. Metabol./endocrine disorders			
21. Anemia/hemoglobinopathy			
22. Blood dyscrasias			
23. Drug addiction			
24. Smoking/alcohol			
25. Infectious diseases			
26. Operations/accidents			
27. Blood transfusions			
28. Other hospitalizations			
29. **No known disease**			

Sensitivities detail positive findings)

30.☐ **None known**
31.☐ Antibiotics
32.☐ Analgesics
33.☐ Sedatives
34.☐ Anesthesia
35.☐ Other

Preexisting Risk Guide

Indicates pregnancy/outcome at risk

36.☐ Age < 15 or > 35
37.☐ < 8th grade education
38.☐ Cardiac disease (class I or II)
39.☐ Tuberculosis, active
40.☐ Chronic pulmonary disease
41.☐ Thrombophlebitis
42.☐ Endocrinopathy
43.☐ Epilepsy (on medication)
44.☐ Infertility (treated)
45.☐ 2 abortions (spontaneous/induced)
46.☐ ≥ 7 deliveries
47.☐ Previous preterm or SGA infants
48.☐ Infants ≥ 4,000 gms
49.☐ Isoimmunization (ABO, etc.)
50.☐ Hemorrhage during previous preg.
51.☐ Previous preeclampsia
52.☐ Surgically scarred uterus
53.☐ ______

Indicates pregnancy/outcome at **high** risk

54.☐ Age ≥ 40
55.☐ Diabetes mellitus
56.☐ Hypertension
57.☐ Cardiac disease (class III or IV)
58.☐ Chronic renal disease
59.☐ Congenital/chromosomal anomalies
60.☐ Hemoglobinopathies
61.☐ Isoimmunization (Rh)
62.☐ Drug addiction/alcoholism
63.☐ Habitual abortions
64.☐ Incompetent cervix
65.☐ Prior fetal or neonatal death
66.☐ Prior neurologically damaged infant
67.☐ ______

Initial Risk Assessment

68.☐ No risk factors noted
69.☐ At risk
70.☐ At **high** risk

Signature

Menstrual History	Onset ___ age	Cycle q. ___ days	Length ___ days	Amount

Last contraceptive ☐ None

Type ______

Last used ______

PAST OBSTETRICAL HISTORY	Grav	Para	Pret	Abort	Live

No.	Month/year	Sex	Weight at birth	Wks. gest.	Hrs. in labor	Type of delivery	Details of delivery: Include anesthesia and maternal or newborn complications. Use Risk Guide numbers where applicable.
1							
2							
3							
4							
5							
6							
7							
8							

FIGURE 17–18. Example of a prenatal record form.

Illustration continued on opposite page

PRESENT PREGNANCY HISTORY

History Since LMP	Patient
1. Headaches	
2. Nausea/vomiting	
3. Abdominal pain	
4. Urinary complaints	
5. Vaginal discharge	
6. Vaginal bleeding	
7. Edema (specify area)	
8. Febrile episode	
9. Rubella exposure	
10. Other viral exposure	
11. Drug exposure	
12. Radiation exposure	
13. Other	

LMP	date	quality
EDC		

16. Medications Since LMP

(Rx, non-Rx, vitamins) ☐ **None**

Describe: ______________________

____

____

____

Initial Physical Examination	Height	Weight	Pregravid weight	B.P.	Pulse

SYSTEM	Normal	ABN	Check and detail all positive findings below. Use reference numbers.
17. Skin			
18. EENT			
19. Mouth			
20. Neck			
21. Chest			
22. Breast			
23. Heart			
24. Lungs			
25. Abdomen			
26. Musculoskeletal			
27. Extremities			
28. Neurologic			
Pelvic Examination			
29. Ext. genitalia			
30. Vagina			
31. Cervix			
32. Uterus (describe)			
33. Adnexa			
34. Rectum			
35. Other			

Bony Pelvis				
	36 Diag. conj.	37 Shape sacrum	38 S.S. notch	39 Ischial spines
	40 Pubic arch	41 Trans. outlet	42 Post sag. diam.	43 Coccyx

44. Classification: ☐ Gynecoid ☐ Android ☐ Anthropoid ☐ Platypelloid

45. Estimation: ☐ Adequate ☐ Borderline ☐ Contracted

Exam by:

FIGURE 17–18 *Continued*

Illustration continued on following page

INTERVAL PRENATAL HISTORY

Flow Chart

Date	Weight this visit	Blood pressure	Urine: Protein	Urine: Sugar	Est. weeks gestation (dates/size)	Fundal height	Fetal heart rate	Edema		PROGRESS NOTES	See Add Prog Note
		/			/						
		/			/						
		/			/						
		/			/						
		/			/						
		/			/						
		/			/						
		/			/						
		/			/						
		/			/						
		/			/						
		/			/						
		/			/						

Year | Pre-gravid

Risk Guide for Pregnancy and Outcome

Preliminary Risk Assessment (detail risk factors from the HHS below)

☐ (0) No risk factors noted
☐ (1) At risk
☐ (2) **High risk**

Continuing Risk Guide

Mo/day	Potential risk factors	Mo/day	**High** risk factors
/	3. Preg. without familial support	/	18. Diabetes mellitus
/	4. Second pregnancy in 12 months	/	19. Hypertension
/	5. Smoking (≥ 1 pack per day)	/	20. Thrombophlebitis
/	6. Rh negative (nonsensitized)	/	21. Herpes (type 2)
/	7. Uterine/cervical malformation	/	22. Rh sensitization
/	8. Inadequate pelvis	/	23. Uterine bleeding
/	9. Venereal disease	/	24. Hydramnios
/	10. Anemia (Hct < 30%:Hgb < 10%)	/	25. Severe preeclampsia
/	11. Acute pyelonephritis	/	26. Fetal growth retardation
/	12. Failure to gain weight	/	27. Premature rupt. membranes
/	13. Multiple pregnancy (term)	/	28. Multiple pregnancy (preterm)
/	14. Abnormal presentation	/	29. Low/falling estriols
/	15. Postterm pregnancy	/	30. Significant social problems
/	16.	/	31. Alcohol and drug abuse
/	17.	/	32.

FIGURE 17–18 *Continued*

distractions allows the patient the confidence to openly discuss areas of concern; this helps to assure a complete and accurate prenatal history. During the first prenatal visit, the medical assistant should relay his or her name and position to the patient to help build a supportive relationship with her as well as to allow the patient to ask for the medical assistant by name when contacting the medical office.

The prenatal record is similar to and contains much of the same information as the health history described in Chapter 3. Particular attention is given to factors that may influence the course of the pregnancy, as will be described in the following paragraphs.

Past Medical History

The *past medical history* focuses on those conditions that could affect the health of the mother and/or fetus such as kidney disease, heart disease, hypertension, venereal disease, phlebitis, diabetes, tuberculosis, endocrine disorders, drug allergies, alcohol and tobacco intake, drug addiction, and so on. In addition, the medical assistant solicits information from the patient regarding past immunizations and childhood diseases to provide the physician with the information needed to assess her antibody protection against such diseases. Rubella, if contracted during pregnancy, can be dangerous to the developing fetus; the earlier in pregnancy the infection occurs, the greater is the chance of birth defects. The infant may be born with heart defects, cataracts, mental retardation, and deafness. Patients who do not have antibody protection against rubella are given a rubella immunization within 6 weeks after delivery. The rubella vaccination is made from a live virus and therefore cannot be given to a pregnant woman because it may be harmful to the fetus. These patients should be told to avoid exposure to children with rubella during their pregnancy.

Menstrual History

A *menstrual history* is obtained from the patient, which includes the date of the onset of menstruation, the menstrual interval cycle, the duration, the amount of flow (recorded as small, moderate, or large), and any gynecologic disorders. The patient should be asked if she was using a method of contraception when she became pregnant. This is especially important if she became pregnant with an intrauterine device (IUD) in place.

Past Obstetric History

A thorough *past obstetric history* is also included as a component of the prenatal record and provides the opportunity to obtain information from the patient relating to previous pregnancies. Information that is obtained and explored includes gravidity, parity, premature births, multiple births, abortions, stillbirths, and any problems relating to infertility.

Gravidity and parity provide data with respect to the pregnancy, and the medical assistant should develop skill in recording this information. *Gravidity* refers to the total number of times a woman has been pregnant, regardless of the duration of the pregnancy and including the current pregnancy. *Parity* refers to the number of children the patient has delivered that reached the age of viability, regardless of whether the child was born alive or dead. Both of these terms refer to the pregnancy rather than the fetus; for example, multiple births (twins, triplets) count as only one pregnancy (gravida) and one delivery (para). *Abortion* (ab) refers to a fetus that did not reach the age of viability. For example, if a woman is pregnant for the first time, the medical assistant would record the information as follows:

gravida I, para 0. After delivery, regardless of whether the infant is born alive or dead (as long as it was carried to the point of viability), she becomes gravida I, para I. If she delivers twins from this pregnancy, the recording is still gravida I, para I, remembering that multiple births count as only one delivery. If she becomes pregnant again and loses the fetus before the age of viability (abortion), the medical assistant would record the information as follows: gravida II, para I, ab I.

If the woman is a multigravida, information is obtained relating to each previous pregnancy, including length of pregnancy, hours of labor, type of delivery (vaginal or cesarean section), and maternal and/or infant complications. The obstetric history assists in identifying areas that may need to be further investigated or monitored during the prenatal period.

Present Pregnancy History

The *present pregnancy history* establishes a baseline for the present health status of the prenatal patient. In addition, the patient is queried regarding any warning signs that may be present such as persistent headaches, visual disturbances, abdominal pain, vaginal bleeding, or discharge that may place the mother and/or fetus in jeopardy. The patient is also asked if she has experienced any of the early signs of pregnancy such as nausea, vomiting, fatigue, or breast changes. Any prescribed or over-the-counter medications being taken by the patient must also be recorded and are assessed by the physician. Certain medications are able to cross the placental barrier and could be harmful to the developing fetus. Therefore, the patient should not take any medications while pregnant without first checking with the physician.

In the space provided under the present pregnancy history, the medical assistant will also need to record the first day of the patient's last menstrual period (LMP). The LMP is used to calculate the due date, or expected date of confinement (EDC), by using Nägele's rule as follows: Add 7 days to the first day of the LMP, subtract 3 months, and add 1 year (EDC = LMP + 7 days − 3 months + 1 year). For example, if the first day of the patient's LMP was June 10, 1989, the EDC, or due date, is March 17, 1990. The problem is set up as follows:

6 10 89	(LMP)
−3 + 7 + 1	(Applying Nägele's rule)
3 − 17 − 90	(Delivery date)

Using Nägele's rule, approximately 4 per cent of patients deliver spontaneously on the EDC and the majority of patients deliver during the period extending 7 days before to 7 days after the EDC. Gestation calculators are commercially available that may also be used to determine the delivery date by lining up an arrow adjacent to the date of the LMP, using a movable inner cardboard wheel (Fig. 17–19). These calculators require less time to determine the EDC than using Nägele's rule and they provide information on the probable size (length and weight) of the fetus on any given date. The accuracy of gestation calculators is comparable to that of Nägele's rule. If the patient is unsure of the date of her LMP, the physician estimates the length of gestation by using other methods such as fundal height measurement or sonography.

Interval Prenatal History

The *interval prenatal history* is also included in the prenatal record form; its purpose is to update the record at each return visit. Essential data are collected and recorded in this section during each return visit, including the weight, blood pressure, urine testing results, fundal height measurement, and fetal heart rate. A general inquiry is made regarding the occurrence of any additional signs of preg-

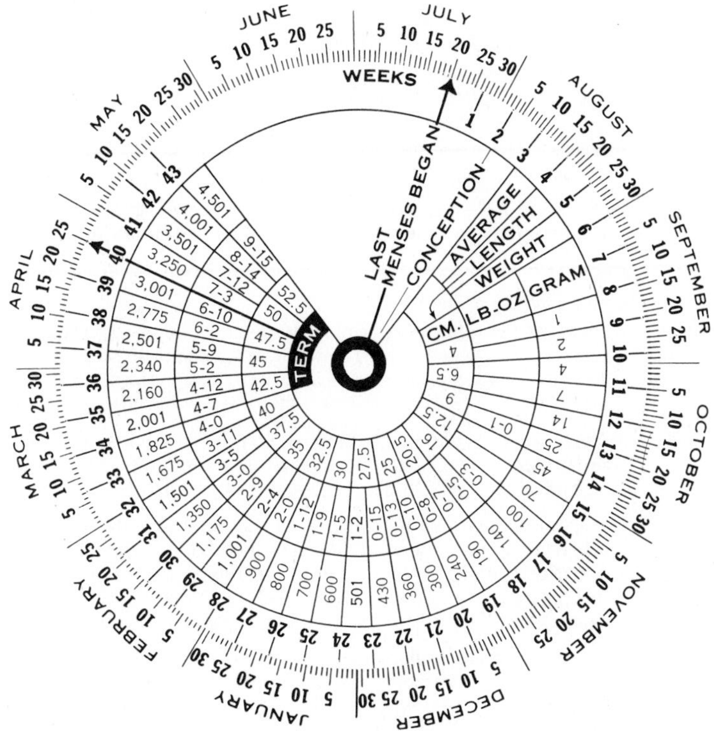

FIGURE 17–19. Gestation calculator. The last menstrual period (LMP) is July 20, and the estimated date of confinement (EDC) is April 25. (Courtesy of Mead Johnson.)

nancy such as quickening or Braxton Hicks contractions, as well as a general inquiry as to how the patient is feeling or the presence of any concerns or symptoms since the last prenatal visit. This information is recorded and assists the medical staff in planning, implementing, and evaluating individual needs. Particular attention is focused on risk factors such as hypertension, thrombophlebitis, and uterine bleeding, which could influence the course of the pregnancy.

Initial Prenatal Examination

The initial prenatal examination is of particular importance because it results in confirmation of the pregnancy and establishes a baseline for the woman's state of health. It includes a thorough gynecologic examination (breast and pelvic) and a general physical examination of the other body systems, although the latter may be performed during a subsequent prenatal visit, depending on the medical office routine. Women often have little or no medical supervision during their childbearing years; therefore, the physical examination is of particular importance in establishing a baseline for the woman's general state of health and in helping to identify high-risk prenatal patients. Conditions such as obesity, hypertension, severe varicosities, and uterine size inappropriate for the due date can be diagnosed by the physician and necessary treatment and/or monitoring can be instituted to help prevent complications.

Once the patient arrives at the medical office and the prenatal record form has been completed, the medical assistant is responsible for taking and recording the patient's vital signs, height, and weight to provide a data base for subsequent prenatal visits. The patient is then asked to completely disrobe and to don an examining gown with the opening in front. The medical assistant must make sure to give complete and thorough instructions so the patient knows exactly what is expected. The patient should be asked if she needs to empty her bladder because an empty bladder facilitates the examination and is more comfortable for her. If the office policy is such that a specimen is needed for urine testing at the initial prenatal visit, the patient will be required to void. Special precautions should be

TABLE 17-2. Initial Prenatal Examination

PROCEDURE	PURPOSE AND IMPLICATIONS
Vital signs (Chapter 2) Temperature Pulse Respiration Blood pressure	To provide a baseline for subsequent prenatal visits. The blood pressure drops slightly during the first and second trimesters and returns to normal or slightly above normal during the last trimester. An elevation in the blood pressure during the pregnancy is used in conjunction with other patient signs and symptoms to assess the presence of a possible pathologic condition. An elevation in the blood pressure may be indicative of possible pre-eclampsia or other hypertensive disorders.
Weight (Chapter 3)	To provide a baseline weight measurement for comparison with all future weight measurements at subsequent prenatal visits. The medical assistant will be plotting the patient's weight on a graph or flow sheet at each prenatal visit, and any deviations from expected progressions will be evaluated by the physician. Measuring and recording the maternal weight gain or loss are helpful in assessing fetal development and to some extent the mother's nutrition and state of health. A sudden unexplained weight gain may be indicative of possible pre-eclampsia of pregnancy.
Physical examination (Chapter 3)	To establish a baseline for the woman's general state of health to be certain the patient is entering pregnancy in the best possible physical condition. The physical examination includes an examination of the patient's eyes, ears, nose, and throat; chest, lungs, and heart; breasts; abdomen; reproductive organs; rectum; and extremities. Of particular importance are the breast, abdominal, and pelvic examinations, which are outlined in a separate category.
Breast examination (Chapter 17)	To check for cysts or lumps and the breast changes that take place during pregnancy, such as tenderness and fullness and darkening of the nipple and areola. Patient position: horizontal recumbent.
Abdominal examination	To detect any masses or lumps other than the developing fetus. The abdomen is inspected for scars or striations, and the initial measurement of the fundal height is generally made to provide a baseline for future fundal height measurements. Patient position: horizontal recumbent.
Pelvic examination (Chapter 17)	To provide data to confirm the pregnancy and to determine the length of gestation. To identify pelvic characteristics and any abnormalities that may result in complications during the pregnancy or delivery. The pelvic examination generally includes the following: a. Inspection of the external genitalia b. Speculum examination of the vagina and cervix c. Pap smear d. Specimen for gonorrhea culture e. Vaginal specimen if an infection is suspected f. Bimanual examination Patient position: dorsal lithotomy.
Rectovaginal examination (Chapter 17)	To assess the strength and irregularity of the posterior vaginal wall and the posterior cervix. The anus is inspected for hemorrhoids and fissures and the rectum is inspected for any herniation and masses. Patient position: dorsal lithotomy.
Pelvic measurements (Chapter 17)	To assure that the size and shape of the pelvis are within normal limits to allow the full-term fetus to pass safely through the pelvic inlet to provide for the normal vaginal route of delivery; if not, a cesarean section will be required. Some physicians delay taking the pelvic measurements until later in the pregnancy. At that time, the prenatal patient's perineal muscles are more relaxed, allowing the pelvic measurements to be taken with less patient discomfort and more accuracy. The pelvic measurements are taken using the hands and an instrument specifically designed for this purpose, known as a *pelvimeter.* The process of measuring the capacity and diameter of the maternal pelvis is known as *pelvimetry.* Patient position: horizontal recumbent and lateral (side).

taken in assisting the prenatal patient onto and off the examination table. The footstool should be placed in a convenient position next to the table and the medical assistant should help the patient onto and off the table to assure her safety and comfort. This is especially important as the pregnancy progresses and the patient becomes more awkward and off-balance. The medical assistant is responsible for setting up the tray required for the examination. The set-up includes the equipment and supplies required for each procedure included. During the prenatal examination, the medical assistant is responsible for positioning the patient as required for each aspect of the examination as well as assisting the physician as necessary. Table 17–2 lists the procedures commonly included in the prenatal examination and the purpose, implications, and (when applicable) the patient position for each. Most of the procedures included in the initial prenatal examination are presented elsewhere in the text; the number of the chapter that contains the step-by-step procedure has been included (Table 17–2).

At the conclusion of the initial prenatal examination and after the patient is dressed, the physician talks with her regarding instructions on diet, weight gain, rest, sleep, clothing, employment, exercise, recreation, intercourse, bowel function, dental care, smoking, alcohol, and drugs. Many offices have a prenatal guidebook designed especially for this purpose that is given to each patient to use as a reference. Some offices also utilize a series of teaching films that the patient views during the return prenatal visit while waiting to see the physician. The physician usually prescribes a daily vitamin supplement to be taken during the prenatal period to help ensure that the mother and fetus obtain an adequate supply of vitamins and minerals.

During the first visit, the patient is also given a laboratory request to have the required specimens collected and tested at an outside medical laboratory. Some offices collect blood and urine specimens at the medical office; these are then picked up or mailed to an outside laboratory for testing. However, most offices find it more convenient to have the specimens collected at an outside laboratory. The prenatal laboratory tests, generally referred to as the prenatal profile, are discussed in more detail on the following pages.

When the physician is finished talking with the patient, the medical assistant is responsible for scheduling the next prenatal visit and for making sure the patient understands the instructions for maintaining health and preventing disease during the pregnancy. He or she should tell the patient to report the occurrence of any of the warning signs of problems in the pregnancy and not to take any medications without first checking with the physician. The patient should also be encouraged to contact the medical office should any questions or problems arise.

Laboratory Tests

A number of laboratory tests are ordered by the physician to assist in the overall initial assessment of the state of health of the prenatal patient. The physician gives the patient a laboratory request at the first prenatal visit for tests that will be collected and evaluated at an outside laboratory. Several of the tests, such as the Pap smear and gonorrhea culture, require the physician to collect the specimens at the medical office and then have them transported to an outside laboratory for evaluation. The blood specimen required for the hematologic tests must be obtained through a venipuncture to provide sufficient quantity for the number of tests ordered. The medical assistant should stress to the patient the importance of having these tests completed as soon as possible to provide the physician with the test results by the time of the next scheduled prenatal visit. Based on the results of the prenatal examination and the laboratory tests, the physician may order further tests, if needed, to assess the patient's condition. The following tests are generally included in the prenatal laboratory work-up.

Urine Tests

Urinalysis. A complete urinalysis is performed, including a physical, chemical, and microscopic analysis of the urine; a clean-catch midstream urine specimen is generally required for the test. If bacteria are found in the urine specimen, the physician usually requests a urine culture and sensitivity test to determine the possible presence of a urinary tract infection. A pregnancy test may also be performed on the urine specimen, if ordered by the physician.

Smears and Cultures

Papanicolaou Smear. A Pap smear is prepared for the detection of abnormalities of cell growth to diagnose precancerous or cancerous conditions of the cervix and uterus. This test can also be used for hormonal assessment and to assist in the detection of vaginal infections.

Cervical Specimen for Gonorrhea Culture. This specimen is taken from the endocervical canal to rule out gonorrhea. If a gonorrheal infection is present at the time of delivery, the *Neisseria gonorrhoeae* organism could infect the infant's eyes and cause *ophthalmia neonatorum,* which could result in blindness. A patient who has contracted gonorrhea requires treatment with an appropriate antibiotic. A gonorrhea culture on prenatal patients is generally mandated by state law.

Specimen for Trichomoniasis or Candidiasis. If an excessive irritating vaginal discharge is present, the physician usually obtains a specimen to rule out trichomoniasis and candidiasis. It is important to control candidiasis before delivery to prevent the development of a yeastlike infection of the mucous membrane of the mouth or throat of the infant, known as thrush.

Blood Tests

Complete Blood Count (CBC). The CBC is a basic screening test used to assist in assessing the patient's state of health. It includes a hemoglobin, hematocrit, white blood count, red blood count, differential white cell count, and red blood cell indices; of particular importance with respect to the prenatal patient are the hemoglobin and hematocrit evaluations, which are described here.

Hemoglobin and Hematocrit. Low hemoglobin or hematocrit values are seen in cases of anemia. Prenatal patients have a tendency to develop anemia because there is an increased demand for and correlating increased production of red blood cells during pregnancy; therefore, the physician carefully reviews the results of these tests. If the hemoglobin or hematocrit value is low, further hematologic evaluation is usually required. If necessary, therapy is instituted usually consisting of an iron supplement and nutritional counseling. The hemoglobin and hematocrit values are checked again at approximately 32 weeks of gestation as a precaution against anemia before delivery.

Rh Factor and ABO Blood Type. These tests are performed to anticipate any ABO or Rh incompatibilities. If the patient is Rh−, the father's blood type must also be evaluated. If the father's blood type is Rh+, the possibility of an Rh incompatibility may exist. This warrants the performance of Rh antibody titer test as well as repeat antibody titers throughout the pregnancy to determine whether the mother's antibody level is increasing. An increased Rh antibody level could be dangerous to the developing fetus.

Serology Test for Syphilis. The microorganism that causes syphilis, *Treponema pallidum,* is able to cross the placental barrier and infect the fetus; this could result in intrauterine death or could cause the fetus to be born with congenital syphilis. Children with congenital syphilis are often born with deformities and may become blind, deaf, paralyzed, or insane. The tests most commonly employed to detect the presence of syphilis are the Venereal Disease Research Laboratories test (VDRL) and the rapid plasma reagin (RPR). The test results are reported as nonreactive, weakly reactive, or reactive; weakly reactive and reactive are considered positive for the presence of the syphilis antibodies. These tests are considered screening tests, and a positive result warrants more specific testing to arrive at a diagnosis for syphilis. A prenatal serology test for syphilis is usually mandated by state law and should be performed early in the pregnancy before fetal damage occurs. A patient who has contracted syphilis requires treatment with an appropriate antibiotic.

Rubella Titer. This test assesses the level of antibody against rubella present in the patient and is used to determine whether or not the woman has immunity to rubella. If the patient lacks immunity, a rubella immunization should be administered within 6 weeks following delivery.

Rh Antibody Titer (on Rh-blood Specimens). This test detects the amount of circulating Rh antibodies against red blood cells. These antibodies can occur in a pregnant woman who is Rh− and is carrying an Rh+ fetus; therefore, an Rh antibody titer is performed in all Rh− blood specimens. Repeat antibody titer levels are also performed during the pregnancy to determine whether the woman's antibody level is increasing. As previously indicated, an increased Rh antibody level could be dangerous to the developing fetus.

Other Tests

Tine Test or Chest Roentgenogram. The tine test (or other type of tuberculin skin test) is used to screen individuals for tuberculosis. The current trend is to order a chest x-ray examination only if the tine test results are positive to avoid any possible x-ray exposure to the growing fetus. If a chest x-ray is ordered, a lead shield is placed over the patient's abdomen to avoid exposure of the fetus. The patient should be screened early in the pregnancy for the presence of tuberculosis, because it is a chronic and debilitating disease that may increase the chance of abortion.

Return Prenatal Visits

Subsequent prenatal visits provide the opportunity for a continuous assessment of the state of health of the mother and fetus. During each visit, essential data are collected and recorded in the prenatal record, resulting in an updated record at each visit, as is discussed in this section. If signs or symptoms of a pathologic condition are present, the physician performs selected aspects of the physical examination as necessary to diagnose and treat the condition. In addition, diagnostic and laboratory tests may be ordered to assist in diagnosis and treatment.

The return prenatal visit also provides the opportunity for the physician and the medical assistant to lend support to the mother and to provide her with ongoing prenatal education to help reduce apprehension and anxiety and to ensure that the mother is well informed and prepared during her pregnancy, childbirth, and the postpartum period. The medical assistant plays an important role in prenatal education and should take the necesssary time with each patient to provide appropriate information and to allow the patient the opportunity to ask questions.

For convenience, the 9 months of pregnancy are divided into three trimesters, each consisting of 3 months. During the first 6 months, or first two trimesters, of the pregnancy, the patient is seen once a month at the medical office. The patient is then seen every 2 weeks during the seventh and eighth months and then each week during the ninth month until delivery. The patient exhibiting complications is seen more frequently for closer monitoring.

The patient is asked to collect a first-voided morning urine specimen on the day of each return visit to be brought to the medical office for testing. Many physicians also require the specimen be a clean-catch midstream collection. A responsibility of the medical assistant is to instruct the patient in the proper collection techniques and care and handling of the specimen until it reaches the office. The medical assistant is responsible for testing the specimen for glucose and protein using a reagent strip and for recording results in the prenatal record. A positive reaction to glucose may indicate the development of diabetes mellitus or a prediabetic condition, whereas a positive reaction to protein may be indicative or preeclampsia. Further testing is usually needed to arrive at a final diagnosis and to institute treatment.

During the return visit the physician performs one or more of the following procedures, depending on the stage of the pregnancy: (1) palpation of the woman's abdomen to measure fundal height, (2) measurement of the fetal heart rate, (3) palpation of the woman's abdomen to determine fetal presentation and position, and (4) a vaginal examination. These procedures are discussed in detail in the following paragraphs.

Fundal Height Measurement. The pregnant uterus rises gradually into the abdominal cavity, and the fundus is palpable between the eighth and thirteenth weeks of the pregnancy. The first fundal height measurement, which is usually performed during the first prenatal visit, is used as a guideline for all subsequent measurements. The physician measures the fundal height by placing one end of a flexible, nonstretchable centimeter tape measure on the superior aspect of the symphysis pubis and measuring to the crest or top of the uterine fundus (Fig. 17–20). The measurement is then recorded on a graph or flow chart in the patient's prenatal record. By 20 weeks the fundus reaches the lower border of the umbilicus, and between 36 and 37 weeks it reaches the tip of the sternum. During the first and second trimesters, measuring the fundal height provides a gross estimate of the duration of the pregnancy; the fundal height measurement is considered accurate to within 4 weeks using McDonald's rule:

Calculation of the duration of the pregnancy using McDonald's rule:

Height of the fundus (in centimeters) $\times$ 8/7 = duration of the pregnancy in weeks
Example: 21 cm $\times$ 8/7 = 24 weeks

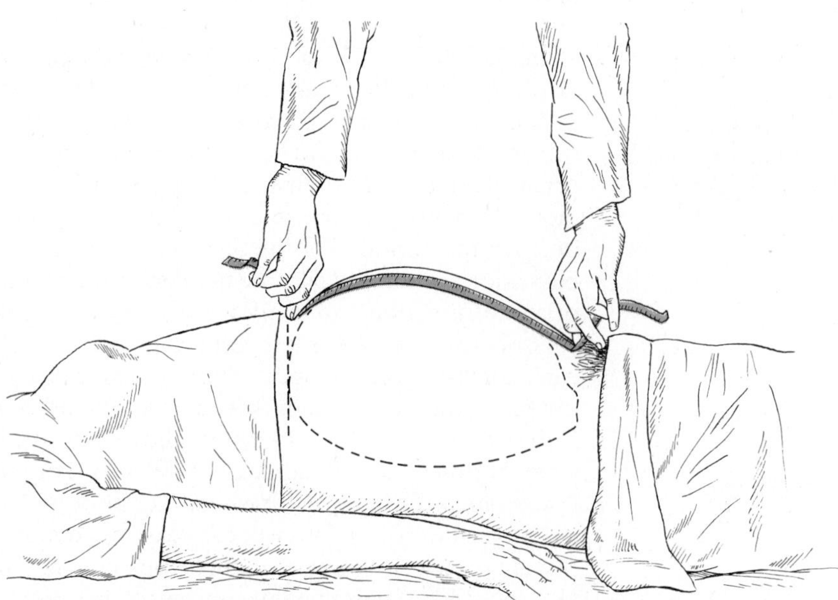

FIGURE 17–20. Measurement of fundal height. The physician places one end of a centimeter tape measure on the superior aspect of the symphysis pubis and measures to the top of the uterine fundus.

Height of the fundus (in centimeters) × 2/7 = duration of the pregnancy in lunar months
Example: 21 cm × 2/7 = 6 months

Because fetal weights vary considerably during the third trimester, it is difficult to use fundal height measurements as an estimate of the duration of the pregnancy in the last trimester.

In addition to assessing the duration of the pregnancy, the fundal height measurements permit variations from normal to become apparent and are used to

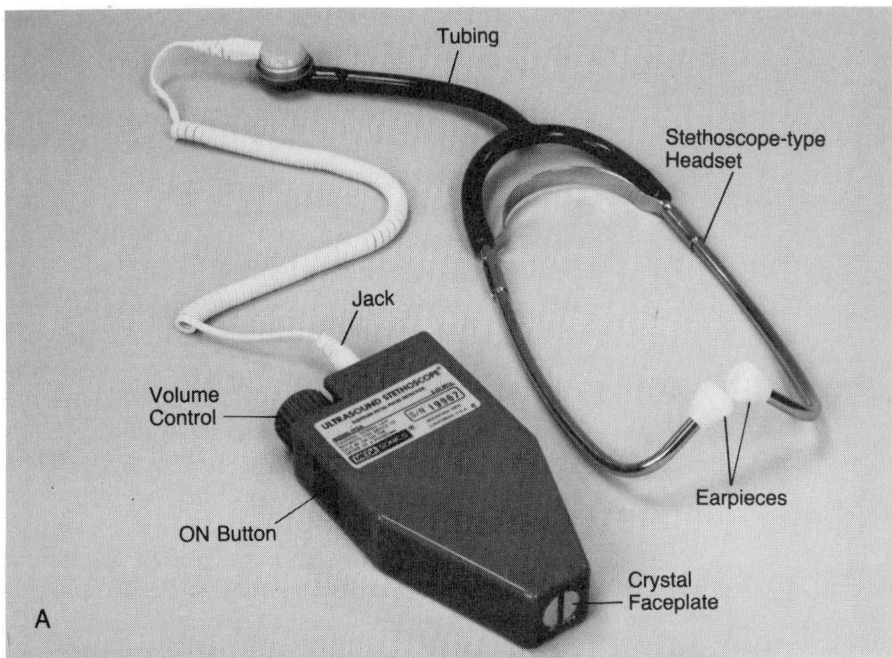

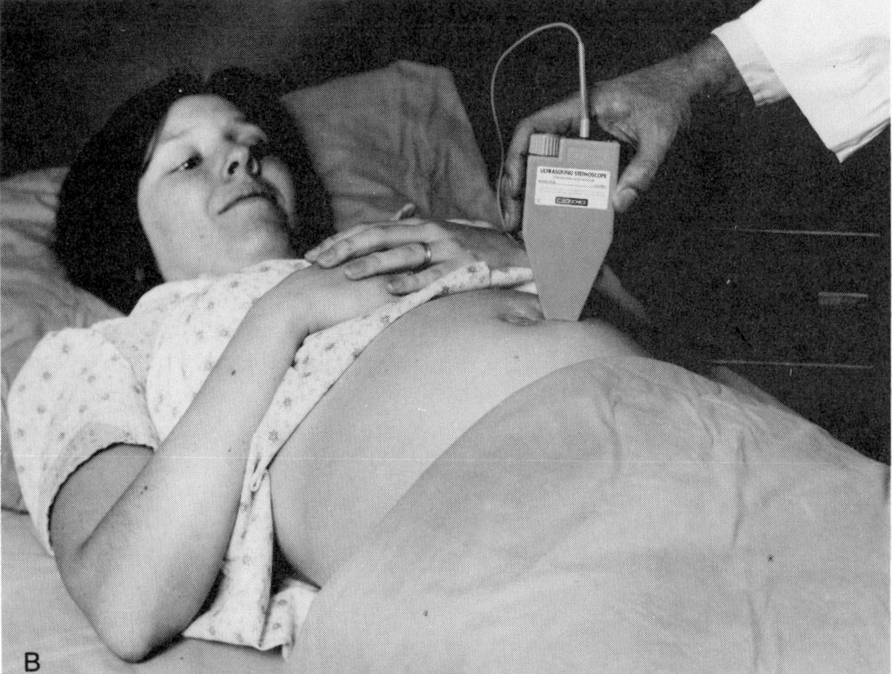

FIGURE 17–21. *A,* The parts of a Doppler device. *B,* The crystal faceplate of the Doppler device is moved across the abdomen to detect the fetal pulse. The speaker-amplifier (located in the background) broadcasts the fetal heart rate to allow for hearing by more than one person. (Courtesy of Media Sonics.)

assess whether or not fetal development is progressing normally. Growth that is too rapid or too slow must be evaluated further by the physician as a possible indication of high-risk conditions such as multiple pregnancies, polyhydramnios, ovarian tumor, intrauterine growth retardation (IUGR), intrauterine death, or an error in estimating the fetal progress.

Fetal Heart Tones. The normal fetal heart rate falls between 120 and 160 beats per minute with a regular rhythm. A very slow or rapid fetal heart rate usually indicates fetal distress. The fetal heart tones (FHT) can usually be heard with a fetoscope between the eighteenth and twenty-second weeks of gestation. The *fetoscope* is an auscultatory instrument that is similar to a stethoscope but is preferred over the stethoscope because it uses bone conduction, which increases hearing ability. A newer type of instrument used to measure fetal heart tones is the Doppler fetal pulse detector, which detects the fetal pulse rate through the conversion of ultrasonic waves into audible sounds of the fetal pulse. The Doppler device consists of an instrument containing a crystal faceplate at its narrow end. Attached to the instrument by means of a jack is a stethoscope-type headset for listening to sounds (Fig. 17–21*A*). Because air is a poor conductor of sound waves, an ultrasound coupling agent must first be spread on the mother's abdomen in the area to be examined to increase conductivity of the sound waves between the abdomen and the crystal faceplate. The earpieces of the headset are then placed in the examiner's ears and the crystal faceplate is slowly moved across the abdomen to detect the fetal pulse. A speaker-amplifier is available for use with the Doppler device that broadcasts the fetal heart rate to allow for hearing by more than one person (Fig. 17–21*B*). With the use of the Doppler device, the fetal heart tones can first be heard between the tenth and twelfth weeks of gestation.

Fetal Presentation and Position. The abdomen is also palpated to determine fetal presentation and position, which can be assessed by 30 weeks of gestation by using the four maneuvers of Leopold. *Leopold's maneuvers* are a series of abdominal palpations used to detect the body parts of the fetus while in utero (Fig. 17–22). Conditions such as multiple gestation, breech position, hydramnios, or other abnormalities may be suspected through use of Leopold's maneuvers and will be confirmed through use of other measures such as sonography. Near the end of the pregnancy, Leopold's maneuvers are used to help determine whether engagement of the presenting part has taken place. The presenting part of the fetus sinks into the pelvis and becomes engaged at approximately 38 weeks gestation.

Vaginal Examination. In the absence of vaginal bleeding, vaginal examinations may be performed at any time during the pregnancy; however, in a normal pregnancy, there is usually no need to perform a vaginal examination until the patient nears term. The vaginal examination is usually begun approximately 2 to 3 weeks from the EDC and is performed to confirm the presenting part and to determine the degree, if any, of cervical dilation and effacement. The purpose of dilation and effacement is to permit the passage of the infant from the uterus into the birth canal (Fig. 17–23).

The medical assistant has many important responsibilities in the return prenatal examination, which are outlined on the following pages under the Procedure for Assisting With a Return Prenatal Visit. She or he is responsible for assembling the equipment and supplies required for the examination, for acquiring relevant information to update the prenatal record, for preparing the patient for the examination, and for assisting the physician during the examination. The physician depends on the medical assistant to have the urine test results and certain measurements such as blood pressure and weight completed and recorded in advance to allow him or her the opportunity to review these measurements before examining the patient.

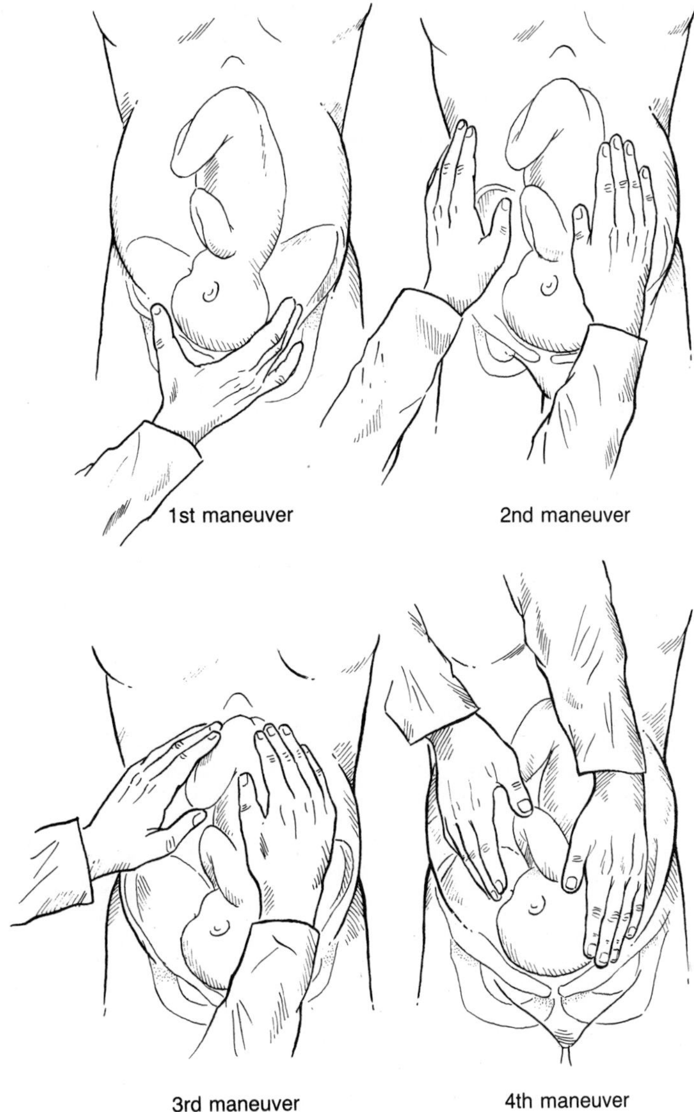

FIGURE 17–22. Leopold maneuvers are a series of abdominal palpations used to detect the body parts of the fetus while in utero.

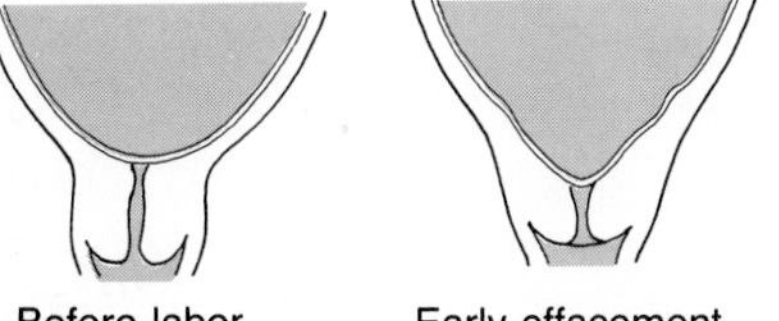

FIGURE 17–23. Effacement and dilation occur to permit the passage of the infant into the birth canal. The cervical canal will shorten from its normal length of 1 to 2 cm to a structure with paper-thin edges in which there is no canal at all. The cervix will dilate from an opening a few millimeters in size to an opening large enough to allow the passage of the infant (approximately 10 cm).

PROCEDURE 17-6

ASSISTING WITH A RETURN PRENATAL EXAMINATION

1. **PROCEDURAL STEP.** Wash the hands.

2. **PROCEDURAL STEP.** Set up the tray for the prenatal examination. The equipment and supplies needed depend on the procedures included in the examination, which are as follows:

Procedure	*Equipment/Supplies*
a. Fundal height measurement	Flexible, nonstretchable centimeter tape measure
b. Measurement of fetal heart tones	Fetoscope or Doppler fetal pulse detector and an ultrasound coupling agent
c. Checking fetal presentation and position	No special equipment/supplies required
d. Examination of the legs, feet, and face for edema and the development of varicosities	No special equipment/supplies required
e. Taking a specimen for the diagnosis of a vaginal infection	Vaginal speculum, sterile swabs, and the appropriate supplies such as slides, transport media, and culture media needed to collect and identify the invading organism
f. Vaginal examination	Clean glove and lubricant

3. **PROCEDURAL STEP.** Identify the patient and obtain the urine specimen, which she has collected at home. Determine whether the patient has taken the necessary precautions to preserve the specimen before bringing it to the medical office.
PRINCIPLE. Specimens that have been left standing out produce inaccurate test results.

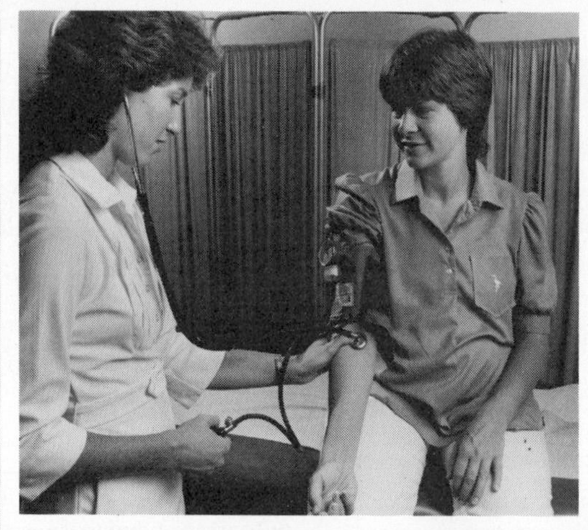

4. **PROCEDURAL STEP.** Ask the patient if she has experienced any problems since the last prenatal visit, and record any information in the appropriate section in her prenatal record.
PRINCIPLE. The physician further investigates any unusual or abnormal signs or symptoms relayed by the patient.

5. **PROCEDURAL STEP.** Take the patient's blood pressure, and record the results in the prenatal record. If the blood pressure is elevated, allow the patient the opportunity to relax, then take the blood pressure again.
PRINCIPLE. Taking an elevated blood pressure again gives the opportunity to determine if the elevation was due to emotional excitement.

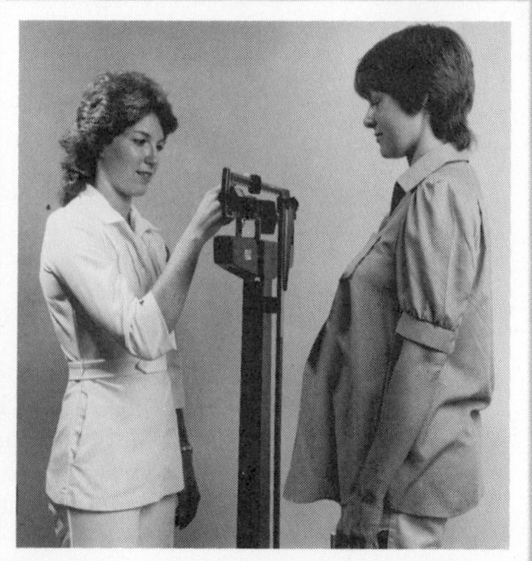

6. **PROCEDURAL STEP.** Weigh the patient and record results on her weight flow sheet or graph provided in the prenatal record.
PRINCIPLE. Maternal weight gain or loss assists in assessing fetal development as well as the mother's nutrition and state of health.

7. **PROCEDURAL STEP.** Ask the patient if she needs to empty her bladder before the examination.
PRINCIPLE. An empty bladder makes the examination easier and is more comfortable for the patient.

8. **PROCEDURAL STEP.** Instruct and prepare the patient for the examination. Have her remove her outer clothing, to expose the abdominal area. If the physician will be performing a vaginal examination, the patient must also remove her panties, otherwise she may leave them on. If the medical assistant senses that the patient may have trouble undressing, assistance should be offered.
PRINCIPLE. Prenatal patients, especially near term, may sometimes require assistance in removing clothing.

9. **PROCEDURAL STEP.** Test the urine specimen for glucose and protein using a reagent strip and record results in the patient's chart. *Note:* The urine specimen may be tested at any time before the physician examines the patient; however, a convenient time to test the specimen is while the patient is disrobing.
PRINCIPLE. The prenatal patient's urine must be tested at each visit to assist in the early detection and prevention of disease.

10. **PROCEDURAL STEP.** Place the footstool close to the examining table. Assist the patient onto the table. Place her in a horizontal recumbent position and properly drape her. Provide support and reassurance to the patient to help her relax during the examination.
PRINCIPLE. The medical assistant should make sure to provide for the safety of the prenatal patient while she is getting onto and off the examining table. The patient should be properly draped to provide for warmth and comfort.

11. **PROCEDURAL STEP.** Place the patient's chart in a convenient location for review by the physician. Inform the physician that the patient is ready to be examined.
PRINCIPLE. The physician will first want to review the measurements taken by the medical assistant and compare them with his or her findings during the prenatal examination.

12. **PROCEDURAL STEP.** Assist the physician as required for the prenatal examination. The medical assistant may be responsible for the following:

a. Handing the physician the tape measure for the determination of the fundal height and recording the measurement in the patient's prenatal record.
b. Handing the physician the fetoscope or Doppler fetal pulse detector for measurement of the FHT and recording the fetal heart rate in the patient's prenatal record. With the use of the Doppler device, the medical assistant may also be responsible for spreading the ultrasound coupling agent on the patient's abdomen.
c. Assisting the patient into the dorsal lithotomy position if a vaginal specimen is to be taken for the detection of a vaginal infection. The medical assistant will also need to hold the appropriate medium and/or slide (labeled with the patient's name, the date, and the source of the specimen) so that the physician can place the specimen on it. In addition, the

Continued

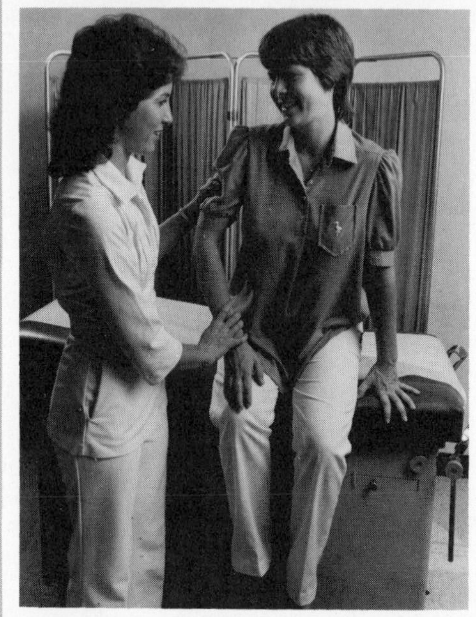

medical assistant is usually responsible for completing the laboratory request if the specimen will be transported to an outside medical laboratory for evaluation. If the specimen is to be examined at the medical office, the medical assistant needs to prepare it as necessary for identification of the invading organism. Make sure to follow the principles of medical asepsis during specimen collection to prevent infection with a pathogen.

d. Assisting the patient into the dorsal lithotomy position if a vaginal examination is performed and assisting the physician with the application of the glove and the application of lubricant to the glove for the examination. Be careful not to allow the tube of lubricant to touch the physician's fingers, to prevent contamination of the contents of the tube.

13. **PROCEDURAL STEP.** After the examination, assist the patient into a sitting position and allow her the opportunity to rest for a moment. If a vaginal examination was performed, offer the patient tissues to remove excess lubricating jelly from the perineum. Assist her off the examining table, using the footstool to prevent falls. Instruct the patient to get dressed, offering assistance if needed.

PRINCIPLE. The patient may become dizzy after being on the examining table and should be allowed to rest before getting off.

14. **PROCEDURAL STEP.** Provide prenatal patient teaching and/or further explanation of the physician's instructions as required to meet individual patient needs.

15. **PROCEDURAL STEP.** Clean the examining room in preparation for the next patient and, if necessary, prepare specimens for transport to an outside medical laboratory, including the completed laboratory request.

Record data below.

DATE	TIME	PATIENT'S NAME	RECORDING

Six-Weeks Postpartum Visit

The *puerperium* includes the period of time in which the body systems are returning to their prepregnant or nearly prepregnant state, which usually extends for 4 to 6 weeks after delivery. During this time period, numerous changes take place within the woman's body. The involution of the uterus (i.e., the process by which it returns to its normal size and state) occurs; this includes healing of any injuries sustained to the birth canal during delivery.

During the puerperium, the patient experiences a vaginal discharge shed from the lining of the uterus, known as *lochia.* Lochia consists of blood, tissue, white blood cells, mucus, and some bacteria. The color of the lochia is an indication of the progress of the healing of the uterus. For the first 3 days after delivery, the lochia consists almost entirely of blood and because of its red color is termed *lochia rubra.* By approximately the fourth day postpartum, the amount of blood decreases and the discharge becomes pink or brownish in color and is known as *lochia serosa.* By the tenth day postpartum, the amount of flow should decrease and the lochia should become yellowish-white; this is known as *lochia alba.* Lochia usually continues in consistently decreasing amounts (from moderate to scant to occasional spotting) and becomes more pale in color until the third week following delivery, when it usually disappears altogether. However, it would not be considered unusual for the discharge to last the entire 6 weeks. The patient should be instructed to contact the medical office under the following circumstances: if the amount of discharge increases rather than decreases; if the discharge is absent within the first 2 weeks after delivery; if it changes to red after having been yellowish white, which indicates bleeding; or if it takes on a foul odor, which indicates infection. Menstruation usually begins approximately 2 months after delivery in the non-nursing mother and 3 to 6 months after delivery in the nursing mother.

During the puerperium, the patient should be encouraged to avoid fatigue, to avoid lifting heavy objects, and to consume a nutritious, well-balanced diet that helps to maintain health and promote healing during this period.

The physician will want to see the patient at the medical office at the end of the 6-week period. The purpose of the 6-weeks postpartum visit is to evaluate the general physical condition of the patient, to make sure there are no residual problems from childbearing, and to provide the patient with education regarding methods of birth control and infant care. The patient is queried during this visit regarding the presence of any problems or abnormalities relating to vaginal discharge, urinary or bowel function, or breast-feeding in the nursing mother. This information is recorded in the patient's chart. The postpartum visit provides an excellent opportunity for the medical assistant to instruct the patient in the technique for performing a breast self-examination and to educate her in the importance of returning to the medical office periodically for a Pap test.

During the postpartal examination, the physician evaluates the patient's general appearance, performs breast and pelvic examinations, and checks to determine whether the muscle tone has returned to the muscles of the abdominal wall. During the puerperium, atypical cells may be sloughed off into the cervical and vaginal mucus as part of the normal healing process. Because of this, the Pap test is not included in the postpartum visit. If the patient has problems with hemorrhoids or varicosities, the physician discusses any further treatment required. If the patient does not have antibody protection to rubella, as has been evidenced through the prenatal laboratory tests, she receives rubella immunization at this time (if it has not previously been administered in the hospital). In addition, hemoglobin and hematocrit are usually performed on the postpartum patient to screen for anemia due to blood loss during delivery and the puerperium.

The responsibilities of the medical assistant during the postpartum visit include measuring and recording the patient's vital signs and weight, preparing the patient for the examination, setting up the tray, and assisting the physician with the examination. The patient is required to completely disrobe for this examination and to don an examining gown with the opening placed in front. Table 17–3 lists the procedures commonly included in the 6-weeks postpartum visit and the purpose of each.

TABLE 17–3. Six-Weeks Postpartum Examination

PROCEDURE	PURPOSE
Vital signs (Chapter 2) Temperature Pulse Respiration Blood pressure	To make sure the vital signs fall within normal limits and that the blood pressure has returned to its normal prepregnant level. Elevated blood pressure may indicate essential hypertension or renal disease.
Weight (Chapter 3)	To determine if the patient's weight has returned to its prepregnant measurement. If not, nutritional counseling may be indicated.
Breast examination (Chapter 17)	To make sure the breasts are not sore or tender and there are no cysts or masses present. In the non-nursing mother, the breasts will be examined to determine if they have returned to their prepregnant size. In the nursing mother, the nipples will be examined for cracks, redness, soreness, and fissures.
Pelvic examination (Chapter 17)	To make sure involution of the uterus is complete and to determine if the cervix has healed. To make sure the episiotomy and any injuries sustained by the birth canal have healed. To make sure there is no abnormal vaginal discharge present.
Rectovaginal examination (Chapter 17)	To make sure the pelvic floor has regained its muscle tone. To determine whether hemorrhoids are present.
Evaluation of the patient's general physical condition (Chapter 3)	To make sure the body systems have returned to their prepregnant state.

Study Questions

1. What is the purpose of prenatal care?
2. What procedures are performed during the initial prenatal examination?
3. What is the purpose of return prenatal visits?
4. What is the purpose of the 6-weeks postpartum examination?

COMPETENCIES

After completing this unit, you should be able to demonstrate the proper procedure to perform the following:

1. Instruct an individual in the preparation and procedure required for a fecal occult blood test.
2. Develop a fecal occult slide test, and interpret and record the test results.
3. Prepare the patient for and assist the physician with a proctoscopy.
4. Instruct a patient in the preparation required for a sigmoidoscopy.
5. Prepare the patient for and assist the physician with a sigmoidoscopy.

LEARNING OBJECTIVES

After completing this unit, you should be able to do the following:

1. Define the terms listed in the vocabulary.
2. Explain the purpose of performing a fecal occult blood test.
3. Describe the patient preparation required for the fecal occult blood test, and explain the purpose of each type of preparation.
4. Explain the purpose of performing the following: digital examination of the anus and rectum, proctoscopy, and sigmoidoscopy.
5. Explain why the knee-chest position is preferred for a proctoscopy and sigmoidoscopy.
6. Describe the patient preparation that may be required for a proctoscopy and sigmoidoscopy.

• VOCABULARY •

biopsy (bi' op-se)—The surgical removal and examination of tissue from the living body. Biopsies are generally done to determine whether a tumor is benign or malignant.

endoscope (en' do-skōp)—An instrument, consisting of a tube and an optical system, that is used for direct visual inspection of organs or cavities.

melena (mĕ-le' nah)—The darkening of the stool due to the presence of blood in an amount of 50 ml or greater.

occult blood (o-kult' blud)—Blood occurring in such a small amount that it is not visually detectable to the unaided eye.

peroxidase (pĕ-rok' sy-dās) (as it pertains to the guaiac slide test)—A substance that is able to transfer oxygen from hydrogen peroxide to oxidize guaiac, causing the guaiac to turn blue.

proctoscope (prok' to-skōp)—An endoscope that is specially designed for passage through the anus to permit visual inspection of the rectum.

proctoscopy (prok-tos' ko-pe)—The visual examination of the rectum using a proctoscope.

sigmoidoscope (sig-moi' do-skōp)—An endoscope that is specially designed for passage through the anus to permit visualization of the rectum and sigmoid colon.

sigmoidoscopy (sig" moi-dos' ko-pe)—The visual examination of the rectum and sigmoid colon using a sigmoidoscope. (also called proctosigmoidoscopy).

Colon Procedures

Fecal Occult Blood Testing

Blood in the stool may be indicative of a number of pathologic conditions, including hemorrhoids, diverticulosis, nonmalignant polyps, upper gastrointestinal ulcers and colorectal cancer. Some of these conditions produce visible red blood on the outside of the stool, making it easy to detect. Blood entering the stool from the upper gastrointestinal tract in an amount of 50 ml or greater causes the stool to exhibit *melena,* meaning it appears black and tarlike. The dark color is a result of the oxidation of the iron component of the blood (heme) by intestinal and bacterial enzymes. If blood is present in a minute quantity, however, it will not be detectable by the unaided eye. This hidden or nonvisible blood is termed *occult blood* and its presence can be determined only through chemical or microscopic analysis.

Colorectal cancer is one of the most common forms of cancer in individuals over the age of 40. During the early asymptomatic stages, almost all neoplasms of the colon and rectum bleed a small amount on an intermittent basis, and this takes the form of occult blood. Assessing the presence of occult blood is of particular importance in the early diagnosis and treatment of colorectal cancer, which, in turn, increases the patient's survival rate. In most cases, when more pronounced symptoms of colorectal cancer start appearing (such as visible bleeding, a change in bowel habits, abdominal pain, and anemia) the condition has reached an advanced stage. It is recommended that screening for occult blood be performed every 2 years on patients 40 years or older and every year on patients considered to be at high risk of developing colorectal cancer.

Routine screening of stool specimens for occult blood is frequently performed in the medical office using chemical testing. The guaiac slide test is most often used and is commercially available with brand names of Hemoccult and Coloscreen (Fig. 17–24). Fecal blood loss in excess of 5 ml/day results in a positive reaction. Patients may normally lose blood in amounts up to 3 ml/day in the feces, owing to minor insignificant abrasions of the nasopharynx and gastrointestinal tract. Thus, to allow for normal blood loss, the test does not show a positive reaction until it reaches 5 ml.

The guaiac slide test is a simple and inexpensive method to screen for the presence of occult blood; however, care must be taken to reduce the occurrence of false-positive or false-negative results. This test is designed to assess the presence of blood in stool specimens collected from three consecutive bowel movements or three bowel movements spaced closely in time. The purpose of using three specimens is to provide for the detection of blood from gastrointestinal lesions

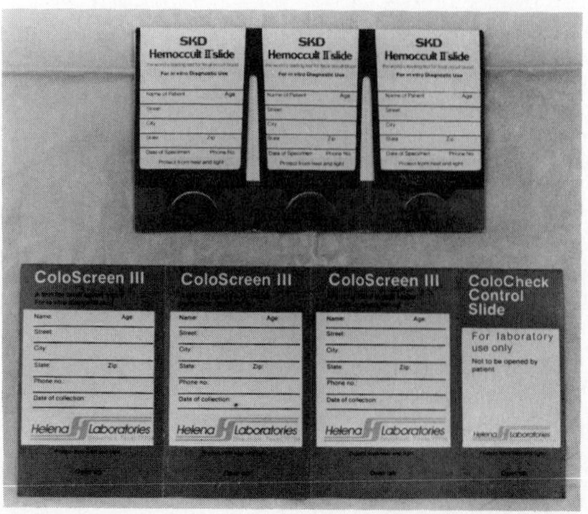

FIGURE 17–24. Examples of fecal occult blood testing kits: Hemoccult (top) and Coloscreen (bottom).

that exhibit intermittent bleeding, meaning they do not bleed every day. Because three stool specimens are required, most physicians prefer that the patient collect and process the specimens at home and return the prepared slides to the medical office for analysis. The medical assistant is responsible for providing the patient with instructions on patient preparation, collection, and processing of the specimens as well as proper care and storage of the slide test until it is returned to the medical office.

Patient preparation plays an important role in ensuring accurate test results. The patient must follow a special diet, beginning 2 days before the test and continuing until all three slides have been prepared. The patient is placed on a high-fiber, meat-free diet. Meat contains animal blood that could lead to a false-positive test result. A high-fiber diet is used because it encourages bleeding from lesions that may only bleed occasionally. In addition, the fiber adds bulk, which promotes bowel elimination and ensures adequate specimen collection. Certain medications cause irritation of the gastrointestinal tract, which may result in a small amount of bleeding; examples include aspirin, indomethacin, phenylbutazone, and corticosteroids. In addition, a vitamin C supplement (ascorbic acid) in excess of 250 mg/day or an iron supplement may cause false-negative results and should also be discontinued before testing. Table 17–4 lists the specific patient preparation requirements and the purpose of each requirement.

Although the primary use of the guaiac slide test is to screen for colorectal cancer, other important uses include screening for occult blood for the detection of an upper gastrointestinal ulcer or for disorders causing gastric and intestinal irritation. A positive test result on the guaiac slide test indicates blood in the stool, although the cause of the bleeding must still be determined. Therefore, further diagnostic procedures must be performed before the physician can make a final diagnosis; these may include proctosigmoidoscopy, colonoscopy, and upper and lower gastrointestinal x-ray studies.

TABLE 17–4. Patient Preparation for Fecal Occult Blood Testing

Beginning 2 days before obtaining the first stool specimen, the patient should follow the diet modifications listed below. The diet should be followed until all three slides have been prepared.

Meats. Eat no red or rare meat (beef and lamb) or processed meats and liver. Small amounts of well-cooked pork, poultry, and fish are permitted. Red meat contains animal blood that could cause a false-positive test result.

Vegetables. Eat moderate amounts of vegetables, both raw and cooked. Especially advised are lettuce, spinach, corn, and celery. Do not consume horseradish, turnips, broccoli, and cauliflower. These foods contain peroxidase, which could cause a false-positive test result.

Fruits. Eat moderate amounts of apples, bananas, oranges, peaches, pears, and plums. Do not consume melons because they contain peroxidase.

Miscellaneous High Fiber Foods. Eat moderate amounts of whole wheat bread, bran cereal, and popcorn. Foods high in fiber provide roughage to promote bowel elimination and encourage bleeding from lesions that only bleed occasionally.

Medications. Do not take any medications that contain aspirin, iron, or vitamin C (ascorbic acid) in excess of 250 mg/day. In addition, based upon the patient's medication therapy, the physician may stipulate additional medication restrictions. Certain medications cause irritation of the gastrointestinal tract, which may result in a small amount of bleeding. (Aspirin and other non-steroidal anti-inflammatory drugs should be avoided for at least 7 days prior to and continuing through the test period.)

Special Guidelines

Inform the physician and do not consume any of the food items listed above if they are known, from past experience, to cause severe gastrointestinal discomfort or serious diarrhea.

Make sure the diet modifications have been followed for 2 days (48 hours) before collecting the first stool specimen.

Do not initiate the test during a menstrual period or in the first three days after a menstrual period, or when bleeding from hemorrhoids is present. These conditions would result in false-positive test results.

Store the slides at room temperature and protect them from heat, sunlight, and fluorescent light to prevent deterioration of the active reagents on the slides.

PROCEDURE 17-7

PATIENT INSTRUCTIONS FOR THE HEMOCCULT SLIDE TEST

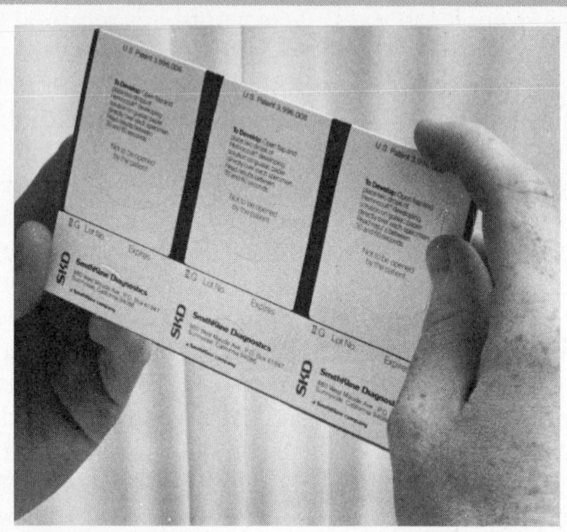

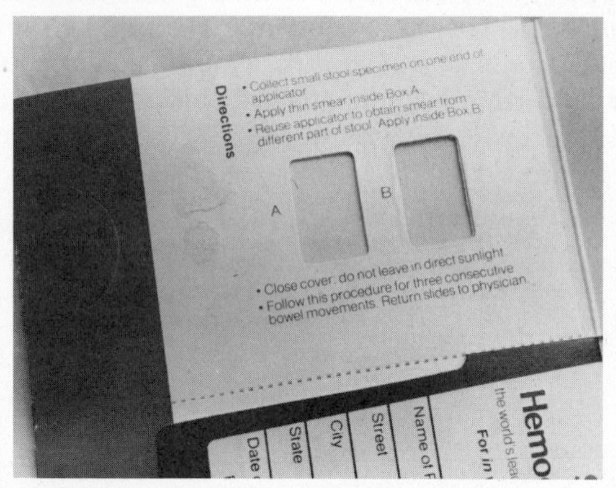

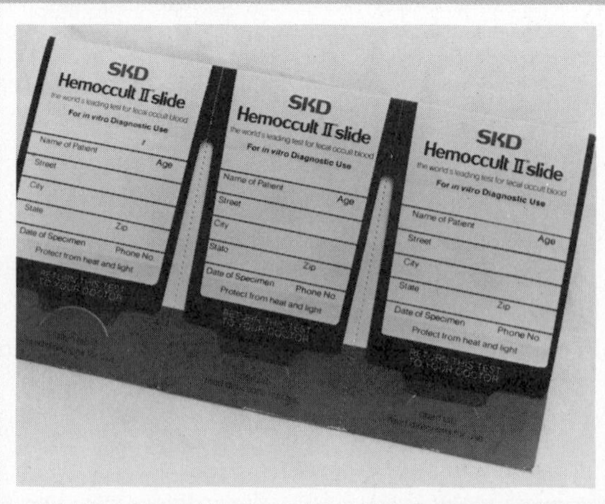

1. **PROCEDURAL STEP.** Obtain a Hemoccult slide testing kit. Check the expiration date located on each cardboard slide.

PRINCIPLE. Out-dated slides may lead to inaccurate test results.

2. **PROCEDURAL STEP.** Identify the patient and explain the purpose of the test. Tell the patient that the test should not be conducted during a menstrual period or when hemorrhoidal bleeding is present.

PRINCIPLE. Bleeding from other (identifiable) sources will invalidate the test results.

3. **PROCEDURAL STEP.** Instruct the patient in the proper preparation for the test. Refer to Table 17–4 for the specific guidelines the patient should follow. Tell the patient to begin the diet modifications 2 days before collecting the first stool specimen. Encourage the patient to adhere to the diet modifications.

PRINCIPLE. The diet modifications may discourage patient compliance. Therefore, the medical assistant should reinforce the importance of adhering to the diet requirements. Improper patient preparation may lead to inaccurate test results.

4. **PROCEDURAL STEP.** Provide the patient with the envelope containing the Hemoccult slide test kit. The kit consists of three identical cardboard slides attached to one another; each slide contains two squares, labeled A and B. Three wooden applicator sticks and written instructions are also included in the testing kit.

PRINCIPLE. Three slides are provided so that three stool specimens can be collected. The two squares in each slide (A and B) contain filter paper impregnated with guaiac, a chemical necessary for detection of blood in the stool.

5. **PROCEDURAL STEP.** Instruct the patient in the completion of the information required on the front flap of each card. This includes the patient's name, address, phone number, age, and the date of the specimen collection. A ball-point pen should be used to indicate this information.

6. **PROCEDURAL STEP.** Provide instructions on the proper care and storage of the slides. The patient should be told that the slides must be stored at room temperature and protected from heat, sunlight, and strong fluorescent light.

PRINCIPLE. Adverse storage conditions may result in deterioration of the active reagents impregnated on the filter paper, leading to inaccurate test results.

7. **PROCEDURAL STEP.** Instruct the patient in the initiation of the test by telling him or her to begin the diet modifications and then to collect a stool specimen from the first bowel movement after the 2-day (48-hour) preparatory period.

8. **PROCEDURAL STEP.** Instruct the patient in the proper collection and processing of the stool specimen as follows:

a. Using a wooden applicator, obtain a sample of the stool from the commode. The sample may be collected with the aid of a container or toilet tissue.
b. Open the front flap of the first cardboard slide (located on the left in the series of three).
c. Spread a very thin smear of the specimen over the filter paper in the square labeled A.
d. Using the same wooden applicator, obtain another specimen from a different area of the stool.
e. Spread a thin smear of the specimen over the filter paper in the square labeled B.
f. Close the front flap of the cardboard slide and indicate the date in the space provided.
g. Discard the wooden applicator in a waste container.

PRINCIPLE. Two squares are included in each slide to allow for specimen collection from different parts of the stool, because occult blood is not always equally distributed throughout the stool, as when bleeding occurs from the lower gastrointestinal tract. Thick specimens prevent adequate light penetration through the filter paper making it difficult to interpret the test results.

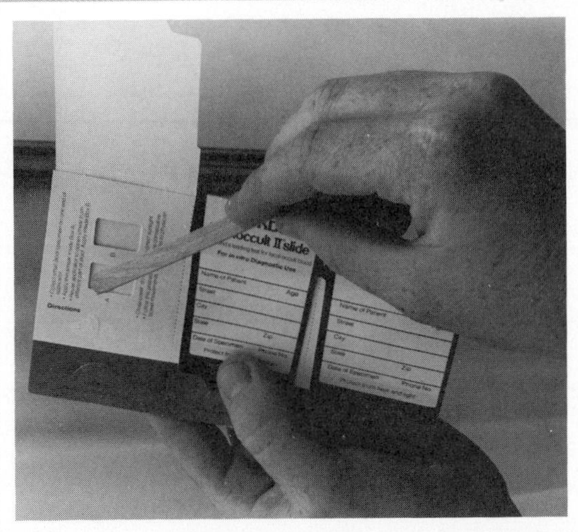

9. **PROCEDURAL STEP.** Instruct the patient to continue the testing period until all three specimens have been obtained and processed as outlined below.

a. Repeat Procedural Step 8 after the next bowel movement, using the cardboard slide located in the middle of the series of three.
b. Repeat Procedural Step 8 after the third bowel movement, using the cardboard slide located to the right in the series of three.
c. Allow the completed slides to air-dry overnight.

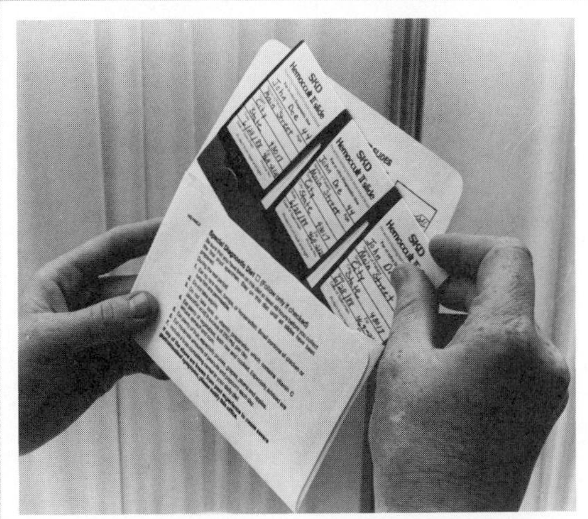

10. **PROCEDURAL STEP.** Instruct the patient to place the cardboard slides in the envelope, seal carefully, and return them as soon as possible to the medical office.

11. **PROCEDURAL STEP.** Provide the patient with an opportunity to ask questions; make sure the patient understands the instructions required for patient preparation, collection, and processing of the stool specimen and for storage of the slides.

PRINCIPLE. Improper patient preparation and technique may lead to inaccurate test results.

12. **PROCEDURAL STEP.** Record in the patient's chart. Include the patient's name and date and documentation that the Hemoccult test and instructions were given to the patient.

Note: The Coloscreen guaiac slide test utilizes a procedure similar to that of Hemoccult.

Record data below.

DATE	TIME	PATIENT'S NAME	RECORDING

PROCEDURE 17-8
DEVELOPING THE HEMOCCULT SLIDE TEST

1. **PROCEDURAL STEP.** Assemble the equipment, which includes the **prepared cardboard slides,** the **Hemoccult developing solution,** and the **reference card that accompanies the product instruction book.** The reference card provides an illustration of positive and negative test results, which can be used as a guide in interpreting results. *Note:* The slides may be prepared and developed immediately or prepared and stored for up to 14 days (at room temperature) before developing.

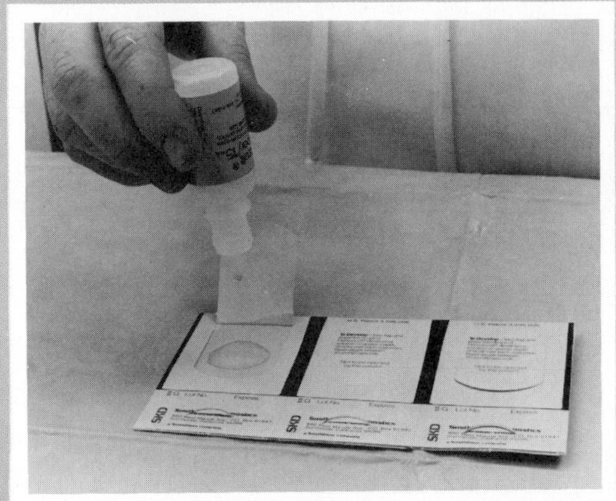

2. **PROCEDURAL STEP.** Check the expiration date on the developing solution bottle. The developing solution contains hydrogen peroxide and should be stored away from heat and light, and tightly capped when not in use.
PRINCIPLE. Outdated solution should not be used, as it may lead to inaccurate test results. The solution should be stored properly because it is flammable and evaporates easily.

3. **PROCEDURAL STEP.** Open the back flap of the cardboard slides. Apply two drops of the developing solution to the guaiac test paper underlying the back of each smear. Do not allow the solution to come in contact with the skin or eyes.
PRINCIPLE. The developing solution will be absorbed through the filter paper and into the stool specimen. This solution could cause irritation to the skin and eyes; should contact occur, immediately rinse the area with water.

4. **PROCEDURAL STEP.** Read the results within 60 seconds. Fecal blood loss in excess of 5 ml/day results in a positive reaction, which is indicated by any trace of blue appearing on or at the edge of the fecal smear. If no detectable color change occurs, the result is considered negative. (See the front inside cover for an illustration of a positive and negative reaction.)
PRINCIPLE. In the presence of hydrogen peroxide, the heme compound in hemoglobin oxidizes guaiac, causing it to turn blue within 60 seconds after adding the developer. The reading time is important because the color reaction may fade after 2 to 4 minutes.

5. **PROCEDURAL STEP.** Perform the quality control procedure.
PRINCIPLE. Quality control procedures ensure the accuracy and reliability of the test results.

6. **PROCEDURAL STEP.** Properly dispose of the Hemoccult slides to prevent transfer of microorganisms.
PRINCIPLE. The stool contains an abundant normal flora, and in some instances microorganisms making up the normal flora are capable of becoming pathogenic.

7. **PROCEDURAL STEP.** Wash the hands and record the results. Include the patient's name, the date and time, the brand name of the test (Hemoccult), the test results (recorded as positive or negative), and your initials.

Continued

Record data below.

DATE	TIME	PATIENT'S NAME	RESULTS

Quality Control for the Guaiac Slide Test

Quality control methods must be employed with the guaiac slide test to ensure reliable and valid results. The quality control procedure should be performed after the patient's slide test has been developed, read, and interpreted. The Hemoccult slide test contains an on-slide performance monitor consisting of positive and negative monitor areas. This monitor is located on the developing side of the filter paper under the back flap of the cardboard slide. The positive monitor area contains a control chemical that has been impregnated into the filter paper during the manufacturing process. The medical assistant should apply one drop of the developing solution between the positive and negative performance areas. The results must be read within 10 seconds after application of the developer. If the slide and developer are functional, the positive area will turn blue, whereas the negative area will show no color change. Failure of the expected control results to occur indicates an error and the test results are not considered valid; possible causes include the use of outdated cards or developing solution, an error in technique, or subjecting the slides to heat, sunlight, or strong fluorescent light. ColoScreen uses a similar control method; the main difference is that the medical assistant must wait 30 seconds before reading the results.

Proctoscopy and Sigmoidoscopy

Proctoscopy and sigmoidoscopy are procedures used to examine the lower intestines to diagnose and treat disorders of this part of the body. The physician may perform a proctoscopy or sigmoidoscopy as part of the physical examination or when the patient complains of a disorder of the bowel.

A digital examination of the anal canal and rectum is performed before the proctoscopy or sigmoidoscopy, using a well-lubricated gloved index finger. The physician palpates the rectum for the presence of tenderness, hemorrhoids, polyps, or tumors. Any palpable abnormality will be viewed directly when the endoscope is inserted. The digital examination also helps to relax the sphincter muscles of the anus and prepares the patient for the insertion of the endoscope.

Proctoscopy is the visual examination of the rectum using a *protoscope,* which is a rigid metal tubular instrument 15 cm in length containing a light and an obturator (Fig. 17–25). Proctoscopy may be performed to determine the presence of hemorrhoids, fissures, ulcerations, rectal bleeding, or other rectal disorders. A long cotton-tipped swab or suction equipment may be introduced through the lumen of the proctoscope to remove secretions such as mucus or particles of feces that interfere with proper visualization of the rectal mucosa. A biopsy may be taken from a tumor for examination by inserting biopsy forceps (Fig. 17–25) through the lumen of the proctoscope. Obtaining a biopsy is usually a painless procedure for the patient. Once the specimen is collected, it is placed in a sterile specimen container with a preservative and transported to the laboratory for histologic examination.

Sigmoidoscopy (also termed proctosigmoidoscopy) is the visual examination of the rectum and sigmoid colon using a *sigmoidoscope,* which is a long (25-cm) rigid tubular instrument containing a light (Fig. 17–26). Sigmoidoscopes are available with either reusable metal endoscopes or disposable plastic endoscopes. The outside of the endoscope is calibrated in centimeters and contains a magnifying lens at one end for visualization of the intestinal mucosa; the lens can be moved to one side for introduction of swabs and instruments such as biopsy forceps and suction equipment. The light source is located in the handle of the endoscope; it transmits light through the walls of the endoscope and provides a ring of light at the distal end for proper visualization of the intestinal mucosa. The obturator is a round-tipped device that is placed in the lumen of the sigmoidoscope before it is inserted through the anus and into the rectum. Its function is to close off the opening of the sigmoidoscope and to facilitate easier insertion. Once the sigmoidoscope has been inserted into the rectum, the physician removes the obturator and adjusts the light to permit adequate visualization of the mucosa. The

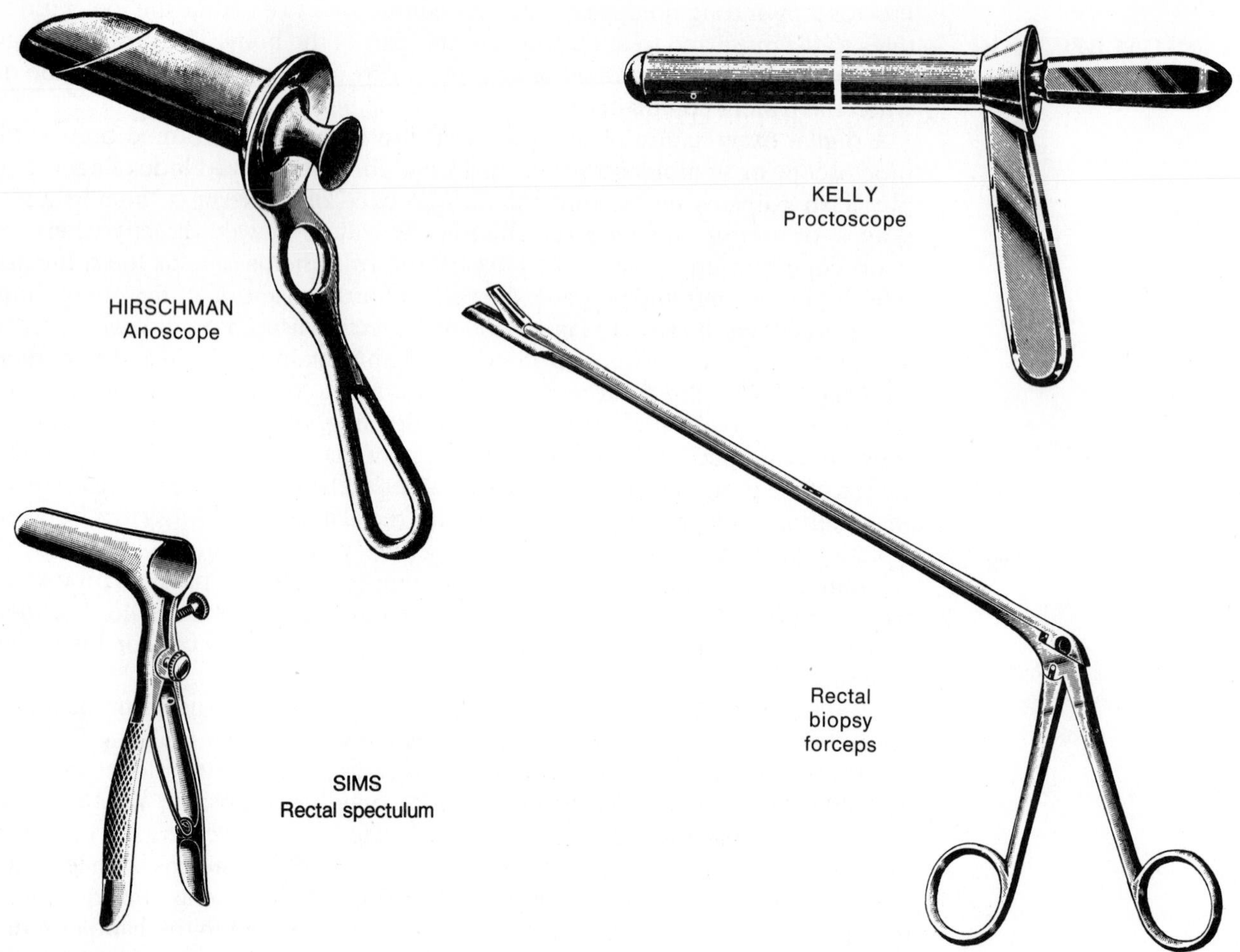

FIGURE 17–25. Rectal instruments that may be utilized in the medical office. (Courtesy of Elmed Incorporated, Addison, Illinois.)

sigmoidoscope is slowly advanced for about 10 inches (25 cm). Air is generally pumped into the colon using an inflation bulb. The function of the air is to distend the lumen of the colon for better visualization. The physician performs the visual examination of the intestinal mucosa as the sigmoidoscope is being inserted and also as it is being withdrawn.

Sigmoidoscopy may be performed to detect the presence of tumors, polyps, ulcerations, hemorrhoids, fissures, rectal bleeding, or other lower intestinal disorders. It is especially valuable as a diagnostic procedure in the early detection of symptomatic and asymptomatic cancer of the rectum and colon. Seventy per cent of all neoplasms occurring in the large intestine lie within the viewing range of the standard 25-cm sigmoidoscope. If a neoplasm is present, a biopsy is usually taken for histologic examination, using biopsy forceps. Early detection of malignant neoplasms leads to early diagnosis and treatment, which in turn increases the cure rate for individuals with this disease.

A newer type of sigmoidoscope is available and consists of a longer (60-cm) endoscope, which is flexible rather than rigid. Because of its flexibility, this sigmoidoscope can be inserted further into the colon than the standard (25-cm) sigmoidoscope previously described; this offers the advantage of an increased range of visualization of the intestinal mucosa.

The physician may want the patient to prepare the bowel prior to the examination. The preparation generally involves eating a light, low-residue meal the evening before the examination. Foods high in residue that should be avoided include raw fruits and vegetables and whole-grain breads and cereals. The patient

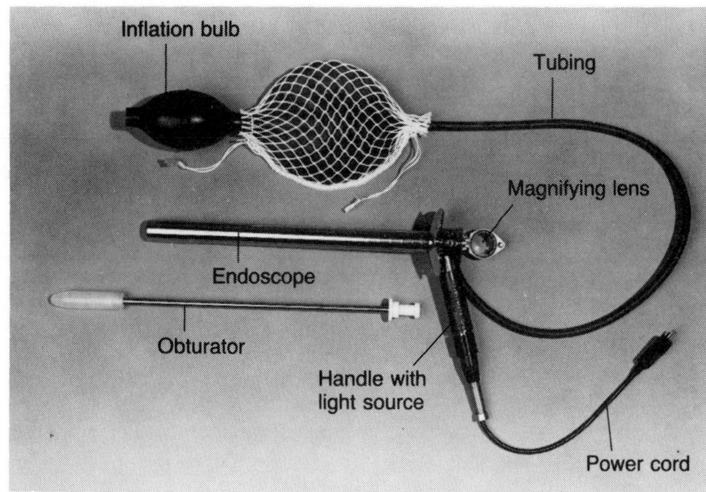

FIGURE 17–26. Reusable sigmoidoscope. This is a long metal tubular instrument containing a light. The obturator is a round-tipped device that is placed in the lumen of the sigmoidoscope before it is inserted into the rectum. Its function is to close off the opening of the sigmoidoscope and to facilitate easier insertion. Once the sigmoidoscope has been inserted into the rectum, the physician will remove the obturator and adjust the light to permit adequate visualization of the mucosa. The sigmoidoscope is slowly advanced for about 10 inches (25 cm). Air is generally pumped into the colon using the inflation bulb. The function of the air is to distend the lumen of the colon, allowing for better visualization.

may also be instructed to take a laxative and/or to perform a saline or warm water cleansing enema the evening before the examination. On the morning of the examination, the patient should consume a light breakfast and perform another cleansing enema until the returns are clear. The fecal material must be removed in order for the physician to visualize the mucosa of the bowel.

Some physicians prefer that the patient not take a laxative or perform an advance cleansing enema because it may change the appearance of the intestinal mucosa of the colon, making diagnosis difficult. In this case, the patient is examined after normal defecation. The medical assistant should consult with the physician to determine his or her preference.

PROCEDURE 17-9
ASSISTING WITH A PROCTOSCOPY AND SIGMOIDOSCOPY

1. **PROCEDURAL STEP.** Wash the hands.

2. **PROCEDURAL STEP.** Assemble the equipment. The tray set-up should include a **nonsterile aseptic glove** for the digital examination, a **proctoscope or sigmoidoscope** as required, **lubricant**, a **drape**, **tissue wipes**, and other equipment, depending on the nature of the examination and the physician's preference (e.g., **long cotton-tipped swabs (12 inches in length), suction equipment, a container of water for siphoning water through the tubing, biopsy forceps, and sterile specimen containers with a preservative**). Check to make sure the electric light bulb of the endoscope is working by plugging in the cord. The cord should be unplugged after checking. Label the specimen containers with the patient's name, the date, and the source of the specimen.

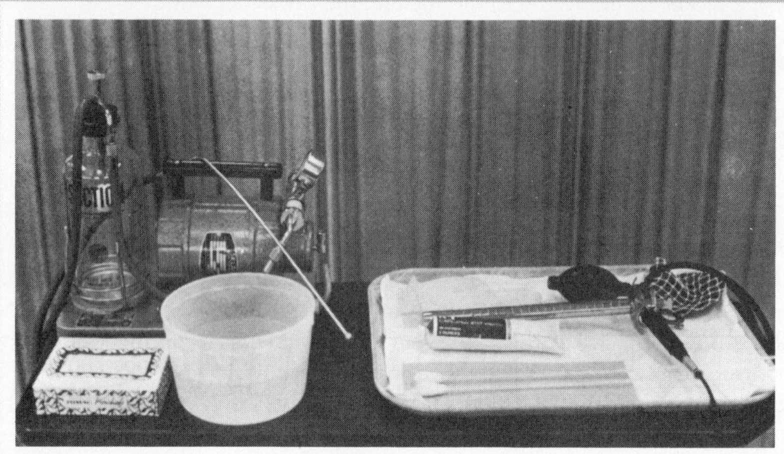

3. **PROCEDURAL STEP.** Ask the patient if he or she needs to empty the bladder before the examination. If a urine specimen is needed, the medical assistant requests that the patient void into a specimen container.
   PRINCIPLE. An empty bladder makes the examination easier and is more comfortable for the patient.

4. **PROCEDURAL STEP.** Instruct and prepare the patient for the examination. Ask him or her to remove all clothing from the waist down and to put on an examining gown with the opening positioned in back. Be sure to give complete and thorough instructions so the patient knows exactly what is expected. If the medical assistant senses that the patient may have trouble undressing, assistance should be offered.
   PRINCIPLE. Complete instructions reduce patient confusion.

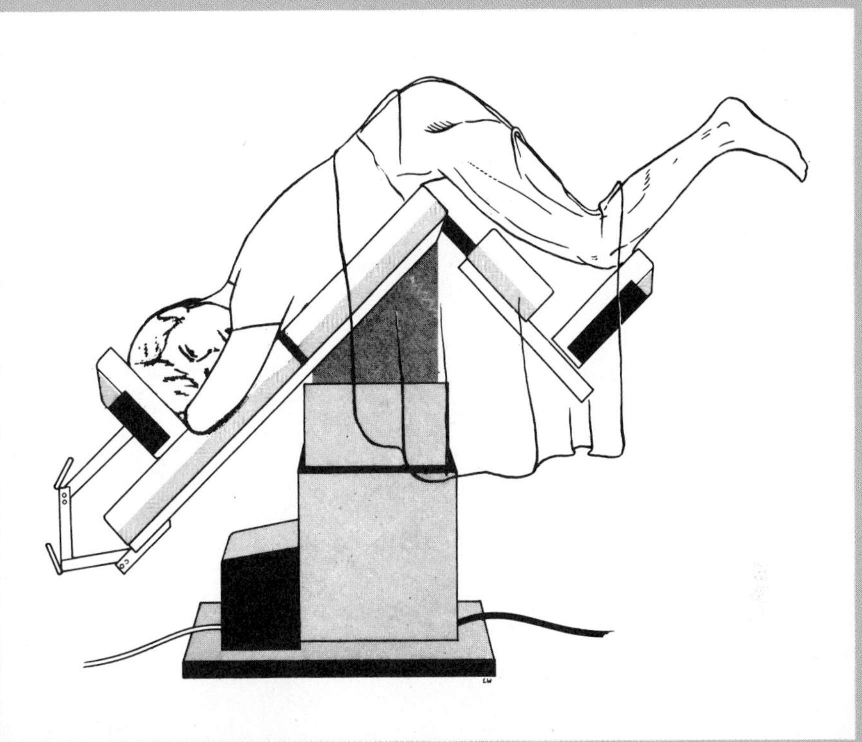

5. **Procedural step.** Assist the patient onto the examining table using the footstool. The preferred position for the examination is the knee-chest position. It is more comfortable and less tiring if the patient rests on the chest instead of the elbows. A pillow may be placed under his or her head for additional comfort. If the patient cannot assume the knee-chest position or has difficulty maintaining it, the physician may recommend that he or she be placed in the Sims position instead. Some physicians have specially designed proctologic tables that tilt the patient into the knee-chest position and provide support in this position. When using a proctologic table, the head and knee boards should be adjusted to fit each patient and then securely locked in place. The patient should be asked to kneel on the knee board, bend at the hips, and place his or her body over the table in a manner that allows the patient's elbows and arms to rest against the head board. The patient should be instructed to rest the head against the arms. The table is then slowly tilted into position. Since the knee-chest position is difficult to maintain, the medical assistant should not assist the patient into this position until the physician is ready to begin the examination.

Principle. The knee-chest position permits the abdominal contents to fall forward and away from the pelvis, making the procedure more comfortable for the patient and making it easier for the physician to insert the endoscope (proctoscope or sigmoidoscope).

Continued

6. **Procedural step.** Properly drape the patient so that only the anus is exposed. Some medical offices use fenestrated drapes with the circular opening placed over the anus.

Principle. Draping the patient reduces exposure and provides warmth.

7. **Procedural step.** Reassure the patient and help him or her to relax the muscles of the anus and rectum by breathing slowly and deeply through the mouth. As the endoscope is inserted, the patient experiences a feeling of pressure and the urge to defecate. This pressure is caused by the insertion of the endoscope, and the patient should be reassured that although it is uncomfortable, it will last for only a short period of time.

8. **Procedural step.** Assist the physician as required during the examination. The medical assistant may be responsible for the following:

a. Lubricating the physician's gloved index finger for the digital examination.
b. Warming the endoscope and placing lubricant on the endoscope before insertion into the rectum. The endoscope should be well lubricated to facilitate insertion.
c. Plugging in the endoscope. *Note:* The endoscope should not be plugged in until the physician is ready to use it, because it will become hot from the heat of the light and may harm the patient.
d. Handing swabs and assisting with the suction equipment as required. The tubing should be cleansed immediately after use by siphoning water through it. This helps keep fecal material from sticking to the sides of the tubing.
e. Assisting with the collection of a biopsy by handing the biopsy forceps to the physician and holding the specimen container to accept the biopsy. Do not touch the inside of the container, because it is sterile.
f. Accepting contaminated instruments and swabs from the physician and properly disposing of them. Take the article from the physician in a manner that does not allow the contaminated part of it to come in contact with your fingers.

9. **PROCEDURAL STEP.** Once the examination is completed, the medical assistant should clean the patient's anal region of any excess lubricant, using tissue wipes. He or she should be allowed to rest in a prone position before sitting up. Wash your hands and assist the patient off the examining table to prevent falls. Instruct him or her to get dressed, offering assistance if needed.

PRINCIPLE. Patients (especially elderly ones) frequently become dizzy after being on the examining table and should be allowed to rest before sitting up.

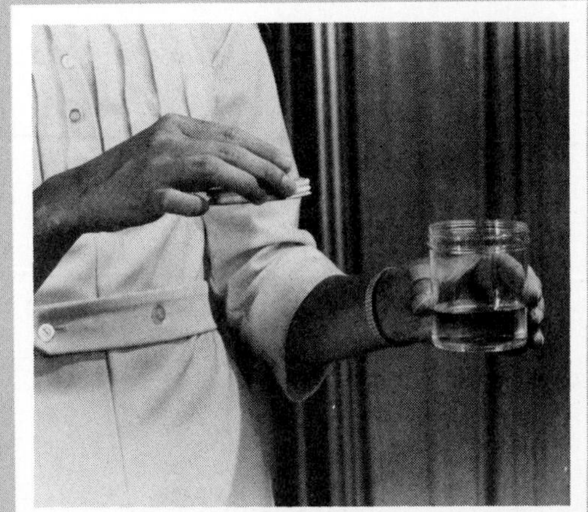

10. **PROCEDURAL STEP.** Record information in the patient's chart as instructed by the physician. Be sure to include your initials next to the recording.

11. **PROCEDURAL STEP.** Transport any specimens that were taken (along with a laboratory request) to the laboratory to be examined by a pathologist.

12. **PROCEDURAL STEP.** Clean the examining room in preparation for the next patient. The proctoscope and sigmoidoscope should be sanitized and disinfected according to the medical office policy.

Record data below.

DATE	TIME	PATIENT'S NAME	RECORDING

Study Questions

1. What is the purpose of performing a fecal occult blood test?
2. What patient preparation is required for a fecal occult blood test?
3. What is the purpose of performing a sigmoidoscopy?
4. What patient preparation is required for a sigmoidoscopy?

Glossary

Abortion (ah-bor′shun) The loss of a pregnancy before the stage of viability.

Abrasion (ah-bra′zhun) A wound in which the outer layers of the skin are damaged; a scrape.

Abscess (ab′ses) A collection of pus in a cavity surrounded by inflamed tissue.

Absorbable suture (ab-sor′ba-b'l soo′-cher) Suture material that is gradually digested by tissue enzymes and absorbed by the body.

Adnexal (ad-nek′sal) Adjacent.

Aerobe (a′er-ōb) An organism that needs oxygen in order to live and grow.

Agglutination (ah-gloo″tĭ-na′shun) The aggregation or uniting of separate particles into clumps or masses.

Alveolus (pl. aveoli) (al-ve′o-lus; al-ve′o-li) A thin-walled air sac of the lungs in which the exchange of oxygen and carbon dioxide takes place.

Ambulation (am″bū-la′shun) The ability to walk as opposed to being confined to bed.

Ameboid movement (ah-me′boid mo͞ov′-ment) Movement used by leukocytes that permits them to propel themselves from the capillaries out into the tissues.

Amplitude (am′plĭ-tūd) Refers to amount, extent, size, abundance, or fullness.

Ampule (am′pūl) A small sealed glass container containing a single dose of medication.

Anaerobe (an-a′er-ōb) An organism that grows best in the absence of oxygen.

Anemia (ah-ne′me-ah) A condition in which there is a decrease in the number of erythrocytes or in the amount of hemoglobin in the blood.

Antecubital space (an″te-ku′bĭ-tal spās) The space located at the front of the elbow.

Antiserum (an″tĭ-se′rum) A serum that contains antibodies.

Anticoagulant (an″tĭ-ko-ag′u-lant) A substance that inhibits blood clotting.

Antiseptic (an″tĭ-sep′tik) A substance that inhibits the growth of, or kills, disease-producing microorganisms but not their spores. An antiseptic is usually applied to living tissue.

Aorta (a-or′tah) The major trunk of the arterial system of the body. The aorta arises from the upper surface of the left ventricle.

Apnea (ap-ne′ah) The temporary cessation of breathing.

Approximation (ah-prok′sĭ-mā′shun) The process of bringing two parts, such as tissue, together, through the use of sutures or other means.

Arrhythmia (ah-rith′me-ah) An irregular rhythm.

Artifact (ar′tĭ-fakt) Additional electrical activity that is picked up by the electrocardiograph that interferes with the normal appearance of the ECG cycles.

Asepsis (a-sep′sis) Free from infection or pathogens.

Aspirate (as′pĭ-rāt) To remove by suction.

Atypical (a-tip′ĭ-kal) Deviation from the normal.

Audiometer (aw″de-om′ĕ-ter) An instrument used to measure hearing.

Auscultation (aw″skul-ta′shun) The process of listening to the sounds produced within the body to detect any signs of disease.

Autoclave (aw′to-klāv) An apparatus for the sterilization of materials, using steam under pressure.

Automated method (aw-to-ma′ted mĕth′-ud) (for testing laboratory specimens) A method of laboratory testing in which the series of steps in the test method is performed by an automated analyzer.

Avoirdupois (av′er-dŭ-poiz″) A system of weight used in English-speaking countries for weighing heavy articles. This system is not used to weigh drugs and precious stones and metals.

Axilla (ak-sil′ah) The armpit.

Bacilli (bah-sil′i) (singular, bacillus) Bacteria that have a rod shape.

Bandage (ban′dij) A strip of woven material used to wrap or cover a part of the body.

Baseline (bās′līn) The flat horizontal line that separates the various waves of the ECG cycle.

Bilirubin (bil″ĭ-roo′bin) An orange-colored bile pigment produced by the breakdown of heme from the hemoglobin molecule.

Bilirubinuria (bil″ĭ-roo″bĭ-nu′re-ah) The presence of bilirubin in the urine.

Biopsy (bi′op-se) The surgical removal and examination of tissue from the living body. Biopsies are generally done to determine whether a tumor is benign or malignant.

Blood antibody (blud an′tĭ-bod″e) A protein present in the blood plasma that is capable of combining with its corresponding blood antigen to produce an antigen-antibody reaction.

Blood antigen (blud an′tĭ-jen) A protein present on the surface of red blood cells that determines the blood type of an individual.

Bounding pulse (bownd-ing puls) A pulse with an increased volume that feels very strong and full.

Bradycardia (brad″e-kar′de-ah) An abnormally slow heart or pulse rate (below 60 beats per minute).

Braxton Hicks contractions (braks′ton hiks kon-trak′shuns) Intermittent and irregular painless uterine contractions that occur throughout pregnancy. They occur more frequently toward the end of the pregnancy and are sometimes mistaken for true labor pains.

Buffy coat (buf′e kōt) A thin, light-colored layer of white blood cells and platelets that lies between a top layer of plasma and a bottom layer of red blood cells when an anticoagulant has been added to a blood specimen.

Canthus (kan′thus) The junction of the eyelids at either corner of the eye.

Capillary action (kap′ĭ-ler″e ak′shun) That action which causes liquid to rise along a wick, a tube, or a gauze dressing.

Cardiac cycle (kar′de-ak si′k′l) One complete heart beat.

Centigrade or Celsius thermometer (sen′tĭ-grād or sel′se-us ther-mom′e-ter) A thermometer on which the freezing point of water is 0 and the boiling point of water is 100 degrees.

Cerumen (sĕ-roo′men) Ear wax.

Charting (chart′ing) The process of making written entries about a patient in the medical record.

Cilia (sil′e-ah) Slender hairlike processes.

Clinical diagnosis (klin′e-k′l di″ag-no′sis) A tentative diagnosis obtained through the evaluation of the health history and the physical examination, without the benefit of laboratory or diagnostic tests.

Cocci (kok′si) (singular, coccus) Bacteria that have a round shape.

Colony (kol′o-ne) A mass of bacteria growing on a solid culture medium that have arisen from the multiplication of a single bacterium.

Colposcope (kol′po-skōp) A lighted instrument with a binocular magnifying lens used for the examination of the vagina and cervix.

Colposcopy (kol-pos′ko-pe) The visual examination of the vagina and cervix using a colposcope.

Compress (kom′pres) A soft, moist, absorbent cloth that is folded in several layers and applied to a part of the body in the local application of heat or cold.

Conduction (kon-duk′shun) The transfer of energy, such as heat, from one object to another.

Conjunctiva (kon″junk-ti′vah) The mucous membrane that lines the eyelids and covers the eyeball, except for the cornea.

Contagious (kon-ta′jus) Capable of being transmitted directly or indirectly from one person to another.

Contaminate (kon-tam′ĭ-nāt) To soil or to make impure. An aseptic object is contaminated when it touches something that is not clean.

Contrast medium (kon′trast me′de-um) A substance that is used to make a particular structure visible on a radiograph.

Contusion (kon-too′zhun) An injury to the tissues under the skin causing blood vessels to rupture, allowing blood to seep into the tissues; a bruise.

Convection (kon-vek′shun) The transfer of energy, such as heat, in the form of currents.

Conversion (kon-ver′zhun) Changing from one unit of measurement to another.

Crisis (kri′sis) A sudden falling of an elevated body temperature to normal.

Cryosurgery (kri″o-ser′jer-e) The therapeutic use of freezing temperatures to treat chronic cervicitis and cervical erosion; also known as cryotherapy.

Cubic centimeter (kyo͞o′bĭk sĕn′tə-mē′-tər) The amount of space occupied by 1 milliliter (1 ml = 1 cc).

Culture (kul′tūr) The propagation of a mass of microorganisms in a laboratory culture medium.

Culture medium (kul′tūr me′de-um) A mixture of nutrients on which microorganisms are grown in the laboratory.

Cyanosis (si″ah-no′sis) A bluish discoloration of the skin and mucous membranes.

Cytology (si-tol′o-je) The science that deals with the study of cells, including their origin, structure, function, and pathology.

Dermis (der′mis) The true skin; its main thickness, with an active blood supply.

Detergent (de-ter′jent) An agent that purifies or cleanses.

Diagnosis (di″ag-no′sis) The scientific method of determining and identifying a disease.

Diapedesis (di″ah-pĕ-de′sis) The ameboid movement of blood cells (especially leukocytes) through the wall of a capillary and out into the tissues.

Diastole (di-as′to-le) The phase in the cardiac cycle in which the heart relaxes between contractions.

Diastolic pressure (di″ah-stol′ik presh′-ur) The point of lesser pressure on the arterial walls, which is recorded during diastole.

Differential diagnosis (dif′er-en′shal di″ag-no′sis) A determination of which of two or more diseases with similar symptoms is producing the patient's symptoms.

Dilation (of the cervix) (di-la′shun) The stretching of the external os from an opening a few millimeters in size to an opening large enough to allow the passage of an infant (approximately 10 cm).

Dilation and curettage (di-la′shun and ku″rĕ-tahzh′) The process of expanding the opening of the uterus to permit scraping of its walls: also called D and C.

Disinfectant (dis″in-fek′tant) A substance used to destroy disease-producing microorganisms but not necessarily their spores. Disinfectants are usually applied to inanimate objects.

Donor (do′ner) One who furnishes something such as blood, tissue, or organs to be used in another person.

Dose (dōs) The quantity of a drug to be administered at one time.

Dyspnea (disp′ne-ah) Labored or difficult breathing.

ECG cycle (ECG si′k′l) The graphic representation of a cardiac cycle.

EDC Estimated date of confinement, or due date; so named because a long period of bed rest following childbirth used to be the norm.

Edema (ĕ-de′mah) The retention of fluid in the tissues, resulting in swelling.

Effacement (ĭ-fās′ment) The thinning and shortening of the cervical canal from its normal length of 1 to 2 cm to a structure with paper-thin edges in which there is no canal at all. Effacement occurs late in pregnancy or during labor, or both. The purpose of effacement along with dilation is to permit the passage of the infant into the birth canal.

Electrocardiogram (e-lek″tro-kar′de-o-gram″) The graphic representation of the electrical activity of the heart.

Electrocardiograph (e-lek″tro-kar′de-o-graf″) The instrument used to record the electrical activity of the heart.

Electrode (e-lek′trōd) A conductor of electricity, usually made of metal, that is used to promote contact between the body and the electrocardiograph (also known as a sensor).

Electrolyte (e-lek′tro-līt) A chemical substance that promotes conduction of an electrical current.

Endocervix (en″do-ser′viks) The mucous membrane lining the cervical canal.

Endoscope (en′do-skōp) An instrument, consisting of a tube and an optical system, that is used for direct visual inspection of organs or cavities.

Enema (en′ĕ-mah) An injection of fluid into the rectum to aid in the elimination of feces from the colon.

Engagement (en-gāj′ment) The entrance of the fetal head or the presenting part into the pelvic inlet.

Epidermis (ep′ĭ-der′mis) The outermost, nonvascular layer of the skin.

Erythema (er″ĭ-the′mah) Redness of the skin caused by congestion of capillaries in the lower layers of skin.

Erythrocyte (ĕ-rith′ro-sīt) Red blood cell.

Eupnea (ūp-ne′ah) Normal respiration.

Exfoliated cells (eks-fo″le-a′ted selz) Cells that have been sloughed off from the surface of tissues into the secretions bathing those tissues.

Exhalation (eks″hah-la′shun) The act of breathing out.

External os (eks-ter′nal os) The opening of the cervical canal of the uterus into the vagina.

Exudate (eks′u-dāt) A discharge produced by the body's tissues.

Fahrenheit thermometer (far′en-hīt ther-mom′ĕ-ter) A thermometer on which the freezing point of water is 32 degrees and the boiling point of water is 212 degrees.

False negative (fôls neg′ah-tiv) A test result denoting that a condition is absent when, in actuality, it is present.

False positive (fôls poz′ĭ-tiv) A test result denoting that a condition is present when, in actuality, it is absent.

Familial (fə-mĭl′yəl) Occurring or affecting members of a family more frequently than would be expected by chance.

Fastidious (fas-tid′e-us) Extremely delicate; difficult to culture, therefore involving specialized growth requirements.

Fasting (fast′ing) Abstaining from food or fluids (except water) for a specified amount of time prior to the collection of a specimen.

Fetal heart rate (fe′tal hart rāt) The number of times the fetal heart beats per minute.

Fetal heart tones (fe′tal hart tōnz) The heart beat of the fetus as heard through the mother's abdominal wall.

Fetoscope (fe′to-skōp) An instrument for auscultation of the heart of the fetus.

Fetus (fe′tus) The child in utero, from the third month after conception to birth; during the first two months of development, it is called an embryo.

Fever (fe′ver) A body temperature that is above normal. Synonym for pyrexia.

Fibroblast (fi′bro-blast) An immature cell from which connective tissue can develop.

Fluoroscope (floo′or-o-skōp″) An instrument used to view internal organs and structures directly.

Fluoroscopy (floo″or-os′ko-pe) Examination of a patient using the fluoroscope.

Forceps (fōr′seps) A two-pronged instrument for grasping and squeezing.

Frenulum linguae (fren′u-lum ling′gwe) The midline fold that connects the undersurface of the tongue with the floor of the mouth.

Fundus (fun′dus) The dome-shaped upper portion of the uterus between the fallopian tubes.

Furuncle (fu′rung-k′l) A localized staphylococcal infection that originates deep within a hair follicle; also known as a boil.

Gene (gēn) A unit of heredity.

Gestation (jes-ta′shun) The period of intrauterine development from conception to birth; the period of pregnancy. The average pregnancy lasts about 280 days or 40 weeks from the date of conception to childbirth.

Glycogen (gli′ko-jen) The form in which carbohydrate is stored in the body.

Glycosuria (gli″ko-su′re-ah) The presence of sugar in the urine.

Gravid (grav′id) Pregnant.

Gravida (grav′ĭ-dah) A woman who is or has been pregnant.

Gravidity (grah-vid′ĭ-te) The total number of pregnancies a woman has had regardless of duration, including a current pregnancy.

Gynecology (gi″nĕ-kol′o-je) The branch of medicine that deals with the disease of the reproductive organs of women.

Hematology (he″mah-tol′o-je) The study of blood and blood-forming tissues.

Hematoma (he″mah-to′mah) A swelling or mass of coagulated blood caused by a break in a blood vessel.

Hemocytometer (he″mo-si-tom′ĕ-ter) An instrument used to count blood cells.

Hemoglobin (he″mo-glo′bin) The iron-containing pigment of erythrocytes that transports oxygen in the body.

Hemolysis (he-mol′ĭ-sis) The breakdown of erythrocytes with the release of hemoglobin into the plasma.

Hemostasis (he″mo-sta′sis) The arrest of bleeding by natural or artificial means.

High-density lipoprotein (HDL) (hi den′sĭ-te lip″o-pro′tēn) A lipoprotein consisting of protein and cholesterol, which removes excess cholesterol from the cells.

High-risk (hī-risk) Having an increased possibility of suffering harm, damage, or death.

Homeostasis (ho″me-o-sta′sis) The state in which body systems are functioning normally and the internal environment of the body is in equilibrium; the body is in a healthy state.

Host (hōst) An animal or plant that provides nourishment for a microorganism to grow and multiply.

Hyperglycemia (hi″per-gli-se′me-ah) An abnormal increase in the glucose level in the blood.

Hyperopia (hi″per-o′pe-ah) Farsightedness.

Hyperpnea (hi″perp-ne′ah) An abnormal increase in the rate and depth of respiration.

Hyperpyrexia (hi″per-pi-rek′se-ah) An extremely high fever.

Hypertension (hi″per-ten′shun) High blood pressure.

Hypoglycemia (hi″po-gli-se′me-ah) An abnormally low level of glucose in the blood.

Hypopnea (hi-pop′ne-ah) An abnormal decrease in the rate and depth of respiration.

Hypotension (hi″po-ten′shun) Low blood pressure.

Hypoxia (hi-pok′se-ah) A reduction in the oxygen supply to the tissues of the body.

Immunity (ĭ-mu′nĭ-te) The resistance of the body to the effects of a harmful agent such as a pathogenic microorganism or its toxins.

Immunization (active, artificial) (im″u-nĭ-za′shun) The process of becoming immune or of rendering an individual immune through the use of a vaccine or toxoid.

Impacted (im-pak′ted) Being wedged firmly together so as to be immovable.

Incision (in-sizh′un) A clean cut caused by a cutting instrument.

Incubate (in′ku-bāt) In microbiology, the act of placing a culture in a chamber (incubator), which provides optimal growth requirements for the multiplication of the organism, such as the proper temperature, humidity, and darkness.

Incubation period (in″ku-ba′shun pir′ē-ud) The interval of time between the invasion by a pathogenic microorganism and the appearance of first symptoms of the disease.

Induration (in″du-ra′shun) An area of hardened tissue.

Infant (in′fant) A child from birth to one year of age.

Infection (in-fek′shun) The condition in which the body, or part of it, is invaded by a pathogen.

Infectious disease (in-fek′shus dĭ-zēz′) A disease caused by a pathogen that produces harmful effects on its host.

Infiltration (in″fil-tra′shun) The process by which a substance passes into and is deposited within the substance of a cell, tissue, or an organ.

Inflammation (in″flah-ma′shun) A protective response of the body to trauma and the entrance of foreign matter. The purpose of inflammation is to destroy invading microorganisms and to repair injured tissue. Local symptoms occurring at the site of inflammation include pain, swelling, redness, and warmth.

Inhalation (in″hah-la′shun) The act of breathing in.

Inhalation administration (in″hah-la′-shun ăd-min″is-tra′shun) The administration of medication by way of air or other vapor being drawn into the lungs.

Inoculate (ĭ-nok′u-lāt) The introduction of microorganisms into a culture medium.

Inoculum (ĭ-nok′u-lum) The specimen used to inoculate a medium.

Inspection (in-spek′shun) The process of observing a patient to detect any signs of disease.

Instillation (in′stĭ-la-shun) The dropping of a liquid into a body cavity.

Intercostal (in″ter-kos′tal) Between the ribs.

Internal os (in-ter′nal os) The internal opening of the cervical canal into the uterus.

Interval (in′ter-val) The length of a wave or the length of a wave with a segment.

Intradermal injection (in″trah-der′mal in-jek′shun) Introducing medication into the dermal layer of the skin.

Intramuscular injection (in″trah-mus′-ku-lar in-jek′shun) Introducing medication into the muscle layer of the body.

Intravenous injection (in″trah-ve′nus in-jek′shun) Introducing medication into the bloodstream directly through a vein.

In vitro (in ve′tro) Occurring in glass. Refers to tests performed under artificial conditions, as in the laboratory.

In vivo (in ve′vo) Occurring in the living body or organism.

Irrigation (ir″ĭ-ga′shun) The washing of a body canal by a flowing solution.

IUD (intrauterine device) A mechanical device inserted into the uterine cavity for the purpose of contraception.

Ketonuria (ke″to-nu′re-ah) The presence of ketone bodies in the urine.

Ketosis (ke″to′sis) An accumulation of large amounts of ketone bodies in the tissues and body fluids.

Laboratory test (lab′o-rah-tor″e test) The clinical analysis and study of materials, fluids, or tissues obtained from patients to assist in diagnosing and treating disease.

Laceration (las″ĕ-ra′shun) A wound in which the tissues are torn apart, leaving ragged and irregular edges.

Length (length) A unit of linear measurement used to measure distance.

Leukocyte (loo′ko-sīt) White blood cell.

Leukocytosis (loo″ko-si-to′sis) An abnormal increase in the number of white blood cells (above 10,000 per cu mm of blood).

Leukopenia (loo″ko-pe′ne-ah) An abnormal decrease in the number of white blood cells (below 5,000 per cu mm of blood).

Ligate (li′gāt) To tie off and close a structure such as a severed blood vessel.

Lipoprotein (lip″o-pro′tēn) A complex molecule consisting of protein and a lipid fraction such as cholesterol. Lipoproteins function in transporting lipids in the blood.

Load (lōd) The articles that are being sterilized.

Local anesthetic (lo′kal an″es-thet′ik) A drug that produces a loss of feeling and an inability to perceive pain in only a specific part of the body.

Lochia (lo′ke-ah) A discharge from the uterus after delivery, consisting of blood, tissue, white blood cells, and some bacteria.

Low-density lipoprotein (LDL) (lo den′sĭ-te lip″o-pro′tēn) A lipoprotein consisting of protein and cholesterol, which picks up cholesterol and delivers it to the cells.

Lysis (li′sis) The gradual return of the body temperature to normal.

Manometer (mah-nom′ĕ-ter) An instrument for measuring pressure.

Manual method (man′u-al mĕth′ud) A method of laboratory testing in which the series of steps in the test method is performed by hand.

Mayo tray (mā′ō trā) A broad, flat metal tray placed on a stand and used to hold sterile instruments and supplies once it has been covered with a sterile towel.

Medical record (mĕd′ĭk′l rek′erd) A written record of the important aspects regarding a patient, his care, and the progress of his illness (also known as "the chart").

Melena (mĕ-le′nah) The darkening of the stool due to the presence of blood in an amount of 50 ml or greater.

Meniscus (mĕ-nis′kus) The curved upper surface of a liquid in a container. The surface is convex if the liquid does not wet the container and concave if it does.

Microbiology (mi″kro-bi-ol′o-je) The scientific study of microorganisms and their activities.

Microorganism (mi″kro-or′gah-nizm) A microscopic plant or animal.

Micturition (mik″tu-rish′un) The act of voiding urine.

Mordant (mor′dant) A substance that fixes a stain or dye.

Mucous membrane (mu′kus mem′brān) A membrane lining body passages or cavities that open to the outside.

Multigravida (mul″tĭ-grav′ĭ-dah) A woman who has been pregnant more than once.

Multipara (mul-tip′ah-rah) A woman who has completed two or more pregnancies to the age of viability regardless of whether they ended in live infants or stillbirths.

Myopia (mi-o′pe-ah) Nearsightedness.

Needle biopsy (ne′d′l bi-op-se) A type of biopsy in which tissue from deep within the body is obtained by the insertion of a biopsy needle through the skin.

Nephron (nef′ron) The functional unit of the kidney.

Nonabsorbable suture (non-ab-sor′ba-b′l soo′cher) Suture material that is not absorbed by the body and either remains permanently in the body tissue and becomes encapsulated by fibrous tissue or is removed.

Nonpathogen (non-path′o-jen) A microorganism that does not normally produce disease.

Normal flora (nor′mal flo′rah) Harmless, nonpathogenic microorganisms that normally reside in many parts of the body but do not cause disease.

Normal range (nor′mal rānj) (for laboratory tests) A certain established and acceptable parameter or reference range within which the laboratory test results of a healthy individual are expected to fall.

Normal sinus rhythm (nor′mal si′nus rith′m) Refers to an electrocardiogram that is within normal limits.

Nullipara (nuh-lip′ah-rah) A woman who has not carried a pregnancy to the point of viability.

Objective symptom (ob-jek′tiv simp′-tom) A symptom that can be observed by an examiner.

Obstetrics (ob-stet′riks) That branch of medicine concerned with the care of the woman during pregnancy, childbirth, and the postpartal period.

Occult blood (ŏ-kult′ blud) Blood occurring in such a small amount that it is not visually detectable to the unaided eye.

Oliguria (ol″ĭ-gu′re-ah) Decreased or scanty output of urine.

Ophthalmologist (of″thal-mol′o-jist) A medical doctor who specializes in diagnosing and treating disorders of the eye.

Ophthalmoscope (of-thal′mo-skōp) An instrument for examining the interior of the eye.

Optician (op-tish′an) A professional who grinds lenses and places them in frames.

Optimum growth temperature (op′tĭ-mum grōth tem′per-ah-tūr) The temperature at which an organism grows best.

Optometrist (op-tom′ĕ-trist) A licensed nonmedical practitioner who is skilled in measuring visual acuity and is qualified to prescribe corrective lenses.

Oral administration (o′ral ăd-mĭn″ĭs-trā-shun) Administration of medication by mouth.

Orthopnea (or″thop-ne′ah) The condition in which breathing is easier when an individual is in a standing or sitting position.

Otoscope (o′to-skōp) An instrument for examining the external ear canal and tympanic membrane.

Oxyhemoglobin (ok″sĭ-he″mo-glo′bin) Hemoglobin that has combined with oxygen.

Palpation (pal-pa′shun) The process of feeling with the hands to detect signs of disease.

Para (par′ah) A term used to refer to past pregnancies that reached viability regardless of whether the infant was dead or alive at birth.

Parity (par′ĭ-te) The condition of having borne offspring who had attained the age of viability regardless of whether they were live infants or stillbirths.

Pathogen (path′o-jen) A disease-producing microorganism.

Pediatrician (pe″de-ah-trish′an) A medical doctor who specializes in the care and development of children and the diagnosis and treatment of diseases of children.

Pediatrics (pe″de-at′riks) The branch of medicine dealing with the care and development of children and the diagnosis and treatment of diseases of children.

Pelvimetry (pel-vim′ĭ-tre) Measurement of the capacity and diameter of the maternal pelvis, which helps to determine if it will be possible to deliver the infant through the vaginal route.

Percussion (per-kush′un) The process of tapping the body to detect signs of disease.

Percussion hammer (per-kush′un ham′-er) A hammer with a rubber head, used for testing reflexes.

Perinatal (per″i-na′tal) Relating to the period shortly before and after birth.

Perineum (per″ĭ-ne′um) The external region between the vaginal orifice and the anus in a female and between the scrotum and the anus in a male.

Peroxidase (pĕ-rok′sĭ-dās) (as it pertains

to the guaiac slide test) A substance that is able to transfer oxygen from hydrogen peroxide to oxidize guaiac, causing the guaiac to turn blue.

pH The degree to which a solution is acidic or basic.

Phagocytosis (fag″o-si-to′sis) The engulfing and destruction of foreign particles, such as bacteria, by special cells called phagocytes.

Pipet (pi-pet′) A glass tube used to measure and/or tranfer small quantities of a liquid by sucking it into the tube (can also be spelled pipette).

Plasma (plaz′mah) The liquid part of the blood consisting of a clear yellowish fluid that makes up approximately 55 per cent of the total blood volume.

Polycythemia (pol″e-si-the′me-ah) A disorder in which there is an increase in the red cell mass.

Polyuria (pol″e-u′re-ah) Increased output of urine.

Position (po-zish′un) The relation of the presenting part of the fetus to the maternal pelvis.

Postoperative (pōst-op′er-ah-tiv) After a surgical operation.

Postpartum (pōst-par′tum) Occurring after childbirth.

Pre-eclampsia (pre″e-klamp′se-ah) A major complication of pregnancy of unknown cause characterized by increasing hypertension, albuminuria, and edema. If this condition is neglected or not treated properly, it may develop into eclampsia, which could cause maternal convulsions and coma. Eclampsia generally occurs between the twentieth week of pregnancy and the end of the first week postpartum.

Prenatal (pre-na′tal) Before birth.

Preoperative (pre-op′er-ah-tiv) Preceding a surgical operation.

Presbyopia (pres″be-o′pe-ah) A decrease in the elasticity of the lens due to aging, resulting in a decreased ability to focus on close objects.

Prescription (pre-skrip′shun) Order for a drug or other therapy written by a physician.

Presentation (prez″en-ta′shun) The part of the fetus that is closest to the cervix and will be delivered first. A cephalic presentation is a delivery in which the fetal head is presenting against the cervix. A breech presentation is a delivery in which the buttocks or feet are presented instead of the head.

Primigravida (pri″mĭ-grav′ĭ-dah) A woman who is pregnant for the first time (gravida I).

Primipara (pri-mip′ah-rah) A woman who has carried a pregnancy to viability regardless of whether the infant was dead or alive at birth (para I).

Proctoscope (prok′to-skōp) An endoscope that is specially designed for passage through the anus to permit visual inspection of the rectum.

Proctoscopy (prok-tos′ko-pe) The visual examination of the rectum using a proctoscope.

Prodrome (pro′drōm) A symptom indicating an approaching disease.

Profile (pro′fīl) A combination of laboratory tests providing related or complementary information used to determine the health status of a patient.

Proteinuria (pro″te-ĭ-nu′re-ah) The presence of protein in the urine.

Puerperium (pu″er-pe′re-um) The period of time (usually four to six weeks) in which the uterus and the body systems are returning to normal following delivery.

Puncture (pungk′tur) A wound made by a sharp pointed object piercing the skin.

Pyrexia (pi-rek′se-ah) A body temperature that is above normal. Synonym for fever.

Quality control (kwol′ĭ-te kon-trōl′) The application of methods to ensure that test results are reliable and valid and that errors are detected and eliminated.

Quickening (kwik′en-ing) The first movements of the fetus in utero as felt by the mother, which usually occur between the sixteenth and twentieth weeks of gestation and are felt consistently thereafter.

Radiation (ra″de-a′shun) The transfer of energy, such as heat, in the form of waves.

Radiograph (ra′de-o-graf″) A permanent record of a picture of an internal body organ or structure produced on radiographic film. Also known as a roentgenogram.

Radiography (ra″de-og′rah-fe) The taking of permanent records (radiographs) of internal body organs and structures by passing x-rays through the body to act upon a specially sensitized film.

Radiologist (ra″de-ol′o-jist) A medical doctor who specializes in the diagnosis and treatment of disease using radiant energy such as x-rays, radium, and radioactive material.

Radiology (ra″de-ol′o-je) The branch of medicine that deals with the use of radiant energy in the diagnosis and treatment of disease.

Radiolucent (ra″de-o-lu′sent) Describing a structure that permits the passage of x-rays.

Radiopaque (ra″de-o-pāk′) Describing a structure that obstructs the passage of x-rays.

Recipient (re-sip′e-ent) One who receives

something, such as a blood transfusion, from a donor.

Refraction (re-frak′shun) The deflection or bending of light rays by a lens.

Refractive index (re-frak′tiv in′deks) The ratio of the velocity of light in air to the velocity of light in a solution.

Refractometer (clinical) (re″frak-tom′ĕ-ter) An instrument used to measure the refractive index of urine, which is an indirect measurement of the specific gravity of urine.

Renal threshold (re′nal thresh′old) The concentration at which a substance in the blood that is not normally excreted by the kidneys begins to appear in the urine.

Reservoir host (rez′er-vwar hōst) The organism that becomes infected by a pathogen and also serves as a source of transfer of the pathogen to others.

Resistance (re-zis′tans) The natural ability of an organism to remain unaffected by harmful substances in its environment.

Retina (ret-ĭ-nah) The interior structure of the eye, which picks up and transmits light impulses to the optic nerve.

Roentgenologist (rent″gĕ-nol′o-jist) A medical specialist who is qualified in the use of x-rays (but not other kinds of radiant energy) for the diagnosis and treatment of disease.

Routine test (ro͞o-tēn′ test) Laboratory tests performed on a routine basis on apparently healthy patients to assist in the early detection of disease.

Sanitization (san″ĭ-ti-za′shun) A cleaning process to reduce the number of microorganisms to a safe level as determined by public health requirements.

Scalpel (skal′pel) A surgical knife used to divide tissues.

Scissors (siz′erz) A cutting instrument.

Sebaceous cyst (se-ba′shus sist) A thin closed sac or capsule containing fatty secretions from a sebaceous gland.

Segment (seg′ment) The portion of the ECG between two waves.

Sequela (se-kwel′lah) A morbid (secondary) condition occurring as a result of a less serious primary infection.

Serum (se′rum) The clear, straw-colored part of the blood that remains after the solid elements have been separated out of it.

Sigmoidoscope (sig-moi′do-skōp) An endoscope that is specially designed for passage through the anus to permit visualization of the rectum and sigmoid colon.

Sigmoidoscopy (sig″moi-dos′ko-pe) The visual examination of the rectum and sigmoid colon using a sigmoidoscope (also called proctosigmoidoscopy).

Smear (smēr) Material spread on a slide for microscopic examination.

Soak (sōk) The direct immersion of a body part in water or a medicated solution.

Sonography (so-nog′rah-fe) A diagnostic aid in which high-frequency sound waves are directed toward a woman's abdomen. Sonography is used to detect the presence of pregnancy and to assess fetal maturity.

Specific gravity (spĕ-sif′ik grav′ĭ-te) The weight of a substance as compared with the weight of an equal volume of a substance known as the standard.

Specimen (spec′i-men) A small sample of something taken to show the nature of the whole. In urinalysis, the specific gravity refers to the measurement of the amount of dissolved substances present in the urine, as compared with the same amount of distilled water.

Speculum (spek′u-lum) An instrument for opening a body orifice or cavity for viewing.

Sphygmomanometer (sfig″mo-mah-nom′ĕ-ter) An instrument for measuring arterial blood pressure.

Spirilla (spi-ril′ah) (singular, spirillum) Bacteria that have a spiral shape.

Sponge (spunj) A porous, absorbent pad, such as a 4″ × 4″ gauze pad or cotton surrounded by gauze, used to absorb fluids, to apply medication, or to cleanse an area.

Spore (spōr) A hard, thick-walled capsule formed by some bacteria that contains only the essential parts of the protoplasm of the bacterial cell.

Sprain (sprān) Trauma to a joint, which causes injury to the ligaments.

Stature (stat′ūr) The height of the body in a standing position.

Sterile (ster′il) Free from all living microorganisms.

Sterilization (ster″il-ĭ-za′shun) The process of destroying all forms of microbial life.

Stertorous respiration (ster′to-rus res″-pĭ-ra′shun) Noisy and snoring respiration.

Stethoscope (steth′o-skōp) An instrument for amplifying and hearing sounds produced by the body.

Strain (strān) An overstretching of a muscle due to trauma.

Streaking (strēk′ing) In microbiology, the process of inoculating a culture to provide for the growth of colonies on the surface of a solid medium. Streaking is accomplished by skimming a wire inoculating loop containing the specimen across the surface of the medium, using a back-and-forth motion.

Streptolysin (strep-tol′ĭ-sin) An exotoxin produced by beta hemolytic streptococci which completely hemolyzes red blood cells.

Subcutaneous injection (sub″ku-ta′ne-us in-jek′shun) Introducing medication beneath the skin, into the subcutaneous or fatty layer of the body.
Subjective symptom (sub-jek′tiv simp′-tom) A symptom that is felt by the patient but is not observable by an examiner.
Sublingual administration (sub-ling′-gwal ăd-mĭn″ĭs-trā′shun) Administration of medication by placing it under the tongue, where it dissolves and is absorbed through the mucous membrane.
Subnormal (sub-nor′mal) A body temperature that is below normal.
Supernatant (soo″per-na′tant) The clear liquid that remains at the top after a precipitate settles.
Suppuration (sup″u-ra′shun) The process of pus formation.
Surgical asepsis (ser′jĭ-kal a-sep′sis) Those practices that keep objects and areas sterile or free from microorganisms.
Susceptible (sŭ-sep′tĭ-b′l) Easily affected; lacking resistance.
Sutures (soo′cherz) Material used to approximate tissues with surgical stitches.
Swaged needle (swājd ne′d′l) A needle with suturing material permanently attached to the end of the needle.
Symptom (simp′tom) Any change in the body or its functioning that indicates that a disease is present.
Systole (sis′to-le) The phase in the cardiac cycle in which the ventricles contract, sending blood out of the heart and into the aorta and pulmonary trunk.
Systolic pressure (sis-tol′ik presh′ur) The point of maximum pressure on the arterial walls, which is recorded during systole.
Tachycardia (tak″e-kar′de-ah) An abnormally fast heart or pulse rate (over 100 beats per minute).
Tachypnea (tak″ip-ne′ah) An abnormal increase in the respiratory rate.
Thermolabile (ther″mo-la′bil) Easily affected or changed by heat.
Thready pulse (thrĕd′ē puls) A pulse with a decreased volume that feels weak and thin.
Thrombocyte (throm′bo-sīt) Platelet.
Tonometer (to-nom′ĕ-ter) An instrument for measuring pressure within the eye.
Topical administration (top′i-kal ăd-mĭn″ĭs-trā′shun) Applying a drug to a particular spot, usually for a local action.
Toxemia (tok-se′me-ah) A pathologic condition occurring in pregnant women that includes preeclampsia and eclampsia. If preeclampsia goes undiagnosed or is not satisfactorily controlled, it can develop into eclampsia, characterized by convulsions and coma.
Toxin (tok′sin) A poisonous or noxious substance.
Toxoid (tok′soid) A toxin (poisonous substance produced by a bacterium) that has been treated by heat or chemicals to destroy its harmful properties. It is administered to an individual to prevent an infectious disease by stimulating the production or antibodies in that individual.
Trimester (tri-mes′ter) Three months or one-third of the gestational period of pregnancy.
Tympanic membrane (tim-pan′ik mem′-brān) A thin, semi-transparent membrane located between the external ear canal and middle ear that receives and transmits sound waves. Also known as the ear drum.
Urinalysis (u″rĭ-nal′ĭ-sis) The physical, chemical, and microscopic analysis of urine.
Urinometer (u″rĭ-nom′ĕ-ter) A device for measuring the specific gravity of urine.
Vaccine (vak′sen) A suspension of attenuated (weakened) or killed microorganisms administered to an individual to prevent an infectious disease by stimulating the production of antibodies in that individual.
Venipuncture (ven″ĭ-punk′tūr) Puncturing of a vein.
Vertex (ver′teks) The summit, or top, especially the top of the head.
Vesiculation (vĕ-sik″u-la′shun) The formation of vesicles (fluid-containing lesions of the skin).
Vial (vi′al) A closed glass container with a rubber stopper.
Void (void) To empty the bladder.
Vulva (vul′vah) The region of the external genital organs in the female.
Weight (wāt) The measure of heaviness of a substance.
Wheal (hwēl) A small raised area of the skin.
Wound (wo͞ond) A break in the continuity of an external or internal surface caused by physical means.
Volume (vol′ūm) The amount of space occupied by a substance.

APPENDIX A

1984 DACUM ANALYSIS OF THE MEDICAL ASSISTING PROFESSION

COMMUNICATE

Listen and observe

Respond to verbal and nonverbal cues

Organize and express ideas in a concise, precise and logical manner

Compose written communications using correct spelling, grammar and format

Use medical terminology accurately

Demonstrate courtesy, tact, and timing

Display empathy

Adapt communication to individual's ability to understand

Determine if communication was understood

Effectively interact with others

Adapt communication to individual's cultural orientation

DISPLAY PROFESSIONALISM

Maintain confidentiality

Maintain ethical and legal standards

Perform within the scope of training and education

Perform within personal capabilities

Accept responsibility for professional actions

Project and promote a positive image of the profession

Keep personal biases from interfering with performance of duties

Support the professional organization

Maintain and increase knowledge and skills

Promote positive public relations

*Monitor legislation applicable to the profession

Courtesy of the American Association of Medical Assistants, Inc.
* Denotes advanced level.

PERFORM ADMINISTRATIVE DUTIES

Type and transcribe accurately

Develop and maintain filing systems

Operate and maintain office equipment

Apply computer concepts to office practices

Prepare and maintain medical records

Screen and process mail

Schedule and monitor appointments

Use procedural and diagnostic coding

Process insurance data and claims

Adhere to current government regulations

Develop and maintain billing and collection system

Maintain office inventory

Arrange meetings and travel

*Organize and prepare reports and manuscripts

*Maintain employee/employer benefit records

*Manage business financial transactions

*Evaluate and update office procedures

PERFORM CLINICAL DUTIES

Maintain and use aseptic techniques

Operate and maintain clinical equipment

Obtain and record patient data

Assess and respond to patient's needs

Prepare examination and treatment area

Prepare patients for examinations and diagnostic procedures

Assist physician with examinations and treatments

Collect and process laboratory specimens

Perform routine diagnostic tests

Administer specified medications

Maintain patient medication records

Maintain inventory of supplies and medications

Exercise efficient time management

MANAGE EMERGENCY SITUATIONS

Recognize emergency situations

Maintain emergency equipment and supplies

Operate emergency equipment

Implement emergency procedures

Administer first aid including CPR

Maintain control of emergency situations

Provide reassurance and support

Document incidents

PROVIDE INSTRUCTION

Inform patients of office policies

Educate patients regarding health care

Consult with patients regarding insurance benefits and coverage

Assist patients in obtaining services from community health resources

*Provide orientation for office personnel

*Supervise student practical experiences

*Train new personnel

*Develop clinical and administrative procedure manual

MANAGE FACILITIES AND PERSONNEL

Enforce safety and security procedures

Provide attractive, clean, orderly, and comfortable surroundings

Maintain personnel and payroll records

Develop and coordinate work schedules

*Supervise personnel

*Delegate responsibilities

*Screen and interview applicants

*Develop job descriptions

*Develop and implement personnel policies

*Conduct routine performance evaluations

APPENDIX B

MEDICAL ABBREVIATIONS

$\overline{aa}$	of each
AAL	anterior axillary line
AAMA	American Association of Medical Assistants
Ab	abortion
Abd	abdomen
ABE	acute bacterial endocarditis
ABG	arterial blood gases
ABO	blood groups
abs	absent
ac	acute
ac	before meals
ACD	anterior chest diameter
ACTH	adrenocorticotropic hormone
AD	right ear
ADH	antidiuretic hormone
ad lib	as desired
adm	admission
Adr	adrenalin
ADT	alternate-day treatment
AF	atrial fibrillation
AGA	appropriate for gestational age
agg	agglutination
AGN	acute glomerular nephritis
A/G	albumin-to-globulin ratio
AHA	American Heart Association
AHD	arteriosclerotic heart disease atherosclerotic heart disease
AI	aortic insufficiency
AIDS	acquired immunodeficiency syndrome
AJ	ankle jerk
AL	left ear
alb	albumin
ALD	alcoholic liver disease
ALL	acute lymphocytic leukemia
ALP	alkaline phosphatase
AM	before noon
AMA	against medical advice American Medical Association
AMI	acute myocardial infarction
AMRA	American Medical Records Association
amt	amount
AODM	adult-onset diabetes mellitus
AOM	acute otitis media
AP	apical pulse
A & P	anterior and posterior auscultation and palpation auscultation and percussion
APB	atrial premature beat
aq	water
AR	apical-radial (pulse) at risk
ARC	AIDS-related complex American Red Cross
ARD	acute respiratory disease
ARF	acute renal failure acute respiratory failure acute rheumatic fever
AS	left ear
ASA	acetylsalicylic acid
ASAP	as soon as possible
ASCAD	arteriosclerotic coronary artery disease
ASCVD	arteriosclerotic cardiovascular disease atherosclerotic cardiovascular disease
ATR	Achilles tendon reflex
AU	in each ear
AVH	acute viral hepatitis
AVR	aortic valve replacement
A & W	alive and well
BA	backache bronchial asthma
Ba	barium
Bab	Babinski (reflex)
BAC	blood alcohol concentration
BaE	barium enema
BaM	barium meal

BBB	bundle branch block
BBT	basal body temperature
BC	birth control
BC/BS	Blue Cross/Blue Shield
bd	twice a day
BE	bacterial endocarditis barium enema
BG	blood glucose
BHS	beta-hemolytic streptococcus
bid	twice a day
BIL	bilirubin
bil	bilateral
BJ	biceps jerk
B & J	bone and joint
BJM	bones, joints and muscles
BK	below knee (amputation)
BM	basal metabolism bowel movement
BMR	basal metabolism rate
BNO	bladder neck obstruction bowels not open
BOM	bilateral otitis media
BP	blood pressure British Pharmacopoeia
BS	blood sugar bowel sounds breath sounds
BSL	blood sugar level
BSN	bowel sounds normal
BSO	bilateral salpingo-oophorectomy
BSR	blood sedimentation rate
BTL	bilateral tubal ligation
BUN	blood urea nitrogen
BW	below waist birth weight body weight
Bx	biopsy
C	Celsius centigrade
c̄	with
C1	first cervical vertebra
C2	second cervical vertebra
CA	cancer carcinoma
Ca	calcium cancer
CAD	coronary artery disease
CAHD	coronary atherosclerotic heart disease
caps	capsules
CAT	computerized axial tomography
CB	chronic bronchitis
CBC	complete blood count
CBD	common bile duct
CBR	complete bed rest
CC	chief complaint
cc	cubic centimeter
CCF	congestive cardiac failure
CCU	coronary care unit
C & D	cystoscopy and dilation
CDC	Center for Disease Control
cerv	cervical, cervix
CH	cholesterol
CHD	childhood disease congenital heart disease congestive heart disease coronary heart disease
Chem	chemotherapy
CHO	carbohydrate
chr	chronic
ck	check
Cl	chloride
CLD	chronic liver disease chronic lung disease
cldy	cloudy
cm	centimeter
CMA	Certified Medical Assistant
CNS	central nervous system
C/O	complains of
COD	cause of death
COPD	chronic obstructive pulmonary disease
CP	cerebral palsy cleft palate
CPN	chronic pyelonephritis
CPR	cardiopulmonary resuscitation
CRD	chronic renal disease chronic respiratory disease
CRF	chronic renal failure
crit	hematocrit
CS	cerebrospinal cesarean section
C & S	conjunctiva and sclera culture and sensitivity
CSF	cerebrospinal fluid
CTS	carpal tunnel syndrome
cu cm	cubic centimeter
cu mm	cubic millimeter

CV	cardiovascular cerebrovascular
CVA	cerebrovascular accident
CVP	central venous pressure
CW	chest wall
Cx	cervix
CXR	chest x-ray
cysto	cystoscopic examination cystoscopy
DB	date of birth
DBM	diabetic management
DBP	diastolic blood pressure
DC	discontinue
D & C	dilatation and currettage
DD	differential diagnosis
DDD	degenerative disc disease
dec	decrease
def	deficiency
deg	degeneration
del	delivery
DI	diabetes insipidus
diab	diabetic
diag	diagnosis
Diff	differential white blood cell count
dil	dilute
dis	disabled disease
disc	discontinue
disp	dispense
DKA	diabetic ketoacidosis
dl	deciliter
DM	diabetes mellitus
DOA	dead on arrival
DOB	date of birth
DOD	date of death
DOE	dyspnea on exertion
dos	dosage
DP	diastolic pressure
DPT	diphtheria, pertussis, and tetanus
DR	delivery room
dr	dram
DSD	dry sterile dressing
dsg	dressing
DT	delirium tremens
DTR	deep tendon reflex
D & V	diarrhea and vomiting
DVA	distance visual acuity
DW	distilled water dry weight
D/W	dextrose in water
Dx	diagnosis
ea	each
EAM	external auditory meatus
EBL	estimated blood loss
EBV	Epstein-Barr virus
ECF	extracellular fluid
ECG	electrocardiogram
Echo	echocardiogram echoencephalogram
E. coli	*Escherichia coli*
ECT	electroconvulsive therapy
EDC	estimated date of confinement
EDD	expected date of delivery
EEG	electroencephalogram
EENT	eyes, ears, nose and throat
EFA	essential fatty acid
eg	for example
EH	enlarged heart essential hypertension
EKG	electrocardiogram
elix	elixir
EMG	electromyography
ENT	ear, nose, and throat
eos	eosinophil
ER	emergency room
ESR	erythrocyte sedimentation rate
EST	electroshock therapy
Ez	eczema
F	Fahrenheit
FA	fatty acid
FB	finger breadth foreign body
FBN	Federal Bureau of Narcotics
FBP	femoral blood pressure
FBS	fasting blood sugar
FD	fatal dose forceps delivery
FDA	Food and Drug Administration
FFA	free fatty acids
FFI	free from infection
FFP	fresh frozen plasma
FH	family history
FHR	fetal heart rate

flex	flexion
FMP	first menstrual period
FOB	fecal occult blood
FP	family practice
freq	frequent
FSH	follicle-stimulating hormone
fx	fracture
G	gravida
g	gram
GA	gastric analysis general anesthesia gestational age
GB	gallbladder
GC	gonococcus gonorrhea
gen	general
ger	geriatrics
GI	gastrointestinal
gm	gram
GP	general practice
gr	grain
GTT	glucose tolerance test
gtt(s)	drop (drops)
GU	genitourinary
GYN	gynecology
H	height hypodermic
h	hour
HA	headache
HAA	hepatitis-associated antigen
H & P	history and physical
HBP	high blood pressure
HC	head circumference
hCG	human chorionic gonadotropin
HCl	hydrochloric acid
HCVD	hypertensive cardiovascular disease
HEENT	head, eyes, ears, nose, and throat
HEW	Health, Education and Welfare
H & H	hemoglobin and hematocrit
HHD	hypertensive heart disease
H & L	heart and lungs
HMO	Health Maintenance Organization
H/O	history of
hpf	high-power field
hs	at bedtime
HT	hypertension
ht	height
HVD	hypertensive vascular disease
Hx	history
IB	immune body
IBC	iron-binding capacity
IBI	intermittent bladder irrigation
IBP	iron-binding protein
IBS	irritable bowel syndrome
IBW	ideal body weight
IC	irritable colon
ICCU	intensive coronary care unit
ICD	International Classification of Diseases (of the World Health Organization)
ICDA	International Classification of Diseases, Adapted
ICU	intensive care unit
ID	intradermal
I & D	incision and drainage
IM	Internal Medicine intramuscular
imp	impression
inf	infant
I & O	intake and output
IPPB	intermittent positive-pressure breathing
ISG	immune serum globulin
IU	international unit
IUD	intrauterine device
IUGR	intrauterine growth rate
IV	intravenous
IVP	intravenous pyelogram
IVSD	interventricular septal defect
JAMA	Journal of the American Medical Association
jaund	jaundice
JODM	juvenile onset diabetes mellitus
JRA	juvenile rheumatoid arthritis
JV	jugular vein
K	potassium
KA	ketoacidosis
KB	ketone bodies
kg	kilogram
kj	knee jerk
KLS	kidney, liver, and spleen
KOH	potassium hydroxide
KUB	kidney, ureter, and bladder
L	liter
l	length

LA left atrium
lactic acid

lac laceration

LAO left anterior oblique

lap laparotomy

lax laxative

LB low back

LBBB left bundle branch block

LBM lean body mass

LBP low back pain

LBW low birth weight

LDL low-density lipoprotein

LE lupus erythematosus

LFT liver function test

liq liquid

LKS liver, kidneys, and spleen

LL left leg

LLQ left lower quadrant

LLE left lower extremity

LMP last menstrual period

LP lumbar puncture

lpf low-power field

LRQ lower right quadrant

LSK liver, spleen, and kidneys

LUQ left upper quadrant

LV left ventricle

L & W living and well

lymphs lymphocytes

m meter
minim

MCH mean corpuscular hemoglobin and red cell indices

MCHC mean corpuscular hemoglobin concentration and red cell indices

MCL midclavicular line

MCV mean corpuscular volume and red cell indices

MD muscular dystrophy
Doctor of Medicine

MDR minimum daily requirement

mEq/L milliequivalents per liter

MG myasthenia gravis

mg milligram

MH marital history
medical history
menstrual history

MHx medical history

MI maturation index
myocardial infarction

ML midline

ml milliliter

MM multiple myeloma

mm millimeter

mm^3 cubic millimeter

mmHg millimeters of mercury

MMR measles, mumps, and rubella

MODM mature-onset diabetes mellitus

MOM milk of magnesia

mono mononucleosis

MP menstrual period

MR metabolic rate
mortality rate

MS mitral stenosis
morphine sulfate
multiple sclerosis

MSL midsternal line

MSU midstream urine specimen

MT medical technologist

multip multipara

MV megavolt
mitral valve

MVP mitral valve prolapse

My myopia

n normal

NaCl sodium chloride

NAD no acute distress
nothing abnormal detected

narc narcotic

NAS nasal

NB newborn

NBW normal birth weight

NC no change
noncontributory

N/C no complaints

ND natural death
normal delivery

NED no evidence of disease

neg negative

NG nasogastric

NGU nongonococcal urethritis

NL normal limits

NM neuromuscular

NMP normal menstrual period

noct nocturnal

non rep do not repeat

NPO nothing by mouth

NR	nonreactive no refill normal range
NS	nonspecific normal saline not significant not sufficient
NSD	normal spontaneous delivery
NSR	normal sinus rhythm
NSU	nonspecific urethritis
N & T	nose and throat
NTG	nitroglycerin
N & V	nausea and vomiting
NVA	near visual acuity
NVD	nausea, vomiting, and diarrhea
NWB	non–weight-bearing
NYD	not yet diagnosed
O	oxygen
O	oral
OA	osteoarthritis
OB	obstetrics
OB-GYN	obstetrics-gynecology
Obs	observed
OC	office call on call oral contraceptive
occ	occasionally
OD	drug overdose right eye
O & E	observation and examination
OGTT	oral glucose tolerance test
OH	occupational history
OHD	organic heart disease
OM	otitis media
OOB	out of bed
OP	operative procedure osmotic pressure outpatient
O & P	ova and parasites
OPV	oral poliovaccine
OR	operating room
ortho	orthopedics
OS	left eye
OT	occupational therapist occupational therapy
OTC	over the counter
OU	both eyes
OURQ	outer upper right quadrant
OV	office visit
P	phosphorus
P	pulse
PA	posteroanterior
P & A	percussion and auscultation
PA	Physician's Assistant
PAC	phenacetin, aspirin, and codeine premature atrial contraction
Pap	Papanicolaou (smear, test)
Para	number of pregnancies
Para I	primipara
PAT	paroxysmal atrial tachycardia
path	pathology
PBI	protein-bound iodine
PC	platelet count
pc	after meals
PCC	Poison Control Center
PCN	penicillin
PCV	packed cell volume
PD	Parkinson's disease
PDR	Physician's Desk Reference
PE	physical examination
peds	pediatrics
PEG	pneumonencephalography
PERRLA	pupils equal, round, regular, react to light and accommodation
PGH	pituitary growth hormone
PH	past history personal history public health
pH	hydrogen ion concentration
PI	present illness pulmonary infarction
PID	pelvic inflammatory disease
PKU	phenylketonuria
PM	post meridiem (after noon) post mortem (after death)
PMB	postmenopausal bleeding
PMN	polymorphonuclear neutrophils
PMP	past menstrual period
PMS	premenstrual syndrome
PMT	premenstrual tension
PNC	penicillin
PND	paroxysmal nocturnal dyspnea
PNS	parasympathetic nervous system
Pnx	pneumothorax
po	by mouth
POB	place of birth

POMR problem-oriented medical record
pos positive
poss possible
postop postoperative
PP postprandial
PPB positive pressure breathing
PPBS postprandial blood sugar
PPD purified protein derivative
PPH postpartum hemorrhage
PPT partial prothrombin time
PRC packed red cells
preop preoperative
PRERLA pupils round, equal, react to light and accommodation
primip woman bearing first child
prn as the occasion arises, as necessary
procto proctoscopy
prog prognosis
PROM premature rupture of membranes
pro-time prothrombin time
PSRO Professional Standards Review Organization
PT physical therapy
prothrombin time
pt patient
PTA prior to admission
PTB prior to birth
PTD prior to discharge
PUD peptic ulcer disease
PVC premature ventricular contraction
PVD peripheral vascular disease
PWD partial weight-bearing
q each; every
q AM every morning
qd every day
qh every hour
q(2,3,4)h every 2, 3, or 4 hours
qid four times a day
qns quantity not sufficient
qod every other day
qs of sufficient quantity
RA right arm
right atrium
RAF rheumatoid arthritis factor
RAO right anterior oblique
RBC red blood cell
RBC/hpf red blood cells per high power field
RBCM red blood cell mass
RBCV red blood cell volume
RBF renal blood flow
RBS random blood sugar
RCM right costal margin
RCV red cell volume
RDA recommended daily allowance
REM rapid eye movement
resp respiration
Rh rhesus (factor)
Rh− rhesus negative
Rh+ rhesus positive
RHD rheumatic heart disease
RHF right heart failure
RI respiratory illness
RL right leg
RLE right lower extremity
RLQ right lower quadrant
RMSF Rocky Mountain spotted fever
R/O rule out
ROS review of systems
RP radial pulse
RQ respiratory quotient
RUQ right upper quadrant
RV right ventricle
RVH right ventricular hypertrophy
Rx prescription
S subjective data (POMR)
s̄ without
SA sinoatrial
S & A sugar and acetone (urine)
SBE shortness of breath on exertion
subacute bacterial endocarditis
SBO small bowel obstruction
SBP systolic blood pressure
SCD sudden cardiac death
sudden coronary death
SD spontaneous delivery
sudden death
S/D systolic to diastolic
SDS sudden death syndrome
sed rate sedimentation rate
segs segmented neutrophils
seq sequela
SF scarlet fever
spinal fluid

SFT	skin-fold thickness
SG	specific gravity
SH	social history
SIDS	sudden infant death syndrome
sig	labeled
sigmoid	sigmoidoscopy
sl	slight
SM	simple mastectomy
SMA 12/60	Sequential Multiple Analyzer (12-test serum profile)
SOAP	subjective data, objective data, assessment, and plan
SOB	shortness of breath
sol	solution
solv	solvent
SOM	serous otitis media
SOP	standard operating procedure
SOS	if necessary
SP	systolic pressure
SPA	suprapubic aspiration
spec	specimen
sp gr	specific gravity
spont ab	spontaneous abortion
SR	sedimentation rate
SS	signs and symptoms
ss	one-half
Staph	Staphylococcus
stat	immediately
STD	sexually transmitted diseases skin test dose
std	standard
Strep	Streptococcus
STS	serologic test for syphilis
subcut	subcutaneous
sum	to be taken
sup	superficial
supp	suppository
surg	surgery
Sx	signs symptoms
sym	symptoms
T	temperature
T_3	tri-iodothyronine
T_4	thyroxine
T & A	tonsillectomy and adenoidectomy
tab	tablet
TAT	tetanus antitoxin
TB	tuberculin tuberculosis
TBF	total body fat
TBLC	term birth, living child
TBW	total body water
TC	throat culture tissue culture total capacity total cholesterol
th	thoracic
ther	therapy
therap	therapeutic
THR	total hip replacement
TIA	transient ischemic attach
tid	three times a day
tinct	tincture
TLC	tender loving care
TM	tympanic membrane
TND	term normal delivery
TOP	termination of pregnancy
TOPV	trivalent oral poliovirus vaccine
TP	total protein
TPM	temporary pacemaker
TPN	total parenteral nutrition
TPR	temperature, pulse, and respiration
Tq	tourniquet
Tr	trace
tr	tincture
Trig	triglycerides
tbsp	tablespoon
TSH	thyroid stimulating hormone
TSP	total serum protein
tsp	teaspoon
TUR	transurethral resection of the bladder
tus	cough
TV	tidal volume total volume Trichomonas vaginitis
T & X	type and crossmatch
U	unit
UA	urinalysis
UC	ulcerative colitis
U/C	urine culture
UCG	urinary chorionic gonadotropin
UCHD	usual childhood diseases

UE	upper extremity
UGI	upper gastrointestinal
ULQ	upper left quadrant
ung	ointment
UOQ	upper outer quadrant
UR	upper respiratory
urg	urgent
URI	upper respiratory infection
urol	urology
URQ	upper right quadrant
URT	upper respiratory tract
URTI	upper respiratory tract infection
US	ultrasound
USP	United States Pharmacopoeia
UT	urinary tract
UTI	urinary tract infection
UV	ultraviolet
V	vein
vac	vaccine
vag	vagina vaginal
VC	vena cava
VD	venereal disease
VDRL	Venereal Disease Research Laboratory
VE	vaginal examination
VF	ventricular fibrillation
VH	vaginal hysterectomy viral hepatitis
VHD	valvular heart disease
vis	vision
vit	vitamin
vit cap	vital capacity
VP	venipuncture venous pressure
VPC	ventricular premature contraction
VRI	viral respiratory infection
VS	vital signs
VV	varicose veins
WB	weight bearing whole blood
WBC	white blood cell
WC	white cell
WDWN	well developed, well nourished
WN	well nourished
WNF	well-nourished female
WNL	within normal limits
WNM	well-nourished male
WO	written order
w/o	without
WP	weakly positive
WR	weakly reactive
wt	weight
X	magnification
XM	crossmatch
XR	x-ray
y	years
yd	yard
YOB	year of birth

Suggestions for Further Reading

Abbott Diagnostics Educational Services: "Chlamydia Implications and Complications." Abbott Diagnostics Educational Services, January, 1987.

American Academy of Pediatrics: *Report of the Committee on Infectious Diseases.* Evanston, Illinois, 1972.

American College of Radiology: *X-Ray Examinations . . . A Guide to Good Practice.* Distributed by the U.S. Department of Health, Education, and Welfare, Rockville, Maryland.

American Medical Association: *Medicolegal Forms with Legal Analysis.* Chicago, 1973.

American National Red Cross: *Standard First Aid and Personal Safety.* New York, Doubleday & Company, Inc., 1982.

Ames Company: *Modern Urine Chemistry, A Guide to the Diagnosis of Urinary Tract Diseases and Metabolic Disorders.* Revised reprint. Elkhart, Indiana, 1982.

AMSCO (American Sterilizer Company): *Sterilization Aids.* Prepared by the Education and Research Department of AMSCO, Erie, Pennsylvania, 1984.

AMSCO: *Tips for Improving Your Sterilization Techniques.* Prepared by the Education and Research Department of AMSCO, Erie, Pennsylvania, 1984.

Asperheim, Mary: *Pharmacology: An Introductory Text.* 6th edition, Philadelphia, W. B. Saunders Company, 1987.

Bates, Barbara: *A Guide to Physical Examination and History Taking.* 4th edition, Philadelphia, J. B. Lippincott Company, 1987.

Bauer, John, and Ackerman, Gelson: *Clinical Laboratory Methods.* 9th edition, St. Louis, C. V. Mosby Company, 1982.

Beaumont, Estelle: "Blood Pressure Equipment." *Nursing 75, 5*:56, January, 1975.

———: "Diagnostic Kits." *Nursing 75, 5*:28, April, 1975.

Bennington, James L: *Saunders Dictionary and Encyclopedia of Laboratory Medicine and Technology.* Philadelphia, W. B. Saunders Company, 1984.

Black, Curtis, Popovich, Nicholas, and Black, Marilyn: "Drug Interactions in the GI Tract." *American Journal of Nursing, 77*:1426, September, 1977.

Blainey, Carol: "Site Selection in Taking Body Temperature." *American Journal of Nursing, 74*:1859, October, 1974.

Bontragen, Kenneth H., and Anthony, Barry T.: *Textbook of Radiographic Positioning and Related Anatomy.* 1st edition, Denver, Multimedia Publishing, Inc., 1982.

Broadribb, Violet, and Corliss, Charlotte: *Maternal-Child Nursing.* Philadelphia, J. B. Lippincott Company, 1973.

Brunner, Lillian S., and Suddarth, Doris S.: *Lippincott Manual of Nursing Practice,* 4th edition, Philadelphia, J. B. Lippincott Company, 1986.

Buckner, Joyce: "Interpersonal Skills: Necessary Conditions for Professional Helpers." *The Professional Medical Assistant, IX*:17, March/April, 1976.

Burdick Corporation: *Electrocardiography: A Better Way.* Milton, Wisconsin, 1976.

Busis, Sidney: "Pointers for Detecting Hearing Loss." *Patient Care, 11*:174, 1977.

Chabner, Davi-Ellen: *The Language of Medicine.* 3rd edition, Philadelphia, W. B. Saunders Company, 1984.

Chaffee, Ellen, and Greisheimer, Esther: *Basic Physiology and Anatomy.* 4th edition, Philadelphia, J. B. Lippincott Company, 1980.

Clark, J. B., Queener, S. G., and Karb, V. B.: *Pharmacological Basis of Nursing Practice.* 2nd edition, St. Louis, C. V. Mosby Company, 1986.

Cooper, Marian: *The Medical Assistant.* 5th edition, New York, McGraw-Hill Book Company, 1986.

Czech, Melanie: "A Mastery Learning Program for Self–Blood Glucose Monitoring." The Diabetes Educator, Spring, 1984.

DeLorenza, Barbara: *The Pharmaceutical Word Book.* Philadelphia, W. B. Saunders Company, 1985.

Deter, Dwight: "Home Glucose Monitoring: The Key to Optimal Diabetes Control." *Physician Assistant,* August, 1985.

Dienhart, Charlotte: *Basic Human Anatomy and Physiology.* 3rd edition, Philadelphia, W. B. Saunders Company, 1979.

Dison, Norma: *Clinical Nursing Techniques.* 4th edition, St. Louis, C. V. Mosby Company, 1979.

Dorland's Illustrated Medical Dictionary. 27th edition, Philadelphia, W. B. Saunders Company, 1988.

DuGas, Beverly: *Introduction to Patient Care.* 4th edition, Philadelphia, W. B. Saunders Company, 1983.

Ebbesen, Peter: *AIDS: A Basic Guide for Clinicians.* Philadelphia, W. B. Saunders Company, 1984.

Enelow, Allen, and Swisher, Scott: *Interviewing and Patient Care.* 2nd edition, New York, Oxford University Press, 1979.

Ethicon, Inc.: *Suture Use Manual.* Somerville, New Jersey, 1978.

Facklam, Richard: "Isolation and Identification of *Streptococci.*" Center for Infectious Diseases, Bacterial Diseases Division, 1984.

Fazio, Victor: "Early Diagnosis of Anorectal and Colon Carcinoma." Hospital Medicine, January, 1979.

Fischbach, Frances: *Laboratory Diagnostic Tests.* Philadelphia, J. B. Lippincott Company, 1988.

Fischer, Paul, Addison, Lois, Curtis, Peter, and Mitchell, Jane: *The Office Laboratory.* Norwalk, Connecticut, Appleton-Century-Crofts, 1983.

French, Ruth: *The Nurse's Guide to Diagnostic Procedures.* 5th edition, New York, McGraw-Hill Book Company, 1981.

Frobisher, Martin, and Fuerst, Robert: *Microbiology in Health and Disease.* 15th edition, Philadelphia, W. B. Saunders Company, 1983.

Fuller, Joanna: *Surgical Technology, Principles and Practice.* 2nd edition, Philadelphia, W. B. Saunders Company, 1986.

Garb, Solomon: *Laboratory Tests in Common Use.* 7th edition, New York, Springer Publishing Company, 1981.

Geolot, Denise, and McKinney, Nancy: "Administering Parenteral Drugs." *American Journal of Nursing,* 75:788, May, 1975.

Goldman, Myer: *A Nurse's Guide to the X-Ray Department.* London, Churchill Livingstone, 1972.

Govoni, Laura, and Hayes, Janice: *Drugs and Nursing Implications.* 5th edition, New York, Appleton-Century-Crofts, 1986.

Hahn, Robert L., Hahn, Ann Burgess, and Oestreich, Sandy Jeanee K.: *Pharmacology in Nursing.* 15th edition, St. Louis, C. V. Mosby Company, 1982.

Henry, John: *Todd-Sanford-Davidsohn Clinical Diagnosis and Management by Laboratory Methods.* 17th edition, Philadelphia, W. B. Saunders Company, 1984.

Hill, George: *Outpatient Surgery.* 3rd edition, Philadelphia, W. B. Saunders Company, 1988.

Hirsh, Robert: "Can Your Examining Rooms Pass This Test?" *Medical Economics,* p. 191, June 13, 1977.

———: "Can Your Office Soundproofing Pass This Test?" *Medical Economics,* p. 131, June 27, 1977.

Hobson, Lawrence: *Examination of the Patient.* New York, McGraw-Hill Book Company, 1975.

Hogstel, Mildred: "How to Give a Safe and Successful Cleansing Enema." *American Journal of Nursing, 77*:816, May, 1977.

Huang et al: *Coronary Care Nursing.* Philadelphia, W. B. Saunders Company, 1983.

Hunter, Robert: AAMA, For Whose Benefit? *The Professional Medical Assistant, VI*:1, November/December, 1973.

Ingalls, A. Joy, and Salerno, M. Constance: *Maternal and Child Health Nursing.* 6th edition, St. Louis, C. V. Mosby Company, 1987.

Jacob, Stanley, Francone, Clarice, and Lassow, Walter: *Structure and Function in Man.* 5th edition, Philadelphia, W. B. Saunders Company, 1982.

Johnson, Richard, and Swartz, Mark: *A Simplified Approach to Electrocardiography.* Philadelphia, W. B. Saunders Company, 1986.

Kee, M. L.: *Laboratory and Diagnostic Tests with Nursing Implications.* Norwalk, Connecticut, Appleton-Century-Crofts, 1983.

Kingsley, Victor: *Basic Microbiology for the Health Sciences.* Philadelphia, W. B. Saunders Company, 1982.

Kinn, Mary, and Derge, Eleanor: *The Medical Assistant, Administrative and Clinical.* 6th edition, Philadelphia, W. B. Saunders Company, 1988.

Kirkindall, W. M., et al.: *Recommendations for Human Blood Pressure Determination by Sphygmomanometers.* New York, American Heart Association, 1980.

Lambert, Martin: "Drug and Diet Interactions." *American Journal of Nursing, 75*:402, March, 1975.

Lancour, Jane: "How to Avoid Pitfalls in Measuring Blood Pressure." *American Journal of Nursing, 76*:773, May, 1976.

Lang, Susan, Zawacki, Ann, and Johnson, Jean: "Reducing Discomfort From IM Injections."*American Journal of Nursing, 76*:800, May, 1976.

Lawton, M. Murray, and Foy, Donald: *A Textbook for Medical Assistants.* 4th edition, St. Louis, C. V. Mosby Company, 1980.

Leifer, Gloria: *Principles and Techniques in Pediatric Nursing.* 4th edition, Philadelphia, W. B. Saunders Company, 1982.

LeMaitre, George, and Finnegan, Janet: *The Patient in Surgery: A Guide for Nurses.* Philadelphia, W. B. Saunders Company, 1980.

Levinson, Daniel: *A Guide to the Clinical Interview.* Philadelphia, W. B. Saunders Company, 1987.

Lewis, LuVerne: *Fundamental Skills in Patient Care.* 4th edition, Philadelphia, J. B. Lippincott Company, 1988.

Linné, Jean, and Ringsrud, Karen: *Basic Laboratory Techniques for the Medical Laboratory Technician.* 2nd edition, New York, McGraw-Hill Book Company, 1979.

Liu, Paul: *Blue Book of Diagnostic Tests.* Philadelphia, W. B. Saunders Company, 1986.

Loebl, Suzanne, Spratto, George, and Wit, Andrew: *The Nurse's Drug Handbook.* 2nd edition, New York, John Wiley & Sons, 1980.

Marlow, Dorothy: *Textbook of Pediatric Nursing.* Philadelphia, W. B. Saunders Company, 1977.

McInnes, Mary: *The Vital Signs.* 3rd edition, St. Louis, C. V. Mosby Company, 1979.

Mechner, Francis: "Examination of the Eye, Part 1." *American Journal of Nursing, 74*:2039, November, 1974.

Memler, Ruth L., and Wood, Dena: *Human Body in Health and Disease.* 6th edition, Philadelphia, J. B. Lippincott Company, 1987.

Meschan, Isadore: *Radiographic Positioning and Related Anatomy.* 2nd edition, Philadelphia, W. B. Saunders Company, 1978.

Metz, Robert, and Benson, Jones: *Management and Education of the Diabetic Patient.* Philadelphia, W. B. Saunders Company, 1988.

Miller, Benjamin, and Keane, Claire: *Encyclopedia and Dictionary of Medicine, Nursing, and Allied Health.* 4th edition, Philadelphia, W. B. Saunders Company, 1987.

Moore, William, and Hamill, Peter: *Contemporary Growth Charts: Needs, Construction and Application.* Columbus, Ohio, Ross Laboratories, 1976.

Morgan, James: *The Art and Science of Medical Radiography.* St. Louis, The Catholic Hospital Association, 1977.

Mueller, Carolyn: "Perfecting Physical Assessment: Part 1." *Nursing 77, 7*:28, May, 1977.

_______: "Perfecting Physical Assessment: Part 2." *Nursing 77, 7*:38, June, 1977.

_______: "Perfecting Physical Assessment: Part 3." *Nursing 77, 7*:44, July, 1977.

_______: "Vital Signs—How to Take Them More Accurately and Understand Them More Fully." *Nursing 76, 6*:31, April, 1976.

Nealon, Thomas: *Fundamental Skills in Surgery.* 3rd edition, Philadelphia, W. B. Saunders Company, 1979.

Oppenheim, Irwin: *Textbook for Laboratory Assistants.* 3rd edition, St. Louis, C. V. Mosby Company, 1981.

Oppenheim, Mike: "Suppose You Were Getting That Physical Exam." *Medical Economics,* p. 249, June 13, 1977.

Pelczar, Michael, and Reid, Roger: *Microbiology.* 5th edition, New York, McGraw-Hill Book Company, 1986.

Perkins, John: *Principles and Methods of Sterilization in Health Sciences.* Springfield, Illinois, Charles C Thomas, 1976.

Pfizer Laboratories: *How to Give an Intramuscular Injection.* New York, 1976.

Phelps, Jeana: "Radiation Protection and the Medical Assistant." *The Professional Medical Assistant, X*:32, July/August, 1977.

Phibbs, Brendan: *The Cardiac Arrhythmias.* 3rd edition, St. Louis, C. V. Mosby Company, 1978.

Phillips, Raymond, and Feeney, Mary: *The Cardiac Rhythms.* 2nd edition, Philadelphia, W. B. Saunders Company, 1980.

Phipps, W., et al.: *Medical Surgical Nursing: Concepts and Clinical Practice,* 2nd edition, St. Louis, C. V. Mosby Company, 1983.

Potter, Patricia A., and Perry, Anne G.: *Clinical Nursing Skills and Techniques.* St. Louis, C. V. Mosby Company, 1986.

Poulos, Jean: "Diagnostic Tests: A Guide to Patient Instruction." *The Professional Medical Assistant, VIII*:15, May/June, 1975.

Raphael, Stanley: *Lynch's Medical Laboratory Technology.* 4th edition, Philadelphia, W. B. Saunders Company, 1983.

Robertson, Carolyn: "How to Teach Patients to Monitor Blood Glucose." *RN,* December, 1985.

Rosdahl, Caroline: *Textbook of Basic Nursing.* 4th edition, Philadelphia, J. B. Lippincott Company, 1985.

Sana, Josephine M., and Judge, Richard D.: *Physical Assessment Skills for Nursing Practice.* 2nd edition, Boston, Little, Brown & Company, 1982.

Scherer, Jeanne: *Introductory Clinical Pharmacology.* 2nd edition, Philadelphia, J. B. Lippincott Company, 1982.

Sellars, Dorothy: "A Basic Understanding of Immunology for the Medical Assistant." *The Professional Medical Assistant, X*:8, July/August, 1977.

Shuman, Charles: "Self-Monitoring of Blood Glucose by the Diabetic Patient." *Practical Cardiology, 6*:27, June, 1980.

Shuman, Delores: "Doing It Better, Tips of Improving Urine Testing Techniques." *Nursing 76, 6*:23, February, 1976.

Skyler, Jay, et al.: "Home Blood Glucose Monitoring as an Aid in Diabetes Management." *Diabetes Care,* May/June, 1978.

Sloboda, Sharon: "Understanding Patient Behavior." *Nursing 77, 7*:74, September, 1977.

Smith, Alice: *Microbiology and Pathology.* 12th edition, St. Louis, C. V. Mosby Company, 1980.

Sorrentino, Sheila: *Mosby's Textbook for Nursing Assistants.* 2nd edition, St. Louis, C. V. Mosby Company, 1987.

Speicher, Carl, and Smith, Jack: *Choosing Effective Laboratory Tests.* Philadelphia, W. B. Saunders Company, 1983.

Stein, Emanuel: *The Electrocardiogram: A Self-Study Course in Clinical Electrocardiography.* Philadelphia, W. B. Saunders Company, 1976.

Stevens, Matthew, and Phillips, Robert: *Comprehensive Review for the Radiologic Technologist.* 4th edition, St. Louis, C. V. Mosby Company, 1983.

Taber, C.: *Taber's Cyclopedic Medical Dictionary.* 16th edition, Philadelphia, F. A. Davis Company, 1989.

Thompson, Eleanor: *Pediatric Nursing: An Introductory Text.* 5th edition, Philadelphia, W. B. Saunders Company, 1987.

Tietz, Norbert: *Clinical Guide to Laboratory Tests.* Philadelphia, W. B. Saunders Company, 1983.

U.S. Department of Health, Education, and Welfare: *NCHS Growth Curves for Children.* Hyattsville, Maryland, National Center for Health Statistics, 1977.

U.S. Department of Health, Education, and Welfare: *Collection, Handling and Shipment of Microbiological Specimens.* Atlanta, Georgia, Centers for Disease Control, 1973.

Van Meter, Margaret: "What Every Nurse Should Know About EKG's." *Nursing 75, 5*:19, April, 1975.

Waechter, Eugenia: *Nursing Care of Children.* 10th edition, Philadelphia, J. B. Lippincott Company, 1985.

Westfall, Elizabeth: "Electrical and Mechanical Events in the Cardiac Cycle." *American Journal of Nursing, 76*:23, February, 1976.

Whaley, Lucille F., and Wong, Donna L.: *Nursing Care of Infants and Children.* 2nd edition, St. Louis, C. V. Mosby Company, 1983.

Widmann, Frances: *Goodale's Clinical Interpretation of Laboratory Tests.* 9th edition, Philadelphia, F. A. Davis Company, 1983.

Wieck, Lynn, et al.: *Illustrated Manual of Nursing Techniques.* 3rd edition, Philadelphia, J. B. Lippincott Company, 1986.

Wittman, Karl S., and Thomas, John C.: *Medical Laboratory Skills.* New York, Gregg Division/McGraw-Hill Book Company, 1977.

Wood, Lucille, and Rambo, Beverly: *Nursing Skills for Allied Health Services.* 3rd edition, Philadelphia, W. B. Saunders Company, 1982.

Wyeth Laboratories: *Intramuscular Injections,* Philadelphia, 1973.

Index

Note: Page numbers in *italics* indicate boxed material and illustrations. Page numbers followed by *t* indicate tables.

Abbreviations, commonly used, 230*t*
  medical, 581–589
Abdomen, examination of, 74
ABO blood type, in prenatal care, 542
Abortion, definition of, 531, 537
Abrasion, definition of, 163, 182, *183*
Abscess, definition of, 163, 200
  surgical incision and drainage of, 200
Absorbable suture, definition of, 163, 187
Acquired immunodeficiency syndrome (AIDS), 8–12
  infection precautions in, 9–12
    for cleaning and decontaminating body fluid spills, 12
    for infective waste, 12
    for laboratory, 10–11
    for sterilization and disinfection, 11–12
  transmission of, 9
ACU Chek II glucose meter, blood glucose measurement using, procedure for, *396–400*
Acuity, visual, 81–90. *See also* Visual acuity.
Adhesive skin closures, 187–188
Adnexal, definition of, 516
Aerobe, definition of, 3, 4
Age, application of heat and cold and, 108
  body temperature and, 19
  drug action and, 231
  pulse rate and, 33
Agglutination, blood typing and, 356–357
  definition of, 293, 353
  of red blood cells, 356
AIDS-related complex (ARC), 9
Alcohol, to control microorganisms, 160
Allergic reaction, to drug, 232
Alveolus, definition of, 38
Ambulation, assistive devices for, 124–137
    canes as, 134–135
    crutches as, 124–133. *See also* Crutch(es).
    walkers as, 136–137
  definition of, 105, 124
Ameboid movement, definition of, 364
Amplitude, definition of, 441
Ampule, definition of, 217, 239
  in parenteral drug administration, 239, *241*
Anaerobe, definition of, 3, 4
Anaphylactic reaction, to drug, 232
Anemia, 373
  definition of, 364
Aneroid manometer, 44
Anesthetic, local, definition of, 163
  for minor office surgery, 193–194
Angiocardiogram, 491
Angiogram, cerebral, 492
Anorexia, 65
Antecubital space, definition of, 31
Anterior chamber, of eye, definition of, 81
Antianemic drug, action of, 221
Antianxiety drug, action of, 221
Antiarrhythmic drug, action of, 221
Antiarthritic drug, action of, 221
Antibiotic, action of, 221
Antibody(ies), and antigen, reaction between, 356
  blood, 355
    definition of, 353
Anticoagulant, action of, 221
  definition of, 333
Anticonvulsant, action of, 221
Antidepressant, action of, 221
Antidiarrheal, action of, 221
Antidote, action of, 221
Antiemetic, action of, 221
Antigen-antibody reaction, 356
Antigens, blood, 354–355
  definition of, 353
Antihistamine, action of, 221
Antihypertensive, action of, 222
Antiseptics, action of, 222
  definition of, 139, 140
  to control microorganisms, 159–161
Antiserum, definition of, 353
Antitussive, action of, 222
Antiulcer drug, action of, 222
Anuria, definition of, 295
Aorta, definition of, 31
Aortogram, 491
Apical pulse, 33
  measurement of, *36–37*
Apnea, definition of, 38, 40
Apothecary system, 225–226
  conversion charts for, 228*t*
  notation guidelines for, 225–226
Applicator, cotton-tipped, for patient examination, 71
Aqueous humor, definition of, 81
Arms, examination of, 74
Arrhythmias, 34, 469–473
  atrial fibrillation as, *470*, 472
  atrial flutter as, 469–472, *470*
  atrial premature contraction as, 469, *470*
  definition of, 31
  paroxysmal atrial tachycardia as, 469, *470*
  premature ventricular contraction as, *471*, 472
  ventricular fibrillation as, *471*, 473
  ventricular flutter as, *471*, 473
  ventricular tachycardia as, *471*, 472–473
Artery, pulse taking at, 33
Artifact(s), definition of, 441
  ECG, 453–457
    alternating current as, 455, *456*
    muscle as, 453–456
    wandering baseline as, 455, *456*
Asepsis, definition of, 3
  medical, 2–12
    application of, 5–6
    definition of, 5
    handwashing in, *6–8*
  surgical, definition of, 165–167
Aspirate, definition of, 217
Atrial depolarization, 444
Atrial fibrillation, *470*, 472
Atrial flutter, 469–472, *470*
Atrial premature contraction (APC), 469, *470*
Atrial tachycardia, paroxysmal, 469, *470*
Atrioventricular node (AV node), 443
Audiometer, definition of, 51, 79, 97
Auditory canal, external, 98
Auditory meatus, external, 98
Augmented ECG leads, 448

Auricle, 98
Auscultation, definition of, 51
  in physical examination, 72
Autoclave, 146–157
  article for, preparing and wrapping, 148–150
  definition of, 139
  faulty operation of, 155
  improper sterilization by, causes of, 154–155
  loading of, 151, *152*
  sterilization indicators for, 151–154
  sterilizing articles in, procedure for, *156–157*
  storage after, 155
Automated analyzers, in laboratory testing, 288–289
Automatic capability, electrocardiograph with, 452, *453*
Autotrophs, definition of, 4
Avoirdupois, definition of, 217, 225
Axilla, definition of, 16
Axillary crutch, 124, 125
  measurement for, 125
  procedure for, *126*
Axillary temperature, procedure for taking, 17, 18

Bacilli, 411, 412
  definition of, 407, 411
Bacitracin susceptibility test, 427–429
Bacteria, 411–412
  in urine, 325
Balance-beam scale, for patient examination, 71
Bandage(s), 208–213
  definition of, 163
  tubular gauze, 212
    application of, *213–215*
  turns for, 210–212, *211*
  types of, 209
Bandage scissors, 169
Bands, 381
Barium enema, 488–489
Barium meal, 488
Baseline, definition of, 441
  in ECG cycle, 444
    wandering, 455, *456*
Basophils, 381
Benzalkonium chloride, to control microorganisms, 160
Bilirubin, 368
  definition of, 364
  in urine, 309
Bilirubinemia, definition of, 293
Bilirubinuria, 309
Bimanual pelvic examination, 527
Biopsy, cervical punch, 205–207
  definition of, 163, 201, *553*
  needle, 201–202
    definition of, 163, 201
Bipolar ECG leads, 448
Bladder, urinary, 294
Blood, antibodies in, 355
    definition of, 353
  antigens in, 354–355
    definition of, 353
  banking of, 352–361
  capillary specimen of, 369–370
  components of, 354
  function of, 354
  glucose in, measurement of, 395–396
      procedures for, *396–402*
    self monitoring of, 403–405
    tests for, 391*t*, 393
  in urine, 310
  occult, definition of, 553, 554
    fecal, testing for, 554–555, *556–560*
Blood *(Continued)*
  specimens of, hemolysis in, prevention of, 335–336
    types of, 336
  spills of, cleaning and decontaminating, 12
  typing of, agglutination and, 356–357
    slide test method for, *357–361*
  whole, separation of plasma from, 351
    separation of serum from, 347–348, *349–351*
Blood chemistry tests, 389–405
  blood glucose measurement with glucose meter as, 395–402
  for blood glucose, 391*t*, 393
  for blood urea nitrogen, 390*t*, 393
  for cholesterol, 389, 390*t*, 393
  for fasting blood sugar, 391*t*, 393
  glucose tolerance test as, 391*t*, 394–395
  in prenatal care, 542–543
  self-monitoring of blood glucose as, 403–405
  two-hour postprandial blood sugar as, 391*t*, 393–394
Blood count, complete, 365
Blood group system, Rh, 356
Blood pressure, 42–49
  factors affecting, 45
  measurement of, equipment for, 43–44
    procedure for, *46–48*
  mechanism of, 43
  normal, 43
Blood urea nitrogen (BUN), tests for, 390*t*, 393
Body, protective mechanisms of, 4–6
  size of, drug action and, 232
Body fluids, spills of, cleaning and decontaminating, 12
Body systems, review of, 60
Boiling, to control microorganisms, 146
Bottle, specimen, for patient examination, 71
Bounding pulse, definition of, 31, 34
Brachial artery, pulse taking at, 33
Bradycardia, 34, 64
  definition of, 31
  sinus, 469
Braxton Hicks contractions, definition of, 531
Breasts, examination of, 74, 517
  self examination of, procedure for, *518*
Bronchodilator, action of, 222
Bronchogram, 491
Buffy coat, definition of, 333
Bundle of His, 443

Candidiasis, specimen for, in prenatal care, 542
  vaginal, 524
Cane, 134
  instructing patient in use of, *135*
Canthus, definition of, 80
Capillary action, definition of, 163
Capillary blood specimen, 369–370
  Autolet method to obtain, *372–373*
  Lancet method to obtain, *371*
Capsule, definition of, 220
Cardiac arrhythmias, 469–473. *See also* Arrhythmias.
Cardiac cycle, 444–445
  definition of, 441
Cardiotonic drug, action of, 222
Carotid artery, pulse taking at, 33
Cassette, in radiography, 479
Casts, in urine sediment, 322*t*, 325
Cathartic, action of, 222
Cells, exfoliated, definition of, 516
    in Pap test, 519
  in urine sediment, 321*t*, 324–325
Cellular casts, in urine, 322*t*, 325

Celsius thermometer, definition of, 16
Centigrade thermometer, definition of, 16
Cerebral angiogram, 492
Cerumen, definition of, 97
Cervical punch biopsy, 205–207
Cervical specimen, for gonorrhea culture in prenatal care, 542
Cervix, dilation of, definition of, 531
Charting, definition of, 51
  in medical record, 60–63
    entries in, 61–62
    guidelines for, 62–63
Chemical agents, to control microorganisms, 159–161
Chemical cold pack, application of, *119*
Chest, examination of, 74
  roentgenogram of, in prenatal care, 543
Child, immunizations for, 510–511
  intramuscular injections for, 508–509, *520*
  understanding of, 497
Chill, 65
Chlamydia, vaginal, 526
Cholangiogram, 492
Cholecystography, 489–490
Cholesterol tests, 389, 390*t*, 393
Choroid, definition of, 81
Cilia, definition of, 3
Ciliary body, definition of, 81
Circulation, impaired, application of heat or cold for, 108
Circulatory system, 64–65
Clamps, towel, *171*, 173
Clean-catch midstream urine specimen, 296–298
Clinical laboratory, medical office and, relationship between, 270–271
Clinitest, measuring urine glucose using, *316–318*
Cocci, 411, 412
  definition of, 407, 411
Cold, application of, by chemical cold pack, *119*
    by cold compress, *118–119*
    by ice bag, *116–117*
    factors affecting, 108
    purpose of, 108
  local effect of, 107
Cold compress, application of, *118–119*
Cold pack, chemical, application of, *119*
Colon procedures, 553–567
  fecal occult blood testing as, 554–555, *556–560*
  guaiac slide test as, 561
  proctoscopy as, 561–563, *564–567*
  sigmoidoscopy as, 561–563, *564–567*
Colony, definition of, 407
Color, of patient, in respiration measurement, 40
  of urine, 300–301
Color comparison method, for hemoglobin measurement, 386–387
Color vision, assessment of, 90–91
  procedure for, *91–92*
Colposcope, definition of, 163
Colposcopy, 204–205
  definition of, 163, 204
Complete blood count (CBC), 365
  in prenatal care, 542
Compound microscope, 413
Compress, definition of, 105
Conduction, definition of, 16, 17
Conduction system, of heart, 443
Conjunctiva, definition of, 51, 81
Constipation, 65
Contagious disease, definition of, 407, 410
Contaminate, definition of, 3, 139, 163
Contraceptive, oral, action of, 222
Contractions, Braxton Hicks, definition of, 531
Contrast medium, 479–480
  definition of, 475
Controlled drugs, 230
Controlled substances, classification of, 231*t*
Contusion, definition of, 163, 182, *183*
Convalescent period, in infectious disease, 411
Convection, definition of, 16, 17
Conversion, definition of, 217, 227
Convulsion, 65
Cornea, definition of, 81
Cotton-tipped applicator, for patient examination, 71
Cough, 65
Cradle position, for carrying infant, 498
Cravat, 209, *210*
Crisis, definition of, 16, 19
Crutch(es), 124–133
  axillary, 124, 125
    measurement for, 125, *126*
  gaits using, 127
    four-point, *129–130*
    instructing patient in, procedure for, *128–133*
    swing, *132–133*
    three-point, *131–132*
    tripod position in, *128*
    two-point, *130–131*
  guidelines for, 127
  Lofstrand, 124–125
Crutch palsy, 125
Cryosurgery, 207–208
  definition of, 163, 207
Cryotherapy, 207–208
Crystals, urinary, *319–320*, 323*t*, 325
Cubic centimeter, definition of, 217
Culture(s), 425–426
  definition of, 407
  in prenatal care, 542
Culture medium, 425
  definition of, 407
Curette, *172*, 173
Cutting needle, 188
Cyanosis, 65
  definition of, 38, 40
Cycle, cardiac, definition of, 441
Cyst, sebaceous, definition of, 164, 199
  removal of, 199–200
Cystogram, 492
Cytology, definition of, 516

Darkness, for microorganism growth, 4
Darkroom, 485
Decline period, in infectious disease, 411
Decongestant, action of, 222
Dehydration, 64
Deltoid, as intramuscular injection site, 254
Depolarization, 444
Dermis, definition of, 217
Detergent, definition of, 139
Diagnosis, definition of, 51, 52
Diagnostic procedures, recording of, 61
Diapedesis, definition of, 364, 368
Diaphoresis, 64
Diarrhea, 65
Diastole, definition of, 42, 43
Diastolic pressure, definition of, 42, 43
Dilation, and curettage, definition of, 516
  of cervix, definition of, 531
Diplococci, 412
Disinfectant(s), definition of, 16, 139, 140
  for control of microorganisms, 159–161
Disinfection, AIDS precautions in, 11–12
Dissecting scissors, 169
Diuresis, definition of, 295
Diuretic, action of, 222
Donor, definition of, 353

Dorsalis pedis artery, pulse taking at, 33
Dose, definition of, 217
Drainage, surgical incision and, of localized infections, 200–201
Draping, in patient examination, 66, 69, 70
Dressing, sterile, changing of, *184–186*
Dressing forceps, *169*
Droplet infection, definition of, 410
Drug(s). *See also* Medication.
  actions of, factors affecting, 231–232
  classification of, based on action, 221–222
    based on preparation, 218–221
  commonly utilized, 219–220*t*
  controlled, 230
  interaction of, 232
  liquid preparation of, 218, 220–221
  powdered, reconstitution of, 241, *242*
  pulse rate and, 34
  solid preparations of, 220–221
Dry heat oven, for control of microorganisms, 158–159
Dyspnea, 65
  definition of, 38, 40
Dysuria, definition of, 295

Ear(s), 98–103
  examination of, 74
  instillation in, procedure for, *102–103*
  irrigation of, 98–99, *99–101*
  structure of, 98
EDC, definition of, 531
Edema, 65
  definition of, 105
Effacement, definition of, 531
Elastic bandage, 209
Electrocardiography, 440–473
  alternating current artifact in, *455*, 456–457
  capabilities of, 450–453
  cardiac arrhythmia detection by, 469–473. *See also* Arrhythmias.
  definition of, 441, 442
  Holter monitor, 462–468
  interpretation of, 453
  leads for, 447–449, *458–462*
  marking and mounting in, 457
  paper for, 445
  standardization of, 446
Electrode, definition of, 441
Electrolyte(s), definition of, 441
  in electrocardiograph, 447
  in plasma, 369
Electronic thermometer, 28
  procedure for using, *28–30*
Elixir, definition of, 218
Emetic, action of, 222
Emotional states, body temperature and, 18
  pulse rate and, 33
Emulsion, definition of, 218
Endocervix, definition of, 516
Endoscope, definition of, 553
Enema, barium, 488–489
  definition of, 475
Engagement, definition of, 531
Enuresis, definition of, 295
Environment, body temperature and, 19
Eosinophils, 381
Epidermis, definition of, 217
Epistaxis, 65
Epithelial cells, in urine, 321*t*, 324–325
Erythema, definition of, 105, 106
Erythrocytes, definition of, 353
  function of, 354, 368
  structure of, 368

Escherichia coli, 412
Eupnea, definition of, 38, 40
Examination room, preparation of, 70–71
Exercise, physical, body temperature and, 198
  pulse rate and, 33
Exfoliated cells, definition of, 516
  in Pap test, 519
Exhalation, 39
  definition of, 38, 39
Expectorant, action of, 222
External auditory canal, 98
External auditory meatus, 98
External ear, 98
External os, definition of, 516
Extremities, lower, examination of, 75
  upper, examination of, 74
Exudate, definition of, 105, 107
Eye(s), 81–96. *See also* Visual acuity.
  examination of, 74
  instillations in, 95, *95–96*
  irrigation of, *93–94*
  structure of, 81

Fahrenheit thermometer, definition of, 16
False negative test result, definition of, 407
False positive test result, definition of, 407
Familial, definition of, 51
Familial disease, definition of, 54
Fastidious, definition of, 407
Fasting, definition of, 267
  for laboratory tests, 279–280
Fasting blood sugar (FBS), 391*t*, 393
Fatty casts, in urine, 322*t*, 325
Fecal occult blood testing, 554–555, *556–560*
Femoral artery, pulse taking at, 33
Fetal heart rate, definition of, 531
Fetal heart tones, definition of, 531
  in prenatal care, 546
Fetoscope, 546
  definition of, 531
Fetus, definition of, 531
  presentation and position of, in prenatal care, 546
Fever, 65
  definition of, 16, 18
  stages of, 19
Fibers, Purkinje, 443
Fibrillation, atrial, *470*, 472
  ventricular, *471*, 473
Fibrin clot, 347
Fibroblasts, definition of, 163, 182
  in healing process, 182
Flashlight, penlight, for patient examination, 71
Flatulence, 65
Flora, normal, 410
  definition of, 407
Fluoroscope, definition of, 475, 481
Fluoroscopy, 481
  definition of, 475, 481
Flushing, 64
Flutter, atrial, 469–472, *470*
  ventricular, *471*, 473
Football position, for carrying infant, 499
Forceps, 169–173
  definition of, 163
  sterile transfer, 179
    utilization of, *180*
Four-point crutch gait, *129–130*
Frenulum linguae, definition of, 16
Frequency, definition of, 295
Fundus, definition of, 531
  height of, measurement of, 544–546
    McDonald's rule for, 544–545

Furuncle, definition of, 163, 200
  surgical incision and drainage of, 200

Gaits, crutch, 127–133. *See also* Crutch(es), gaits using.
Galvanometer, in electrocardiograph, 447
Gastrointestinal system, 65
Gastrointestinal tract, x-rays of, 488–489
Gauze, Kling, 209
Gene, definition of, 353
Genitalia, examination of, 75
Gestation, definition of, 531
Gestation calculator, 538, *539*
Glass syringe, 237
Glass thermometers, 19–20
Gloves, for patient examination, 71
  sterile, application of, *174–175*
    removal of, *175*
Glucometer II glucose meter, blood glucose measurement using, *401–402*
Glucose, blood, measurement of, with glucose meter, 395–396
    self monitoring of, 403–405
    tests for, 391*t*, 393
  in urine, 308
    measurement of, using Clinitest, *316–318*
Glucose meter, blood glucose measurement with, 395–396
Glucose tolerance test (GTT), 391*t*, 394–395
Gluteus medius intramuscular injection site, 253
Glycogen, definition of, 388
Glycosuria, alimentary, 308
  definition of, 293
Gonorrhea, culture of, cervical specimen for, in prenatal care, 542
  vaginal, 524–526
Gown, for patient examination, 70
Gram stain, in microscopic examination of microorganisms, 434, *435–438*
Granular casts, in urine, 322*t*, 325
Granular leukocytes, 381
Gravid, definition of, 531
Gravida, definition of, 531
Gravidity, definition of, 531, 537
Grid, in radiography, 478
Growth, requirements of microorganisms for, 4
Growth patterns, 500
Guaiac slide test, quality control for, 561
Gynecologic examination, 516–530
  assisting with, procedure for, *528–530*
Gynecology, definition of, 516, 517

Hammer, percussion, definition of, 51
  for patient examination, 71
Hands, examination of, 74
Handwashing, in medical asepsis, *6–8*
Hanging drop preparation, in microscopic examination of microorganisms, 430, *431*
Head, examination of, 74
Headache, 66
Healing, promotion of, through physical therapy, 104–137. *See also* Physical therapy.
Healing process, 182–183
Health history, 52–60
  chief complaint in, 53–54
  family history in, 54
  form for, *55–59*
  introductory data in, 53
  past history in, 54
  personal history in, 60
  present illness in, 54
Health history *(Continued)*
  review of systems in, 60
Heart, conduction system of, 443
  examination of, 74
  structure of, 442–443
Heart rate, fetal, definition of, 531
Heart tones, fetal, definition of, 531
  in prenatal care, 546
Heat, application of, by heating pad, *111–112*
    by hot compress, *114–115*
    by hot soak, *112–113*
    by hot water bag, *109–110*
    factors affecting, 108
    purpose of, 107
  dry, to control microorganisms, 158–159
  local effects of, 106, *107*
  moist, to control microorganisms, 146–157
      by autoclaving, 146–157. *See also* Autoclave.
      by boiling, 146
Heating pad, application of, *111–112*
Height, in patient examination, 66
  measurement of, *67*
  metropolitan tables on, 68*t*
Hematocrit, 373–375
  in prenatal care, 542
Hematology, 362–387, 365–368
  definition of, 364
  tests in, 366*t*–367*t*
Hematoma, definition of, 333
Hematuria, 310
  definition of, 295
Hemoccult slide test, development of, *559–560*
  patient instructions for, *556–558*
Hemocytometer, 376
  definition of, 364
Hemoglobin, concentration of, measurement of, 386–387
  definition of, 364
  in prenatal care, 542
Hemolysis, 368
  definition of, 333, 364, 368
  in antigen-antibody reactions, 356
  prevention of, in blood specimen, 335–336
Hemolytic reaction, in streptococcus testing, 427–429
Hemostasis, definition of, 163
Hemostatic drug, action of, 222
Hemostatic forceps, *170*, 171, 173
Heterotroph, definition of, 4
High-density lipoprotein (HDL), definition of, 388, 389
High-risk, definition of, 531
Holders, needle, *170*, 173
Holter monitor, application of, *466–468*
Holter monitor electrocardiography, 462–468
  activity diary for, *464*
  electrode placement in, *466–468*
Homeostasis, definition of, 267, 268
Host, definition of, 3
Hot compress, application of, *114–115*
Hot soak, application of, *111–113*
Hot water bag, application of, *109–110*
Household system, 226–227
  apothecary and metric equivalents of, 228*t*
Human immunodeficiency virus (HIV), AIDS from, 8–9
Humor, aqueous, definition of, 81
  vitreous, definition of, 81
Hyaline casts, in urine, 322*t*, 325
Hyperglycemia, definition of, 388
Hyperopia, definition of, 80, 82
Hyperpnea, definition of, 38, 40
Hyperpyrexia, definition of, 16, 18
Hypertension, definition of, 42, 45

Hypnotic, action of, 222
Hypodermic syringe, 238
Hypoglycemia, 395
  definition of, 388
Hypopnea, definition of, 38, 40
Hypotension, definition of, 42, 45
Hypoxia, definition of, 38, 40
Hysterosalpingogram, 492

Ice bag, application of, *116–117*
Immunity, definition of, 496, 510
Immunization(s), 510–511
  definition of, 407, 496
Impacted, definition of, 97
In vitro, definition of, 353
In vivo, definition of, 253, 267
Incineration, for control of microorganisms, 158
Incision, definition of, 163, 182, *183*
  surgical, and drainage, for localized infections, 200–201
Incontinence, urinary, definition of, 295
Incubate, definition of, 139, 407
Incubation period, definition of, 407
  in infectious disease, 410
Induration, definition of, 217, 260
Infant, carrrying of, 497–499
  definition of, 496, 531
  measuring length of, *505*
  measuring weight of, *504*
Infection(s), 410–411
  control of, 2–12
  cycle of, 4, *5*
  definition of, 3, 163
  droplet, definition of, 410
  in infectious disease, 410
  localized, surgical incision and drainage of, 200–201
  vaginal, 523–526
Infectious disease(s), definition of, 407, 410
  prevention and control of, 439
  stages of, 410–411
Infective waste, AIDS precautions for, 12
Infiltration, definition of, 163
  of local anesthetic, 193
Inflammation, definition of, 105, 163, 182
  in healing process, 182
Ingrown toenail, removal of, 202–203
Inhalation, 39
  definition of, 38, 39
Inhalation medications, administration of, 217
Injection(s), intradermal, 246–247
    definition of, 217
    procedure for, *248–249*
  intramuscular, 253–259. *See also* Intramuscular injection(s).
  intravenous, definition of, 217
  preparation of, *243–246*
  subcutaneous, 250
    definition of, 217
    procedure for, *251–252*
Inner ear, 98
Inoculate, definition of, 407
Inoculum, definition of, 407
Inspection, definition of, 51
  in physical examination, 72
Instillation, definition of, 79, 80
  ear, *102–103*
  eye, 95, *95–96*
Instructions, to patient, recording of, 62
Instruments, for minor office surgery, 167–173
  sanitization of, *141*
Insulin, action of, 222
Insulin syringe, 238
Integumentary system, 64
Intensifying screens, in radiography, 479
Intercostal, definition of, 31
Internal os, definition of, 516
Interval, definition of, 441
  in ECG cycle, 445
Intradermal injection(s), 246–247
  definition of, 217
  procedure for, *248–249*
Intramuscular injection(s), 253–259
  administration of, *256–257*
  definition of, 217
  into deltoid, 254
  into gluteus medius, 253
  into vastus lateralis, 254, *255*
  into ventrogluteal area, 255
  pediatric, 508–509, *510*
  Z-track method of, 258, *259*
Intrauterine device (IUD), definition of, 163
Intravenous injection, definition of, 217
Intravenous pyelography (IVP), 491
Iodine, to control microorganisms, 161
Iris, definition of, 81
Irrigation, definition of, 79, 80
  of ear, 98–99, *99–101*
  of eye, *93–94*

Jaundice, 64

Kaposi's sarcoma, AIDS and, 8, 9
Ketone bodies, in urine, 309
Ketonuria, 309
  definition of, 293
Ketosis, 309
  definition of, 293
Kidney basin, for patient examination, 71
Kidneys, 294
Kling gauze, 209
Knee-chest position, for physical examination, 69
  for proctoscopy and sigmoidoscopy, 565
Korotkoff sounds, 45

Laboratory, clinical, 266–291
    medical office and, relationship between, 270–271
  infection precautions for, in AIDS, 10–11
  reference, 271
  safety in, 290
Laboratory profiles, 276*t*
Laboratory requests, 271, *273*, 274–277
Laboratory tests, 268–270
  categories of, 281*t*
  definition of, 267
  in prenatal care, 541
  patient preparation and instructions for, 278–280
  purpose of, 269–270
  quality control in, 289–290
  recording of, 62
  reports on, *277*, 278
  representative, from laboratory directory, 272*t*
  specimens for, collection of, handling and
      transporting in, 280–286, *284–286*
    testing of, 286–289
      automated analyzers in, 288–289
      manual method of, 288
Laceration, definition of, 163, 182, *183*
Lag phase, in healing process, 182
Lamp, gooseneck, for patient examination, 71

Lancet method, to obtain capillary blood specimen, *371*
Laxative, action of, 222
Legs, examination of, 75
Length, definition of, 217, 222, 496
  of infant, measurement of, *505*
Lens, of eye, definition of, 81
Leopold's maneuvers, 546, *547*
Leukocytes, categories of, 381
  definition of, 353
  function of, 354, 368–369
  in urine, 310
  structure of, 368–369
Leukocytosis, 368
  definition of, 364
Leukocyturia, 310
Leukopenia, 368
  definition of, 364
Ligaments, suspensory, definition of, 81
Ligate, definition of, 163
Liniment, definition of, 218
Lipoprotein, definition of, 388, 389
Lips, examination of, 74
Lithotomy position, for physical examination, 66
Load, definition of, 139
Local anesthetic, definition of, 163
  for minor office surgery, 193–194
Lochia, 551
  definition of, 531
Lofstrand crutch, 124–125
Lotion, definition of, 220
Low-density lipoprotein (LDL), definition of, 388, 389
Lozenge, definition of, 220
Lubricant, for patient examination, 71
Lungs, examination of, 74
Lymphocytes, 381
Lysis, definition of, 16, 19

Mammogram, 492
Manometer, aneroid, 44
  definition of, 42
  mercury gravity, 44
Mantoux test, 261–262
Manual method, definition of, 267
  of laboratory testing, 288
Maturation phase, in healing process, 182
Mayo tray, definition of, 163
McDonald's rule, for fundal height measurement, 544–545
Meatus, urinary, 294
Mechanical assistive devices, for ambulation, 124–137
Medical abbreviations, 581–589
Medical asepsis, 2–12. *See also* Asepsis, medical.
Medical assisting profession, 1984 Dacum analysis of, 579–580
Medical history, past, in prenatal record, 537
Medical office, clinical laboratory and, relationship between, 270–271
Medical record, charting in, 60–63
  definition of, 51
  entries in, types of, 61–62
  guidelines for, 62–63
Medication. *See also* Drug(s).
  administration of, 216–265
    guidelines for, 232–233
    inhalation, 217
    oral, *234–236*
    parenteral, 236–259. *See also* Parenteral administration, of medications.
    prescription, 229–231
    recording of, 61
Medication *(Continued)*
  administration of, systems of measurement used in, 222–229
    apothecary, 225–226
    conversion between, 227–229
    household, 226–227
    metric, 223–225
  preparation of, guidelines for, 232–233
  restrictions on, for laboratory tests, 280
Medium, culture, 425
  definition of, 407
Medulla oblongata, 39
Melena, definition of, 553, 554
Membrane, mucous, definition of, 407
  tympanic, definition of, 51, 97, 98
Meniscus, definition of, 42, 44, 293
Menstrual history, in prenatal record, 537
Mercury gravity manometer, 44
Metabolism, pulse rate and, 34
Metric system, 223
  conversion charts for, 228*t*
  notation guidelines for, 224
Microbiology, 406–439
  cultures in, 425–426
  definition of, 407, 409
  sensitivity testing in, 429–430
  specimens for, collection of, 419–425
    for throat culture, *422–423*
    handling and transporting of, 419–420, *420–421*
    wound, 424–425
Microhematocrit method, of hematocrit determination, 373
  procedure for, *374–375*
Microorganism(s), and disease, 411–413
  control of, chemical agents used in, 159–161
    physical agents used in, 146–157
  definition of, 3
  growth requirements for, 4
  microscopic examination of, 430–438
    Gram stain in, 434
    hanging drop preparation in, 430, *431*
    smears in, 432, *432–433*
    wet mount method of, 430
Microscope, 413–418
  care of, 416
  compound, 413
  optical system of, 415–416
  support system for, 413–414
  use of, *417–418*
Micturition, 295
  definition of, 293, 295
Middle ear, 98
Moist heat, to control microorganisms, 146–157
Moisture, for microorganism growth, 4
Monocytes, 381
Mordant, definition of, 407
Mouth, examination of, 74
Mucous membrane, definition of, 407
Mucous threads, in urine, 325
Multigravida, definition of, 531
Multipara, definition of, 531
Multistix 10 SG reagent strip, chemical testing of urine using, *314–315*
Muscle artifacts, on ECG, 453–456
Muscle relaxant, action of, 222
Myelogram, 492
Myopia, definition of, 80, 82

Nausea, 65
Neck, examination of, 74
Needle(s), cutting, 188
  noncutting, 188–189

Needles(s) *(Continued)*
parts of, 236–237
reusable, sanitizing, *143*
straight, *188*, 189
swaged, *188*, 189
definition of, 164
Needle biopsy, 201–202
definition of, 163, 201
Needle holders, *170*, 173
Nephron, 294
definition of, 293
Nervous system, 65–66
Neurologic examination, 75
Neutrophils, 381
Nitrite, in urine, 310
Nocturia, definition of, 295
Nonabsorbable suture, definition of, 163, 187
Noncutting needle, 188–189
Nongranular leukocytes, 381
Nonpathogen, definition of, 3, 4
Nose, examination of, 74
Nullipara, definition of, 531
Nutrients, in plasma, 369
Nutrition, for microorganism growth, 4

Obstetric history, in prenatal record, 537
Obstetrics, definition of, 531, 533
Occult blood, definition of, 553, 554
fecal, testing for, 554–555, *556–560*
Office surgery, minor. *See* Surgery, minor office.
Ointment, definition of, 221
Oliguria, 295
definition of, 293, 295
Open wounds, 182
Operating scissors, 168
Ophthalmologist, definition of, 80, 82
Ophthalmoscope, definition of, 51
for patient examination, 71
Optical system, of microscope, 415–416
Optician, definition of, 80, 82
Optimum growth temperature, definition of, 3, 4
Optometrist, definition of, 80, 82
Oral administration, definition of, 217
Oral contraceptive, action of, 222
Oral medications, administration of, *234–236*
Oral temperature, procedure for taking, 17
Orthopnea, definition of, 38, 40
Otoscope, definition of, 51, 97
for patient examination, 71
Oven, dry heat, to control microorganisms, 158–159
Oxygen, for microorganism growth, 4
Oxyhemoglobin, 368
definition of, 364

P wave, 444
Pain, 66
Palpation, definition of, 51
in physical examination, 72
systolic pressure determination by, *49*
Palsy, crutch, 125
Papanicolaou (Pap) test, 518–522
in prenatal care, 542
procedure for, *520*
report form for, *522*
results of, 522
Para, definition of, 531
Parasites, in urine, 325
Parenteral administration, of medications, 236–259
needle and syringe in, 236–239
preparation of medication for, 239–241
Parenteral administration, of medications *(Continued)*
reconstitution of powdered drugs in, 241
Parity, definition of, 531, 537
Paroxysmal atrial tachycardia (PAT), 469, *470*
Pathogens, definition of, 4
protective mechanisms of body against, 4–6
Patient, positioning of, for x-ray, 481–482
preparation of, for examination, 71–72
instructions for, for laboratory tests, 278–280
Pediatric examination, 497–515
carrying infant in, 497–499
growth patterns and, 500, *501–503*
understanding child in, 497
Pediatric intramuscular injections, 508–509, *510*
Pediatric office visits, 497
Pediatrician, definition of, 496, 497
Pediatrics, definition of, 496, 497
Pelvic examination, 517
bimanual, 527
Pelvimetry, 492
definition of, 531
Penlight flashlight, for patient examination, 71
Percussion, definition of, 51
in physical examination, 72
Percussion hammer, definition of, 51
for patient examination, 71
Perinatal, definition of, 3
Perineum, definition of, 516
Peroxidase, definition of, 553
pH, definition of, 3, 293
for microorganism growth, 4
of urine, 306, 308
Phagocytosis, definition of, 364, 369
Pharyngitis, streptococcal, testing for, 426
Phenol, for control of microorganisms, 160
Phenylalanine hydroxylase, lack of, in PKU, 511
Phenylketonuria (PKU) screening test, 511–512
procedure for, *513–514*
Photometer, reflectance, for hemoglobin measurement, 386, *387*
Physical examination, 72–77
assisting with, *76–77*
charting in, 60–63
draping for, 66, 69
health history in, 52–60
height and weight in, 66
patient preparation for, 71–72
positioning for 66, 69
room preparation for, 70–71
Physical exercise, body temperature and, 19
pulse rate and, 33
Physical therapy, assistive devices for ambulation in, 124–137. *See also* Ambulation, assistive devices for.
cold in, 107–108. *See also* Cold.
heat in, 106–107. *See also* Heat.
promoting healing through, 104–137
ultrasound in, 120–123
Physician, assisting, for minor office surgery, 194–195
Pipet, definition of, 364
Plasma, definition of, 267, 333
function of, 354, 369
separation of, from whole blood, 351
Plastic syringe, 237
Platelets, structure and function of, 369
Pneumocystis carinii, AIDS and, 8–9
Pneumoencephalogram, 492
Polycythemia, 373
definition of, 364
Polyuria, 294–295
definition of, 293, 294
Popliteal artery, pulse taking at, 33

Positioning of patient, for physical examination, 66, 69
for x-rays, 481–482
Posterior chamber, of eye, definition of, 81
Postpartum, definition of, 531
Postpartum visit, six weeks, 551–552
Potter-Bucky diaphragm, 478
Powdered drugs, reconstitution of, 241, *242*
P-R interval, 445
P-R segment, 444
Pre-eclampsia, definition of, 531
Pregnancy, body temperature and, 19
tests for, serum, 328
urine, 326–328, *329–331*
Pregnancy history, present, in prenatal record, 538
Premature ventricular contraction (PVC), *471*, 472
Prenatal, definition of, 531
Prenatal care, 531–552
examination in, assisting with, *548–550*
initial, blood tests in, 542–543
chest roentgenogram in, 543
cultures in, 542
laboratory tests in, 541
smears in, 542
tine test in, 543
urine tests in, 541
visits in, first, 533
return, 543–546
Prenatal history, 538–539
Prenatal record, 533, *534–536*, 537–538
Presbyopia, definition of, 80, 82
Preschoolers, distance visual acuity in, measurement of, 88
Prescription, 229–231
definition of, 217
Presentation, definition of, 531
Pressure, diastolic, definition of, 42, 43
steam under, to control microorganisms, 146–157. *See also* Autoclave.
systolic, definition of, 42, 43
determination of, by palpation, *49*
Primigravida, definition of, 531
Primipara, definition of, 531
Probes, *171*, 173
Proctoscope, 561
definition of, 553
Proctoscopy, 561–563
assisting with, procedure for, 564–567
definition of, 553
Prodome, definition of, 407
Prodromal period, in infectious disease, 410
Profile, definition of, 267
Progress notes, recording of, 62
Prone position, for physical examination, 66
for x-ray, 482
Protective mechanisms, of body, 4–6
Protein(s), in urine, 309
plasma, 369
Proteinuria, 309
definition of, 293
Pruritus, 66
Puerperium, 551
definition of, 531
Pulse, 32–36
apical, 33
measurement of, *36–37*
bounding, definition of, 31, 34
definition of, 32
mechanism of, 32
radial, measurement of, *35*
rhythm of, 34
taking of, sites for, 32–33
thready, definition of, 31, 34
volume of, 34
Pulse rate, 33–34
Puncture, definition of, 164, 182, *183*
Pupil, definition of, 81
Purkinje fibers, 443
Pyelography, intravenous, 491
Pyrexia, 19, 65
definition of, 16, 18
Pyuria, definition of, 295

QRS complex, 444
Q-T interval, 445
Quad cane, 134
Quality control, definition of, 267
for guaiac slide test, 561
in laboratory testing, 289–290
Quickening, definition of, 531

Radial pulse, measurement of, *35*
Radiation, definition of, 16, 17
Radiograph, definition of, 475, 477
production of, *486–487*
Radioimmunoassay (RIA), of hCG, in pregnancy diagnosis, 328
Radiologist, definition of, 475, 477
Radiolucent, definition of, 475
Radiolucent structure, 480
Radiopaque, definition of, 475
Radiopaque structure, 480
Rapid streptococcus tests, 427
Rash, 64
Reagent strips, for urine testing, 311
parameters and diagnostic uses for, 312*t*–313*t*
procedures for, *314–318*
Recipient, definition of, 353
Record, medical, definition of, 51
Rectal temperature, procedure for taking, 17, 18
Rectum, examination of, 75
Recumbent position, for physical examination, 66
Red blood cell count (RBC), 380
Red blood cells, in urine, 321*t*, 324
Reference calibration mark, 446
Reference laboratory, definition of, 271
Reflectance photometer, hemoglobin measurement with, 386, *387*
Refraction, definition of, 80, 82
errors of, 82
Refractive index, definition of, 293
Refractometer, definition of, 293
Relaxant, muscle, definition of, 222
Renal epithelial cells, in urine, 321*t*, 325
Renal threshold, definition of, 293
Repolarization, ventricular, 444
Reservoir host, definition of, 3
Resistance, definition of, 407
Respiration, 39–41
abnormalities of, 40
color of patient and, 40
control of, 39
depth of, 40
external, 39
internal, 39
measurement of, *41*
mechanism of, 39
rhythm of, 40
stertorous, definition of, 38, 40
Respiratory gases, carried by plasma, 369
Respiratory rate, 39–40
Respiratory system, 65
Retention, definition of, 295
Retina, definition of, 51, 81
Retractors, *171*, 173
Retrograde pyelogram (RP), 492
Rh antibody titer, in prenatal care, 543

Rh blood group system, 356
Rh factor, determination of, in prenatal care, 542
Rhythm, of pulse, 34
of respiration, 40
Roentgen rays, definition of, 476
Roentgenogram, definition of, 477
Roentgenologist, definition of, 475, 477
Roller bandage, 209
Routine test, definition of, 267
Rubber goods, sanitization of, *144-145*
Rubella titer, in prenatal care, 543

Safety, laboratory, 290
Sanitization, definition of, 139, 140
of instruments, *141*
of reusable needles, *143*
of reusable syringes, *142*
of rubber goods, *144-145*
procedure for, 140
Sarcoma, Kaposi's, AIDS and, 8
Scalpel, 167-168
definition of, 164, 167
Scissors, 168-169
definition of, 164, 168
Sclera, definition of, 81
Screens, intensifying, in radiography, 479
Sebaceous cyst, definition of, 164, 199
removal of, 199-200
Sedative, action of, 222
Segment, definition of, 441
in ECG cycle, 444
Self monitoring, of blood glucose, 403-405
Sensation, impaired, application of heat or cold and, 108
Sensitivity testing, 429-430
Sequela, definition of, 407
Serology test, for syphilis in prenatal care, 542-543
Serum, definition of, 164, 267, 333
pregnancy tests using, 328
separation of, from whole blood, 347-348, *349-351*
Serum separator vacuum tubes, 348
Sex, pulse rate and, 33
Sheaths, temperature, *20*, 21
Sialogram, 492
Sigmoidoscope, 561-562
definition of, 553
Sigmoidoscopy, 561-563
assisting with, 564-567
definition of, 553
Sims position, for physical examination, 69
Sinoatrial node (SA), 443
Sinus bradycardia, definition of, 469
Sinus rhythm, normal, definition of, 441, 469
Sinus tachycardia, definition of, 469
Skin, preparation of, for minor office surgery, 193
Slide agglutination test, for pregnancy, 326, *327*
procedure for, *329-331*
Slide test method, for blood typing, *357-361*
Smear(s), definition of, 407
in microscopic examination of microorganisms, 432
preparation of, 432, *432-433*
in prenatal care, 542
Papanicolaou. *See* Papanicolaou (Pap) test.
Snellen Big E eye chart, *84*, 84-85
Snellen eye chart, *83*, 84-85
Soak, definition of, 105
Soap, to control microorganisms, 160
Solution, definition of, 220
sterile, pouring of, *181*
Sonography, definition of, 531
Sound, *172*, 173

Space, definition of, 139, 140
Specific gravity, definition of, 293
of urine, 301-303
measurement of, urinometer method of, *304-305*
Specimen(s), cervical, for gonorrhea culture, in prenatal care, 542
collection of, recording of, 61-62
definition of, 267, 407
for trichomoniasis or candidiasis, in prenatal care, 542
laboratory, collection of, handling and transporting in, 280-286, *284-286*
testing of, 286-288
microbiology, 419-425. *See also* Microbiology, specimens for.
urine, clean-catch midstream, 296-298
collection of, *297-298*
wound, 424-425
Specimen bottle, for patient examination, 71
Speculum, *172*, 173
definition of, 51
for patient examination, 71
Spermatozoa, in urine, 326
Sphygmomanometer, 43-44
definition of, 42, 43
for patient examination, 70
Spirilla, 411, 412
definition of, 407, 411
Spirit, definition of, 220
Splinter forceps, *169*, 171
Sponge, definition of, 164
Sponge forceps, *170*, 173
Sprain, definition of, 105
Spray, definition of, 220
Squamous epithelial cells, in urine, 321*t*, 325
S-T segment, 444
Stabs, 381
Stadium stage, of fever, 19
Standard ECG leads, 448
Staphylococcus aureus, 412
Staphylococcus epidermidis, 412
Stature, definition of, 496
Steam, under pressure, to control microorganisms, 146-157. *See also* Autoclave.
Steptococcus pyogenes, 426
Sterile, definition of, 164
Sterile dressing, changing, procedure for, *184-186*
Sterile gloves, application of, *174-175*
removal of, *175*
Sterile packages, commercially prepared, 178-179
opening of, *176-177*
Sterile solution, pouring of, *181*
Sterile transfer forceps, 179
utilization of, *180*
Sterilization, AIDS precautions for, 11-12
by autoclave, 146-157. *See also* Autoclave.
definition of, 139, 140
Stertorous respiration, definition of, 38, 40
Stethoscope, definition of, 42, 43
for patient examination, 70
Straight needle, *188*, 189
Strain, definition of, 105
Streaking, definition of, 407
in culture, 426
Streptococci, 412
Streptococcus testing, 426-429
Streptolysin, definition of, 407
Subcutaneous injection(s), 250
definition of, 217
procedure for, *251-252*
Sublingual administration, of drugs, 217
Subnormal temperature, definition of, 16, 18
Supernatant, definition of, 293

Supine position, for physical examination, 66
  for x-ray, 482
Suppository, definition of, 221
Suppuration, definition of, 105, 107
Surgery, minor office, 162–215
  asepsis for, 165–167
  assisting physician in, 194–195
  bandaging for, 208–215
  cervical punch biopsy as, 205–207
  colposcopy as, 204–205
  cryosurgery as, 207–208
  gloving procedures for, *174–175*
  healing process and, 182–183
  ingrown toenail removal as, 202–203
  instruments for, 167–173
  local anesthetic for, 193–194
  needle biopsy as, 201–202
  pouring sterile solution in, *181*
  procedures in, 199–208
  sebaceous cyst removal as, 199–200
  skin preparation for, 193
  sterile dressing change in, *184–186*
  sterile packages for, *176–177*, 178–179
  sterile transfer forceps for, 179, *180*
  surgical incision and drainage of localized infections as, 200–201
  sutures in, insertion of, 187–191
    removal of, 191–192
  tray set up in, 192–193
  wounds in, *183*
Surgical asepsis, definition of, 164, 165–167
Susceptibility, definition of, 3, 407
Suspensory ligaments, definition of, 81
Suture(s), absorbable, definition of, 163, 187
  definition of, 164
  insertion of, 187–191
  nonabsorbable, definition of, 163, 187
  removal of, 191–192
Suture scissors, 168
Swaged needle, *188*, 189
  definition of, 164
Swing crutch gaits, *132–133*
Symbols, commonly used, 230*t*
Symptoms, 63–66
  definition of, 51, 63
  objective, definition of, 51
  recording of, 61
  subjective, definition of, 51, 63–64
Syphilis, serology test for, in prenatal care, 542–543
Syringe(s), glass, 237
  hypodermic, 238
  insulin, 238
  parts of, 237
  plastic, 237
  prefilled disposable, 239
  reusable, sanitization of, *142*
  tuberculin, 238
  types of, 237–239
Syringe method, of venipuncture, 334
  procedure for, *342–346*
Syrup, definition of, 220
Systole, definition of, 42, 43
Systolic pressure, definition of, 42, 43
  determination of, by palpation, *49*

T wave, 444, 445
Tablet, definition of, 221
Tachycardia, 34, 65
  definition of, 31
  paroxysmal atrial, 469, *470*
  sinus, 469
  ventricular, *471*, 472–473
Tachypnea, definition of, 38, 39
Tape measure, for patient examination, 71
Telephone transmission capability, electrocardiograph with, 452
Temperature, body, 17–30
    maintenance of, 17
    patient's normal, 19
    range of, 18
    taking of, methods of, 17, 18, *22–27*
    variations in, 18–19
  for microorganism growth, 4
  optimum growth, definition of, 3, 4
  tolerance to change in, 108
Temperature sheaths, *20*, 21
Temporal artery, pulse taking at, 33
Tenaculum, *172*, 173
Test tube agglutination test, for pregnancy, 327
Therapeutic procedures, recording of, 61
Thermolabile, definition of, 139
Thermometer(s), centigrade or Celsius, definition of, 16
  electronic, 28, *28–30*
  Fahrenheit, definition of, 16
  for patient examination, 71
  glass, 19–20
    cleaning of, 21
Thready pulse, definition of, 31, 34
Three-channel recording capability, electrocardiograph with, 450, *451*
Three-point crutch gait, *131–132*
Throat, examination of, 74
Throat culture, taking specimen for, *422–423*
Thrombocytes, definition of, 353
  function of, 354
  structure of, 369
Thumb forceps, *169*, 170
Tincture, definition of, 220
Tine test, 262
  administration of, *262–264*
  in prenatal care, 543
  reading of, *264–265*
Tissue forceps, *169*, 171
Tissues, for patient examination, 71
Toenail, ingrown, removal of, 202–203
Tolerance, drug action and, 232
Tongue blade, for patient examination, 71
Tonometer, definition of, 51
  for patient examination, 71
Topical medications, administration of, 217
Towel clamps, *171*, 173
Toxemia, definition of, 531
Toxin, definition of, 105
Toxoid, definition of, 496
Tranquilizer, action of, 222
Tray setup, for minor office surgery, 192–193
Treponema pallidum, 412
Triangular bandage, 209
Trichomoniasis, specimen for, in prenatal care, 542
  vaginal, 523
Trimester, definition of, 532
Tripod cane, 134
Tripod position, for crutch gaits, *128*
Tuberculin skin testing, 260–265
  administration of, 260–261
  Mantoux test as, 260, 261–262
  reading of, 261
  tine test as, 260, 262–265
Tuberculin syringe, 238
Tubular gauze bandage, 212
  application of, *213–215*
Tuning fork, for patient examination, 71
Turbidity, of urine, 301
Two-hour postprandial blood sugar (2-hour PPBS) test, 391*t*, 393–394
Two-point crutch gait, *130–131*
Tympanic membrane, definition of, 51, 97, 98

U wave, 444
Ultrasound, in physical therapy, 120–121
  treatment with, administration of, *122–123*
Upright position, for carrying infant, 498–499
Ureters, 294
Urethra, 294
Urgency, definition of, 295
Urinalysis, 292–331
  chemical examination in, 306–310
  definition of, 293, 300
  diagnostic kits for, 307*t*
  in prenatal care, 541
  laboratory request form for, *299*
  microscopic examination in, 319–326
  physical examination in, 300–305
  reagent strips in, 311–318
Urinary bladder, 294
Urinary incontinence, definition of, 295
Urinary meatus, 294
Urinary system, structure and function of, 294
  terms relating to, 295
Urine, analysis of, 300–303. *See also* Urinalysis.
  casts in, 322*t*, 325
  chemical examination of, 306–310
    using reagent strips, 311–318
  collection of, methods of, 295–297
  composition of, 294–295
  crystals in, *319–320*, 325
  epithelial cells in, 321*t*, 324–325
  glucose in, measurement of, *316–318*
  microorganisms and artifacts in, 324
  microscopic examination of, 319–326
  miscellaneous structures in, 325–326
  physical examination of, 300–305
  pregnancy testing using, 326–328, *329–331*
  red blood cells in, 321*t*, 324
  specimen of, clean-catch midstream, 296–297
      collection of, *297–298*
    collection of, 295–299
    first-voided morning, 295
    pediatric collector for, application of, *506–507*
  white blood cells in, 321*t*, 324
Urinometer, 303
  definition of, 293
  specific gravity of measurement using, *304–305*
Urobilinogen, in urine, 309

Vaccine, definition of, 496
Vacuum tube method, of venipuncture, 334
  procedure for, *337–341*
Vaginal examination, in prenatal visits, 546, *547*
Vaginal infections, 523–526
  candidal, 524
  chlamydial, 526
  gonorrheal, 524–526
  trichomonal, 523
Vasoconstrictor, action of, 222
Vasodilator, action of, 222
Vastus lateralis, as intramuscular injection site, 254, *255*
Venipuncture, 332–351
  definition of, 333, 334
  methods of, 334–336
  syringe method of, 334, *342–346*
  vacuum tube method of, 334, *337–341*
Ventricular depolarization, 444
Ventricular fibrillation, *471*, 473
Ventricular flutter, *471*, 473
Ventricular repolarization, 444
Ventricular tachycardia, *471*, 472–473
Ventrogluteal area, as intramuscular injection site, 255
Vertex, definition of, 496
Vertigo, 66
Vesiculation, definition of, 217
Vial, definition of, 217, 239
  in parenteral drug administration, 237, *241*
Vibrio cholera, 412
Viruses, 413
Vision, color, assessment of, 90–91, *91–92*
Visual acuity, 81–90
  definition of, 81
  distance, measurement of, 82, 84–85
    in preschoolers, 88
    procedure for, *86–87*
  near, measurement of, 88–90
Vital signs, 14–49
  blood pressure as, 42–49. *See also* Blood pressure.
  body temperature as, 17–30. *See also* Temperature, body.
  pulse as, 31–37. *See also* Pulse.
  respiration as, 38–41. *See also* Respiration.
Vitreous humor, definition of, 81
Void, definition of, 293
Volume, definition of, 217, 222
  of pulse, 34
Vomiting, 65
Vulva, definition of, 516

Walker, 136
  instructing patient in use of, *137*
Wandering baseline artifacts, on ECG, 455, *456*
Waste, infective, AIDS precautions for, 12
Waste container, for patient examination, 71
Waxy casts, in urine, 322*t*, 325
Weight, definition of, 217, 222
  in patient examination, 66
  measurement of, *67*
  metropolitan tables on, 68*t*
  of infant, measurement of, *504*
Wet mount method, of microscopic examination of microorganisms, 430
Wheal, definition of, 217
White blood cells, in urine, 321*t*, 324
White blood count (WBC), 376
  differential, 380–381, *382–386*
  manual method for, *377–379*
Wintrobe method, of hematocrit determination, 373
Wound specimens, 424–425
Wounds, definition of, 164, 182
  open and closed, 182

X-ray examinations, 474–493
  cholecystography as, 489–490
  contrast media in, 479–480
  darkroom and, 485
  intravenous pyelography as, 491
  of chest, 543
  of gastrointestinal tract, 488–489
  patient positioning for, 481–482
  precautions for, 482–483
X-ray film, processing of, *484*, 485
X-ray machine, 477–479
X-rays, 477
  definition of, 476

Yeast cells, in urine, 25

Z-track method, of intramuscular injection, 258, *259*
Zephiran chloride, to control microorganisms, 160

THE HUMAN BODY

HIGHLIGHTS of STRUCTURE and FUNCTION

SKELETAL SYSTEM

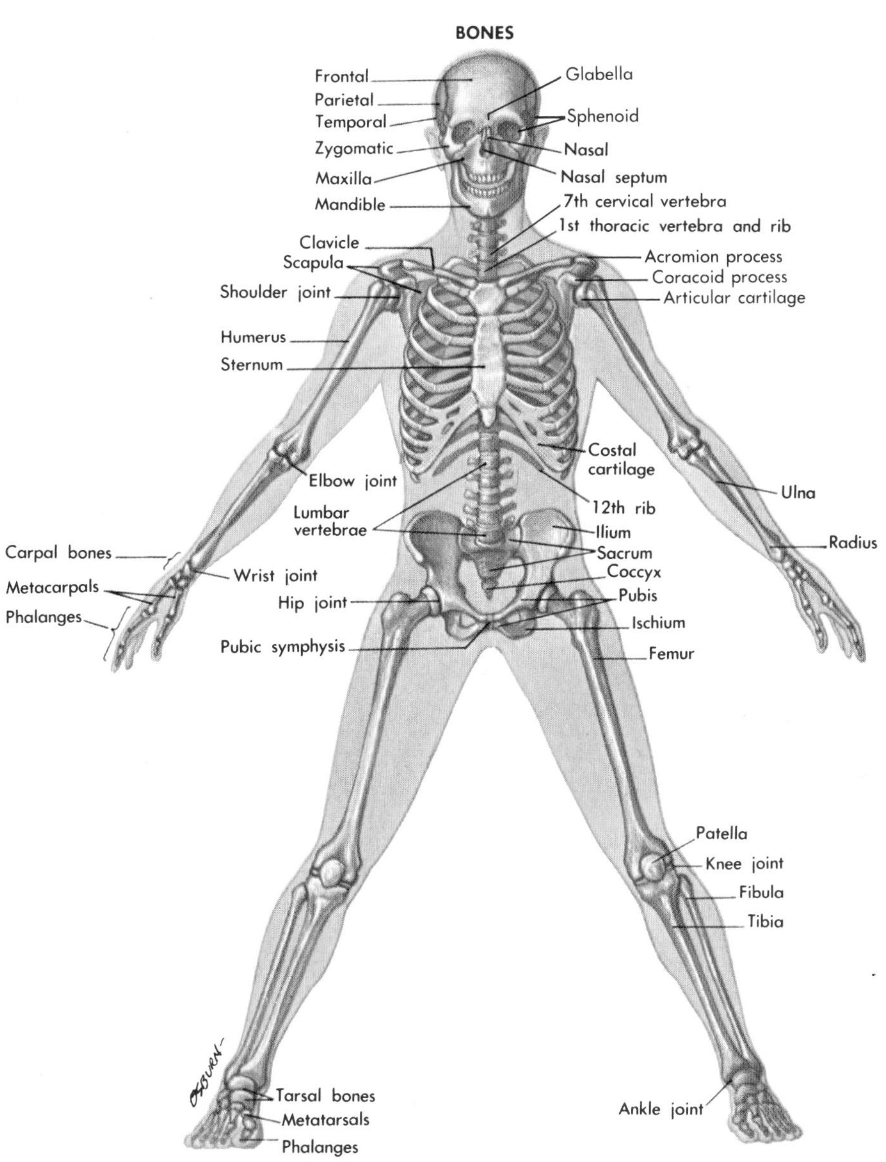

Designed by
WILLIAM A. OSBURN, M.M.A.
Artwork by
ELLEN COLE
ROBERT DEMAREST
GRANT LASHBROOK
WILLIAM OSBURN
W. B. SAUNDERS COMPANY
Philadelphia — London — Toronto

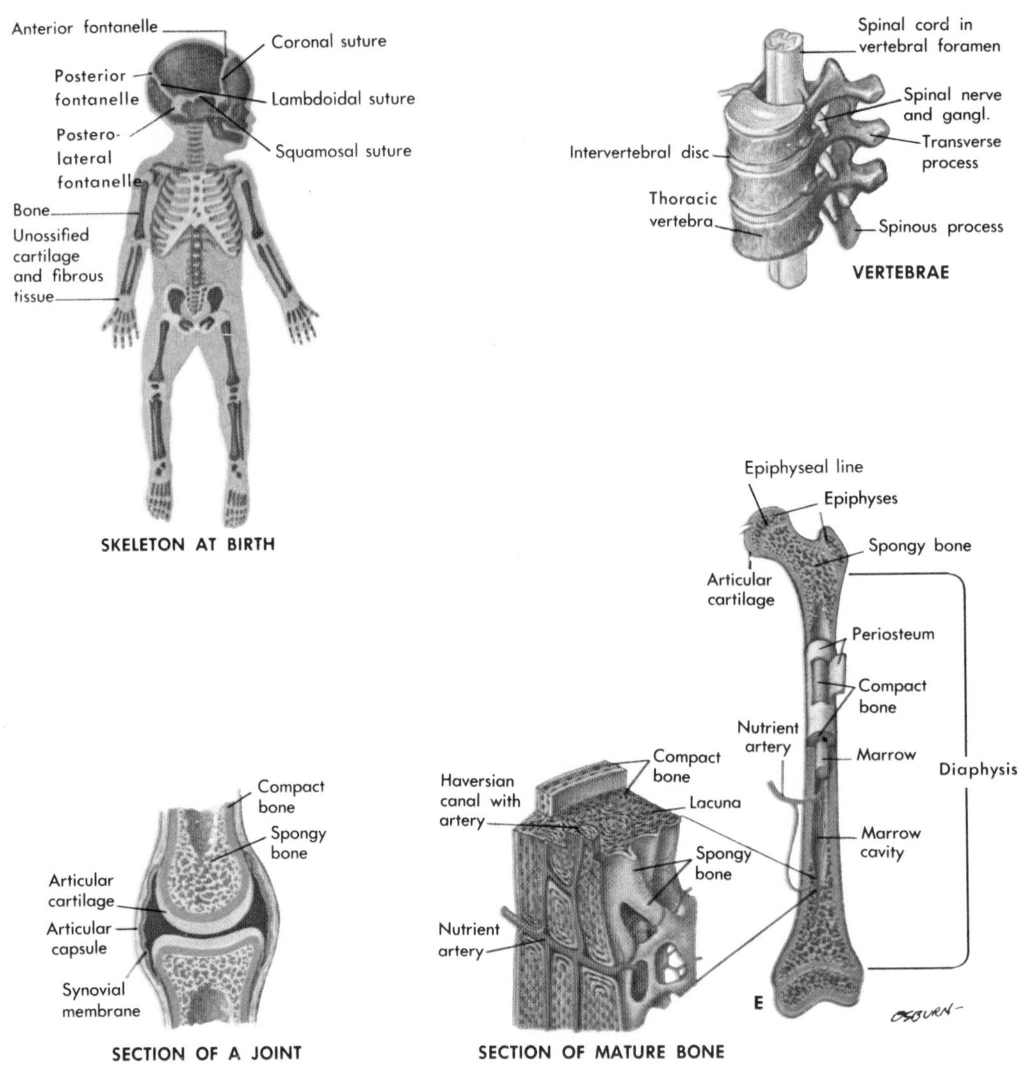
Anterior fontanelle
Coronal suture
Posterior fontanelle
Lambdoidal suture
Postero-lateral fontanelle
Squamosal suture
Bone
Unossified cartilage and fibrous tissue
SKELETON AT BIRTH
Spinal cord in vertebral foramen
Spinal nerve and gangl.
Transverse process
Intervertebral disc
Thoracic vertebra
Spinous process
VERTEBRAE
Epiphyseal line
Epiphyses
Spongy bone
Articular cartilage
Periosteum
Compact bone
Nutrient artery
Marrow
Diaphysis
Marrow cavity
E
Compact bone
Spongy bone
Articular cartilage
Articular capsule
Synovial membrane
SECTION OF A JOINT
Haversian canal with artery
Compact bone
Lacuna
Spongy bone
Nutrient artery
SECTION OF MATURE BONE

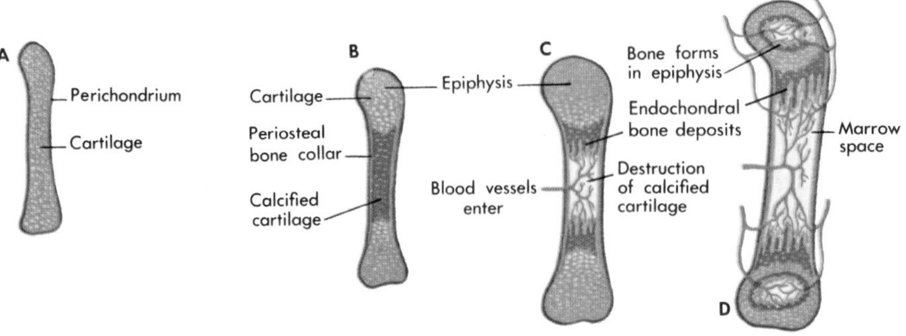
A
Perichondrium
Cartilage
B
Cartilage
Periosteal bone collar
Calcified cartilage
Epiphysis
C
Blood vessels enter
Bone forms in epiphysis
Endochondral bone deposits
Destruction of calcified cartilage
Marrow space
D

DEVELOPMENT OF BONE

SKELETAL MUSCLES

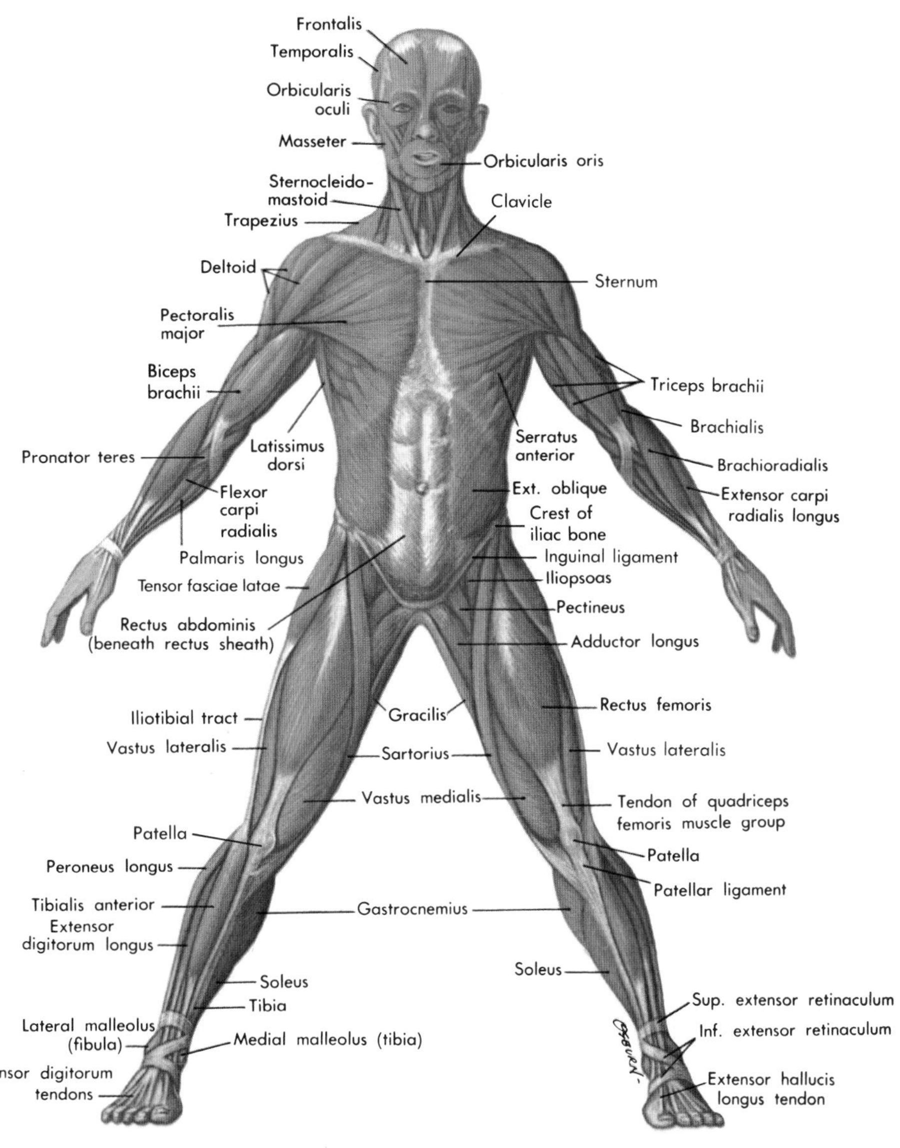

Frontalis
Temporalis
Orbicularis oculi
Masseter
Orbicularis oris
Sternocleido-mastoid
Clavicle
Trapezius
Deltoid
Sternum
Pectoralis major
Biceps brachii
Triceps brachii
Brachialis
Pronator teres
Latissimus dorsi
Serratus anterior
Brachioradialis
Flexor carpi radialis
Ext. oblique
Extensor carpi radialis longus
Crest of iliac bone
Palmaris longus
Inguinal ligament
Tensor fasciae latae
Iliopsoas
Pectineus
Rectus abdominis (beneath rectus sheath)
Adductor longus
Iliotibial tract
Gracilis
Rectus femoris
Vastus lateralis
Sartorius
Vastus lateralis
Vastus medialis
Tendon of quadriceps femoris muscle group
Patella
Patella
Peroneus longus
Patellar ligament
Tibialis anterior
Gastrocnemius
Extensor digitorum longus
Soleus
Soleus
Tibia
Sup. extensor retinaculum
Lateral malleolus (fibula)
Medial malleolus (tibia)
Inf. extensor retinaculum
Extensor digitorum tendons
Extensor hallucis longus tendon

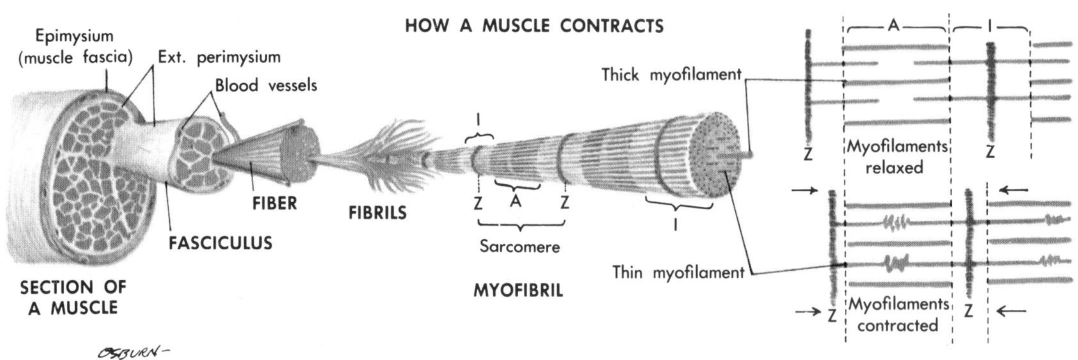

HOW A MUSCLE ATTACHES TO BONE

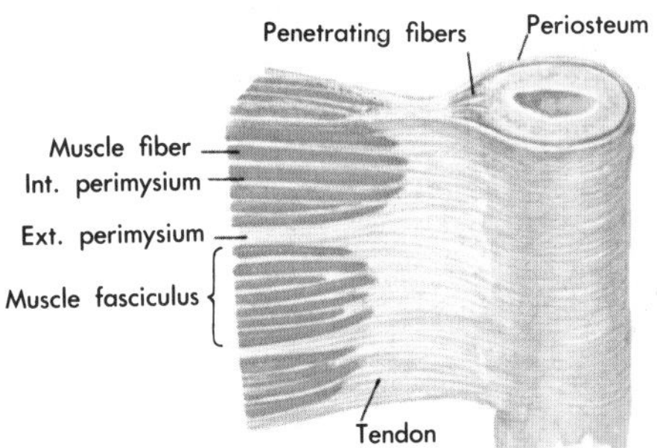

The connective tissue which surrounds the muscle fibers and bundles may (1) form a tendon which fuses with the periosteum, or (2) may fuse directly with the periosteum without forming a tendon.

HOW A MUSCLE PRODUCES MOVEMENT

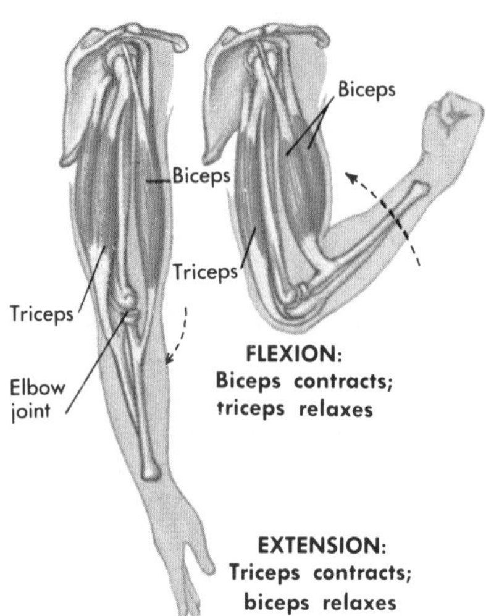

FLEXION:
Biceps contracts; triceps relaxes

EXTENSION:
Triceps contracts; biceps relaxes

RESPIRATION AND THE HEART

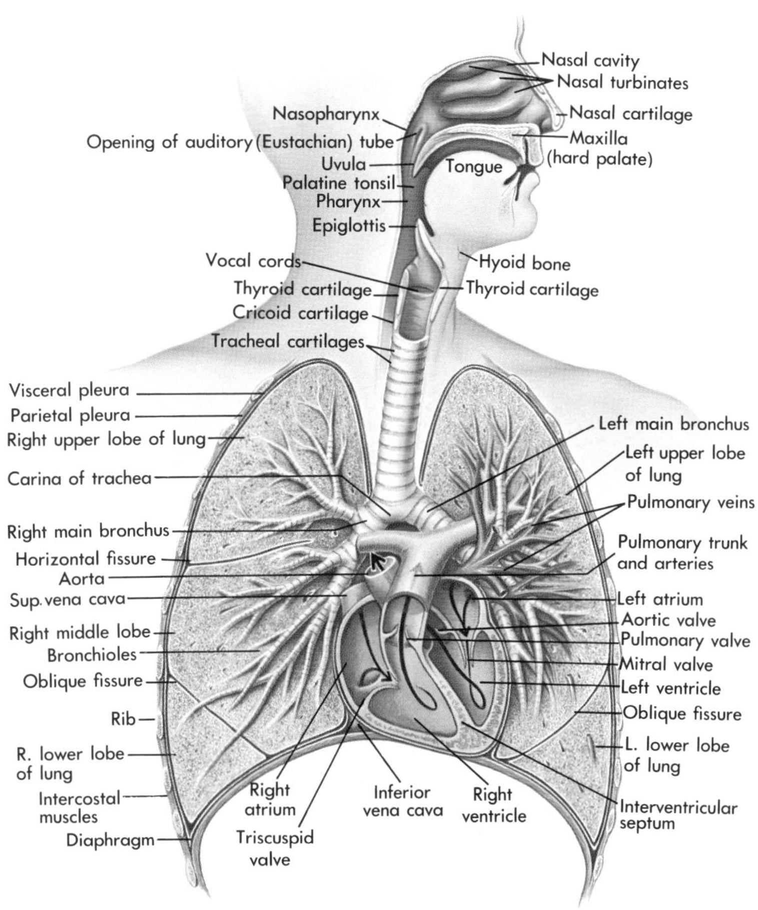

Nasal cavity
Nasal turbinates
Nasal cartilage
Maxilla
(hard palate)
Nasopharynx
Opening of auditory (Eustachian) tube
Uvula
Palatine tonsil
Pharynx
Epiglottis
Tongue
Vocal cords
Thyroid cartilage
Cricoid cartilage
Tracheal cartilages
Hyoid bone
Thyroid cartilage
Visceral pleura
Parietal pleura
Right upper lobe of lung
Carina of trachea
Right main bronchus
Horizontal fissure
Aorta
Sup. vena cava
Right middle lobe
Bronchioles
Oblique fissure
Rib
R. lower lobe
of lung
Intercostal
muscles
Diaphragm
Right
atrium
Triscuspid
valve
Inferior
vena cava
Right
ventricle
Left main bronchus
Left upper lobe
of lung
Pulmonary veins
Pulmonary trunk
and arteries
Left atrium
Aortic valve
Pulmonary valve
Mitral valve
Left ventricle
Oblique fissure
L. lower lobe
of lung
Interventricular
septum

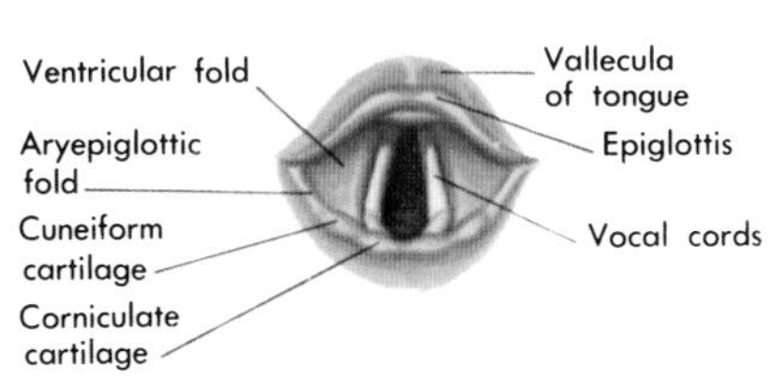

SUPERIOR VIEW OF LARYNX

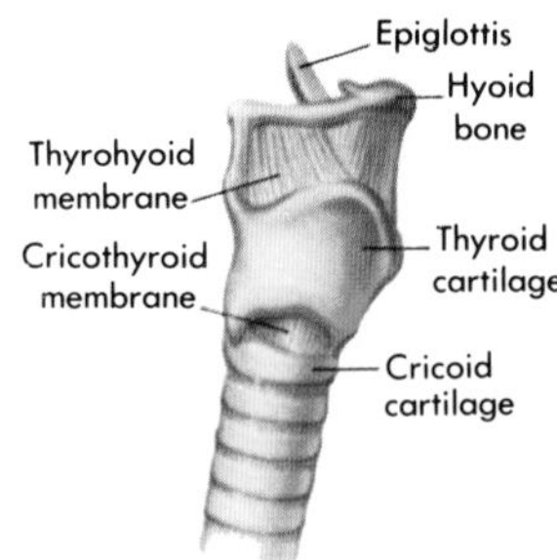

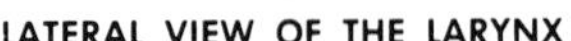

LATERAL VIEW OF THE LARYNX

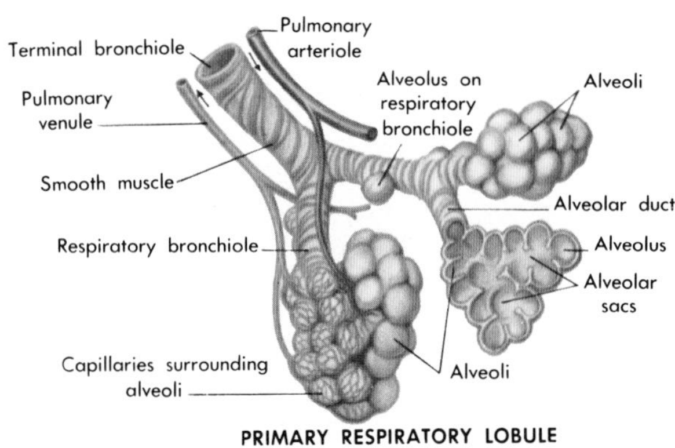

PRIMARY RESPIRATORY LOBULE

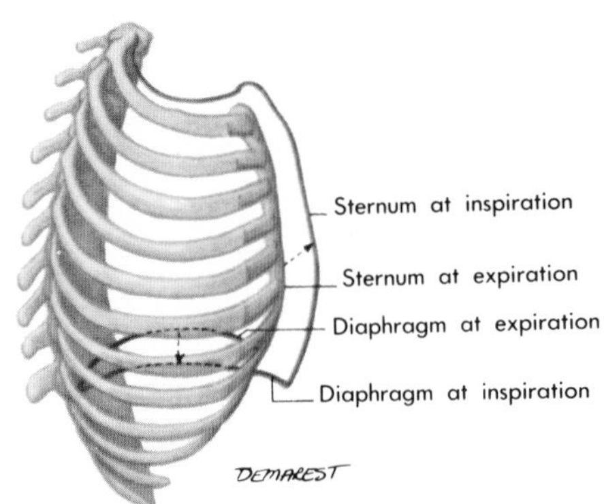

THORACIC RESPIRATORY MOVEMENTS

BLOOD VASCULAR SYSTEM
VEINS

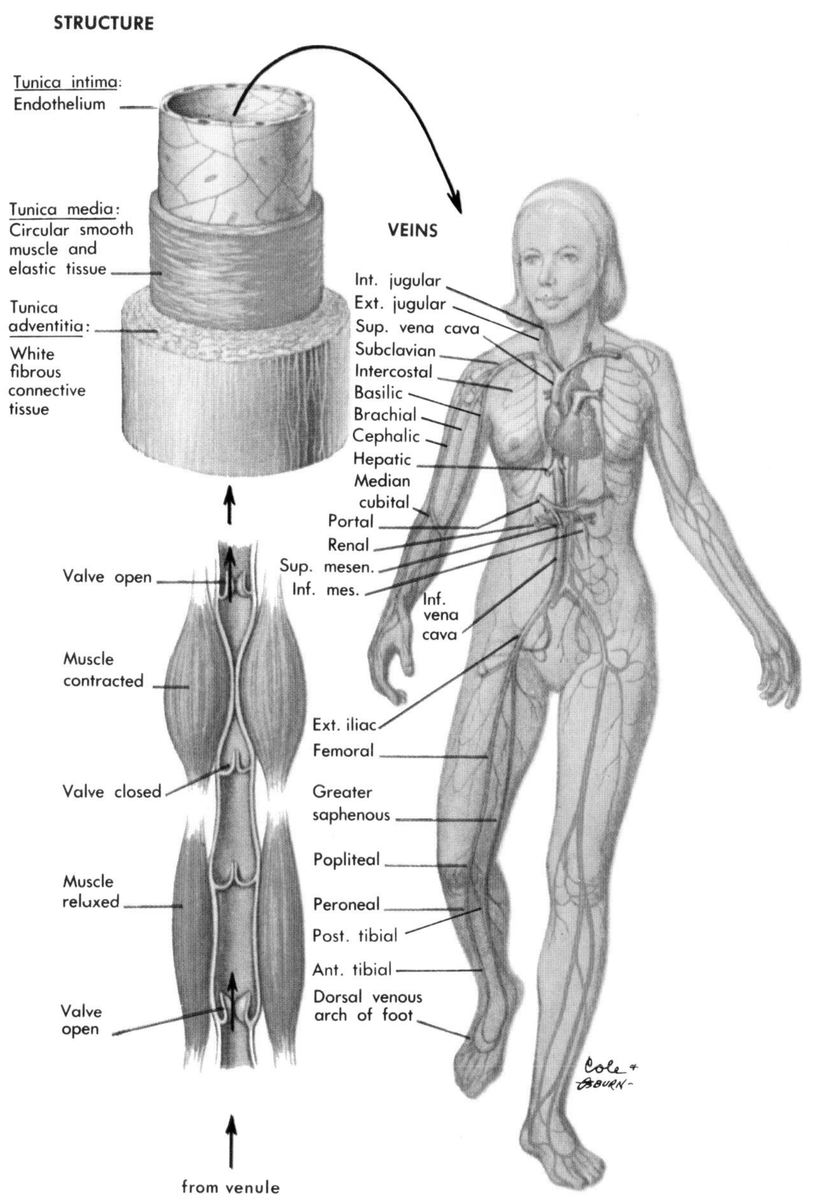
STRUCTURE
Tunica intima:
Endothelium
Tunica media:
Circular smooth muscle and elastic tissue
Tunica adventitia:
White fibrous connective tissue
Valve open
Muscle contracted
Valve closed
Muscle relaxed
Valve open
from venule
VEINS
Int. jugular
Ext. jugular
Sup. vena cava
Subclavian
Intercostal
Basilic
Brachial
Cephalic
Hepatic
Median cubital
Portal
Renal
Sup. mesen.
Inf. mes.
Inf. vena cava
Ext. iliac
Femoral
Greater saphenous
Popliteal
Peroneal
Post. tibial
Ant. tibial
Dorsal venous arch of foot

ARTERIES

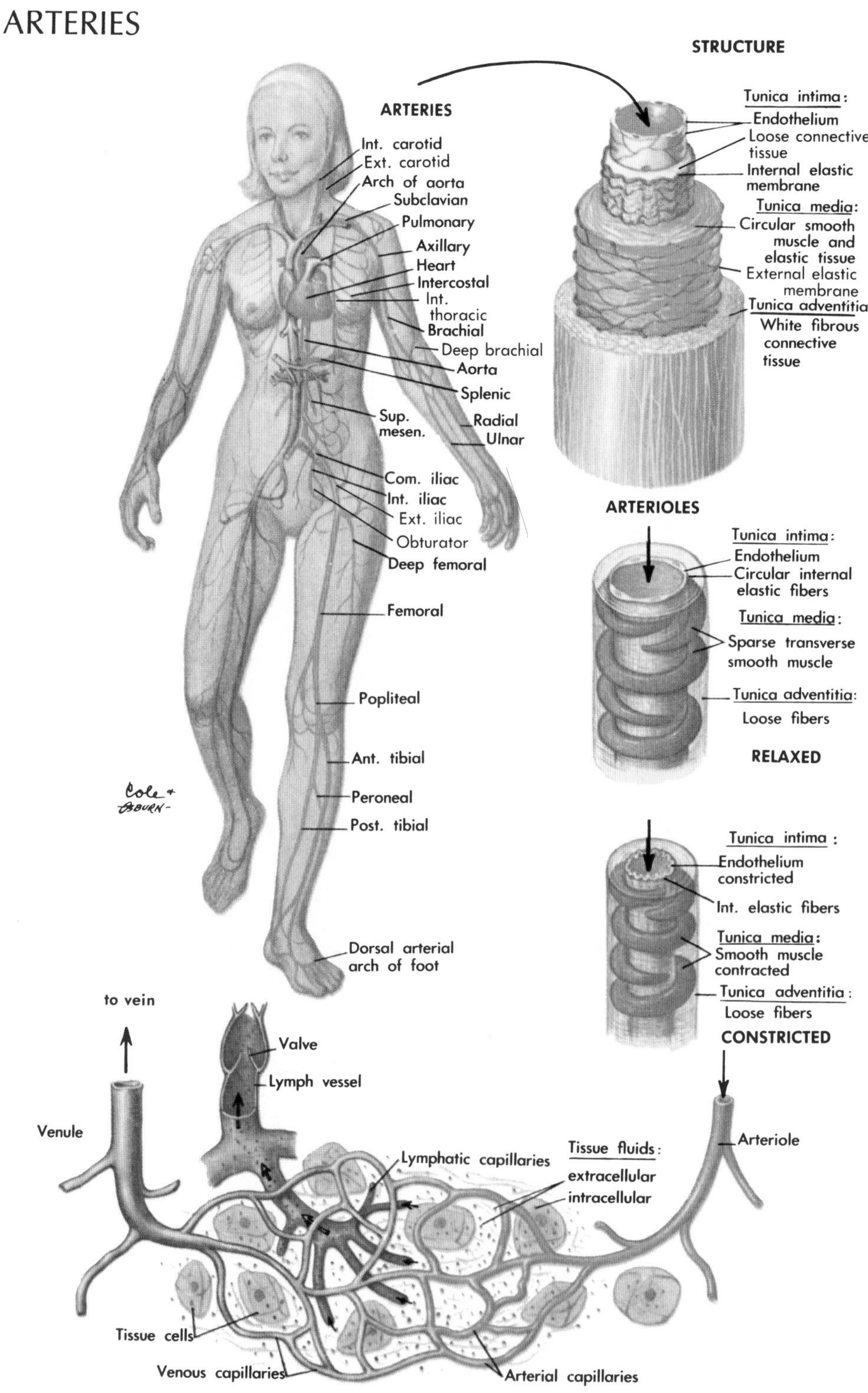
ARTERIES
Int. carotid
Ext. carotid
Arch of aorta
Subclavian
Pulmonary
Axillary
Heart
Intercostal
Int. thoracic
Brachial
Deep brachial
Aorta
Splenic
Sup. mesen.
Radial
Ulnar
Com. iliac
Int. iliac
Ext. iliac
Obturator
Deep femoral
Femoral
Popliteal
Ant. tibial
Peroneal
Post. tibial
Dorsal arterial arch of foot
Cole + Osburn
STRUCTURE
Tunica intima:
Endothelium
Loose connective tissue
Internal elastic membrane
Tunica media:
Circular smooth muscle and elastic tissue
External elastic membrane
Tunica adventitia
White fibrous connective tissue
ARTERIOLES
Tunica intima:
Endothelium
Circular internal elastic fibers
Tunica media:
Sparse transverse smooth muscle
Tunica adventitia:
Loose fibers
RELAXED
Tunica intima:
Endothelium constricted
Int. elastic fibers
Tunica media:
Smooth muscle contracted
Tunica adventitia:
Loose fibers
CONSTRICTED
to vein
Valve
Lymph vessel
Venule
Lymphatic capillaries
Tissue fluids:
extracellular
intracellular
Arteriole
Tissue cells
Venous capillaries
Arterial capillaries

A CAPILLARY BED

Plate 8

DIGESTIVE SYSTEM

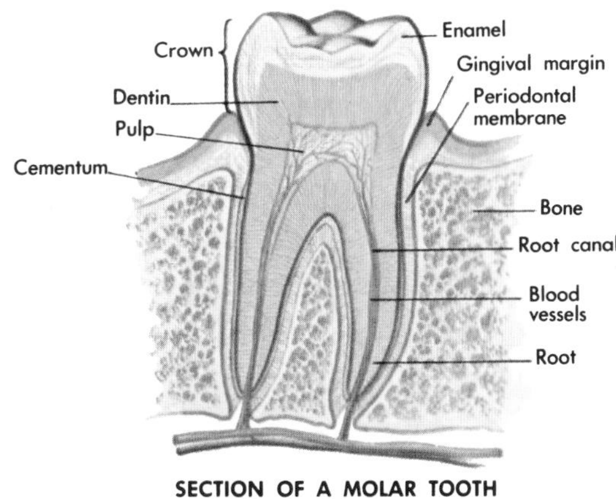

Crown
Dentin
Pulp
Cementum
Enamel
Gingival margin
Periodontal membrane
Bone
Root canal
Blood vessels
Root

SECTION OF A MOLAR TOOTH

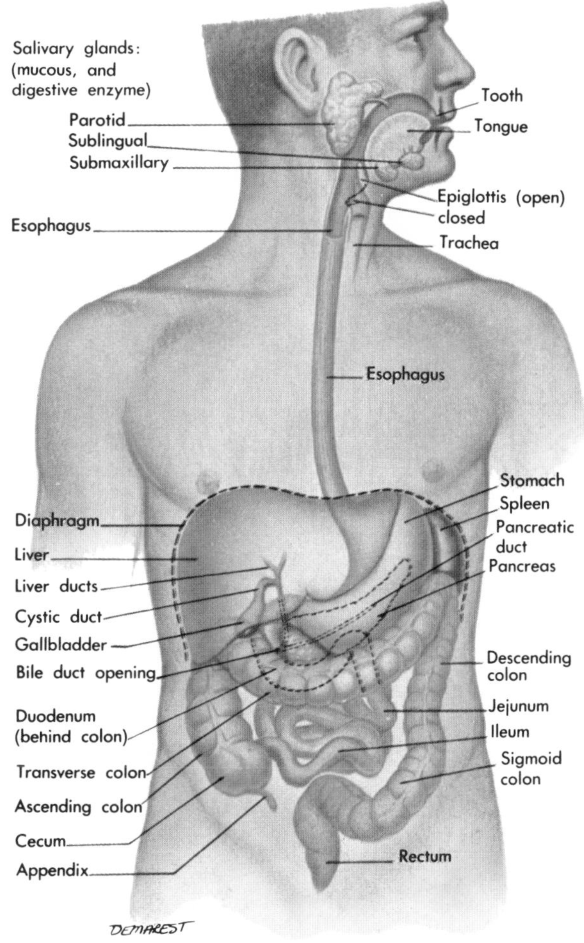

Salivary glands: (mucous, and digestive enzyme)
Parotid
Sublingual
Submaxillary
Esophagus
Tooth
Tongue
Epiglottis (open)
closed
Trachea
Esophagus
Stomach
Spleen
Pancreatic duct
Pancreas
Diaphragm
Liver
Liver ducts
Cystic duct
Gallbladder
Bile duct opening
Duodenum (behind colon)
Transverse colon
Ascending colon
Cecum
Appendix
Descending colon
Jejunum
Ileum
Sigmoid colon
Rectum
DEMAREST

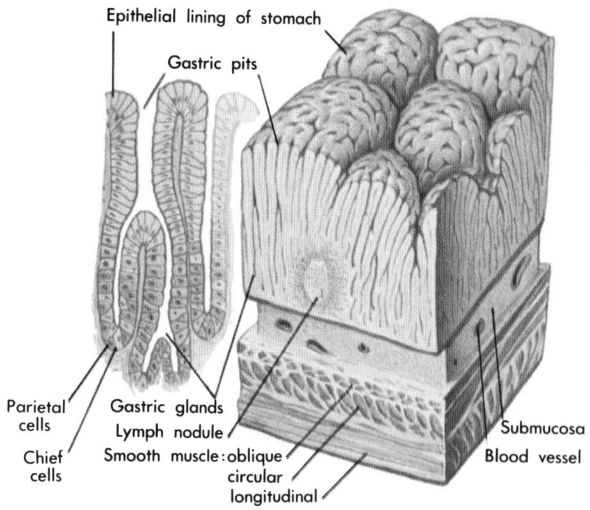

SECTION OF STOMACH WALL

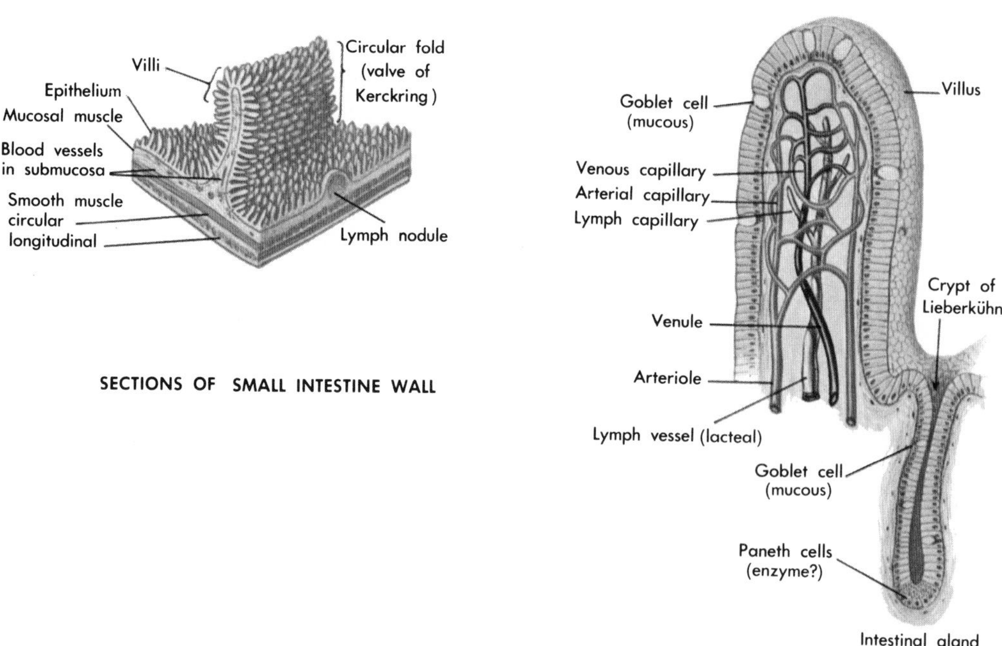

SECTIONS OF SMALL INTESTINE WALL

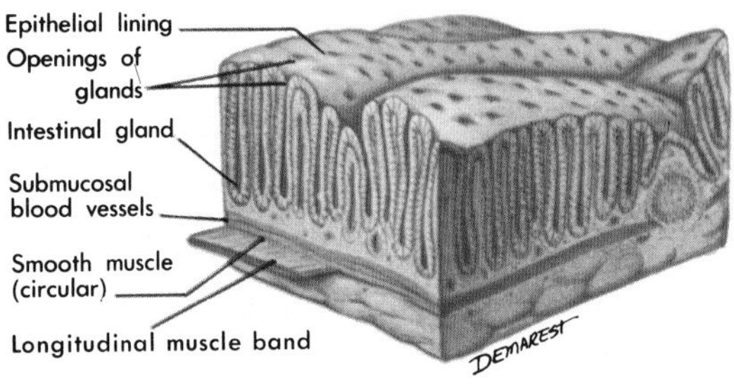

SECTION OF LARGE INTESTINE (COLON)

GENITOURINARY SYSTEM

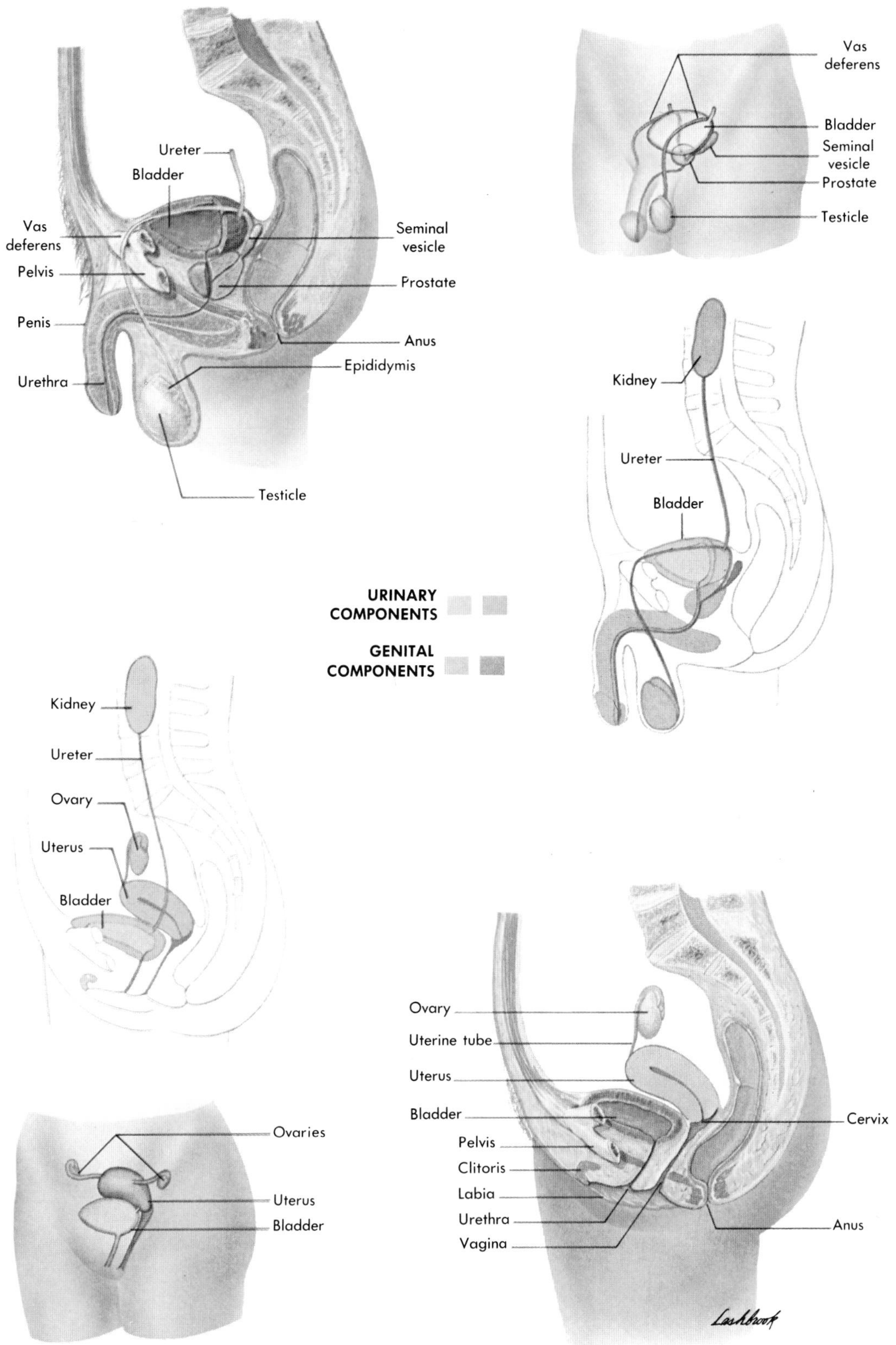

STRUCTURAL HIGHLIGHTS OF THE NERVOUS SYSTEM

GENERAL ARCHITECTURE AND PHYSIOLOGY

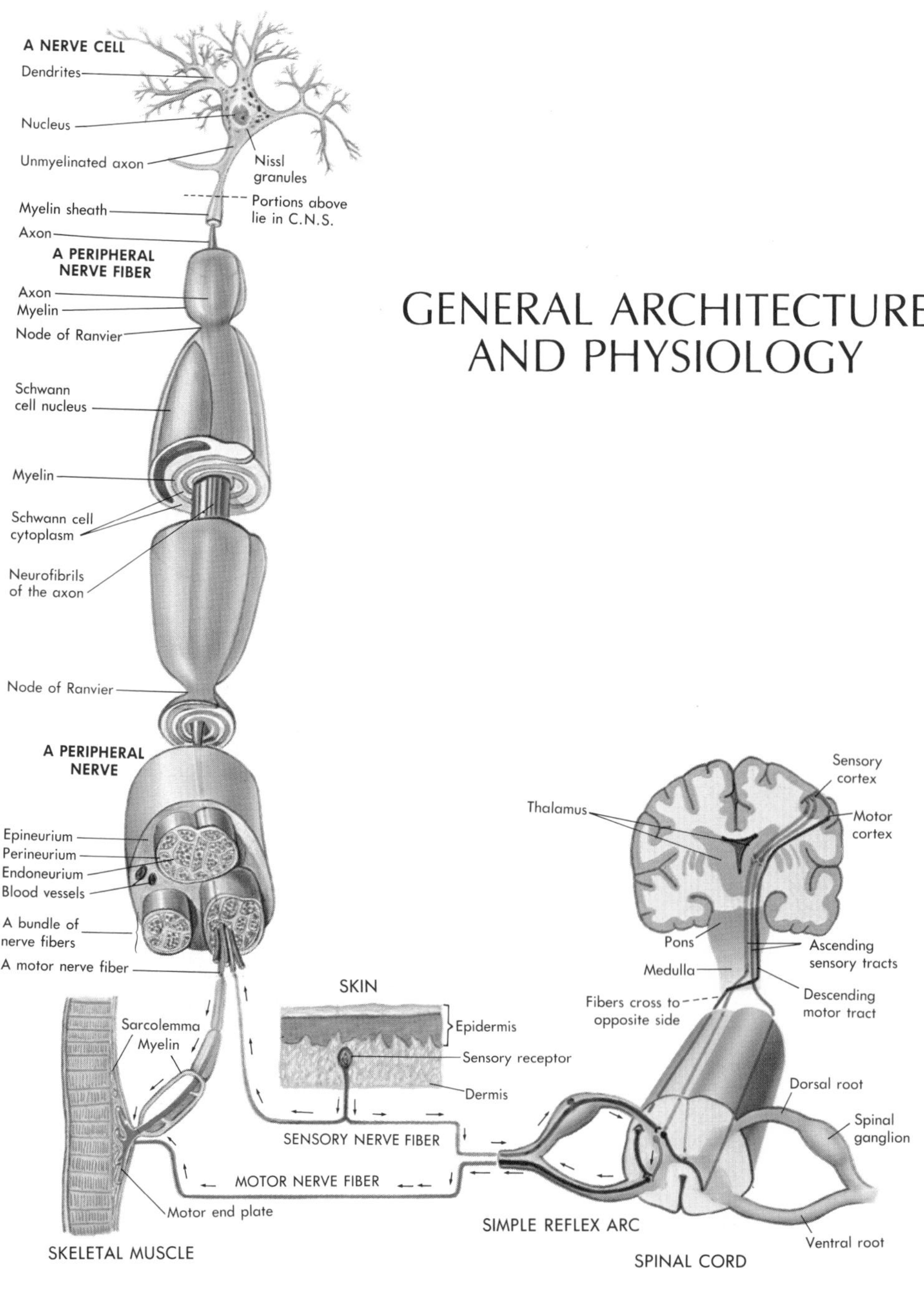

Plate 12

BRAIN AND SPINAL NERVES

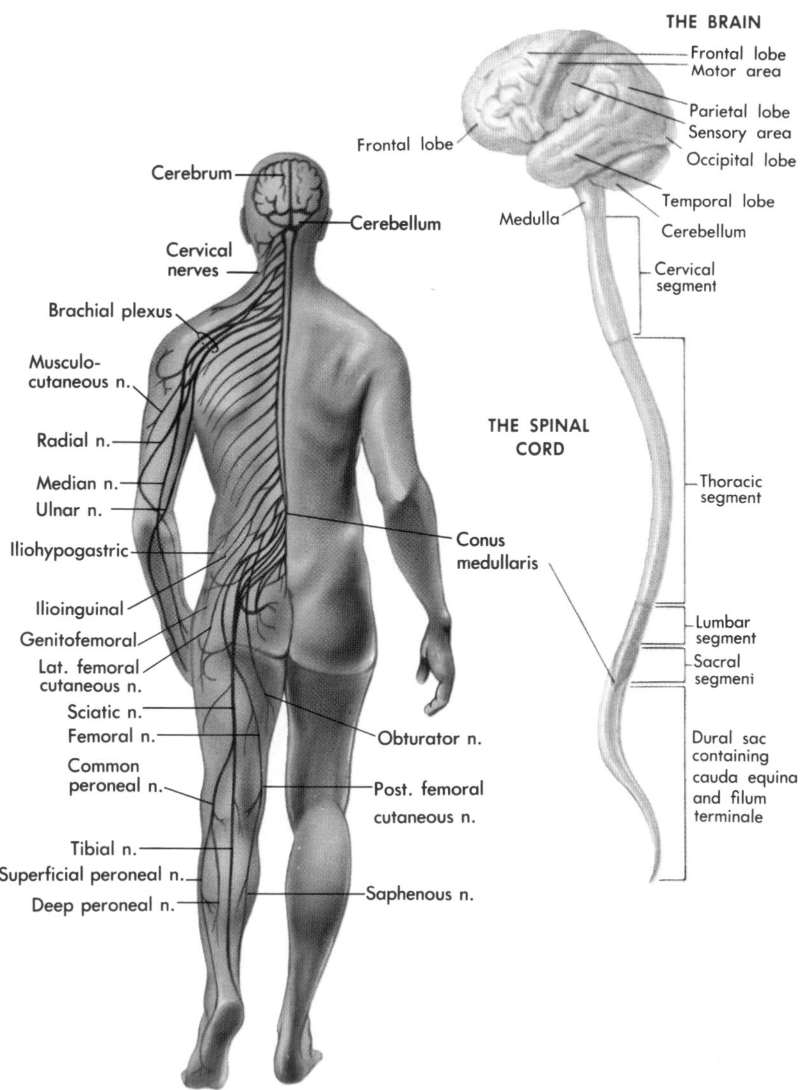
THE BRAIN
Frontal lobe
Motor area
Parietal lobe
Sensory area
Occipital lobe
Temporal lobe
Cerebellum
Frontal lobe
Medulla
Cervical segment
THE SPINAL CORD
Thoracic segment
Lumbar segment
Sacral segment
Dural sac containing cauda equina and filum terminale
Cerebrum
Cerebellum
Cervical nerves
Brachial plexus
Musculo-cutaneous n.
Radial n.
Median n.
Ulnar n.
Iliohypogastric
Ilioinguinal
Genitofemoral
Lat. femoral cutaneous n.
Sciatic n.
Femoral n.
Common peroneal n.
Tibial n.
Superficial peroneal n.
Deep peroneal n.
Conus medullaris
Obturator n.
Post. femoral cutaneous n.
Saphenous n.

THE MAJOR SPINAL NERVES

AUTONOMIC NERVES

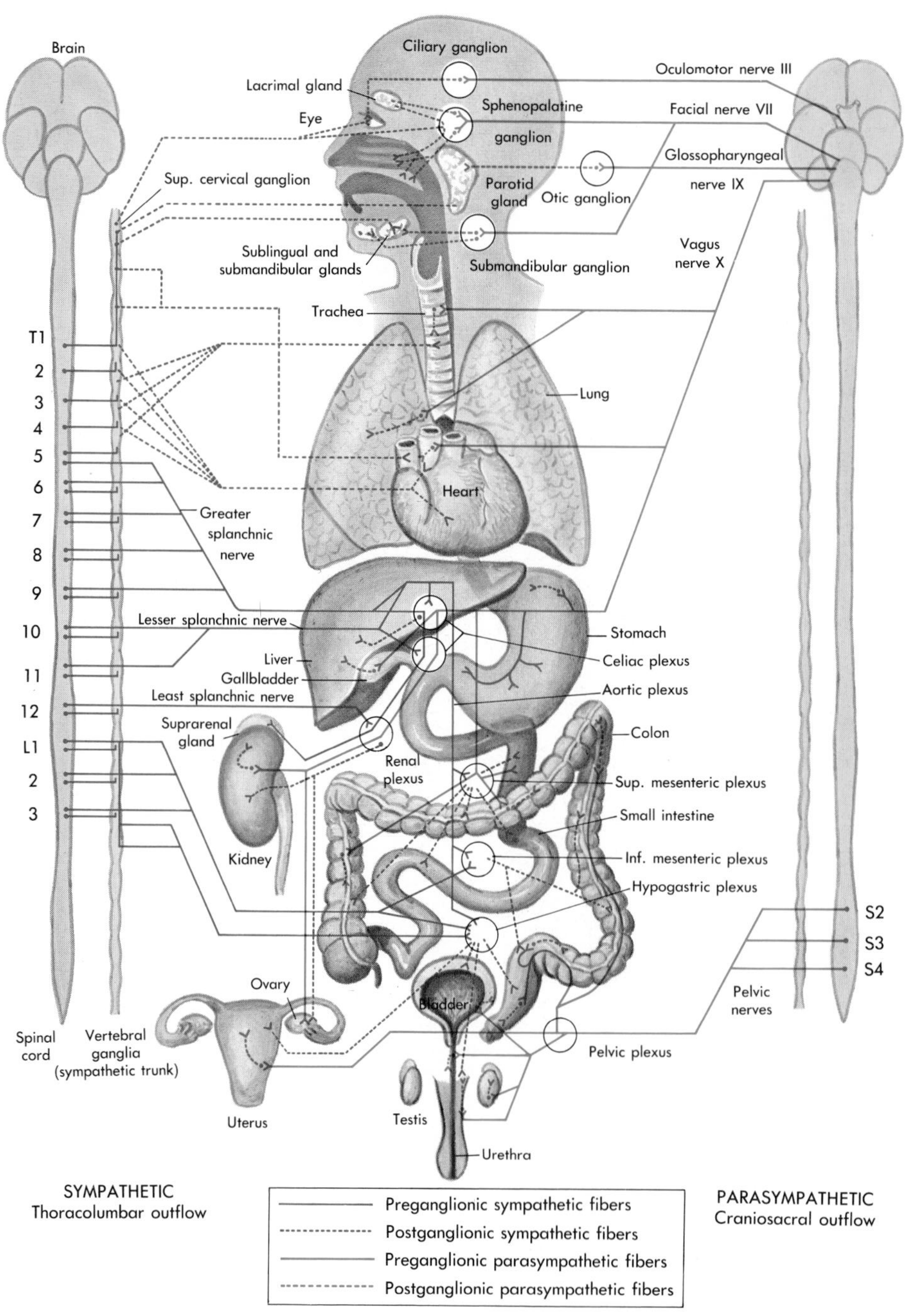

Brain
Ciliary ganglion
Oculomotor nerve III
Lacrimal gland
Eye
Sphenopalatine ganglion
Facial nerve VII
Glossopharyngeal nerve IX
Sup. cervical ganglion
Parotid gland
Otic ganglion
Sublingual and submandibular glands
Submandibular ganglion
Vagus nerve X
Trachea
T1
2
3
4
5
6
7
8
9
10
11
12
L1
2
3
Lung
Heart
Greater splanchnic nerve
Lesser splanchnic nerve
Stomach
Celiac plexus
Liver
Gallbladder
Aortic plexus
Least splanchnic nerve
Suprarenal gland
Colon
Renal plexus
Sup. mesenteric plexus
Small intestine
Kidney
Inf. mesenteric plexus
Hypogastric plexus
S2
S3
S4
Ovary
Bladder
Pelvic nerves
Spinal cord
Vertebral ganglia (sympathetic trunk)
Pelvic plexus
Uterus
Testis
Urethra
SYMPATHETIC
Thoracolumbar outflow
Preganglionic sympathetic fibers
Postganglionic sympathetic fibers
Preganglionic parasympathetic fibers
Postganglionic parasympathetic fibers
PARASYMPATHETIC
Craniosacral outflow

Plate 14

ORGANS OF SPECIAL SENSE

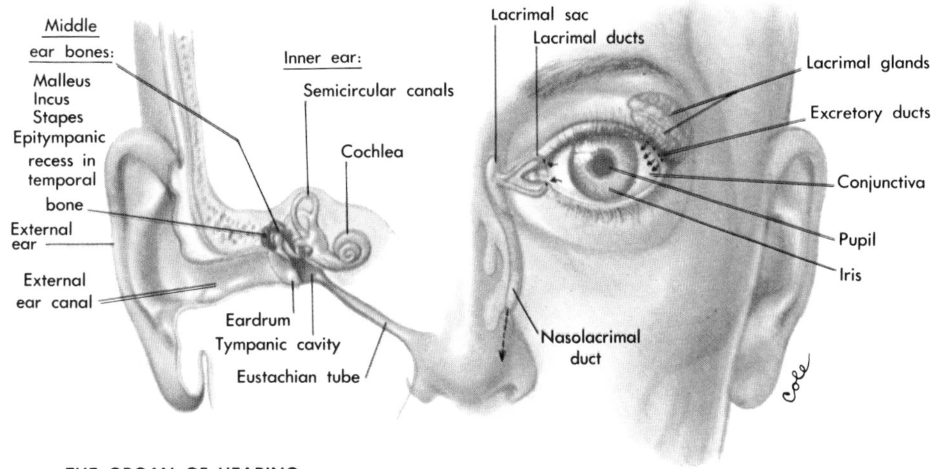

THE ORGAN OF HEARING

THE LACRIMAL APPARATUS AND THE EYE

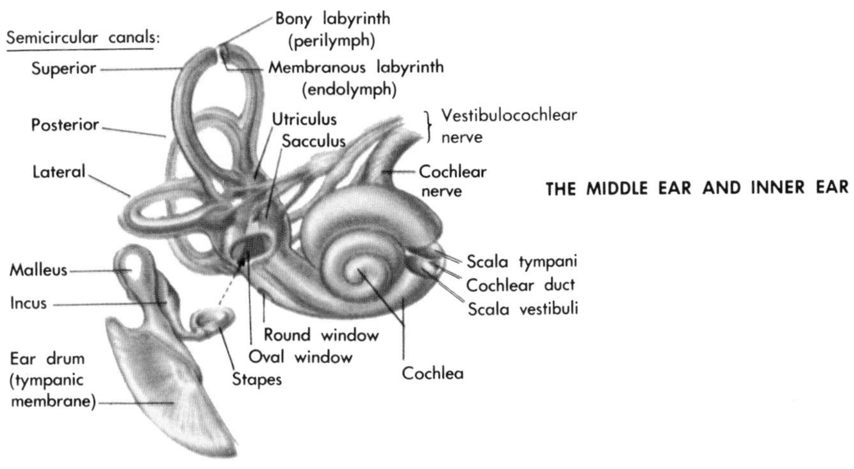

THE MIDDLE EAR AND INNER EAR

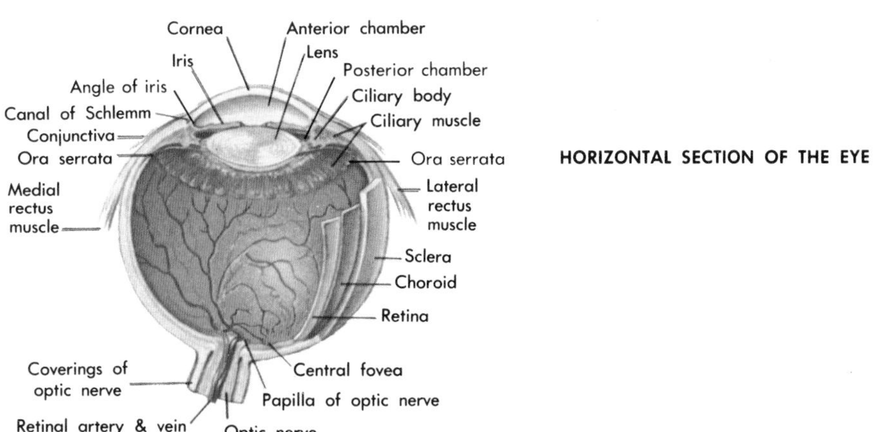

HORIZONTAL SECTION OF THE EYE

PARANASAL SINUSES

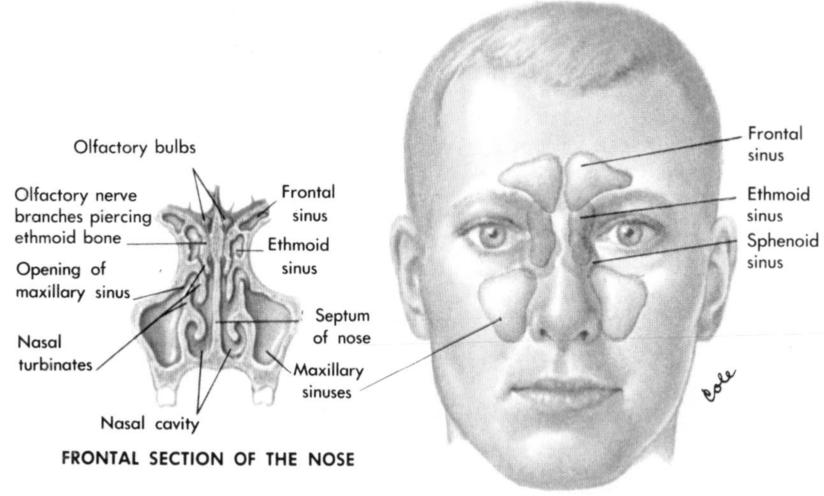

FRONTAL SECTION OF THE NOSE

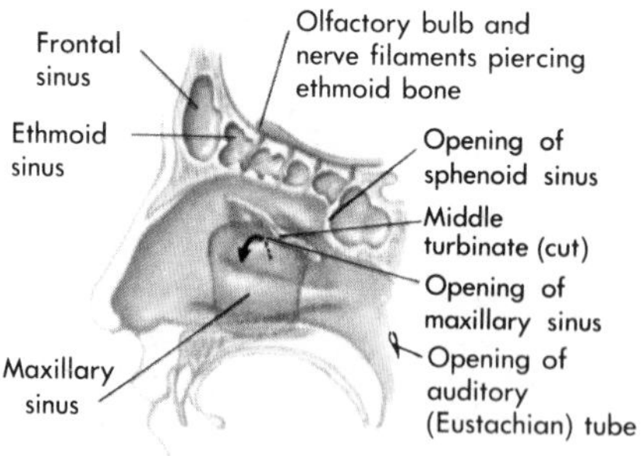

SAGITTAL SECTION OF THE NOSE

Plate 16

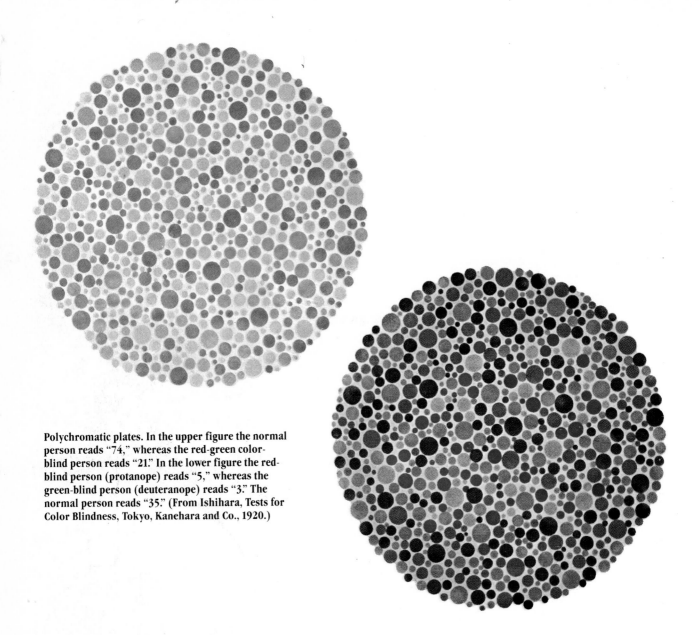

Polychromatic plates. In the upper figure the normal person reads "74," whereas the red-green color-blind person reads "21." In the lower figure the red-blind person (protanope) reads "5," whereas the green-blind person (deuteranope) reads "3." The normal person reads "35." (From Ishihara, Tests for Color Blindness, Tokyo, Kanehara and Co., 1920.)

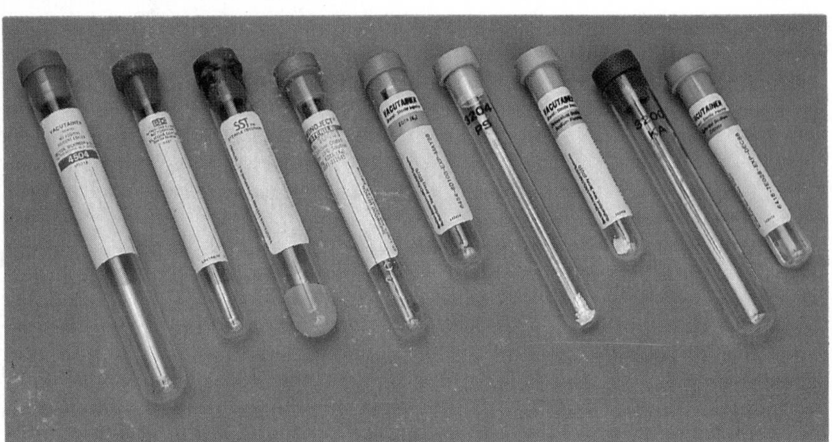

Vacutainer glass vacuum blood collection tubes. The stoppers of the blood collection tubes are color coded for ease in identifying the additive content of each type of tube. The red stoppered and red and slate-gray stoppered tubes contain no additives and are used to obtain clotted blood or serum. The lavender, gray, green, and light blue stoppered tubes contain an anticoagulant and are used to obtain whole blood or plasma.